TEXTBOOK OF FAMILY AND COUPLES THERAPY

Clinical Applications

*To Ed + Stacy Pobe
with much affection
and best
wishes
Pirooz
7/27/04*

TEXTBOOK OF FAMILY AND COUPLES THERAPY

Clinical Applications

Edited by

G. Pirooz Sholevar, M.D.

With

Linda D. Schwoeri, Ph.D.

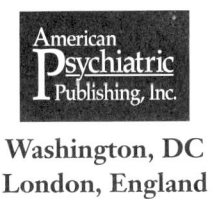

Washington, DC
London, England

Note: The authors have worked to ensure that all information in this book is accurate at the time of publication and consistent with general psychiatric and medical standards, and that information concerning drug dosages, schedules, and routes of administration is accurate at the time of publication and consistent with standards set by the U.S. Food and Drug Administration and the general medical community. As medical research and practice continue to advance, however, therapeutic standards may change. Moreover, specific situations may require a specific therapeutic response not included in this book. For these reasons and because human and mechanical errors sometimes occur, we recommend that readers follow the advice of physicians directly involved in their care or the care of a member of their family.

Books published by American Psychiatric Publishing, Inc., represent the views and opinions of the individual authors and do not necessarily represent the policies and opinions of APPI or the American Psychiatric Association.

Copyright © 2003 American Psychiatric Publishing, Inc.
ALL RIGHTS RESERVED

Manufactured in the United States of America on acid-free paper
07 06 05 04 03   5 4 3 2 1
First Edition

Typeset in Adobe's Janson Text and GillSans

American Psychiatric Publishing, Inc.
1000 Wilson Boulevard
Arlington, VA 22209-3901
www.appi.org

Library of Congress Cataloging-in-Publication Data
Textbook of family and couples therapy / edited by G. Pirooz Sholevar with Linda D. Schwoeri.—1st ed.
    p. ; cm.
Includes bibliographical references and index.
ISBN 0-88048-518-3 (alk. paper)
1. Family psychotherapy. 2. Marital psychotherapy. I. Sholevar, G. Pirooz. II. Schwoeri, Linda.
    [DNLM: 1. Family Therapy—methods. 2. Couples Therapy—methods. 3. Marital Therapy—methods. WM 430.5.F2 T355 2003]
RC488.5 .T44 2003
616.89′156—dc21
                                                        2002071166

British Library Cataloguing in Publication Data
A CIP record is available from the British Library.

*This book is dedicated to
my teachers and mentors:*

*Salvador Minuchin, Murray Bowen, Carl Whitaker,
Jay Haley, and Nathan Ackerman*

and

The next generation of the Sholevar family:

*Darius, Maryam, David, Reza, Timo, Michelle,
Wilkie, Christina, Roxanne, and Cyrus*

G.P.S.

Contents

Contributors. xiii

Part I
Introduction

Chapter 1
Family Theory and Therapy: An Overview 3
G. Pirooz Sholevar, M.D.

Part II
Family Therapy: Theory and Techniques

Introduction to Family Theories 29
G. Pirooz Sholevar, M.D.

Chapter 2
Structural Family Therapy 35
H. Charles Fishman, M.D., and Tana Fishman, D.O.

Chapter 3
Constructing Therapy: From Strategic, to Systemic, to
Narrative Models 55
Scott W. Browning, Ph.D., and Robert-Jay Green, Ph.D.

Chapter 4
Psychodynamic Family Therapy 77
G. Pirooz Sholevar, M.D., and Linda D. Schwoeri, Ph.D.

Chapter 5
Multigenerational Family Systems Theory of
Bowen and Its Application 103
Michael Kerr, M.D.

Chapter 6
Contextual Therapy 127
Catherine Ducommun-Nagy, M.D., and Linda D. Schwoeri, Ph.D.

Chapter 7
Behavioral Family Therapy 147
Ian R. H. Falloon, M.D.

Chapter 8
Psychoeducational Family Intervention 173
Linda D. Schwoeri, Ph.D., and G. Pirooz Sholevar, M.D.

Chapter 9
Social Network Intervention 193
Ross V. Speck, M.D.

Chapter 10
Gender-Sensitive Family Therapy 203
Linda D. Schwoeri, Ph.D., G. Pirooz Sholevar, M.D., and George S. Villarose, M.A.

Chapter 11
Techniques of Family Therapy 225
G. Pirooz Sholevar, M.D., and Linda D. Schwoeri, Ph.D.

Family Theories: Conclusion 251
G. Pirooz Sholevar, M.D.

Part III
Family Assessment

Chapter 12
Initial and Diagnostic Family Interviews 257
G. Pirooz Sholevar, M.D.

Chapter 13
Family Assessment 277
Bruce D. Forman, Ph.D., Jodi Aronson, Ph.D., and Mark P. Combs, Ph.D.

Chapter 14
The Family Life Cycle: A Framework for
Understanding Family Development 303
Joan Zilbach, M.D.

Chapter 15
Functional and Dysfunctional Families 317
W. Robert Beavers, M.D.

Chapter 16
Diagnosis of Family Relational Disorders 341
David J. Miklowitz, Ph.D., and John F. Clarkin, Ph.D.

Part IV
Family Therapy With Children and Adolescents

Chapter 17
Family Therapy With Children and Adolescents: An Overview 367
G. Pirooz Sholevar, M.D.

Chapter 18
Family Therapy With Children: A Model for
Engaging the Whole Family 381
Richard Chasin, M.D., and Tanya B. White, Ph.D.

Chapter 19
Parent Management Training 403
Ellen Harris Sholevar, M.D.

Part V
Couples Therapy

Chapter 20
Couples Therapy: An Overview 417
G. Pirooz Sholevar, M.D.

Chapter 21
Psychodynamic Couples Therapy 439
Derek C. Polonsky, M.D., and Carol C. Nadelson, M.D.

Chapter 22
Behavioral Couples Therapy 461
Steven L. Sayers, Ph.D., and Richard E. Heyman

Chapter 23
The Divorcing Family: Characteristics and Interventions 501
G. Pirooz Sholevar, M.D., and Linda D. Schwoeri, Ph.D.

Chapter 24
The Remarried Family: Characteristics and Interventions 523
Emily B. Visher, Ph.D., and John S. Visher, M.D.

Chapter 25
Marital Enrichment in Clinical Practice 539
Paul Giblin, Ph.D., and Mark P. Combs, Ph.D.

Chapter 26
Sex Therapy at the Turn of the Century:
New Awareness and Response 559
Linda D. Schwoeri, Ph.D., G. Pirooz Sholevar, M.D., and Mark P. Combs, Ph.D.

Part VI
Family Therapy With Different Disorders

Chapter 27
Family Variables and Interventions in Schizophrenia.................. 585
David J. Miklowitz, Ph.D., and Martha C. Tompson, Ph.D.

Chapter 28
Depression and the Family: Interpersonal Context and
Family Functioning 619
G. Pirooz Sholevar, M.D., Linda D. Schwoeri, Ph.D., and Howard Jarden, Ph.D.

Chapter 29
Family Intervention and Psychiatric Hospitalization 637
G. Pirooz Sholevar, M.D., Ira D. Glick, M.D., and Ellen Harris Sholevar, M.D.

Chapter 30
National Alliance for the Mentally Ill (NAMI) and Family Psychiatry:
Working Toward a Collaborative Model 657
G. Pirooz Sholevar, M.D., and Linda D. Schwoeri, Ph.D.

Chapter 31
Alcoholic and Substance-Abusing Families.........................671
G. Pirooz Sholevar, M.D., and Linda D. Schwoeri, Ph.D.

Chapter 32
Family Intervention With Incest................................695
G. Pirooz Sholevar, M.D., and Linda D. Schwoeri, Ph.D.

Chapter 33
Family Therapy With Personality Disorders......................715
G. Pirooz Sholevar, M.D., and Linda D. Schwoeri, Ph.D.

Chapter 34
Impact of Culture and Ethnicity on Family Interventions..............725
Linda D. Schwoeri, Ph.D., G. Pirooz Sholevar, M.D., and Mark P. Combs, Ph.D.

Chapter 35
Medical Family Therapy 747
G. Pirooz Sholevar, M.D., and Christoph Sahar, M.D.

Part VII
Research in Family and Couples Therapy

Chapter 36
The State of Family Therapy Research: A Positive Prognosis...........771
John F. Clarkin, Ph.D., Daniel Carpenter, Ph.D., and Eric Fertuck, Ph.D.

Chapter 37
Couples Therapy Research: Status and Directions...................797
Susan M. Johnson, Ph.D.

Chapter 38
Conclusion and Future Directions................................815
G. Pirooz Sholevar, M.D.

References 821

Index..907

Contributors

Jodi Aronson, Ph.D.
Vice President of Clinical Administration, Employer Service Division, CIGNA Behavior Health, Eden Prairie, Minnesota; Professor of Psychology, Monterrey Institute for Graduate Studies, Del Centro de Estudios Universitarios, Monterrey, NL, Mexico

W. Robert Beavers, M.D.
Clinical Professor of Psychiatry, University of Texas Southwestern Medical Center, Dallas, Texas

Scott W. Browning, Ph.D.
Professor, Department of Clinical Psychology, Chestnut Hill College, Philadelphia, Pennsylvania

Daniel Carpenter, Ph.D.
Chief Information Officer, Division of Expert Knowledge Group, Comprehensive Neuroscience, New York Presbyterian Hospital, White Plains, New York

Richard Chasin, M.D.
Associate Clinical Professor of Psychiatry, Harvard Medical School, The Cambridge Hospital, Cambridge, Massachusetts; Past President, American Family Therapy Association

John F. Clarkin, Ph.D.
Professor of Clinical Psychology and Co-Director, Personality Disorder Institute, Department of Psychiatry, New York Presbyterian Hospital, Weill Medical College of Cornell University, White Plains, New York

Mark P. Combs, Ph.D.
Devereux Foundation, Beneto Center, Malvern, Pennsylvania

Catherine Ducommun-Nagy, M.D.
Clinical Assistant Professor, Graduate Programs in Marriage and Family Therapy, Drexel University, Philadelphia, Pennsylvania; President, Institute for Contextual Growth, Inc.

Ian R. H. Falloon, M.D.
Department of Psychiatry, University of Auckland, Auckland, New Zealand

Eric Fertuck, Ph.D.
Fellow in Psychology, Department of Psychiatry, New York Presbyterian Hospital, Weill Medical College, Cornell University, White Plains, New York

H. Charles Fishman, M.D.
Senior Consultant, Middlemore Hospital, Auckland, New Zealand

Tana Fishman, D.O.
Consultant, Department of General Practice and Primary Health Care, Faculty of Medicine and Health Sciences, University of Auckland, Auckland, New Zealand

Bruce D. Forman, Ph.D.
Vice President for Academic Affairs, Monterrey Institute for Graduate Studies, Del Centro de Estudios Universitarios, Monterrey, NL, Mexico; Private Practice, Fort Lauderdale, Florida

Paul Giblin, Ph.D.
Professor, Institute of Pastoral Studies, Chicago, Illinois

Ira D. Glick, M.D.
Professor, Department of Psychiatry and Behavioral Sciences, and Director of Schizophrenia Research, Stanford University School of Medicine, Stanford, California

Contributors

Robert-Jay Green, Ph.D.
Professor, California School of Professional Psychology at Alliant International University; Director of Family/Child Psychology Training Program, San Francisco Bay Campus, Alameda, California

Richard E. Heyman
Research Associate Professor, Department of Psychology, State University of New York at Stony Brook, Stony Brook, New York

Howard Jarden, Ph.D.
Clinical Director, Devereux Foundation, Beneto Center, Malvern, Pennsylvania

Susan M. Johnson, Ph.D.
Professor of Psychology, Department of Psychiatry, University of Ottawa and Ottawa Couple and Family Institute, Ottawa, ONT, Canada

Michael Kerr, M.D.
Director, Bowen Center for the Study of the Family and Clinical Associate Professor of Psychiatry, Georgetown University School of Medicine, Washington, DC

David J. Miklowitz, Ph.D.
Professor of Psychology, Department of Psychology, University of Colorado, Boulder, Colorado

Carol C. Nadelson, M.D.
Director, Partners Office for Women's Careers; Clinical Professor, Department of Psychiatry, Brigham and Women's Hospital, Harvard Medical School, Boston, Massachusetts

Derek C. Polonsky, M.D.
Clinical Instructor, Department of Psychiatry, Harvard Medical School; Private Practice, Boston, Massachusetts

Christoph Sahar, M.D.
Department of Family Practice, Hunterton Medical Center, Flemington, New Jersey

Steven L. Sayers, Ph.D.
Assistant Professor, Department of Psychiatry, University of Pennsylvania, Philadelphia, Pennsylvania

Linda D. Schwoeri, Ph.D.
Department of Psychiatry, School of Osteopathic Medicine, University of Medicine and Dentistry of New Jersey, Stratford, New Jersey

Ellen Harris Sholevar, M.D.
Associate Professor and Director, Child and Adolescent Psychiatry, Temple University School of Medicine, Philadelphia, Pennsylvania

G. Pirooz Sholevar, M.D.
Clinical Professor of Psychiatry, Jefferson Medical College, Thomas Jefferson University, Philadelphia, Pennsylvania; Robert Wood Johnson Medical School, University of Medicine and Dentistry of New Jersey, Piscataway, New Jersey

Ross V. Speck, M.D.
CORE Professor, Union Institute University, Cincinnati, Ohio

Martha C. Tompson, Ph.D.
Assistant Professor, Boston University, Boston, Massachusetts

George S. Villarose, M.A.
Psychotherapist, Devereux Foundation, Beneto Center, Glenmoore, Pennsylvania

Emily B. Visher, Ph.D.
Adjunct Faculty Emeritus, John F. Kennedy University, Contra Costa County, California

John S. Visher, M.D.
Lecturer in Psychiatry Emeritus, Stanford University School of Medicine, Palo Alto, California

Tanya B. White, Ph.D.
Private Practice; Adjunct Faculty, Massachusetts School of Professional Psychology, Lexington, Massachusetts

Joan Zilbach, M.D.
Training and Supervising Analyst, Boston Psychoanalytic Institute and Society, Boston, Massachusetts

I

Introduction

1

Family Theory and Therapy

An Overview

G. Pirooz Sholevar, M.D.

Introduction

Family theory is a special theoretical and clinical orientation that views human behavior and psychiatric disturbances in their interpersonal context (Lansky 1989). This orientation is most apparent in the practice of family therapy, which is an umbrella term for a number of clinical practices based on the notion that psychopathology resides in the family system rather than individuals. Interventions are designed to effect change in the family relationship system rather than in the individual (Bell 1975; Minuchin 1974a; Olson 1970; Shapiro 1966). Family theory considers family as an interpersonal system with cybernetic qualities. The relationships among the components of the system are nonlinear (or circular); the interactions are cyclic rather than causative. There are complex interlocking feedback mechanisms and patterns of interaction among the members of the system that repeat themselves sequentially. Any symptom can be viewed simply as a particular type of behavior functioning as a homeostatic mechanism that regulates family interactions (Jackson 1965; Minuchin et al. 1975).

The system is nonsummative and includes the individuals as well as their interactions (Olson 1970). A person's problems cannot be evaluated or treated apart from the *context* in which they occur and the *functions* that they serve. This notion further implies that an individual cannot be expected to change unless the family system changes (Haley 1962). Therefore, the treatment addresses behavioral dysfunctions as a manifestation of disturbances within the entire family relational system; the role of the total family in aiding or in sabotaging treatment is the focus, even when a distinct, diagnosable psychiatric illness is present in one of the family members.

Family therapy as a psychotherapeutic modality has the following goals (Steinglass 1995):

1. Exploring the interactional dynamics of the family and its relationship to psychopathology
2. Mobilizing the family's internal strength and functional resources
3. Restructuring the maladaptive interactional family styles
4. Strengthening the family's problem-solving behavior

In the 1970s and 1980s, the field of family therapy viewed itself as preeminent among diverse therapeutic approaches, particularly by focusing on its own unique promise and the limitations of other approaches. In the 1990s, the field reached a level of maturity that also recognized the unique contributions of other intervention models, the complexities of human behavior and adaptation, and the limitations of the family approach. This maturation has helped family therapy to assume a responsible and leading role in the creation of multisystemic and multimodal approaches to many disorders such as alcoholism and substance abuse, medical illness, and the major mental disorders described in many chapters in this volume.

History

The roots of family therapy were established in the early 1900s with the emergence of the child guidance movement (1909) and marriage counseling (1920s). Psychoanalytic treatment was applied in parallel confidential sessions with spouses and provided a strong theoretical foundation for early family and marital investigations. The formal development of family therapy dates back to the late 1940s or early 1950s for different parts of the country. Early pioneers of family therapy included Ackerman; Bowen; Wynne; Bell; Bateson, Jackson, Haley, and Satir; Lidz and Flick; and a semi-independent root of family therapy that emerged in Milan, Italy. In addition to these practitioners, a number of other important figures, including Carl Whitaker, Salvador Minuchin, and Ivan Boszormenyi-Nagy, have enhanced the development of family therapy.

The development of the field of family therapy was facilitated by a number of movements in the field of mental health in general. Sociologists' interest in the study of the family started quite early (Burgess 1926), but their impact on the field of psychiatry followed the emergence of social psychiatry, which emphasized the significance of cultural differences and social settings in the development and amelioration of psychiatric disorders (Leighton 1960; Spiegel 1971). The expansion of psychoanalytic theory and ego psychology encouraged the belief that symptoms were both embedded in the personality and emerged from adaptation to the family environment. In the stage of psychoanalytic theory most influenced by ego psychology, the significance of social and cultural determinants of behavior was emphasized by Horney (1939), Fromm (1941), and Sullivan (1953). The "interpersonal" psychoanalytic school of Sullivan (1953) emphasized the relational and interactional aspects of the human condition. Erikson's (1950) epigenetic theory of human development mapped out the interrelationship between individual maturational processes and the social and cultural environment. The interest in the mother-child relationship was expanded through the work of David Levy (1943) on "maternal overprotection," as well as Frieda Fromm-Reichmann's (1948) conceptualization of the disturbances in the mother-child relationship in the genesis of schizophrenia. John Bowlby's (1949) work on bonding established the theoretical basis for the object relations school of family therapy.

The expansion of group therapy in the United States after 1924 enhanced knowledge about the operation of small-group processes, symptomatic behavior within a group, and ways of correcting individual behavior within a group setting. The emergence of learning theory and behavior therapy underlined the interconnection between symptomatic behavior and the contingencies of the family environment. Dissatisfaction with the traditional practices of child psychotherapy inspired a number of early contributors to family therapy, particularly John Bell (1975) and Nathan Ackerman (1954). Nathan Ackerman, a psychoanalyst, child psychiatrist, and group therapist, was disenchanted with the prevailing practices of child psychotherapists who treated the parents and children in tandem therapy in child guidance clinics (Ackerman 1954). Ackerman's contributions included the concepts of shared unconscious conflicts and defenses, symbiotic relationships, and the use of interpretation, confrontation, and manipulation of metaphors in psychotherapy (Simon 1985).

Murray Bowen (1961, 1966, 1978) was a major early figure and remained an independent thinker in the field of family therapy. He had an ongoing impact on the generations of family therapists that followed. A psychoanalyst by background, he pioneered the investigation and observation of family members together with hospitalized schizophrenic patients.

His observations led to a number of conclusions, some of which have strongly influenced the course of family therapy. Although his work is couched within an intergenerational family systems model and psychodynamic concepts, his influence on all schools of family therapy is readily apparent. His investigations resulted in the recognition of the "undifferentiation" phenomenon and its relationship to the transmission of "anxiety" within the family system. His early term of "undifferentiated ego mass" families has gone through many transformations. Differentiation, his foundational concept, is closely related to his other theoretical concepts, such as anxiety, interpersonal triangulation, marital and family fusion, and family projective system (see Chapter 5, "Multigenerational Family Systems Theory of Bowen and Its Application").

Wynne and his colleagues' investigation of psychodynamic aspects of schizophrenia attempted to identify the characteristic structure and roles in families that produce schizophrenia (Ryckoff et al. 1959; Wynne et al. 1958). Wynne's work is premised on the concept that all humans experience both a fundamental need to relate to others and a lifelong striving to develop a sense of personal identity. This concept resulted in the recognition of the two phenomena of "pseudo-mutuality" and "pseudo-hostility." Pseudo-mutuality is based on an intense need for togetherness, at the cost of not permitting differentiation of the identities of the persons in the relationship and denial of divergence in people's perceptions. Wynne and Singer designed a number of studies to recognize the phenomenon of communication deviance (CD) in the families of young schizophrenic patients; these families were then compared with a group of borderline and "neurotic" adults. The original work of Wynne and Singer, published in the 1960s (Singer and Wynne 1965a, 1965b; Wynne 1968; Wynne and Singer 1963), resulted in a consistent description of CD, which has been applied in a number of longitudinal studies continuing to the present time (see Chapter 27, "Family Variables and Interventions in Schizophrenia"). Lidz and his coworkers conducted an extensive investigation of the families of young adults with schizophrenia, including the relationship between parental/marital dysfunctions and the emergence of psychopathology in young children. Lidz and his colleagues (Lidz et al. 1957) described two family types: "schismatic," based on the display of constant strife; and "eschewed families," which maintain a trade-off of peaceful appearance for various dysfunctions. The schismatic family types (characterized by overt marital hostility) can result in acute schizophrenic breakdown, whereas chronic and "process" types of schizophrenia are the product of eschewed families (characterized by covert accommodation to a dysfunctional spouse) (see Chapter 16, "Diagnosis of Family Relational Disorders," and Chapter 27, "Family Variables and Interventions in Schizophrenia").

The Palo Alto group started its investigations in the 1950s through the efforts of Bateson, Jackson, Haley, Weakland, and subsequently Satir. They described communication patterns, cybernetics, systems theory, and the *double-bind* phenomenon in the early and current life situations of schizophrenic patients. The study of the work of Milton Erickson by Haley and Weakland resulted in a variety of related observations described in *Strategies of Psychotherapy* (Haley 1963) and other publications by Haley. The Mental Research Institute (MRI), a major family therapy center, was established by Jackson in 1959 and was enriched by the addition of Virginia Satir and Jay Haley in 1962. After Jackson's death in 1968, a number of other directors, including Bell, Riskin, Weakland, and Watzalwick, have continued with the early work of the MRI and have established the school of brief strategic therapy based on "paradoxical interventions" (Stanton 1980) (see Chapter 3, "Constructing Therapy: From Strategic, to Systemic, to Narrative Models"). Carl Whitaker became interested in families in 1946 at Emory University. His creativity in the use of unconscious fantasies, countertransference, and the inclusion of all family members in therapy resulted in the development of the experiential school of family therapy. His charismatic use of feeling and expression had the goal of a patient's self-actualization, and he shied away from distinct theoretical formulations. He was particularly gifted at involving young children in family sessions.

The European investigation of family therapy evolved from two centers in particular: the Milan School of Family Therapy, and Object Relations Family Therapy in England. The Milan School of Family Therapy was established by Mara Selvini-Palazzoli in Milan, Italy, in the 1960s, and furthered her investigation of schizophrenia and anorexia nervosa in collaboration with a number of other investigators, namely, Boscolo, Cecchin, and Prata. The group was influenced by the studies by Lidz and Wynne and subsequently the work of the MRI group on paradoxical interventions (see Chapter 3, "Constructing Therapy: From Strategic, to Systemic, to Narrative Models"). The group analytic approach was initiated by a variety of object relations theorists, including Middlefort, Faulkes, Bion, and Skynner. Recently, the object relations approach to families has gained more recognition in the United States (see Chapter 4, "Psychodynamic Family Therapy," for further discussion).

In 1965, Salvador Minuchin moved to the Philadelphia Child Guidance Clinic and, along with Jay Haley, established the Structural School of Family Therapy, which is applied extensively to families with young children with behavioral disorders. They defined "psychosomatic families"—that is, the families of patients with anorexia nervosa and other psychosomatic disorders (Minuchin et al. 1978) (see Chapter 2, "Structural Family Therapy").

In 1962, an underappreciated attempt at family therapy with adolescents and children was made by the Multiple Impact Therapy (MIT) group in Galveston, Texas. More recent contributions to family therapy with children have come from the work of Patterson et al. (1982, 1992), Forehand and McMahon (1981a), Alexander and Parsons (1973), Joan Zilbach (1986), and David and Jill Scharff (1987). The first two groups of contributors have added immeasurably to our knowledge of delinquent behavior. Zilbach has provided a systematic way of including young children in families. David and Jill Scharff's formulations and recommendations are particularly applicable to families with adolescents (see Chapter 17, "Family Therapy With Children and Adolescents: An Overview"; Chapter 18, "Family Therapy With Children: A Model for Engaging the Whole Family"; and Chapter 19, "Parent Management Training").

Twin and adoption studies beginning in the 1960s revealed the likely genetic, anatomical, and biochemical contributions to the etiology of schizophrenia. Paradoxically, some of these studies, such as the Finnish adoptive project (Tienari et al. 1983), also revealed an important family and environmental role in influencing the genetic transmission. These findings facilitated the application of family interventions to major psychiatric disorders. Following initial disappointment with investigation of schizophrenia in psychiatric hospitals, family therapy moved to outpatient settings that isolated family therapy from medical facilities. More recently, family interventions have been reintroduced in inpatient settings as a cost-effective measure to reduce both the length of stay and the risk of relapse (Glick and Kessler 1980; Glick et al. 1993) (see Chapter 28, "Depression and the Family: Interpersonal Context and Family Functioning," and Chapter 29, "Family Intervention and Psychiatric Hospitalization").

Indications and Contraindications

An apparent and clear *indication* for family therapy is the presence of open and stressful conflicts in a family, with or without symptomatic behaviors in one or more family members. Family therapy also can be applied to covert problems in the relationships within the family, which can give rise to dysfunctional behavior on the part of one or more family members. Family therapy may also be indicated when other family members encourage the perpetuation and continuation of the disorder. The recognition of covert family problems in the face of overt dysfunctions in one or more family members is the specific contribution of the field of family therapy. More recently recognized uses of family interventions are in the treatment of major psychiatric disorders such as schizophrenia, depression, alcoholism, conduct disorders, and somatoform disorders. Family-based interventions with this group of disorders are mostly psychoeducational in nature and are combined with other treatment modalities such as pharmacotherapy. Family therapy or other treatment modalities should be chosen on the basis of the nature and adequacy of family communication, structure, boundaries, conflicts, stresses, and resources. Recent application of family treatment to hospitalized, psychotic, and depressed patients has exhibited the beneficial effects of combining multiple treatment modalities, particularly with psychopharmacotherapy. Psychodynamic family therapy is increasingly used for interventions with narcissistic and borderline personality disorders (see Chapter 4, "Psychodynamic Family Therapy"; Chapter 27, "Family Variables and Interventions in Schizophrenia"; Chapter 28, "Depression and the Family: Interpersonal Context and Family Functioning"; and Chapter 33, "Family Therapy With Personality Disorders").

Contraindications to family therapy are relative rather than absolute. They include discussion of long dormant, charged, or explosive family issues before the family has made a commitment to treatment. Another relative contraindication is the engagement of the family in a discussion of stressful situations when one or more members of the family is severely destabilized and requires hospitalization.

Models of Family Therapy

The extreme diversity of models of family therapy has raised questions about the common ground among family therapies. Each model may focus on different dimensions of the family system, making the models appear significantly unlike each other. The emphasis of pioneers on different family dimensions in therapy was to some degree reflective of the unacknowledged differences among the patient populations treated by the early family therapists. The subsequent divergent paths adopted by family therapists continued to ignore the likely conclusion that different approaches to family therapy are closely linked with family characteristics commonly observed in different disorders and that therefore different models may have differential applicability to certain family types and disorders. For example, families with relatively acute or chronic disorders who have negotiated a relatively successful separation from the previous generation may benefit differentially from different models of family treatment, in contrast to families who have failed in such negotiations. Psychoeducational family therapy with severely disturbed patients has demonstrated the effectiveness of the model with a treatment-resistant population. This model has provided an intelligent framework for multimodal intervention by a multidisciplinary team that can offer the family members the opportunity to join the treatment team.

The strong bias against the use of individual diagnosis, medication, or hospitalization by some family therapists may reflect their nonmedical background and their lack of experience with certain patient populations. For example, family therapists primarily trained in the treatment of acute behavioral disorders in families with young children may have little understanding of families with chronically ill and seriously disabled adult patients in need of intermittent hospitalization and ongoing use of pharmacological agents. This lack of perspective has been combined with strong antiprofessional, antibiological, and antimedical attitudes in certain family therapists.

The evidence strongly suggests that different models of family therapy have *differential application* to various patient populations. The intergenerational family therapy models of Bowen and Boszormenyi-Nagy are particularly applicable to families whose members have long-standing and chronic disorders, and who have not negotiated adequate separation between the generations. Structural and strategic family therapy are particularly applicable to families in a crisis situation in which there has been adequate separation from previous generations and a reasonably satisfactory precrisis adjustment in the nuclear family. Behavioral family therapy is particularly applicable to marital therapy and children with chronic conduct disorders. Psychodynamic and experiential family therapies are exceptionally helpful for families with narcissistic vulnerability; members of such families often have a broad range of personality and "neurotic" disorders but have also managed to maintain a relatively adequate level of functioning, although with little enjoyment in their life. Social network therapy is particularly applicable to seriously and chronically disabled families with concomitant disintegration in the family and their social network.

Different models of family therapy utilize *different theoretical concepts and techniques*. Some models can be grouped together based on their similarities. The intergenerational models include Bowen's family systems theory and contextual family therapy by Boszormenyi-Nagy. The communicational/systems models include structural and strategic family therapy. The strategic model includes several variations as its subgroup. The communicational/systems models are closely related to behavioral family therapy. The psychodynamic and experiential models are closely aligned.

Psychodynamic Family Therapy

Psychodynamic family therapy emphasizes individual maturation, personality development, early childhood experiences, and resolution of symptoms and conflicts in the context of the family system. It pays special attention to the "unconscious" life of the family members and inadequate resolution of prior developmental passages by the family or its members. Traumatic events in the life of the current or previous families are considered a significant source of dysfunctional feedback resulting in symptoms, inhibitions, lack of pleasure, or immaturities. Common theoretical concepts include "shared unconscious conflicts," intrafamilial transference reactions, dyadic and triadic family transferences in treatment situations, projective identification, and a host of object relations psychoanalytic concepts. The concept of "holding environment" in object relations theory is particularly relevant in the establishment of a highly empathic relationship between the therapist and the family members to allow for the emergence of dormant conflicts from the past (Scharff 1995; Scharff and Scharff 1987) (see Chapter 4, "Psychodynamic Family Therapy").

The psychodynamic model is most applicable with multiple long-standing but subtle symptomatic behaviors that are intricately interwoven with personality traits. Such behaviors include the inability to enjoy life, narcissistic vulnerability, and personality constrictions. Narcissistic relationships exhibit themselves by mutual blaming, preoccupation, and sensitivity to shame and guilt, which lend themselves well to psychodynamic family therapy (Lansky 1981, 1986). The borderline disorders occurring in families with excessive use of projective identification, trading of dissociations, and fear of abandonment are appropriate for psychodynamic family interventions. Psychodynamic family therapy can be combined readily and beneficially with individual therapy, conducted simultaneously or in tandem. Ackerman, Stierlin, Shapiro, Zinner, Sonne, and Framo are major contributors in this area. More recently, a comprehensive application of object relations theory to family therapy has taken place as a result of the work of Zinner and Shapiro (1974) and Scharff and Scharff (1987) (see Chapter 4, "Psychodynamic Family Therapy"). A recent application of the psychodynamic model is the exciting and empirically validated approach of emotionally focused therapy (Johnson and Whiffen 1999; Johnson et al. 2001), based on the application of attachment theory to differentiate between "defensive" and "attachment" affects to enhance the therapeutic process (see Chapter 20, "Couples Therapy: An Overview").

Experiential Family Therapy

Experiential family therapy focuses on the expression of feelings, conscious or preconscious fantasies, intrafamilial transference reactions, and the therapist's use of his or her experience in the family to expand the feeling range of the family. Clear communications, role flexibility, exploration, and spontaneity are highly encouraged. Carl Whitaker and Virginia Satir are the major pioneers of this approach (Gurman and Kniskern 1981b).

Family Systems Theory (Bowen)

Bowen's Family Systems Theory is one of the most influential schools in family therapy. Many of Bowen's concepts have been adopted in different forms by other schools of family therapy. The foundational concept of Bowen is "differentiation" from the family of origin and the establishment of a true self in the face of familial triangulation. Differentiation and maturity are accomplished when a person can "define himself" within the context of the family relationship. The failure of this process occurs in the cases of "undifferentiation" and "cut-off" phenomenon. The basic contributor to undifferentiation is "triangulation" by the parents who are emotionally divorced and position their child between themselves to reduce the "anxiety" in their relationship. The major concepts are "differentiation," "anxiety" within the system, "triangulation," "transmission of illness across generations," "emotional versus cognitive processes," "family projective system," and "overadequate-inadequate couple." The genogram of the family is an especially useful tool in this model. The interventions of Bowen are based on the technique of "funneling through the therapist" (Bowen 1978), by which the therapist responds to the family's undifferentiation and their attempts to triangulate him or her. The family is encouraged to make "family voyages" to their families of origin and resist the attempt of the senior generation at triangulating them again in their conflicts (see Chapter 5, "Multigenerational Family Systems Theory of Bowen and Its Application").

Contextual Therapy (Boszormenyi-Nagy)

This intergenerational model of family therapy developed by Ivan Boszormenyi-Nagy (1987c, 1987d) addresses the concepts of loyalty, indebtedness, entitlement, and the ethical basis of the family relationships. The symptom is seen as the by-product of disorder in the above dimensions (see Chapter 6, "Contextual Therapy").

Communicational and Systems Approaches to Family Therapy

The systems approach to family therapy combines the principles of general systems theory and cybernetics, which together emphasize the circular causality and feedback mechanisms to maintain family homeostasis. The family strives to maintain its homeostasis in the face of environmental forces that require change. Rigid families attempt to maintain homeostasis at all costs, which results in the lack of adaptability to environmental demands.

Under such circumstances, the heightened tension results in the emergence of symptomatic interactions and maladaptive behavior in one or more members. Rigid family boundaries and homeostatic mechanisms also reduce the flexibility necessary to adapt to the internal requirements for the passage through life cycles. Structural and strategic family therapies are the major *communicational/systems approaches* to family therapy.

Structural Family Therapy

Structural family therapy was developed by Salvador Minuchin and his colleagues (Minuchin 1974a). The collaborations with Haley and Montalvo further enriched this approach. The foundational theoretical concept in structural family therapy is that of "boundary." The polar family types of "enmeshed families" and "disengaged families" describe families whose members are excessively intrusive or unavailable to one another. The structural model of family intervention emphasizes the establishment of boundaries within the family through the decisive and sensitive actions of the therapist, further enforced by the assignment of family tasks and homework. The methods of "joining" the family are particularly emphasized to enhance the impact of the therapist in the sessions; these methods are described in Chapter 3, "Constructing Therapy: From Strategic, to Systemic, to Narrative Models." The therapist makes multiple maneuvers to join the family and shift family members' positions in order to disrupt dysfunctional patterns and strengthen parental hierarchies. Clear and flexible boundaries are established in the session, and the family is encouraged to search for new types of interaction. Structural family therapy has been applied to psychosomatic disorders, particularly anorexia nervosa and eating disorders in children and adolescents. Its effectiveness with psychosomatic disorders and behavioral problems has been documented in numerous case reports and observations, as well as in family outcome studies (Minuchin et al. 1978) (see Chapter 2, "Structural Family Therapy").

Strategic Family Therapy

Strategic family therapy emphasizes the need for a strategy developed by the family therapist to intervene in the ongoing efforts of the family to maintain their homeostasis by adhering rigidly to dysfunctional family patterns and symptoms. Strategic family therapy, like psychodynamic family therapy, has a well-articulated approach to address the resistance within family systems. The expectation of the resistance, particularly in response to interventions, requires innovative methods. One technique ("paradoxical intervention") attempts to reduce resistance and bring about change in the family structure and interactions by discouraging change. The paradoxical interventions facilitate the therapist's joining the family with minimal resistance to restructure the family interactional system.

Strategic interventions are based on identifying the family "rules" or metacommunicational patterns underlying the symptomatic behaviors. The interventions are applied through "directives" and assignment of homework to be practiced between the sessions. The homework can be a logical and "straightforward" approach to the symptomatic behavior, or it can be "paradoxical" by recommending something that the family has been doing all along. Paradoxical approaches reduce family resistance and undermine the family interactional pattern by going along with family communicational pathways. The *strategic approach* of Haley (1973) and Madanes (1981) emphasizes the importance of strengthening the parental alliance to deal effectively with the symptomatic and often challenging behavior of the children. The power struggles between family members and subsequently between the therapist and the family are the focus of treatment. The Mental Research Institute (Stanton 1986) emphasizes brief treatment and a highly creative use of paradoxical interventions. The *systemic school* of Milan uses a history-taking method to uncover the function of the symptoms and alter family interactions through "positive connotation," "reframing," "directives," and paradoxical interventions.

The strategic approaches gave rise to a number of new therapeutic approaches in the 1990s. In stark contrast to traditional strategic approaches, the new models emphasize *collaboration* between the therapist and the family. *Solution-focused therapy* concentrates on the exceptional solution repertoires already practiced infrequently by the patients to de-emphasize their problem-saturated outlook and enlarge the application of such solutions.

Narrative therapy focuses on patients' restrictive internal narratives and helps them to coauthor new and empowering ones. The disempowering influence of the stereotypical cultural beliefs on the families is recognized and resolved through exploratory efforts. The narrative approach is highly collaborative with the families, in contrast with early strategic models (see Chapter 3, "Constructing Therapy: From Strategic, to Systemic, to Narrative Models," and Chapter 20, "Couples Therapy: An Overview").

Behavioral Family Therapy

Behavioral family therapy applies the principles of positive and negative reinforcement to the family unit with the goal of enhancing reciprocity and minimizing coercive family processes. Coercive family processes generally assume the forms of punishment, avoidance, and power play. The enhancement of communication and problem-solving skills in the family are emphasized, and the family is discouraged from a tendency to punish one another. Contracting and behavioral exchange are enhanced in the family. Contemporary behavioral family therapy is based on social learning theory and has been particularly applied in the form of the Parent Management Training interventions (see Chapter 7, "Behavioral Family Therapy," Chapter 19, "Parent Management Training," and Chapter 22, "Behavioral Couples Therapy").

New models of behavior therapy have moved closer to the psychodynamic model by emphasizing the acceptance of symptomatic behavior before attempting to change it and carry out collaborative work with the patients.

Psychoeducational Family Intervention

Psychoeducational intervention uses diathesis-stress theory as its foundational concept and attempts to enhance family adaptation primarily through informing the family and the patient in detail about the nature of psychopathology in psychiatric disorders. It provides detailed information about treatment process and outcome and has been applied extensively to major mental illnesses such as schizophrenia, depression, alcoholism, and anxiety disorders. It consists of a series of in-depth instructional sessions by experts on the phenomenology, etiology, and diagnosis of the disorders. The family is informed about clinical research findings, housing arrangements, crisis management, financial assistance, and other resources.

Psychoeducational family therapy can be easily combined with other treatment modalities, particularly pharmacotherapy, crisis intervention, hospitalization, partial hospitalization, residential treatment, and behavioral and cognitive psychotherapies. The psychodynamic and exploratory psychotherapies are postponed until the later phases of treatment when the patient and the family have been stabilized.

Psychoeducational approaches make extensive use of the recent empirical findings such as expressed emotion, communication deviance, affective styles, and problem solving. By reducing the stressful family processes, the level of stress on the patient is reduced, with concomitant reduction in recurrence of illness and rehospitalization (see Chapter 8, "Psychoeducational Family Intervention").

Gender-Sensitive Family Therapy

The *gender-sensitive and feminist* approach to family therapy has alerted family therapists to hidden biases against women in structural therapy and psychoanalytic family therapy. It pays special attention to the issues of gender, money, and division of household tasks in conducting family therapy. Such biases generally exhibit themselves by therapist's insensitivity to inequity in the family roles and issues that generally underlie the family dysfunction. Lack of attention to these issues by the therapist can perpetuate existing family problems based on unbalanced gender roles, rather than enhance flexibility and fairness (see Chapter 10, "Gender-Sensitive Family Therapy").

Social Network Therapy

Social network therapy, developed by Ross Speck (Speck and Attneave 1971; Speck and Rueveni 1969), is applicable to families in which the family dysfunction and disintegration are closely related to the dysfunction and disintegration of the family's social network. It assesses the health and effectiveness of the social network, particularly the more recent constrictions in the family network prior to the immediate crisis. The size, homogeneity, and heterogeneity of the social network are assessed. The intervention techniques facilitate the emergence of activists within the family social network to enhance leadership, communication, relatedness, functioning, and expansion of the network. These changes can result in uncovering and resolving problems involving members of the family or the network.

Social network therapy can provide the necessary and appropriate theoretical framework for recently developed family preservation and wraparound services (see Chapter 9, "Social Network Intervention").

The Family Life Cycle

The concept of family life cycle was introduced in family theory by Duvall (1962), who proposed that the family moves through a series of developmental stages. Haley (1973) applied the concept of family life cycle to the understanding of clinical problems of families by relating dysfunction to the difficulties in moving from one developmental stage to another. Terkelson (1980) and Carter and McGoldrick (1980b) have defined critical emotional issues for the family at different stages of the life cycle.

Zilbach's (1988) model presents marriage as the first stage in the family life cycle. The anticipated eight stages of family life cycle are 1) marriage, 2) the beginning family, 3) the childbearing family, 4) the family with school-aged children, 5) the family with teenagers, 6) the family as a launching center, 7) the family in its middle years, and 8) the aging family. The concept of family life cycle has been utilized differentially, by different clinicians. In communicational approaches to family therapy, the life cycle assumes a primary position in the explanation of dysfunctional family patterns. Psychodynamic family therapists focus on subtle, complex, reciprocal, and interlocking developmental forces within the individual and the family. Intergenerational family therapists are concerned with deviant family role assignments that result in the stagnation and role immaturity of the younger generation. The family life cycle model has been studied recently and extensively in relation to families with chronically ill members, different cultural groups, and gay and lesbian couples (see Chapter 14, "The Family Life Cycle: A Framework for Understanding Family Development").

Family Therapy With Children and Adolescents

All schools of family therapy provide theoretical concepts specifically applicable to family therapy with children and adolescents. Inadequate separation and individuation processes in enmeshed family organizations do not provide for sufficient distance and objectivity to allow differentiation of the children. Subsequently, the children exhibit significant difficulty in relating to the school and social system, which further curtails their maturity. "Overinvolvement" between a child and a parent, "projective family mechanisms," and triangulation are major sources of the lack of differentiation in which immaturities and illness are transferred across generations. Projective identification describes the projection of unresolved parental conflicts onto a child who assumes an identity based on a historically assigned role that interferes with appropriate identity formation. Traumatic events such as child neglect and physical or sexual abuse in the early history of the family or parents can result in the repetition of such traumatic situations. "Parentification" assigns a parental role to the children and deprives them of age-appropriate experiences. Helm Stierlin (1974) has described the modes of binding, delegating, and expulsion as three ways that families negotiate a pathological separation in order to overcome the fear of prolonged fusion.

In family therapy with children, improvement in the child's behavior through enhanced school performance and peer-group relationships frequently encourages the parents to enter treatment for themselves to address additional goals of resolution of marital dysfunction or parental psychopathology (see Chapter 17, "Family Therapy With Children and Adolescents: An Overview").

The tensions between the fields of child psychiatry and family therapy were summarized in 1974 in two papers that examined the state of "the undeclared war between child psychiatry and family therapy" (Malone 1974;

McDermott and Char 1974). Child psychiatrists accused systemic family therapists of a lack of appreciation for the individual child and his or her unique developmental and intrapsychic characteristics. In the last decade, there has been empirical evidence for the necessity of combining multimodal treatment interventions with a range of childhood disorders such as attention-deficit/hyperactivity disorder (ADHD), childhood depression, and suicidality.

The Birth of Family Psychiatry

Progress in genetic research, biological psychiatry, and pharmacotherapy has broadened our knowledge about the etiological factors in the inception, maintenance, and recurrence of major mental illnesses and emotional disorders. This progress also has substantiated the combined role of a variety of biological, interpersonal, and psychological factors. A true field of family psychiatry has emerged. Contemporary family psychiatry provides a framework to address both the biological and interpersonal variables in major mental illnesses. Among other findings, the diathesis-stress theory (Rosenthal 1970) and the Finnish adoption studies (Tienari 1987) have provided significant data emphasizing the combined role of biological and interpersonal variables. Schizophrenia and depression are examples of disorders whose treatment involves a new integrative orientation of family psychiatry.

Diathesis-Stress Theory

The diathesis-stress or vulnerability-stress theory was first proposed by Rosenthal (1970) and further refined by Zubin and Spring (1977). It views the disorder as the product of two sets of variables: vulnerability and stressors. The vulnerability can be the result of genetic and biological factors, although psychological and interpersonal vulnerability can function in a similar fashion. Genetic factors have been studied best in schizophrenia, depression, and alcoholism.

Finnish Adoption Studies

The Finnish adoption studies (Tienari 1987) produced data supportive of the combined and interconnected role of genetic and familial variables in the genesis of schizophrenia. The study examined the level of family functioning, adaptability, and organization of adoptive families by dividing them into five groups ranging from "optimally functioning" to "inadequately functioning." Although all families adopted children with comparable genetic vulnerability, the outcome of the children was significantly correlated with level of family functioning (see Chapter 27, "Family Variables and Interventions in Schizophrenia").

Nonshared Environment in Adolescent Development

A comprehensive and well-designed study has attempted to directly measure the environment to locate differences between siblings' exposure and experience, and the impact of these differences on their development (Reiss et al. 1994; Reiss et al. 2000). It attempts to determine along which parameter siblings differ in their exposure to an experience of the environment and which shared or nonshared differences are associated with differential developmental outcomes in individuals.

This study has included several hundred families, which have been divided into the following six groups: 1) families with monozygotic twins, which were 100% genetically similar; 2) families with dizygotic twins; 3) ordinary siblings in nondivorced families; 4) full siblings in stepfamilies (all 50% related); 5) half siblings in stepfamilies (25% genetically related); and 6) unrelated siblings in stepfamilies (0% related). Nonshared variables could be any social, biological, or physical factors that affect psychological development. The environment measured in the study refers to shared and nonshared environmental components that account for the portion of variance that remains after subtracting the variance accounted for by genetic factors and error.

The emerging data suggest that at least certain nonshared variables have systematic influence on developmental outcomes (Dunn et al. 1990). For example, some data point to the importance of differential parenting between siblings. Children who receive more affection and less control from their mothers are less likely to show signs of internalizing behaviors as rated by mothers. The siblings who received more paternal affection may become more ambitious educationally and occupationally (Baker and Daniels 1990; Reiss et al. 2000).

Family Variables in Schizophrenia

Recent family studies have investigated the variables that can distinguish families with schizophrenic members from those with no schizophrenic members. The studies have looked at indicators of risk and have particularly focused on the three variables of expressed emotion, communication deviance, and affective style (Goldstein 1987). *Expressed emotion* refers to criticizing communications and negative attitudes in the family. *Communication deviance* refers to lack of communication clarity. *Affective style* refers to negative emotional-verbal behavior in family interactions. The studies use the vulnerability-stress model (see Chapter 27, "Family Variables and Interventions in Schizophrenia").

Expressed Emotion (EE)

In 1962, Brown reported that chronic male schizophrenic patients who had returned to live with their families following psychiatric hospitalization were more prone to rehospitalization than patients who went to other living arrangements. He and his colleagues then designed a prospective study to examine the affective atmosphere of the family and proposed the term "expressed emotion" (EE), a composite variable with the values of high and low, as an index of the family's criticism of and overinvolvement with the patient (Brown et al. 1962). A number of subsequent reports of British and American samples have indicated that the percentage of relapse in schizophrenic and depressed patients in families with high EE is four times higher than in low-EE homes (Hahlweg et al. 1989; Hooley et al. 1986; Vaughn and Leff 1976.). The interventions with families high in EE, with specific goals of reducing familial hostility and overinvolvement, have provided experimental evidence that EE is indeed causally related to the course of illness and a decrease in the level of EE results in relapse reduction (Hahlweg et al. 1989).

Communication Deviance (CD)

The family variable of CD was studied by Wynne and Singer (1963), who looked at a group of parents of schizophrenic patients and compared them with parents of nonschizophrenic patients. They found a lack of communication clarity and disturbances in maintaining attention in the parents of schizophrenic patients. Subsequent studies have indicated that CD is related to the severity of psychopathology in offspring, although some of the disturbances are nonschizophrenic in nature. Further studies also have indicated that high CD, together with high EE or negative affective style, can be a risk marker for schizophrenia spectrum disorders (Wynne 1987).

Affective Style (AS)

Affective style (AS) refers to the emotional-verbal behavior of family members during family discussions with patients. It is measured by counting the number of criticisms, guilt inductions, intrusions, and supportive statements made by the relatives.

Family Intervention With Depression

Deficits in social functioning in depressed patients are common and can persist in the absence of clinical symptoms. Depressed patients tend to be aversive with others and also to feel victimized by them. They engage frequently in escalating negative exchanges with their mates. Depressed patients and their spouses tend to verbalize their negative, subjective feelings more frequently than ordinary couples. The marriages of depressed women and men are characterized by friction, poor communication, dependency, lack of affection, overt hostility, silence, withdrawal, and tendency for husbands to view their spouse's unspoken misery as an accusation (Coyne 1987; Haas et al. 1985). An intimate relationship with a spouse may be a protective factor against depression, and a good marital relationship seems to help neutralize the effects of stress-producing situations such as the care of many young children and unemployment (Brown and Harris 1978).

Children of depressed parents are at risk for many psychological problems. The rate of diagnosable psychiatric disturbance in children of depressed parents can be as high as 40%–50% (Coyne 1987). The risk to children is increased if 1) the depressed person's spouse becomes depressed or is unavailable to the child; 2) there are marital problems or a divorce (Coyne 1987); and 3) a supportive relationship with another adult is unavailable.

A model for prevention of depression in children of depressed parents has been empirically tested in the past decade and its positive outcome confirmed (Beardslee et al. 1997, 1998b) (see Chapter 28, "Depression and the Family: Interpersonal Context and Family Functioning").

Psychoeducational Family Intervention

Psychoeducational interventions enhance the capacity of the family to cope with illness in children by informing the family about the etiology, phenomenonology, and treatment process with, for example, schizophrenic and depressed patients. At the same time, psychoeducational family therapy has enabled mental health professionals to intervene with families in ways that prevent further emotional crisis in the family. The application of the psychoeducational model to childhood depression and suicidality has been particularly productive (Brent 1997; Brent et al. 1997; Goldman and Beardslee 1999). The model has been applied preventively to a range of stressful and potentially pathogenic situations for children, such as pediatric cancer and death and dying (Koocher et al. 1996; McCreary et al. 1998; Pettle 1998) (see Chapter 8, "Psychoeducational Family Intervention").

Family Intervention With Alcoholism

The investigation of the structure and dynamics of families of alcoholic patients, conducted over the past two decades, has produced definitions of "the alcoholic family" and the "alcoholic family identity." This family identity is formed when alcohol comes to play a critical role in the day-to-day behavior of the family. Alcohol becomes the central organizing principle in the family, limits the family's flexibility to adjust to changes and crises, and affects the family regulatory mechanisms such as rituals, routines, and celebrations.

The investigations of "alcoholic" families are an example of integrating sound theoretical concepts, such as transmission of an illness across generations and family life cycle, within a prevention framework. This framework identifies the role of protective and risk factors using an empirically refined methodology.

The transmission of alcoholism to the next generation is facilitated by the interruption in the family regulatory mechanisms. These mechanisms include family rituals and "ritual process," which is a systematized form of communication that contributes to the establishment and preservation of the family's identity and collective sense of self (Wolin and Bennett 1984).

Equally productive and influential has been the range of family interventions with adolescent substance abuse, using a multimodal approach (Friedman 1990; Henggeler 1997; Liddle and Dakof 1995a, 1995b) (see Chapter 31, "Alcoholic and Substance-Abusing Families").

Family Classification and Diagnosis

The *Diagnostic and Statistical Manual of Mental Disorders* series, including DSM-IV and DSM-IV-TR, has rekindled the interest in an empirically based family classification and diagnostic system (American Psychiatric Association 1980, 1987, 1994, 2000). A family classification system has been proposed by the Group for the Advancement of Psychiatry (GAP). The GAP (1991) Committee on the Family has proposed a document consistent with DSM-IV to specify diagnostic criteria for family and couple relational disorders. Their criteria focus around specific family problems such as sexual or physical abuse, divorce, sexual disorders, failure to thrive, and separation anxiety (see Chapter 16, "Diagnosis of Family Relational Disorders").

Family Intervention in Psychiatric Hospitals

The goals of the family-oriented model of inpatient intervention are to prevent rehospitalization, maintain fragile ties between the family and the patient, and reach the highest functional level for the identified patient and the family. The inpatient family intervention (IFI) model accepts the patient's illness as the focus of treatment while recognizing the importance of family variables. Based on a stress-diathesis model and guided by recent research on EE, the relatively "causative" biological factors are placed in perspective along with familial and environmental influences. Medication is considered a natural ally of family intervention (Glick et al. 1985b, 1993). A psychoeducational model of IFI has been proposed by Glick et al. (1985b, 1993). Sholevar (1983, 1986b) has proposed a psychodynamic model of family intervention particularly applicable to hospitalized adolescents (see Chapter 29, "Family Intervention and Psychiatric Hospitalization").

Research in Family Therapy

Research in family therapy has been active from the early days of the clinical practice. Initially, there were uncontrolled studies of family interventions with poorly described families. This period was followed by controlled investigation of family intervention with different disorders or family structures. The more recent studies have expanded to family intervention with individually diagnosed illnesses.

Recent advances in marital therapy and family therapy research have been summarized in this book by Johnson (Chapter 37, "Couples Therapy Research: Status and Directions") and by Clarkin, Carpenter, and Fertuck (Chapter 36, "The State of Family Therapy Research: A Positive Prognosis"). Their research from couples therapy has provided a bridge between different couples therapy models and the empirically and clinically based initiatives. They have also underlined the need for defining and describing the nature of intimate relationships to help refine research methodology (Johnson and Lebow 2000). In addition to family outcome studies, there has been an interest in the investigation of family system concepts as they relate to treatment methodology and outcome. The question "Is family therapy effective?" has been made more specific by examining the impact of specific treatment formats and strategies with specific family problems, individual diagnoses, and the mediating therapeutic goals. The comparison of family therapy with other treatment modalities or in combination with other treatment approaches has focused on the *level of responsiveness* of different problems to different treatment modalities, rather than attempting to make family therapy appear to be the superior treatment approach. In the area of child and adolescent disorders, the treatment of conduct disorders and delinquency has produced encouraging results. The Parent Management Training of Patterson and his colleagues (Forehand et. al. 1981;

Patterson and Forgatch 1987; Patterson et al. 1992) and the Functional Family Therapy of Alexander and Barton (1976) have proved very effective.

Investigations with families of schizophrenic patients have been very impressive in the past decade. The treatment has been manualized and clearly exhibits the usefulness and effectiveness of family therapy as part of the overall treatment of these seriously disturbed patients (Bellack and Mueser, in press). The interventions have focused on lowering EE and increasing family coping capacity by using psychoeducational and cognitive-behavior strategies.

Conclusion

The turn of the century marks the coming of age of the field of family therapy. There is a clear movement toward horizontal and vertical integration within the divergent models of family theory, as well as between family theory and biological, psychological, and social theories in the context of the broader cultural perspective. The effectiveness of other therapeutic modalities and the role of psychobiological and genetic factors are acknowledged and beneficially incorporated by family investigators. This integrative approach is in its early phase but is sufficiently advanced to allow the collection and examination of data according to a comprehensive model that can guide investigation and clinical practice. The multidimensional investigation of schizophrenia and depression and the application of psychoeducational family therapy to these disorders are productive examples of the contemporary approach (see Chapter 27, "Family Variables and Interventions in Schizophrenia"; Chapter 28, "Depression and the Family: Interpersonal Context and Family Functioning"; and Chapter 8, "Psychoeducational Family Intervention"). The multidimensional approach has enhanced the investigative power of the field of family therapy, as well as other mental health fields such as biological psychiatry. The effective collaboration has extended beyond the mental health fields and has embraced the medical field—particularly in "medical family therapy" with chronic disorders (see Chapter 35, "Medical Family Therapy").

The application of refined research methodology and advanced data analysis methods has sharpened the focus of clinical observation and theory building. This productive collaboration has paved the road in family intervention with alcoholism, schizophrenia, depression, adolescent substance abuse, and conduct disorders. The intelligent recognition of the multiple factors contributing to such complex disorders has given rise to several models of multisystemic interventions that are deeply grounded in family theory (see Chapter 17, "Family Therapy With Children and Adolescents: An Overview").

Family Theory and Therapy: An Overview

The past two decades (1980–2000) can be distinguished from the earlier three decades (1950–1980) by the enhanced integration of biopsychosocial therapies, which has allowed the application of family theory to the recognized disorders affecting different patient populations. This orientation has in turn allowed for formulation of special intervention procedures such as the psychoeducational family approach with schizophrenia (see Chapter 27, "Family Variables and Interventions in Schizophrenia," and Chapter 8, "Psychoeducational Family Intervention"). The emphasis on scientific examination of clinical variables and the impact of interventions have enabled the field to take great pride and joy in its accomplishments and refrain from making unsubstantiated claims. The investigations of expressed emotions are a fitting example of such productive collaboration between investigators and clinicians from different countries and cultures (see Chapter 27, "Family Variables and Interventions in Schizophrenia"). Chapter 36, on family therapy research, by John Clarkin, Daniel Carpenter, and Eric Fertuck, and Chapter 37, on couples therapy research, by Susan Johnson review and synthesize the present state of our knowledge.

II

Family Therapy: Theory and Techniques

Introduction to Family Theories

G. Pirooz Sholevar, M.D.

The pioneers of family therapy adopted and developed a dramatic variety of theoretical perspectives. Their orientations were so dissimilar that at times it was hard to recognize any common ground. For example, Ackerman, one of the major contributors to psychodynamic family therapy, was highly influenced by his background in psychoanalysis and child psychotherapy. Bowen, best know for his Multigenerational Family Systems Theory, originally incorporated many psychoanalytic elements in his work before moving toward more biological/systemic orientation and biology-specific terminology. Bowen's biological and medical background was instrumental in his description of the phenomenon of differentiation in family systems.

Communication theory, developed by Bateson, Jackson, and Haley, was another unique perspective of family therapy—one that was rooted in Bateson's anthropological background. Bateson and Haley subsequently worked with the family as a whole by way of the general systems theory described by von Bertalanfy (whose theory was favored to a large degree by all family therapists). Later still, Bateson and Haley employed the science of cybernetics to describe family behavior as an organized whole and the function of feedback mechanisms in the maintenance of the systemic homeostasis.

The work of Don Jackson showed communication theorists how *covert* behaviors and messages could describe phenomena similar to unconscious experiences; analogously, covert behaviors and interactions in the family system could describe events that were not quite conscious. The relationship between covert and conscious experience posited by family theorists was compatible with both psychoanalytic and systems theory. As with Bowen, a biological and medical background was instrumental in Jackson's psychological theory, and particularly in his description of homeostasis in family systems.

Two other influences on the diverse field of family therapy should be mentioned. Behavior therapists ushered in a keen interest in the antecedents and consequences of the behavior and demonstrated the use of concrete and measurable factors in patient-family interactions. Object relations theorists, such as Guntrip and subsequently the Scharffs, brought knowledge of the characteristics of small-group interactions to family therapy.

Divergence in the schools of family therapy has continued to the present time and to some degree has increased. For example, the communicational approach to family therapy has given rise to multiple approaches, including structural, multiple strategic, solution-based, and narrative family therapy. Most of the systems and communicational schools have borrowed many concepts from behavioral and cognitive family therapies.

The following nine chapters in this volume describe the theoretical systems and concepts used by different family therapists. The *structural* and multiple *strategic* schools of family therapy emphasize the family as a system and the functions of communication, feedback, and homeostasis in that system. In addition, structural and strategic therapists emphasize the contemporary social context of the family as the primary focus for functional and dysfunctional interactions. The *structural* school (see Chapter 2, "Structural Family Therapy") emphasizes family structure, organization, boundaries, and the level of proximity or distance within the relationships. Restructuring and the stabilization of new family structures are emphasized. The search for realms of competence by individual family members and the family as a whole is given special attention.

Multiple *strategic* approaches to family therapy (see Chapter 3, "Constructing Therapy: From Strategic, to Systemic, to Narrative Models") emphasize the role of the therapist to direct change within the family system. Cybernetic concepts and the role of feedback in family interactions are principles most evident in the work of Mental Research Institute (MRI) and Haley. Different strategic approaches identify problems using different ways of conceptualizing different mechanisms for bringing about change. The assignment of homework or directives is an essential aspect of this approach. "Resistance" is conceptualized and dealt with in an organized manner in strategic schools, although the strategic therapist's concept of resistance is different from both psychodynamic and behavioral family therapists. The strategic schools' therapeutic strategy is based on the construction of a map by the therapist to help him or her approach the family in a unique and individualized way.

Among the new strategic approaches described in Chapter 3 are *solution-focused* and *narrative* therapies. The phrase "constructing therapy" is used in the chapter title instead of a more literal description of chapter contents like "strategic approaches"; we feel that "constructing therapy" is a more representative title for the group of family therapies that arose in 1990s and at turn of the century.

Narrative therapy encourages families to construct genuinely new, *solution-based* narratives for their lives. Reality and meaning of the narrative are viewed as co-constructions between the therapist and the family that do not necessarily coincide with objective reality. The "tools" of new narratives, meanings, and contexts for their problems empower families to pursue their lives with less contradiction and greater success.

The *systemic* approach pays special attention to the family game (i.e., the way families protect themselves from change through homeostatic rules and patterns of communication). Also important are *positive connotation*, which increases cooperation of the family, and the role of *invariant prescription* (see Chapter 3, "Constructing Therapy: From Strategic, to Systemic, to Narrative Models," for more details). Systemic therapists take family histories to learn about the properties and origins of current family games.

Psychodynamic family therapy (see Chapter 4, "Psychodynamic Family Therapy") has the goal of helping families to reach higher levels of maturity and self-observation, and to enhance relationships and intimacy both among family members and outside the family. The success of this goal is predicated on personality (and ego) expansion as the family members individually and collectively are freed from conflicts and restrictions embedded in the early life of the current generation or previous generations of the family. Personality expansion occurs by reexamining and reintegrating of past and present experiences of the individual and by resolving restrictive forces. Such restrictive mechanisms, particularly *shared family defenses*, attempt to protect the family from their *shared conflicts* and fantasized dangers through overly restrictive practices. These practices in turn deprive family members of developmental progression. Shared conflicts and defenses exhibit themselves in the transference reactions among the family members and between the family and the therapist. Therapists use personal empathy and other aspects of the therapeutic alliance to expand the experiential self of family members. Closely related to the psychodynamic school is the *experiential* approach to family therapy, which emphasizes the role of unexpressed feelings in limiting the developmental progression of the family.

Bowen's school of multigenerational family system theory (see Chapter 5, "Multigenerational Family Systems Theory of Bowen and Its Application") examines failure in families across multiple generations. Parents' involvement with their families of origin through the mechanism of triangulation initiates and maintains *fusion* between generations and results in limited *differentiation* in the next generation. Interactional disturbances in the families are seen as the result of poor differentiation between family members. The lack of differentiation curtails parents' ability to constructively cope with "anxiety" and leads to their attempts to diffuse anxiety by triangulating other family members, particularly their children.

The *contextual therapy* of Boszormenyi-Nagy (see Chapter 6, "Contextual Therapy") combines many psychoanalytic concepts with the existential philosophy of Hegel. In addition to psychological concepts, contextual therapists pay special attention to the *ethics* of caring and the concept of *fairness* as the context for relationships. Major theoretical concepts of contextual therapy include self-delineation and validation, the relational ethics of fairness, constructive and destructive entitlement, and visible and "invisible loyalties" of patients and parents to the previous generation.

Contemporary *behavioral family therapy* and social learning theory (see Chapter 7, "Behavioral Family Therapy") adheres to the principles of reciprocity and resolution of punitive interactions as the basis for the school's conceptualizations and interventions. Social learning theory is a major current theoretical perspective for the behavioral approach and has been particularly used in couples therapy and in treatment of conduct disorders.

Psychoeducational family interventions (see Chapter 8, "Psychoeducational Family Intervention") view the families as a major resource for members with chronic mental illnesses and helps enhance families' coping capacity by providing in-depth and practical information about the nature of the illness, its symptomatology, and treatment methodology. The emphasis on stress-diathesis theory has made psychoeducational and behavioral methods particularly applicable to the treatment of major mental disorders such as schizophrenia, depression, and anxiety disorders.

Social network therapy (see Chapter 9, "Social Network Intervention"), developed by Ross Speck, pays special attention to the role of the broader social network in the maintenance and disintegration of adequate family functioning. The social network approach is also a comprehensive methodology for the process of family reintegration. In addition to psychological measures, this approach activates the community and makes the enormous resources of the social network available to its members. The methodology can provide a theoretical frame for new initiatives such as family preservation.

Gender-sensitive and *feminist* approaches to family therapy (see Chapter 10, "Gender-Sensitive Family Therapy") have alerted therapists to hidden biases against women in the general systems theory and psychoanalytic family therapy. In addition to gender, gender-sensitive and feminist family therapists may pay attention to the distribution of power and money and the division of household tasks. Biased therapists may be insensitive to inequities in family roles and other issues that generally underlie family dysfunction. Inattention to gender issues can perpetuate problems based on unbalanced gender roles.

2

Structural Family Therapy

H. Charles Fishman, M.D.
Tana Fishman, D.O.

Introduction

One day in the mid-1970s, a 14-year-old girl was referred to the psychosomatic research project at the Philadelphia Child Guidance Clinic with a suspected case of anorexia nervosa. The physicians at Children's Hospital told the researchers that they suspected the youngster was losing weight because of psychological factors; they had performed numerous medical tests that were negative. As part of the subsequent research project, an interactional task was administered to all the members of the family: they were requested to listen to and reply to a tape recorder that asked the family to plan a meal out loud, to talk about what each member liked or did not like about one another, and to talk about a recent conflict. They were also asked to interpret a very conflict-laden Thematic Apperception Test (TAT).

The taped interactional patterns of the family were then rated by researchers, who did not know whether this was a "normal" family or a symptomatic family, for patterns of enmeshment, triangulation, rigidity, overprotectiveness, and diffusions of conflicts. The researchers found that this family did *not* evidence patterns of a psychosomatic family. They were not enmeshed, overly involved, rigid, or conflict avoiding. The researchers called the doctors at the hospital and said, "This child, as far as we could ascertain, is not losing weight on a psychological basis." The doctors at the hospital redoubled their diagnostic efforts and discovered that the youngster, indeed, had a medical illness in the form of a pineal tumor!

In this chapter we will discuss the central points of four areas of *structural family therapy* (SFT): history, theory, techniques, and applications. SFT is a large body of knowledge and as such cannot be covered in a single chapter. However, we hope to provide a clear picture of the uniqueness of the model as well as some of the promise it holds for the future.

A Very Brief History

The following section gives a brief history of structural family therapy. Anecdotes have always divulged the finer moments in family therapy. The ability to find interactional markers precise enough to discriminate between physical and psychological symptoms is almost *science*, and psychotherapy does not travel that path very often. This capacity to describe family systems in consensually agreed upon ways is one of the most powerful aspects of SFT.

Edgar Levenson (1972) described the progression of psychotherapy over the last 80 years as moving through three stages, or paradigms. The first paradigm was the psychoanalytic model, stemming from the work of Sigmund Freud. In this model, the problem was seen within the individual. What needed to change was the inner working of the individual. Interestingly, these inner workings were metaphorically described using terms borrowed from the "high" technology of the time, the steam engine: repression, sublimation, and displacement.

The second paradigm, which came into prevalence during World War II, was the communication model. It was based on cybernetics—if one communicated and followed the resulting feedback, one's problems would be resolved. The metaphors for this model were the telephone and the guided missile system. For example, a missile that received appropriate feedback would hit its target.

The third paradigm was the organismic model, which looked at the world as an organization or system and analyzed the relationships within that system. The metaphor came not from engineering but from biology.

Family therapy is based on this third, and organismic, model. If an individual has a problem, the problem is not based within his or her individual psyche, nor does it reside in the communications between two people. It resides instead in the interactions in the individual's social ecology.

The direct precursor of SFT is the work on the "double bind" interactions found in schizophrenic families. Gregory Bateson, in his double-bind theory (Bateson et al. 1956), proposed that specific interactions could influence a disease. He postulated that conflicting injunctions from parents put their schizophrenic child in a bind, and that further injunctions from them forbidding the child from leaving the social field increased the bind and led to the emergence of schizophrenic symptoms.

The work of Bateson et al. (1956) opened the door to a new dimension in the organismic model by describing interactions on a micro level. Such a jump was essential for the further development of the organismic paradigm. It allowed clinicians to see the patient as embedded in a system that maintained behavior and enabled them to describe the system (and to plan treatment) using a theory that was grounded in observations.

This system for describing interactions in all systems, not just those with schizophrenic members, was the initial contribution of SFT. While the model has evolved far beyond this initial concept, it was, nonetheless, the concept of structure that allowed observations of interactions to be organized.

Frank Pittman (1993) claims that it was Salvador Minuchin who "structured" the field of family therapy. The concept of structure in this field was a breakthrough: it provided a lens through which the clinician's observations of family interaction could be organized.

In a discussion with Pittman about how the idea of SFT emerged, Minuchin said,

> I was influenced by medicine. In describing families, I was looking for something like the structure of an organ—something that had perceivable architecture. Of course, the concept has been misinterpreted. The concept of structure has been criticized as describing a static system. My concept at the beginning was that structure describes structures that are *changing*.
>
> I was always interested in context. In Israel, there was a tremendous mélange of cultures—Yemenite kids playing with European and South American youngsters alongside Turkish children. I was struck by the differences in their cultural contexts—yet there were similarities in their family interactional patterns. (S. Minuchin, personal communication, 1992)

The SFT model was formally applied for the first time at a residential treatment facility for adolescents outside New York City, the Wiltwyck School for Boys. The work in that project (Minuchin et al. 1967) was the first formal inquiry into family functioning from a structural perspective. This groundbreaking work in the 1960s did not focus on the intrapersonal dynamics of the delinquent but rather on the family environment that had produced and supported the adolescent's behavior. This innovative study was designed to include both experimental and control group families. The results confirmed the hypothesis that SFT can positively influence a delinquent's behavior. After treatment, patterns of executive functioning improved significantly in experimental families. Mothers used less behavioral control yet were more effective. Mothers also displayed more affectionate behavior, and yet there were fewer instances of aggression or control in the family. Overall, this work supported the value of intervening in family systems and the essentiality of working within the contemporary context. The study also demonstrated the usefulness of working with structure as a marker to direct therapy. Minuchin and his colleagues showed that as the structure of these families was modified, each person's experience in the family changed. As a result the adolescent found a new position in the family and altered his behavior.

Two books in the 1970s served to confirm SFT as a major model for family therapy. In 1974 Salvador Minuchin published *Families and Family Therapy* (Minuchin 1974a) and formally introduced the SFT model to the clinical world. The concepts of reading structure, mapping the family system, and complementarity became common parlance in the family therapy world.

In 1978, Minuchin, along with Bernice Rosman and Lester Baker, published the book *Psychosomatic Families* (Minuchin et al. 1978), which described the conceptualization and results of a research project with anorexic teenagers and their families and introduced the concept of the "psychosomatic family." Follow-up findings in the book confirmed the effectiveness of SFT. Among the 52 children who completed the treatment program, a 2- to 7-year follow-up showed that 86% were asymptomatic with good psychosocial functioning. By 1980 SFT was firmly established as a model. To further elaborate this model, Minuchin and Fishman published *Family Therapy Techniques* (Minuchin and Fishman 1981), which provided the specific therapeutic techniques that the structural family therapist now uses to transform systems.

Theoretical Concepts

Systems Theory

Like most family therapies, the theoretical base for SFT is systems theory stemming from the work of Ludwig von Bertalanffy (1968), Norbert Wiener (1950), and Gregory Bateson (1972; Bateson et al. 1956). The three postulates of systems theory—circular causation (causation is circular), equipotentiality (every part of a system maintains the other), and complementarity (every behavior is the complement to every other)—are the central underpinnings of the clinical work of SFT.

Homeostasis

The second fundamental concept of SFT is the notion of homeostasis. SFT holds that the system, while *slowly* changing and becoming more complex, can, nevertheless, be seen as having a steady state, a systemic homeostasis. This observation is, of course, an artifact of the length of time we are observing the system. If we take an extremely long time period in a family's life, there are obviously great changes. But within the real time in which we live our lives and do therapy, we can perceive a steady state in terms of the organization of the system. Transforming the system's homeostasis is the goal of therapy—the dysfunctional homeostasis is seen as maintaining the difficulties.

Importance of the Contemporary Context

The third fundamental concept of SFT is the notion that the problem is maintained by the contemporary social context—the family, the extended family, friends, agencies, and any other social or physical forces that impinge on the client and family. The focus on the contemporary context is based also on a belief regarding the self. Salvador Minuchin and H. Charles Fishman (1979) proposed that the self is multifaceted; behavior and emotion expressed by a given individual not only are the result of history, temperament, and biology but also are called forth by demand characteristics of the present context. In a clinical setting, as we change the patient's social context, the problem is ameliorated as different facets of the patient's self are expressed.

Structure

The fourth theoretical underpinning of SFT is the concept of structure. As defined by Minuchin (1974a), "family structure is the invisible set of functional demands that organizes the ways in which family members interact. A family is a system that operates through transactional patterns. Repeated transactions establish patterns of how, when, and with whom to relate, and these patterns underpin the system." For example, a mother tells her child to pick up his socks and he obeys. This interaction defines who she is in relation to him and who he is in relation to her. Repeated interactions constitute a transactional pattern.

An operational definition of structure shows structure as the proximity and distance between members in a system. The functionality and dysfunctionality of this proximity and distance are determined on the basis of the developmental stage of the family members. This mother telling her son to pick up his socks may be appropriate when the boy is three but not when he is twenty.

Stemming from the concept of structure is the concept of boundaries. Boundaries describe the patterned transactions between members of a system to the exclusion of others. The structural family therapist posits that a functional organization within the family must have appropriate boundaries between subsystems: the parental, the siblings, the family unit as a whole, and the individual.

Emanating from this concept is a very useful family diagnostic nosology that describes dysfunction: *enmeshed*, for a family (or a subsystem) that is overly close; *disengaged*, where members of a family are too distant from one another. Other concepts that follow are *triangulation*, in which one person is torn between two other people. An example of this would be when parents disagree and then ask the child, "Is Mommy right or is Daddy right?"

As we have mentioned earlier, many assessments are gauged against developmental norms. Enmeshment is the inappropriate closeness of family members against a backdrop, of course, of developmental appropriateness. Disengagement is used to signify too much distance between family members again against a backdrop of developmental staging.

The use of a normative model of family functioning has become a controversial aspect of the SFT model. Critics say that a normative model is culturally incorrect—that the model only describes one kind of family—the prototypical middle-class American family.

While there is little research into this question of cultural correctness, the SFT model remains extremely useful. This model, which employs structure and boundaries, is the same model utilized by other disciplines, such as business. For example, it is vocationally dangerous to complain to your boss's supervisor about your boss. In SFT language, this would be called a cross-generational violation.

Nonetheless, there must be more research to determine whether in other cultures the tenets of SFT are valid. At the very least, in our culture, in a large variety of social contexts, SFT is both valid and invaluable. The fact that the therapist can ascertain structural dysfunction on the basis of observation in the room allows the practitioner to direct therapy toward patterns that are observable. Success, and at times failure, are readily apparent.

Techniques

In discussing techniques, we start with those that differentiate SFT from other models.

Enactment

Enactment refers to the construction of an interpersonal scenario during the session in which a dysfunctional transaction among family members is played out. Its significance for therapy resides in the fact that the transaction is not described in the past; it occurs in the context of the session in the present, and in relation to the therapist. As such, the therapist is in the position of observing the family members' verbal and nonverbal ways of signaling to each other. The therapist can then intervene in the process, increasing its intensity, prolonging the time of the transaction, introducing other family members, initiating alternative transactions, and in general introducing experimental probes. These interventions may give the therapist and the family information about the nature of the problem, the flexibility of the family solutions, and the possibility of an alternative therapeutic framework.

Beyond this, the therapist can have the family enact "changed" transactional patterns during the therapy session that can then serve as a template for the functional interactions outside the therapy.

The explicit use of enactment is facilitated by the therapist decentralizing himself or herself in the session and allowing the family to enact dysfunctional interactional patterns. Then, as therapy proceeds, the therapist challenges the family toward the enactment of more functional interactional patterns.

We think of this central concept as akin in some ways to Gestalt Therapy in that it is experiential. The major difference between the two is that the gestalt experience takes place with strangers, while the changed experience with SFT occurs with the most important people in a person's life—the family. Thus, the changes that are introduced in SFT will have a greater probability of being maintained postsession than in gestalt, in which only one family member or strangers had been involved.

This concept of the "therapy of experience" is central to the theory of change in SFT. Through the use of therapeutic techniques, change occurs by the family members having different experiences with one another in the therapy room and new interactional patterns emerge.

An obvious advantage of enactment is that it allows the therapist to take an objective position. The therapist can skillfully resist participating in the family interactions and can instead observe the interactions as they emerge. In so doing, the therapist can get invaluable information about the system.

A common concern that therapists have is whether one can possibly observe the family in the session and get accurate information. The mere presence of the therapist may distort the system unrecognizably.

This is where the technique of enactment becomes so valuable. Enactment allows for the emergence of semi-naturalistic interactions in the session. Thus, the therapist can observe the family almost "in vivo." Indeed, to the extent that the therapist is decentralized, he or she is able to see the interactional family sequences that are more or less what they are at home—in terms of, for example, enmeshment and triangulation.

Use of Self

In SFT, the therapist acknowledges that the self is an essential ingredient in the therapeutic process. The therapist uses himself or herself as a tool for producing therapeutic change. From this perspective, the self is utilized in a highly discriminating manner to move the family toward the therapeutic goals. For example, the therapist may be disciplined to be decentralized so that an enactment may emerge between family members. In this situation, the therapist is consciously becoming peripheral and setting the stage for interactions between the members of the system to emerge. On the other hand, when the therapist unbalances the system—that is, therapeutically sides with one family member over another—the therapist is actively using his or her personal power to perturb the system.

While these techniques will be described later in this chapter, it is important to emphasize that one of the powers of SFT is the therapist's willingness to use himself or herself in this differential way. We believe strongly in the fact that the power of psychotherapy is in the human relationship. People change in many ways. Jay Haley (personal communication, 1975) said that people change for their therapists. In large part, a corollary to this idea is the belief that the therapist recognizes the power of this relationship and utilizes this human connection to mobilize the family system. As such, the therapist is aware that there is a freedom to use a large array of family therapy techniques, but always in the context of the personal relationship between the clinician and the family.

The structural therapist is aware that this is a potentially hazardous position. There are dangers of induction, of somehow being influenced by the family to unknowingly follow the family's dysfunctional patterns. Nevertheless, the structural therapist needs to take the honest position that while the use of self is an essential ingredient, the self must be used in a thoughtfully directed manner. The therapist must be cognizant of the goals and the indications for specific techniques.

The clinician must always be following feedback from the family as the session proceeds. For that reason, "Training for Spontaneity" was an alternative title under consideration for Minuchin and Fishman's (1981) book *Family Therapy Techniques*. The notion was that a well-trained therapist, one with a refined use of self, would have mastered the techniques needed to be truly spontaneous. Such a self would be a well-honed instrument of change, available to intervene accordingly.

Structural Family Therapy   43

Goals of Therapy

The structural family therapist has specific structural goals for each session as well as for the overall course of treatment. These goals will clearly demonstrate the amelioration of all symptomatology in the system along with changed dysfunctional transactional patterns. Beyond that, however, the therapist works with the family toward the stabilization of the new structures that have been introduced in the therapy.

We see this as a direct contrast to Haley's (1976) approach, in which treatment ceased once the symptom was ameliorated rather that being continued until the new structures were stabilized. The structural family therapist, while being available to support the new organization of the family system, is aware of the danger of therapy becoming "interminable." It is necessary to ask if one is continuing therapy not so much to stabilize new structures, but because of a loss of therapeutic control.

Joining

Joining is the central technique of entering the family system in order to create the new system, the therapeutic system. One joins by confirmation of the individuals. The therapist confirms the individuals, acknowledges their pain, and presents himself or herself as a healer.

There are a number of different positions the therapist can utilize in joining with the family, including the close position, the median position, and the disengaged position. In the position of proximity to the family, or the *close position*, the therapist affiliates with the members, perhaps even entering into a coalition with some members against others. Although part of the unbalancing technique, it also affords an extremely powerful way of joining with the person with whom one has established a coalition. Probably the most useful tool for affiliation, however, is confirmation. In using confirmation, the therapist validates the reality of the individuals as he or she joins. The therapist searches out positives and makes a point of recognizing and rewarding them. Also, by identifying areas of pain, difficulty, and stress and acknowledging these areas rather than avoiding them, the therapist responds with sensitivity. This greatly facilitates joining.

In the *median position*, the therapist joins as an active, neutral listener. The therapist helps people tell their stories. This modality of joining, which is called *tracking*, is drilled into the therapist by objective schools of psychodynamic theory. While it is a useful way of gathering data, it is never as neutral or as objective as the user thinks because it can hamper the therapist's freedom of movement. While the family members are avidly telling the story, the therapist might find his or her attention locked into the content. While tracking the communication, the therapist may indeed be unaware that the family life was being enacted before the therapist's eyes.

The therapist could also join the family from the *disengaged position*, in which the clinician stands as an expert creating a therapeutic context that brings family members a sense of competence, a hope of change. In this way, the therapist functions not as an actor, but as a director. Perceiving patterns, the therapist creates a scenario facilitated by the enactment of familiar movements by forcing members to engage with each other in novel ways. While these techniques are change producing, they are also methods of joining that increase the therapist's leadership.

As an expert, the therapist monitors the family's worldviews. The clinician accepts and supports some family values and myths, while avoiding and deliberately ignoring others.

Paying attention to communicational patterns that express and support the family experience, the therapist extracts the phrases that are meaningful to the family. These phrases can be used to support the family reality or to construct an expanded worldview that will allow for flexibility and change.

Regulating Intensity

Intensity involves the therapist's selective regulation of the degree of impact of the therapeutic message. Family members have developed, through time, their preferred patterns of transaction and the explanations necessary to defend their preference. Preferences become values and then laws. The therapist, in attempting to challenge the way in which family members punctuate reality, sends a message that exceeds the threshold of selected deafness by which they protect their habitual patterns.

Intensity can be achieved by increasing the affective component of a transaction, by increasing the time in which family members are involved in such transactions, or by using frequent repetition of the same message in different transactions.

Regulating the degree of therapeutic intensity according to the feedback from the family is one of the structural family therapist's most powerful tools. By following the body language and the verbal feedback, the therapist uses the intensity to address the homeostatic threshold that keeps the system from changing. During the course of the session, the therapist selectively monitors the intensity of the message by reading the feedback from the system. The clinician then intervenes accordingly.

Searching for Competence

Families and individuals are often searching for a personal realm of competence when they come to therapists. The search for the locus of pathology in therapy is related to a conceptualization of what is expected to change. Families tend to come to therapy convinced that the pathology resides in one individual. This fact creates the necessity for alternative explanations. The therapist's search for competent areas in the individuals and family provide for powerful alternatives that enhance the therapeutic process.

On the basis of the concept of the "multifaceted self," the therapist challenges the system but confirms the individuals. In so doing, the therapist is confronting the family's view of one another. According to Minuchin and Fishman (1981),

> Families in which there are unresolved conflicts tend to become stereotyped in the repetitive mishandling of interpersonal transactions, with the result that the family members narrow their observation of each other and focus on the deficits in the family. (pp. 245–246)

In the course of therapy, as the transactional patterns change, people come to see one another differently, and a more functional self emerges.

The therapist, in the process of supporting these new aspects of self, believes that the self is like a diamond with many facets. If one shines a light on the diamond, certain facets will be seen, depending on the direction, strength, and quality of the light. If you change the light, different facets of the diamond will be reflected. The context of people, systems, and relationships surrounding the multifaceted self is like the light shining on the diamond. It is this context that brings out certain facets of the self and not others; if the context changes, other facets of the self will be expressed. In the clients we see, some of the facets are problematic. Thus, when we want to bring about change in our clients, we must transform their contemporary context such that their more functional facets will be brought out. That is, true even in the most encapsulated intrapersonal problems, such as multiple personality disorder or posttraumatic stress disorder.

Constructions

The construction of new interpretive frameworks is an important feature of structural therapy. There is a matching between the belief systems and the transactional patterns of families; therefore, changes in one are reflected as modifications in the other. Construction is the therapist's organization of this data in such a way that it provides the family members with a different framework for experiencing themselves and one another. The therapist presents the conflictive and stereotyped reality of the family as a reality that has alternate interpretations. This new reality also has alternate solutions.

With structural therapy the issue is not only constructing a new reality for the family. The therapist must also go beyond the conceptual and work with the family as their interactional patterns change as a result of the new reality. The goal is not only to get people to think differently about their problems but also to help shepherd them into interacting differently as a result of the new construction.

Use of Paradox

A paradox is a construction in which the family truth is embedded in a larger truth that contradicts it. The result is a conflict between truth and truth that the therapist organizes to confuse family members into a search for alternatives.

The structural family therapist uses paradox relatively infrequently. The belief is that we do better if we develop a collaborative relationship with the family. Ideally, we want the families to be our co-therapists. Nevertheless, there are times when the use of paradox can be an important way to move a system that is immobile: the dissonant information plus the changed position of the clinician to one of greater distance can mobilize a system.

According to Peggy Papp, the therapist usually expects, with direct interventions that are compliance based, the family to respond to the advice, explanations, suggestions, and tasks. Tasks are to be

> taken literally and followed as prescribed. They are aimed at directly changing family rules or roles. They include coaching parents on how to control children, redistributing jobs amongst family members, establishing disciplinary rules, regulating privacy, establishing age hierarchy, and providing information that the family lacks. (Minuchin and Fishman 1981, p. 248)

> Paradoxical interventions that are defiance based are interventions that will accomplish the opposite of what it is seemingly intended to accomplish. It depends for success on the family's defying the therapist's instructions or following them to the point of absurdity and recoiling....A reversal is an intervention in which the therapist directs someone in the family to reverse her attitude or behavior around a crucial issue in the hope that it will elicit a paradoxical response from another family member. It requires the conscious cooperation of the family member who is being instructed by the therapist and the defiance of the family member who is receiving the results of the instruction....Reversals can be used effectively in helping parents handle rebellious children. Remarkable results can be achieved in a short period of time if the parents are willing to follow the therapist's coaching. (Minuchin and Fishman 1981, p. 248)

Education

Education is an intervention on the cognitive level in which the therapist conveys a model of normative family functions based on the therapist's experience and axioms. Education differs from construction in that constructions are idiosyncratic in regard to the individual family situation, whereas education deals with generic issues of family functioning. It includes notions such as the meaning and importance of boundaries, optimal functioning in developmental stages, and transitional crises in family development.

There are certain principles of adolescent development that frequently can redirect families to focus on more essential issues. Statements illustrating these principles include "order your priorities," "only fight the big battles," or, as David Treadway said, "no child ever died of a messy room" (personal communication, 1987). One issue that is frequently misunderstood is that younger adolescents need considerable supervision completing school tasks. Developmentally they cannot conceptualize long-term goals—such as if they study hard, they will grow up and have a more comfortable life. An additional important issue is making sure that adolescents and parents understand that families are laboratories for learning negotiation skills.

The clinician must be aware, however, that the therapist and the family educator are different. While adding information can be valuable, the major task of the therapist is to transform the system so that the family can utilize knowledge. Usually it is a dysfunctional system that is maintaining the problem, not ignorance.

Boundary Making

Boundary making is an essential concept of SFT and distinguishes it from other therapies. Of course, boundaries are intellectual constructions. Interpersonal boundaries are a construction to help the therapist describe a patterned transaction among certain family members with the exclusion of other members. Boundaries define the members excluded, as well as those "framed in," and are described as residing on a continuum from enmeshed to disengaged.

Boundary making is the process by which the therapist controls membership of family members in a subsystem. It may be done by increasing proximity and experimentation among subsystem members with the exclusion of others (making boundaries), or by facilitating participation of subsystem members with other family and extrafamilial subsystems (diffusing boundaries).

Unbalancing

Unbalancing is a method of disrupting an entrenched family hierarchical organization. "Steady state" (homeostasis) is the capacity of a system (biological or social) to maintain its equilibrium within a certain functional range. Through unbalancing, the therapist introduces disequilibrium.

Unbalancing refers to the therapist's use of self as a member of the therapeutic system to disequilibrate the family organization. The clinician does so by joining and supporting an individual or family subsystem at the expense of other family members. This affiliation modifies the accustomed hierarchical organization of the family, introducing the possibility of new alternatives.

Unbalancing is a difficult technique for many of us. We have been trained to be equal and fair at all times. There are times, however, that in order to catapult a system toward change, one must side with one family member over another. This intervention can be immensely powerful because the prestigious person in the system, the therapist, dared to take sides. Suddenly, the other family members in the system see the allied member with new respect; their position has new credibility. This can greatly add to the intensity of the session and overcome the homeostatic threshold that keeps the system intractable.

It should be noted that during the course of a session, the therapist's unbalancing usually involves multiple alliances, not just an alliance with a single family member. The clinician skillfully alternates unbalancing, which ironically reintroduces a sense of fairness to the therapy.

Working With Complementarity

Complementarity refers to the characteristic of systems that holds that causation is circular. As in the Chinese metaphor of yin-yang, each part of the system complements every other. This concept can be difficult for families. Family members think linearly. A profound change in the perspective of the family members results from a transformation of their epistemology of change, from linear causality to complementarity. It is a change from "he is the symptom bearer," to "we are all involved." This relation of part to whole has major implications for the way of experiencing self in relation to others. This notion is embedded in the very foundation of family therapy: You, the family, must come to therapy and change so that your symptomatic member(s) will improve.

Complementarity, of course, is a basic principle of systems theory. Used as a technique, complementarity can be immensely powerful. For example, a young couple had separated because of marital difficulties. Each had a long litany of complaints about the other; they had each been in individual therapy, in which they had honed their criticisms. The psychiatrist Salvador Minuchin told the couple: You cannot change the other person directly. You can change yourself as the complement to your spouse. To the degree that you change, your partner will change. This use of complementarity underlines the fact that each of you is creating the other's behavior by your own behavior. Ironically, only if your spouse changes will you know that you have changed. We have little objectivity regarding our own degrees of change.

Applications

In this section we discuss applications of the principles discussed above, which are the foundation of structural family therapy. There are also new techniques and applications that have developed over the years in response to the needs of patients, families, and society. One of these new applications consists of involving the family by using the concept of the homeostatic maintainer and isomorphism. A second application applies SFT to the present medical climate of case management; objective observation becomes a critical marker of change. A third application is the work on adolescents—the clinical area in which SFT "cut its teeth." The fourth application revolves around advances produced by the SFT model in the areas of eating disorders—anorexia, bulimia, and compulsive eating. The fifth, and last, application that we discuss is the work we did with disadvantaged families and their communities.

Homeostatic Maintainer and Intensive Structural Therapy

An extrapolation of basic SFT theory is the concept of the homeostatic maintainer (HM). The HM is a tool that allows the therapist to organize perceptions about the dysfunctional system by illuminating the forces that are maintaining the status quo. The concept provides information about which individuals and which isomorphic interactional patterns are responsible for maintaining the system. By "isomorphism" we mean "equal structures" that are mirrored in different contexts. For example, the pattern of triangulation between two conflictual parents and their child is mirrored in the triangulation of the father between his elderly mother and father.

Isomorphism has been criticized as a concept because of the early claims that there exists an inevitable identical isomorphism between the family and the other systems in which it is embedded. This, of course, is not necessarily the case. There exists a bilateralism in systems. That is, there can be *different* isomorphs that exist concurrently between the family and the broader systems. These patterns do not necessarily reflect the same patterns of the family.

The tool of HM and the concept of isomorphism can be very useful when combined. The tool of HM can help the clinician identify the specific people involved in maintaining the homeostasis. Isomorphism can help identify the interactional patterns within which the HM's behavior is embedded. Furthermore, the use of the isomorphic patterns removes the theoretically untenable position of identifying a single person as maintaining a problem (systems theory holds that, on the basis of the equipotentiality of systems, all members of a system bear responsibility for maintenance of a problem).

The use of these ideas is central to a model called Intensive Structural Therapy. This model, elaborated in Fishman (1993), provides a clinical framework to include the family's broader context in treatment. We believe that this new direction is so critical because the family of today is changing and becoming increasingly more dependent on the broader context. Why this change? There are myriad reasons; a few seem obvious. For the typical American employee, who is paid an hourly wage, real income has not increased since 1973 (Schor 1991). As a result, families are working much harder and have less leisure. In 1987, the average employed person worked the equivalent of an extra month per year as compared with total hours worked in 1969 (Schor 1991). Richard Luov, in his book *Childhood's Future*, quotes a study that states the average American parents spend four minutes a day meaningfully talking to each other. Contact with their children merits even less time—30 seconds a day—in meaningful conversation between parent and child (Luov 1990).

And those people who are working are the lucky ones. There is severe unemployment and ensuing dislocation. At the same time, the various support facilities available to families are facing ever-diminishing finances. In addition, with changing political priorities over the last 12 years in the United States, there has been a dismantling of some vital social support services.

These social changes force the family to be more dependent on outside pressures. As a result, we must develop specific interventions and protocols for specific contexts.

Case Management and Interactive Markers

Case management and the use of interactive markers in managed care are other areas in which SFT is proving to be invaluable. SFT provides a clear conceptual system for clinicians to organize their treatment; in so doing, it provides goals and treatment effectiveness markers. The clinician is able to quantify for managed care consults. Structural change is used as a marker of effectiveness and allows the therapist to base the therapy on external observations. In those situations when the therapist is asked to work with patients and their families with problems such as incest, child abuse, and delinquency, the question sometimes demanded is how, on the basis of the therapy, can we assure the family, and in many cases the authorities, that the problem will not reoccur.

The logicians tell us that we cannot prove a negative. We can prove that something can happen, but not that something *won't* happen. Thus there needs to be some objective markers to ascertain when there has been a change. A clinician working toward the amelioration of dysfunctional interactions can get an estimation of the probabilities that a certain behavior, such as child abuse, may not reoccur if the dysfunctional interactional patterns have changed.

Of course, since medicine and psychology are sciences of probability, there cannot be complete certainty. But the fact that these objective patterns have changed gives some reassurance. Conversely, in situations in which the therapy is not successful and the interactional patterns have not changed, the therapist can have cause to be pessimistic. Markers of effectiveness are especially valuable in situations in which there is a fear that a dangerous behavior may reoccur. Indeed, when workers do not have a clear and objective basis on which to determine change in systems, conclusions are made on partial information. Such conclusions can lead to extremely deleterious consequences for the child and family and may even impact future generations.

Adolescents

As we mentioned earlier, the SFT model was initially developed in working with adolescents at the Wiltwyck School in the 1960s. The work of Jose Szapocznik and his group in Miami, using a family task based on the Wiltwyck project to evaluate family change, and using a similar population of adolescent youngsters, has provided evidence of the effectiveness of SFT as compared with the psychodynamic psychotherapy. Their work using SFT is supported by compelling empirical data (Letich 1993). Szapocznik et al. (1989a, 1989b) randomly assigned 69 boys from ages 6 to 12 who were referred for emotional and behavioral problems, as well as their families, to one of three treatment conditions: SFT, psychodynamic child therapy, and a recreational activities control group.

The SFT and individual psychodynamic child therapy were more effective than the control condition in retaining subjects in treatment. SFT and individual psychodynamic child therapy were equally effective in decreasing the presenting symptoms, as evidenced by both parent ratings of child behavior and child self-report. The researchers found that the biggest difference was in the effect the treatments had on the boys' families. Families of the boys in SFT continued to improve both during the course of therapy and up to the 1-year follow-up. By contrast, the families of the boys in the psychodynamic group deteriorated during the course of therapy and continued to deteriorate up to the one-year follow-up (Szapocznik et al. 1989a, 1989b).

Eating Disorders

Psychosomatic families are characterized by enmeshment, overinvolvement, rigidity, and conflict avoidance. As a result of the research on the psychosomatic family mentioned earlier, SFT is considered by many to be the treatment of choice for eating disorder patients. Its use of the contemporary context directs the therapist to involve all of the significant individuals in the patient's life. The technique of enactment empowers the therapist, in cases of very ill anorexic individuals, to challenge the parents to get their child to eat. This intervention addresses the split between the parents and forces the parents to work together while successfully getting nutrients into their child. Through this SFT intervention, the problem is corrected on two levels—the structural rift in the family and the patient's inanition. The system is addressed *and* the symptom is on the road to being corrected. Furthermore, the clinician is able to monitor closely the effectiveness of the therapeutic changes in the family process—challenged by the enactment.

Disadvantaged Families and Their Communities

Structural therapy has been useful in community work partly because it is a model of psychotherapy that does not depend solely on talking. At its core, SFT involves people experiencing one another differently. For this reason, SFT is extremely useful in work with populations for whom English is a second language or in which there is not a tradition of introspection.

In the mid-1990s, we were involved in a project involving troubled adolescents and their families. This project, located in New Jersey, used both a structural family therapist and a paraprofessional to whom we gave the title "Community Resource Specialist" (CRS). The CRS enhanced the effectiveness of the therapy (groups using the CRS showed a 66% rate of improvement, while the control group improved by only 28%). The design for the project resulted from the fact that the family infrastructure in many of our cities and rural areas had decayed, making family therapy more difficult. The family problems were not solely the result of structural difficulties, however. Through the work of the CRS, we enhanced the family therapy by partnership with someone who was an integral part of the community. The therapeutic initiative involved both the interior of the family system (the family structure) and its exterior (i.e., its relationship to its community).

In this model, the CRS helped a child get a mentor, or helped one of the parents get a job. This person, who was an integral member of the community, helped to strengthen the family's infrastructure by better connecting it to the community that the CRS knew so well. In addition, the structural family therapist worked to transform the interior of the family.

Recent Developments

The application of Structural Family Therapy to eating disorders has continued into the late 1990s (Fishman 1996). There has been further refinement of SFT in the treatment of couples (Minuchin and Nichols 1998). Structural (and psychodynamic) Family Therapy received a "broadside" from the feminists in the 1990s (Minuchin and Nichols 1998); however, their criticism seemed related to the misapplication of structural views rather than to faulty theoretical concepts (see Chapter 10, "Gender-Sensitive Family Therapy"). More importantly, Structural Family Therapy was applied to divergent cultural groups in the late 1990s (Kurtines and Szapocznik 1996; Minuchin and Nichols 1998; Navarre 1998).

Conclusion

Structural family therapy is an extremely effective model of family therapy. Its greatest advantage is the fact that by following structural process, the clinician is using a theory that is grounded in observation. For psychiatry, this has great advantages. Assessment and nosology are based on visible interactional processes and not solely on psychiatric symptoms—which are usually dependent on self-report. Diagnosis can then describe a dysfunctional context, and this description can be used to prescribe interventions. In addition, there are well-defined therapeutic techniques. The clinician, however, often uses interventions from other models of family therapy and even psychopharmacology to create and stabilize change; nonetheless, the markers of effectiveness are determined by structural assessment.

In family therapy there is always a balancing act that the psychiatrist must play between the need to transform the system and the need to maintain close surveillance of changes in the self of the patient. Family therapists believe, in the words of Dr. Larry Dossey, in the concept of the "nonlocal mind"—that "mind" is determined by the contemporary social context. We must, however, not lose sight of the individual. We must attend closely through empathy, respect, and confirmation to the evolving selves of our patients.

Chapters on Related Topics

The following chapter describes concepts related to structural family therapy:

- Chapter 3, "Constructing Therapy: From Strategic, to Systemic, to Narrative Models"

3

Constructing Therapy

From Strategic, to Systemic, to Narrative Models

Scott W. Browning, Ph.D.
Robert-Jay Green, Ph.D.

Introduction

The purpose of this chapter is to examine five models of family therapy that loosely form a subgroup within the field of family therapy. These models cannot be considered bound by an overarching descriptive label. Most significantly, they share, to a greater or lesser extent, the seminal concepts put forth in the writings of both Gregory Bateson (1972, 1979) and Milton Erickson (Haley 1967). Therefore, these models encompass some theoretical and technical commonalties. In addition, they have a common forum, the *Journal of Strategic and Systemic Therapies* and also have a central position in the pages of such mainstream journals as *Family Process* and the *Journal of Marital and Family Therapy*.

As will become apparent below, a schism has developed between the five models of therapy discussed in this chapter, even though the resulting therapies may look remarkably similar. The schism may be a result of the different emphases of Bateson and Erickson. Bateson brought to the field an intellectual understanding of families as "systems." He influenced the field to examine patterns of communication in the family. However, as an anthropologist and theoretician, Bateson did not address the practical applications that clinicians felt were necessary to institute change in the lives of their clients. For praxis, the field looked to the brilliant interventions of Erickson. His clinical work revealed to therapists the myriad of possible approaches to assist families in becoming "unstuck." Numerous therapy models have been, and continue to be, constructed using the ideas of Bateson and Erickson as a foundation.

The five theories discussed in this chapter are 1) Strategic/Problem-Solving—Jay Haley and Cloe Madanes; 2) Brief Strategic/Interactional—The Mental Research Institute (MRI); 3) Solution-Focused—Steve de Shazer and the Milwaukee Group; 4) Milan Systemic—The Milan Associates; and 5) Narrative—Michael White and David Epston.

These five therapeutic models suffer from an identity problem in the field at large. Arguments have been presented that they can be viewed as both distinct from one another (Fish and Piercy 1987; Fraser 1986; Goldenberg and Goldenberg 2000; Held 1986; MacKinnon 1983; Piercy et al. 1996) and essentially similar (Brown and Christensen 1999; Fraser 1986; Stanton 1981). Because they share some techniques and theoretical constructs, the five approaches have suffered from the perception that they represent a variation on a theme, rather than unique models. In clarifying their relationships, the different theories can be conceptualized as related species on an evolutionary tree, with Bateson and Erickson as progenitors.

To an outsider to the two species, similarities are more obvious than differences. However, while each "branch" is the offspring of both Bateson and Erickson, the degree of kinship varies. For example, the lineage of Problem-Solving Therapy is more clearly tied to Erickson, whereas an examination of the Milan Systemic approach shows an obvious kinship with Bateson.

The primary differences between the five models of family therapy to be articulated in this chapter are

- The responsibility of the therapist for directing change
- The degree to which an identified problem is the focus of treatment
- The specific techniques and assumptions about how change occurs

These differences constitute a theoretical continuum on which each of the theories falls.

Therapists generally support either the notion that they work to promote behavioral change via direct suggestion or that they assist their clients in developing an alternative view from which change follows. The dichotomy between behavioral change and understanding is the critical difference between the "therapist as director" stance of the problem-focused (Haley

1967) and interactional approaches (Fisch et al. 1982), and the noninterventionist stance taken by Boscolo and Cecchin (Cecchin 1987) and the Galveston group (H. Anderson et al. 1986). The therapeutic models of the Milwaukee group (de Shazer 1991b) and narrative therapy (White and Epston 1990) employ techniques and theoretical constructs that place them in a middle ground between the directorial and noninterventionist extremes.

The writings of Bateson and Erickson represent opposite extremes of the schism between clinical understanding and directed change, between hierarchical control by the therapist and therapist-client equality. Whereas Erickson clearly endorsed the use of his directive methods in the clinical setting, Bateson regretted the incorporation of his ideas into change-promoting strategies. His heart remained that of an anthropologist, one who observes, records, and acknowledges his or her role in a system but does not intervene as an active agent of change.

Each of the five models of family therapy discussed in this chapter offers ideas about how change occurs, a body of techniques, and ways to utilize the client's worldview. These components will be discussed below.

Essential Ideas

Certain ideas are central to understanding the models. None of these therapeutic models are based on a comprehensive theory of human behavior and development. Instead, they rely on a nucleus of concepts that serves as a foundation for treatments whose main concern are the daily problems of living. First, however, we review some of the basic ideas put forth by Erickson and Bateson.

Milton Erickson

Erickson broke with established psychiatric method, which offered elaborate theories in order to understand human behavior but few guidelines about how to produce change. Insight, so important a tool in psychoanalytic treatment, was viewed as unnecessary by Erickson. He believed that his clients had the knowledge to solve their own problems and that they only lacked the ability to access that knowledge. Opening clients up to their own solutions involved helping them change their problem behavior in order to create new contexts for understanding this behavior. Viewed in the light of a new situation, the problem behavior no longer made sense (Feldman 1985). When a small change occurred, it set forth reverberations that Erickson believed would generate more change. Hence, he often suggested small steps for clients to take as "homework" to be completed between sessions.

Believing that therapy could work quickly, Erickson took charge of finding ways to change his clients beliefs and interactions. Thus, his methods addressed "resistance" differently than traditional models of therapy. Rather than analyzing or confronting resistance, Erickson chose to utilize it in order to achieve a clinical goal. The use of paradoxical directives and positive reframes, common features in the early strategic models, came from Erickson's practice of using hypnosis with resistant clients (Haley 1981). Paradoxical interventions directed the client to continue, increase, or schedule symptoms. Resistance to change was encouraged in situations in which the client may still be unconvinced of the usefulness of change. Positive reframing labeled as desirable or beneficial some aspect of resistance or some behavior viewed negatively by the client. Hence, failure to change was redefined as cooperation, and competitive struggles between therapist and client were avoided.

The profound impact of Erickson's ideas on family therapy is indisputable. However, his often indirect and counterintuitive methods left some therapists feeling uncomfortable. Many saw him as doing something *to* the family without informed consent rather than working *with* the family openly and collaboratively. This distinction became all the more problematic as the field continued to debate the issue of therapeutic control.

Gregory Bateson

Bateson was primarily interested in how humans communicate. He introduced the concept of cybernetics to the field of family therapy. Cybernetics is a scientific explanation of organization and pattern. Of particular interest is how feedback allows a system to self-correct. Applied to the family, this work examined how patterns of communication were homeostatic, stabilizing family interaction and individual symptoms. Bateson also focused on the role of feedback in producing change in family systems. He proposed the concept of circular, rather than linear, causality. Circular causality focuses on reciprocal cause and effect among elements of a system in the present, whereas linear causality focuses on simple, one-way, cause-and-effect relations (from past to present). Circular causality is a central tenet of family systems thinking.

The focus on circularity moved family therapists away from the historical, linear, cause-and-effect mentality of most other therapeutic models (most notably, psychoanalytic) into the realm of the current system. Rather than supposing that a problem came from some traumatic past event, as a linear theorist would, the systems thinker would consider a problem as part of an ongoing pattern of mutually causal elements in the present. The emphasis shifted away from what *caused* symptoms in the client's past to what reciprocal interactions *maintained* symptoms in the present.

The implications of Bateson's ideas for psychotherapy were profound. The notion that there was an objective reality within which the client existed was discarded. Bateson's ideas made it clear that therapist (observer) and family were both part of a larger intertwined system in which neither could pretend the other did not exist (Bateson 1979). Accepting that the observer (in this case, the therapist) was part of the family's sphere required therapists to conceptualize a family's actions in the unique context of that sphere. The observer could not stand "outside" a system to watch its functioning. Rather, the observer co-constructed an "observing system."

From Strategic to Narrative Models

Strategic/Problem-Solving Therapy

Basic Theory

Jay Haley and Cloe Madanes established a model that bridged Erickson's methods (Haley 1967) with the structural model of Salvador Minuchin (1974a, 1974d). Symptoms, for the problem-solving therapist, were seen as functional in the broader context of the system's organization. According to this model, the therapist observes the structure of the family in order to choose the strategy that is best suited to assist the family in alleviating the presenting problem.

A primary feature of the strategic/problem-solving model is that the therapist takes the main responsibility to set goals and create a plan that will result in the dissolution of the client's problem (Haley 1967, 1977, 1980b). The therapist chooses a strategy by attempting to understand and convey to the family a view of the problem and its solution in operational terms. In other word, the problem and solution must be presented in terms of things that can be said and done differently, as well as couched within an explanation of the problem that makes sense to the family. A family does not progress from dysfunctional to functional in one simple step; rather, Haley (1976a) suggests, the family must first become a "different malfunctioning system." In so doing, the family becomes functional in stages, rather than rushing forward only to have members fail in their new roles.

Diagnostic categories, an important staple of most traditional psychotherapies, are of little importance to the problem-solving therapist. Assessment therefore takes on a different meaning. To assess is to focus on the presenting problem within the whole social unit responding to an intervention and not just the individual psyche as if it existed in a social vacuum. Instead of arriving at a label for the client, which Haley (1976a) felt would only "crystallize a problem," the therapist must observe and understand the key dimensions of the system in relation to the presenting problem. Assessing these key dimensions includes observing the interactional sequences within the family and determining its hierarchical organization, especially coalitions among family members.

Once sufficiently well versed in the family's interactional sequences and its members' views of the problem, the therapist determines a method of conceptualizing the problem that will serve to move the therapy forward. Madanes (1991) provides six "dimensions" with which to conceptualize the problem:

1. *Voluntary versus involuntary behavior.* Symptomatic behavior, though typically considered involuntary by the client, is seen by the therapist, except in the case of organic illness, as under the control of the client.
2. *Helplessness versus power.* Behavior that is perceived as helpless by the family may in fact be understood, as in the case of a child's tantrum, to be quite powerful.
3. *Metaphorical versus literal sequences.* A symptom expressed by one family member, such as a child's refusal to use the toilet, may well serve a function for the family.
4. *Hierarchy versus equality.* When the problem in the family involves a dual hierarchy, the therapist must reposition the family into a correct hierarchy.
5. *Hostility versus love.* In the eyes of strategic therapists, people are generally benevolent; therefore, will the therapist choose to redefine problematic behavior as an attempt to help rather than hurt?
6. *Personal gain versus altruism.* Rather than being an expression of selfishness, symptomatic behavior may be an unsuccessful attempt to show or receive love.

Basic Techniques

To achieve the goals of therapy, the problem-solving therapist begins by being very clear about goals. An exploratory interview is recommended. If a client is hospitalized, the therapist assumes that hospitalization is the problem (Haley 1980b).

The initial interview is a time of planning, listening, and directing. Haley (1977) sees the interview as progressing through five stages: 1) social, 2) problem-focus, 3) interaction-tracking, 4) goal-setting, and 5) task-setting. Throughout this process, conclusions remain tentative, and the therapist does not offer his or her observations about the family. The therapist will seek to engage the least involved parent rather than focusing on the parent who is already involved.

Everyone attending the sessions following the initial interview is asked to share his or her experience of the problem in order to emphasize that each person's view is valuable. In addition to discussing the problem, the therapist facilitates enactments of the problem in the sessions, in order to directly shift interactions in vivo. On receiving a clear statement of the problem from all people involved, the therapist moves toward gathering information about the change requested. The clarity of the goal is a determining factor in the success or failure of this treatment. Therefore, the therapist actively pursues a solvable goal that emerges from the definition of the problem stated by the family.

The technique of giving directives and homework assignments, of principal importance in the writings of both Haley (1967, 1980a, 1980b, 1987) and Madanes (1980, 1984), is respectfully attributed to Erickson (Haley 1967). Directives are designed to get clients to make changes, intensify the therapeutic relationship, and gather information. Moreover, simply by discussing the possibility of assigning and complying with a directive, the client and therapist are utilizing the language of behavioral change.

Directives can be straightforward or counterintuitive. Straightforward directives are best presented in an unorthodox manner. Otherwise, such a directive may be perceived as just one more piece of useless "good advice." The directive should take into account what pattern or behavior has failed in the past so as not to repeat it, and the directive must, on some level, be based on a rationale that makes sense to the client. Directives are intended to propel the family to consider changing a pattern or behavior that is maintaining the presenting problem.

Both Jay Haley and Cloe Madanes continue to introduce innovative directive techniques to the field. Haley (1984), in his book *Ordeal Therapy*, discusses the notion that when continuing to perform an ordeal (e.g., scrubbing the floor) is more of a bother than keeping a symptom (e.g., procrastination), a client will choose the less difficult option. Madanes (1990) recently created a 16-step model for dealing with sex offenders and their victims in a family context, which culminates in a ritual in which the offender and the entire family make amends to the victim.

Brief Strategic/Interactional Therapy

Basic Theory

Brevity is implied in the name of the Mental Research Institute's (MRI's) Brief Therapy Center and is also stated in MRI's original clinical mission; however, MRI's therapy is more appropriately referred to as "interactional" than "brief." Although brief strategic/interactional therapy is an active model that can achieve rapid results, the presupposition that it can only be used as a short-term model is inaccurate.

Problems in the clinical sense consist of undesired behavior in the present. Because this model pays little attention to determining historical factors, a session often begins with the question "What is the problem that brings you in?" Chubb, Nauts, and Evans (1984) suggest that a problem defined in terms of feelings is not a clearly defined problem. Unlike "joining" in the problem-solving model, which involves social talk, the interactional model holds that the client and therapist join around solving the problem. In discussing the presenting problem, the therapist is interested not only in what the problem is but why clients believe it to be a problem. In other words, no assumption is made that a given behavior would necessarily be problematic for all clients. The reason one person may desire to change his or her work habits is often entirely different from the next person's reason for wishing to change the same behavior. So although the MRI model pushes therapists to emphasize the desired and observable behavioral change, that information in and of itself is not a sufficient focus for therapy (Weakland et al. 1974).

To resolve a problem, one must change the behaviors related to it. The interactional therapist needs to understand, with the client's assistance, how the problem fits into the interactional pattern of the individual and his or her world. A nonpathological view of behavior is taken, in which it is assumed that problems often involve getting stuck in an ineffective cycle of doing things. Stated another way, attempted solutions that seem the logical way to solve the problem simply do not work. Therefore, the goal is to help the client to do something different from what he or she is already doing to try to solve the problem (Fisch et al. 1982).

Given the intractable nature of patterns of behavior, the interactional therapist needs to clearly understand the attitudes, motivation, and opinion of the client surrounding the problem. With full understanding of the client's position, any move toward resolution is consistent with that position. For example, a client may report a desire to be more assertive at work in order to request a raise. If, however, exploration of the client's position reveals that he or she associates assertiveness with being "too pushy," assisting the client to become assertive without recognizing the client's discomfort with such a change is likely to result in a failed intervention.

When the client is able to acknowledge a problem of primary concern and does not feel reluctant to change because of the subjective "dangers of improvement" (Fisch et al. 1982, p. 162), the next step involves clarifying all attempted solutions. What has the client tried before to resolve the problem? Asking this question helps the therapist to avoid recommending some action that is simply more of the same. Because the client is caught in a positive feedback loop, with problem and attempted solution amplifying each other, the therapist wants to interdict the old attempted solution or variations of that solution. The assumption is that even a very small change can be expanded upon, so the goal is to find that crucial point where some change is possible.

Basic Techniques

Interactional therapists use a series of techniques to institute change once the initial questioning has led client and therapist to a point where a primary problem is selected for change. Although this appears to follow the method of many clinical interviews, interactional therapists attempt to approach the client with absolute naïveté. In other words, the therapist expresses confusion about how the problem fits into the client's life so that the client's position and theory about the problem become clear. The questioning style is designed to arrive at a problem description in the client's own words—that is, in observable, behavioral terms.

The model dictates that the therapist avoid taking a strong position. Instead, clients are encouraged to select the problem that is of concern to them. The problem presented is not necessarily the one embraced; the therapist considers each problem presented as equally important. It is up to the client to choose the problem to be worked on. There is no suggestion that there is one "real" problem; the message conveyed is that any problem resolved is a successful therapeutic intervention.

A therapist must accept a role that is less dramatically "helpful." This stance, one that insists that clients define the problem from within their worldview, runs counter to the natural inclination of many therapists to select problems and determine goals for therapy. The struggle experienced by clients as they work toward a definition of the "problem" may appear laborious while it is ongoing, but the effort is necessary. The therapist is best able to assist his or her client by providing an objective forum so that each issue can be examined to see if the client is willing to pursue change regardless of other systemic ramifications.

The next step is accomplished by examining the situation and fully understanding each factor that makes it difficult for clients to initiate change, even if they are requesting change. When change is particularly difficult for a client to initiate, some personal theory, myth, or sense of obligation is assumed to be the stumbling block. Determine what that blocking factor is and summarize why you, the therapist, imagine that taking a contrary course of action is difficult. For example, clients convinced that some helpful action on their part can halt another's addiction may be living with the myth that they have not done enough. Rather than attack that myth, the therapist's respect for the client's worldview dictates that an honest appraisal of the stalemate be presented to the client (e.g., "Sally, no matter how hopeless this situation might seem, I believe that you will not be willing to care for yourself until you have tried every available option to stop Ernie's drinking"). In making this statement, the therapist is not utilizing paradox simply as a maneuver to initiate change; rather, the intention is to acknowledge and identify the dilemma that is causing the client to struggle. The client's response indicates his or her level of readiness to work on change. If the client agrees with the therapist's statement, then it is better that the therapist not begin to propose a change that runs counter to the client's belief at the time.

When the problem is sufficiently understood and the dangers of change have been explored, the interactional therapist might utilize the following interventions:

1. *Reframe the problem.* Provide an alternative, yet acceptable, definition of the problem that may help the client take new action.
2. *Prescribe a relapse.* Increase the client's control of the problem by being able to produce the problematic behavior on demand.
3. *Recommend "no change."* Clearly support the client's right to continue the symptom if that choice is less difficult.
4. *Assign homework.* Introduce a new behavior that might make the old pattern no longer necessary.
5. *Conduct paradoxical interventions.* Have a client perform a behavior that, seemingly in conflict with the stated goal, actually opens the situation to change.

As with all interventions within the interactional modality, the rationale used to encourage a client to follow an intervention must "fit" the client's worldview or position.

Solution-Focused Therapy

Basic Theory

Working in Milwaukee, Wisconsin (de Shazer 1988; de Shazer et al. 1986; Nunnally et al. 1986), the Brief Family Therapy Center (BFTC) established their own influential model that continues to evolve. The chief members of the Center—Steve de Shazer, Insoo Berg, Eve Lipchik, Elem Nunnally, and Alex Molnar—were interested in clinical research as well as therapy.

In an effort to come up with an organized method of determining how a client's problem was perpetuated, de Shazer initially worked to integrate

Heider's Balance Theory (Cartwright and Harary 1956) with the work of Milton Erickson. In determining "balance," the interpersonal relationships between people are mapped in order to reveal coalitions. Although the use of balance-theoretical mapping became too time-consuming for clinical practice, the process led de Shazer to conceptualize the "mapping" of complaints and solutions (de Shazer 1982).

de Shazer (1985) strongly supported Erickson's conclusion that the concept of "resistance" is not therapeutically useful. The solution-focused therapist makes the assumption that the client comes to therapy wishing to change. What may appear as "resistance" is interpreted by the solution-focused therapist as a communication that the therapist has not yet discovered this client's unique context for cooperating. In other words, the appropriate solution to the client's problem has not yet been discovered.

The most dramatic shift in the evolving theory came when the focus moved from "problems" to "solutions." When the core team at BFTC studied the process of gaining information about the problem, it became clear that it would be easier to establish a limited number of solutions than to fully understand the enormous pool of potential problems and their causes. In other words, the solution-focused therapist believes that with relatively little information about the problem, one can select from a short menu of solutions and still effect change in the client. de Shazer (1985, p. 7) suggested that "any really different behavior in a problematic situation can be enough to prompt solution." The shift away from problems to solutions also led the team to become interested in how clients solve problems naturally, without therapeutic intervention.

The solution-focused therapist assumes that clients have the solution to their problem within them. The purpose of the therapy is to focus on how the client would know that the problem is solved and on what the client is already doing that is useful and should be continued or increased. The intention of working in this manner is to create a collaborative relationship between therapist and client.

An interesting addition to the field was an effort in the 1990s to address children's issues in family therapy. The field of family therapy has, surprisingly, often not emphasized writings on specific interventions for children; however, the solution-focused models has generated an exception (Selekman 1997).

Also central to the solution-focused model are concepts adapted from Erickson (Haley 1967), which de Shazer credits Watzlawick, Weakland, and Fisch (1974) for explicating: 1) the importance of understanding the particular worldview of the client; 2) an acceptance that clients have tried to solve their problems in a manner they believe is correct and logical; and 3) the belief that only minimal change is necessary because it will have systemic ramifications. The mainstay of de Shazer's recent work is to help clients locate "exceptions to the problem" (times when the problem does *not* occur) and to increase the conditions that lead to such exceptions.

Basic Techniques

The solution-focused model encourages clinicians to expand their assumptions about the client and his or her problem, thus creating an environment where new "maps," and therefore new solutions, can be found. When the complaint is discussed with the therapist, the therapist begins to construct a map, either mentally or on paper, of the complaint. The purpose of the map is to determine assumptions made by the client regarding the problem. For example, if the complaint involves arguing, the therapist might ask about the location of the arguments. If the client reports one consistent location or time of day, the solution may be as simple as moving the argument to another room or changing interaction patterns at that time of day. In other words, the solution-focused therapist looks to transform complaints directly into solutions. By evaluating the complaint from different perspectives, the therapist is constructing different therapeutic realities. Although the process of mapping the complaints is certainly enhanced by having a supporting team available, a variety of listeners makes it easier to generate an unworkable number of alternate realities. Therefore, solution-focused therapists must become skilled at generating alternative hypotheses without a team. A relatively new innovation by Gingerick and de Shazer (1991) is a computer program that assists the clinician in generating alternative views without a team.

de Shazer (1985, p. 30) suggests that 12 factors can be used as "doors leading to solutions." Each of these doors is considered a potential entrance to a solution. There is no "right" or "wrong" door; rather, each offers a possible solution that may be more or less effective. The different doors also allow the therapist to pursue the complaint in a manner that is consistent with the client's assumptions and worldview concerning the problem.

The following example, a family coming to BFTC regarding a child's school problems, will illustrate the 12 factors and the solutions that would be generated. The child, Angie, becomes fearful and physically ill when required to attend school. The following 12 questions are formulations of the 12 factors used to explore Angie's problems.

1. Does someone hold a utopian expectation regarding Angie's school performance?
2. Is there something about the particular physical location of Angie's reaction that is making a difference?
3. Is there a reason this environment should cause this particular reaction?

4. Who or what is to blame for Angie's reaction?
5. Are there others who are significantly involved in assisting this behavior to continue?
6. If we understand the actual behavior, is there a behavioral task that will solve the complaint?
7. What ascribed meanings have been assigned to Angie's behavior?
8. How often does this complaint occur?
9. Is this behavior voluntary or involuntary?
10. Is the behavior due to a physical illness?
11. Is there anything from the past that would explain Angie's behavior?
12. Are there dire predictions of what will happen if Angie never returns to school?

Each of these questions can lead to one or more possible solutions. Depending on the factor endorsed by both family and therapist, some of the possible solutions tried in this situation might be 1) Are there exceptions to the rule? In other words, are there days or conditions in which Angie goes to school without incident, and can these conditions be replicated? 2) Might some minimal change, such as a new teacher, help the situation? 3) Can the problem be reframed in order for the problem to be seen in a new way? 4) Are there successful past changes in behavior (going to school with a friend, for example) that have worked and can be replicated?

In addition to the solutions that might flow from the 12-question style described above, solution-focused therapists also use a series of "formula tasks" that were invented for specific cases but were later found to be useful in a variety of situations. The following three are the most common formula tasks recommended:

1. *The "structured fight" task.* A coin is tossed to decide who will go first. The winner can complain for 10 uninterrupted minutes, followed by 10 minutes of complaining from the other client. Before a next round can start, there must be 10 minutes of silence (de Shazer 1985, p. 122).
2. *The "do something different" task.* When a client reports that they have tried "everything possible" to change their own or another person's behavior, the therapist instructs the client to "do something different" the next time the behavior occurs. In so doing, the therapist is introducing "randomness" into the system (de Shazer 1985, p. 123).
3. *The "pay attention to what you do the next time you overcome the urge to…" task.* Clients often have a storehouse of solutions that they may have found successful on one occasion but are reluctant to incorporate into their regular responses. This intervention challenges the client to explore his or her own resources (de Shazer 1985, p. 132).

A final intriguing technique utilized by solution-focused therapists demonstrates their proclivity to look for strengths in the client. Near the end of the first session, the therapist requests that the client go home and think about the things that are happening that the client does not wish to see changed. In other words, what about the family or individual should remain the way it is? In the midst of complaints, an affirmation of something good happening can be encouraging for a client and can set the problem in a less overwhelming and helplessness-inducing framework for both client and therapist.

Systemic Family Therapy

The work of the Milan Associates is presented below in three sections. The model and its proponents will identify each section. The first section concentrates on the theory and techniques of the original Milan Associates (Luigi Boscolo, Gianfranco Cecchin, and Mara Selvini Palazzoli) (Roberts 1986; Selvini Palazzoli et al. 1978, 1980; Tomm 1984a, 1984b). The second section discusses those team members (Gianfranco Cecchin and Luigi Boscolo) who retained many aspects of the original theory and adopted the name "the New Milan Associates" but have shifted emphasis (Boscolo et al. 1987; Campbell et al. 1991; Cecchin 1987). The third section describes the research efforts of Mara Selvini Palazzoli and her colleagues, including the fourth original team member, Giuliana Prata (Mashal et al. 1989; Selvini Palazzoli 1980; Selvini Palazzoli et al. 1989).

Basic Theory and Techniques: Milan Associates 1974–1979

Mara Selvini Palazzoli formed the Milan Associates. She invited three psychiatrist colleagues to meet weekly in order to explore other methods, rather than psychoanalytic, of treating families with a seriously dysfunctional member (anorexic or psychotic). The primary readings adhered to by this group were the works of Don Jackson, Jay Haley, Paul Watzlawick, and Gregory Bateson. Their plan was to study one theoretical model intensively and then create their own treatment method based on their clinical experience as a team (Sluzki 1999).

The original group created a team format that they followed when seeing families. The format broke the session into five parts: 1) pre-session team discussion; 2) interview with the family; 3) discussion of the interview by team members; 4) conclusion of the interview, including a comment and/or prescription given to family; and 5) postsession team discussion of the family's reaction to the prescription. The team saw all of their cases during this period as a foursome (two therapists in front and two behind the mirror) so that the whole team functioned as the therapist.

The central assumption of the method was that the intervention had to be aimed at the "family game" rather than focusing on a particular family member. In concentrating on the family game, the Milan associates suggested that the family as a whole protects itself from change through homeostatic rules and patterns of communication. The systemic therapist took a stance of neutrality; he or she remained equally attentive and respectful to all family members in order to avoid induction into a coalition for or against a particular change. In fact, the team even included the referring therapist from the beginning, if one was involved in the case, in order to avoid changing any of the relationships surrounding the problem.

"Positive connotation" was an intervention used by Milan Systemic therapists to support the family's symptomatic behavior and increase cooperation (Selvini Palazzoli et al. 1978). This intervention delivered a statement to the family citing all the things the family is doing connected with the presenting problem, and describing how those actions were necessary from the standpoint of preserving family relationships and the well-being of the members. The following is an example of a positive reframe with an anorexic patient and her family:

> It is a good thing that you refuse to eat...it is good because it makes your parents afraid that you will die...when they are afraid that you may die they get together and talk...they talk about what they can do to help you...they are talking much more now than before...it is good that they talk more now because it is necessary that they prepare themselves for when you leave home and are gone forever...so by deciding not to eat, you have decided to help your parents in this way...and so we feel that you should continue in this work for the time being. (Tomm 1984b, pp. 264–265)

The effect of such an intervention is that the family game may be shaken. New meanings and options appear, and the rules of the game are made explicit so that the family can no longer disclaim awareness or choice in perpetuating the problematic pattern.

Systemic therapists do not capriciously identify just any area of family life and positively connote it. Rather, the team explores patterns in the family that may match one or more systemic hypotheses developed by the team in the pre-session. A hypothesis is a conjectural statement linking the symptom to patterns of family interaction and/or to new problems that may emerge if the original symptom disappears. Deciding which hypothesis, if any, should be employed in the development of an intervention involves testing and investigation through a circular style of questioning during the session.

Selvini Palazzoli et al. (1980) discussed how circular questioning is entirely relationship-based. The therapist asks each member to discuss in front of the other family members his or her perceptions of how the family relates via the problem. These questions might inquire about 1) what was happening before the problem started, 2) what would happen if the problem ceased, and 3) who is most affected by the problem. When family members answer such questions, they become aware of how each other sees the situation, as well as the role that the problem is playing in organizing and stabilizing the family. The hypothesis that receives the most verbal affirmation in the session is used as a rationale for an intervention at the conclusion of the session. The intervention may be a positive connotation, a paradoxical prescription, or a therapeutic ritual to be performed between sessions.

The New Milan Associates: Boscolo and Cecchin

Boscolo and Cecchin, members of the original team, continue to work with families and train family therapists using their own model. Although they still tend to utilize interviewing neutrality, circular questioning, and the five-part format, in other ways their approach has changed considerably. Cecchin (1987) described the process by which the systemic therapist looks to the family's descriptions of their problems and the fixed patterns that develop due to these descriptions. The therapist works to introduce a variety of explanations to the family, instead of searching for a correct one. Solutions to the family's problem can develop as a consequence of the style of interviewing, without a final intervention. The New Milan Associates work to gently loosen the family's rigid grip on their view of the problem. Introducing different perceptions and explanations of the problem via circular questioning throughout the interview encourages the family's own ability at innovation and self-correction (Boscolo et al. 1987; Hoffman 1991). The goal of treatment is simply to break the developmental impasse in which the family has become "stuck." After the impasse is broken, therapy terminates quickly, enabling the family to continue evolving in its own direction.

The Invariant Prescription: The Research of Selvini Palazzoli

A deep and unwavering interest in working with families with psychotic members motivated Mara Selvini Palazzoli to continue her clinical research throughout her career. She developed a single "invariant prescription" that allowed her to study a family's reaction to intervention in a more controlled manner. The original Milan team attempted interventions because this method seemed to offer the best possibility for breaking the cycle of the family's "game." However, Selvini Palazzoli expressed reservations about the original model's effectiveness (Selvini Palazzoli 1988), and subsequent researchers (Coleman 1987; Green and Herget 1989a, 1989b, 1991; Mashal et al. 1989) have suggested that the initial astounding success reported in anecdotal case studies has not been supported in more controlled outcome studies. Selvini Palazzoli and her research colleagues (Selvini Palazzoli et al. 1989) suggested that the generic and nonsystematic interventions used by the original Milan team may explain their failure.

Although Selvini Palazzoli abandoned paradoxical interventions, she preserved the strategic directive tendency of the original Milan model. The invariant prescription (Selvini Palazzoli et al. 1989) is assigned only after the therapist has fully explored the family's patterns. The invariant prescription is begun by instructing the parents to inform their children, and other involved family members that they have a secret from their meeting as a couple with the therapist. The spouses then record exactly how other family members respond to this information. These parents are then instructed to go out on dates that are not discussed with the rest of their family. In fact, only a short note is left on the table to announce that the parents "will not be home until later." If asked by the family about their actions or whereabouts, the couple will respond that "it is a matter that only concerns the two of us." The continuing sessions with the parents revolve around the chronicling of family reactions to the parents' private activities. This intervention, which is assigned to all families, is designed to shore up boundaries around the parental subsystem, thus breaking the pattern of the family game that has allowed the symptom to control everyone so that no alliances could be formed.

The recent passing of Mara Selvini Palazzoli (1916–1999) leaves a great void in the field of family therapy. She was innovative and opinioned, yet was always refining and revising her thinking. Clearly, postmodern thinking owes Selvini Palazzoli a great debt; without her emphasis on inclusion of the therapist and his or her own operations in the conceptual understanding of families, narrative postmodern perspectives would have lacked an early foundation. Interestingly, she professed to be "rather anti-postmodern" (Sluzki 1999).

Narrative Therapy

Basic Theory

The theory of Michael White draws on Bateson's (1972, 1979) theories and on the philosophy of Michel Foucault (1973, 1980). White's view is that each therapist incorporates the ideas of the narrative model in different ways; therefore his (White's) ideas cannot exist separately from the practitioners who are influenced by them. In other words, the model is the sum of its practitioners. However, White does readily acknowledge some facets of narrative therapy as his own work, so for the purpose of this chapter, his work will be referred to as a model.

Initially, White emphasized two points, drawn directly from Bateson (1972): "negative explanation" and "restraint." In his classic article "Negative Explanation, Restraint, and Double Description: A Template for Family Therapy," White (1986) argued that a person's behavior was not caused by internal drives or forces, but instead by his or her beliefs and interactional patterns. The term "restraints" refers to beliefs and assumptions that leave clients examining a problem over and over without stumbling on a new solution or noticing temporary changes in the problem. The narrative model shares with the interactional model a recognition that clients often believe they are trying new solutions but are often simply trying more of the same unsuccessful solution. At the suggestion of David Epston, White moved away from the cybernetic metaphor to the metaphor of "narrative" to explain the repetitive patterns within which clients were trapped.

The narrative model emphasizes empowering clients by assisting them in "externalizing" their problems and "reauthoring" their lives (Prest and Carruthers 1991; White 1989, 1995; White and Epston 1990). White points out that families tend to act as if problems are certainties. "Problem-saturated descriptions" and the contexts in which the client exists cause these certainties. It is White's belief that clients become entwined in dominant, problem-saturated stories that in fact shape his or her experience of life. In other words, if a client's dominant story involves feeling worthless, that story will shape both how the client expresses himself or herself and how the client derives meaning from past, present, and future experiences.

Generally, according to White, clients come into therapy engaged with "internalizing discourses." These discourses encourage people to think about and discuss a problem in terms of either another's personality or seemingly intractable notions of oneself. An example of an internalizing conversation might involve a client's describing herself as "worthless" or else her boyfriend as "dysfunctional." Neither description (both called a "fixed entity") offers useful information to the narrative therapist. White recommends "externalizing conversations" as an antidote. For example, rather than simply pursuing the topic of a client's self-hate as internal, White might ask, "How is this self-hate affecting how others see you?"

Once the problem is understood from an external perspective, which separates the problem from the "self" of the client, White believes that the client has begun the process of "deconstruction." What then follows is a "reconstruction" or "reauthoring" of the client's story—a story no longer controlled by the dominant, problem-saturated plot, but instead placed in the context of an alternative plot.

More recently, White (1997) has specified that societal reparations often serve to keep people from discovering their authentic selves. Narrative exploration is meant to free the client of personal and cultural demands that often shape one's values and beliefs. Free of the constraints that come from being bound by societal pressures, the client can identify and consider expanded options.

In keeping with White's belief that narrative concepts evolve as each practitioner utilizes them, a number of authors have articulated alterations and theoretical integration with other models (Eron and Lund 1996; Freedman and Combs 1996; Rosenblatt 1994; Zimmerman and Dickerson 1996).

Basic Techniques

The therapeutic techniques begin with learning how the problem is described and experienced by the family. The narrative therapist wishes to see specifically how the problem is maintained by meanings or definitions that often have their basis in larger sociocultural discoveries and structural injustices.

Once a description or definition of the problem has been formed, a therapist can then examine the externalized problem from two directions. The first is to study how the problem influences the client and the family ("mapping the influence of the problem" on the persons involved). The second, more novel direction examines how the family "influences" and nurtures the problem. These directions might be pursued by including questions that "collapse time" (White 1986), and that highlight how the problem might progress over time (its predicted trajectory for the future). By projecting the family and problem forward in time, the narrative therapist demonstrates that, unless halted, the problem will continue to grow, survive, and affect the family.

Deconstructing a problem enables the client to view the problem as external to any individual self. Rather, the problem is seen as having a life of its own, creating the dominant story by which the individual lives and with which he or she unwittingly cooperates. Once the dominant plot is described and its oppressive influence understood, White emphasizes the importance of developing an alternative plot. The therapist might examine ways in which family members have exerted some influence over the problem and have successfully resisted some of its meanings and effects. These "unique outcomes" become the gateways to alternative narratives. Once an alternative story has been unearthed (e.g., a client's kindness as opposed to aggressiveness), the narrative therapist (primarily using questions) searches for examples of when such an alternative plot was expressed. White highlights and seeks to amplify unique outcomes. The bulk of the work in therapy revolves around understanding ways in which unique outcomes can be embraced so that they coalesce to form a new, more positive, dominant story about the client and his or her life. The simple existence of past unique outcomes may be enough to release the client from an oppressive dominant story. Since identity, claims, and stories are only authenticated through their acknowledgement by others, the therapist may try and engage significant others in the client's life as audiences to these new developments. As the alternative story begins to organize the client's actions and self-perceptions, the process of reauthoring a life has begun. The dominant influence of the problem and the problem-saturated description decline as the new narrative about self and relationships replaces them.

Conclusion

The five approaches to therapy summarized in this chapter share, to varying degrees, a common heritage in the works of Milton Erickson and Gregory Bateson. Hence, they also share a common epistemological assumption: that "reality" and "meaning" ultimately are socially co-constructed phenomena that do not exist separately from a "community of observers" (such as a family or a therapist-client dyad). All of the authors of the various models reviewed in this chapter embrace this basic "antirealistic," social constructivist assumption in their work (Held 1992).

Thus, in contrast to what has been called the "naïve realist" stance of structural, Bowenian, and intergenerational approaches, none of the models reviewed in this chapter propose formal developmental or causal theories (or assessment categories) of family pathology and normality. Neither do any of the models prescribe standard outcome goals for treatment (other than the generic "resolution of the presenting problem," however codefined). Rather, these models of therapy all are infused with what might be called an "applied anthropological" or social constructivist perspective, in contrast to the perspectives inherent in most other approaches to family therapy (e.g., naïve realism or dichotomies of health and illness or functional and dysfunctional). John Weakland, a member of the MRI group, once described these differences in an oral history interview about the field of family therapy:

> I think it was very important for our work that Gregory Bateson and I were both trained anthropologically....Psychiatrists, and even psychologists, to a large extent, tend to view the world in terms of pathology. If something looks strange or different, their first thought is that it is some kind of pathology. Anthropology is different. If you go out into the field in a new so-

ciety, then every damned thing they do is strange. You can't get anywhere just by saying "it's all pathological, it's all crazy." It's *your* job to make sense out of it, no matter how crazy it looks. This produces a very different slant on the observation of behavior. (Bassi 1991, pp. 69–70)

Moreover, the strategic, systemic, and narrative approaches all emphasize *the process* (the "how to") *of therapeutic change in the present* (toward whatever goals the client selects), rather than specifying universally appropriate or normative contents for change (i.e., what behaviors are dysfunctional, or what goals are to be pursued with all clients) (Held 1992). The five approaches discussed in this chapter do not offer a universal causal theory to explain the historical development of problems; they are more concerned with *the way problems are maintained in the present* and with factors that restrain changes from being amplified. In this sense, strategic, systemic, and narrative therapies, like cognitive behaviorism, are oriented toward the client's present and future rather than the past.

Where these five approaches seem to differ most from one another is along the behavior-directive versus behavior-nondirective dimension. In particular, the New Milan Associates and some of the narrative conversation therapists (Andersen 1987; Goolishian and Anderson 1992; Hoffman 1985) eschew all specifically behavioral directives such as homework and paradoxical behavior prescription, relying instead on less direct methods of intervention (e.g., asking questions to elicit new descriptions).

While the models discussed in this chapter have been studied in controlled experiments, and the overall effectiveness of family therapy has been supported, the findings regarding specific models as being more effective than others are still inconclusive (Shadish et al. 1995). Some models have particular strengths, but more often than not, the strength of these models can be exhibited in only limited paradigms (Goldenberg and Goldenberg 2000). Some experimentally controlled studies that have been conducted in this area have yielded generally positive results for the systemic and strategic therapies, but much more research is needed on varying client populations, presenting problems, and specific treatment protocols (Brown and Christensen 1999; Green and Herget 1989a, 1989b, 1991).

In particular, there is growing theoretical and research support for the notion that therapist relationship skills (such as warmth and active structuring) and the positive strength of the therapeutic alliance are important determinants of outcome in systemic and strategic therapies (Green 1988; Green 1992; Green and Herget 1991; Kleckner et al. 1992; Solovey and Duncan 1992). We support the idea that virtually all techniques and stances discussed in this chapter can be utilized in an ethical manner; however, strong ethical and aesthetic objections are being raised about certain strategic and systemic methods (e.g., the sometimes coolly dispassionate stance adopted by some systemic therapists, or the intentional deceit used in some paradoxical methods) (Solovey and Duncan 1992). In light of these recent research reports and ethical questions, we believe that each of the approaches reviewed here must begin investigating the impact of its specific techniques on the development of therapist-client working alliances.

Finally, although the authors of these models have begun doing so, we believe strategic, systemic, and narrative therapists must continue to discuss the social values that inform their treatments, especially their selection and shaping of treatment goals (Green 1992). In light of feminist critiques of therapeutic "circularity" and "neutrality" (e.g., in situations of wife abuse) the models discussed here generally have failed to articulate principles, techniques, and goals that take into account power differentials among family members, particularly between men and women. Some treatment goals and methods may be oppressive to various system members, even if presenting problems are resolved.

Inevitably, the values of both therapist and client inform the selection of treatment goals and the means for achieving those goals (Aponte 1985). To pretend otherwise is folly. The question remains: What values and treatment goals *should* strategic, systemic, and narrative therapists embrace, and what techniques within the five existing models are consistent with those values?

The ideas, constructs, and interventions developed by these theorists who fall within the overarching heritage of Bateson and Erickson continue to survive and thrive in the field of family therapy. The view of these models as interconnected can assist the clinician in case formulation and selection of clinical interventions. Elevating one model and rejecting the others diminishes the benefits that emerge from examination of the strategic, systemic, and narrative spectrum of models.

Chapters on Related Topics

The following chapters describe concepts related to constructing therapy:

- Chapter 2, "Structural Family Therapy"
- Chapter 20, "Couples Therapy: An Overview"
- Chapter 37, "Couples Therapy Research: Status and Directions"

4

Psychodynamic Family Therapy

G. Pirooz Sholevar, M.D.
Linda D. Schwoeri, Ph.D.

Introduction

Psychoanalytic theory was the dominant psychiatric conceptual system in the first seven decades of the twentieth century. The comprehensive body of knowledge supplied by psychoanalytic theory attempts to explain non-pathological and pathological human behavior, particularly human motivation. Therefore, it is not surprising that almost all the major early pioneers in family therapy were psychoanalysts. Encountering the failures in psychodynamic psychotherapy as applied to individuals, family therapists searched for the motivational sources of behavior, as well as resistance to change originating from beyond the autonomous, individual patient. Psychodynamic psychology was particularly suited to the family therapist's search for motivation because it viewed the mental apparatus and mental activity as the end product of the individual's interpersonal relationships in early life. The psychotherapeutic system was also based on the understanding of transference as the externalization of internal elements operating in the interpersonal domain. Since then, psychodynamic family therapy has developed in an evolutionary fashion in an ongoing search for continuities and discontinuities in individual and interpersonal psychologies. The perspective of continuity or discontinuity allows a psychodynamic formulation and rationale for intervention that is equally applicable in individual, couple, or family sessions. Conducting individual and joint sessions concomitantly or serially remains one of the major advantages of psychodynamic family therapy, unmatched by any other family therapy approach.

Definition

Contemporary psychodynamic and psychoanalytic approaches to family therapy share the common view that the family is a social unit with interpersonal rules. The family and its members can be best evaluated when the family is examined *as a whole*. The psychodynamic—and particularly the psychoanalytic—approach explores the significant dimension of the collective unconscious of family life to explain the adaptive or dysfunctional behavior of the family. The success of family members toward optimal adaptation to each other, to the environment, and to the developmental needs of the children is related to the capacities of the family as a whole. The family adaptive capacity in turn is associated with developmental level of family members through the course of their life cycle. A well-functioning family has achieved a high degree of freedom from restrictions imposed by developmental failures in earlier phases of their development. A dysfunctional family, particularly a "neurotic family," is burdened to a greater or lesser extent by its developmental failures. Psychodynamic family therapists assume that married couples choose partners who share similar or complementary developmental failures in early life. The choice of marital partner is closely related to earlier patterns of relations, especially the mother-child and father-child relationship in oedipal and preoedipal configurations. The neurotic choice of a marital object is a significant factor in the establishment of a pattern of interpersonal relationships. This pattern continues to be regulated by the early experiences of the couple rather than the adaptational needs of their subsequent family.

Psychodynamic family therapists utilize the concept of "system" in a manner similar to other family therapists. They attempt to unearth the repetitive interactional patterns in the family, the rules governing the interactions, the roles of family members, the family power hierarchy, and family affect. Therapists consider the overall interactional organization of the system as the *exterior* of the family unit; they will then attempt to explore the complex and subtler characteristics of the individuals and their interactions—that is, the *interior* mental working of the family and its members. The unconscious and conscious mental life of the individuals as the components and elements of the family system receive more recognition in psychodynamic family therapy than in other approaches to family treatment.

Unconscious factors of the family system consist of two subgroups: 1) motivational forces representing desires and wishes, and 2) defensive forces attempting to control the expression of the motivational forces. The motivational forces in different family members join together to form *shared family fantasies* based on *shared family conflicts*. The shared family conflicts are in turn contained by *shared family defenses* that consist of the collective defenses of members. The shared family conflicts are represented in a hierarchy of fantasies moving from the conscious surface to deep unconscious levels. The conscious fantasies are closer to external reality, and the deep unconscious fantasies are more closely associated with traumatic and dangerous situations in early family life. The repetitive interactional patterns in the family are generally the manifestations of shared family defenses. The shared family defenses attempt to contain the family conflicts and therefore prevent the occurrence of traumatic or dangerous situations for family members.

Psychodynamic family therapists share with other contemporary psychodynamic psychotherapists the belief that unconscious dynamics can be best understood in the context of the conscious organization of experience and the total integrating pattern of the personality. However, psychodynamic family therapists further propose that the unconscious life can be best understood within the context of the prevailing interpersonal reality (Ackerman 1958, p. 30).

The developmental failures and lack of developmental achievement in early phases of family life can originate in multiple phases. They include

- Traumatic events in the intergenerational sphere
- Traumatic events in the childhood of the marital partners
- Traumatic events in the early stages of the marriage or family life of the current couple

Psychodynamic family therapists are attentive to both the level of need satisfaction and the functioning of family members and consider these capacities as closely related to each other. The multiple needs of the family members fall particularly in the areas of the need for relationships, dependency, sexual gratification, identity, and the discharge of aggression.

Major approaches to psychodynamic family therapy include the work of the object relations school of psychoanalysis, primarily originating in Great Britain, and the ego psychology–oriented psychoanalysts from the United States. More recently, the self psychology of Kohut has become influential in family treatment of patients with early developmental deficits. The major contributors to psychodynamic family therapy include Ackerman, Lidz, Wynne, Dicks, Nagy, Stierlin, Sager, Framo, Zinner, and Shapiro.

History

An early cornerstone of the psychoanalytic family approach was the *Psycho-Analytic Study of the Family* by Flugel (1921). Flugel's propositions adhered very closely to classical psychoanalytic theory, but Flugel attempted to understand the influence family exerts on the desires and impulses of the child, particularly in the areas of love and hate. Concentrating mostly on family dyads, he examined the role of dyads in negotiating the force of infantile sexuality and oedipal strivings. His therapeutic method examined the patient-analyst relationship in the traditional individual psychotherapeutic situation using transference as a major tool of understanding.

Another early groundbreaking contribution was that of Clarence Oberndorf (1938), who utilized the previously described concept of *folie à deux* and proposed a theory of interactive or emergent neurosis in marriage. He attempted to describe the *interlocking* neurotic aspects of marital relationships. *Folie à deux* was first described in a French paper by Lasegue and Falret (1877). The interlocking neurotic process was unearthed in individual analytic treatment with both spouses, and its clinical manifestation was the appearance of therapeutic impasses in the treatment of each spouse. Oberndorf (and later Mittleman) hypothesized that the close nature of the marital relationship supported corresponding neurotic processes in married couples. Bela Mittleman (1948) elaborated on Oberndorf's concept and noted that because of the intimate nature of marriage, every neurosis in a married person is strongly *anchored* in the marriage relationship. Therefore, Mittleman found it a useful and at times indispensable therapeutic measure to concentrate the analytic discussion on these complementary patterns and "if necessary to have both mates treated" (Mittleman 1944, p. 491).

Henry Dicks' work with married couples at the Tavistock Clinic in England occurred in the 1940s, and the results were published in his classic book *Marital Tensions* (Dicks 1967). His work examined the parallel representation of internal and external objects and their influence on the functioning of the personality. He proposed that the projection of past object representations onto the marital partner resulted in a return to a mode of past object relationship that had been repressed. This concept served as the forerunner of Zinner and Shapiro's work at the National Institute of Mental Health (NIMH) (Zinner 1976; Zinner and Shapiro 1974, 1975) on the process of projective identification. Dicks' elaboration of norms—namely, cultural and personal norms and the unconscious forces shaping the marriage—are reflected in Sager's marital contract theory (Sager 1976).

Christian Midelfort (1957) applied the concept of family unit and family pathology to schizophrenia and emphasized the importance of seeing the family together in order to enhance therapeutic results and effectiveness. Although Midelfort was an important contributor during the founding decade of family therapy from 1952 to 1961, his influence on the field remained limited because of his lack of a broadly based contribution to family therapy literature (Gurman and Kniskern 1981b).

Johnson and Szurek (1952) examined the coexistence and transmission of antisocial psychopathology in the interpersonal sphere. Their approach was the simultaneous psychoanalysis of parents and children. They observed that superego deficiencies and "lacunae" were formed in children in response to antisocial tendencies in the parents. These parents transmitted their poorly integrated delinquent impulses to the children and unconsciously sanctioned their antisocial acting-out behavior. The formulation of Johnson and Szurek shifted the focus of inquiry to the externalization of internal conflict in the interpersonal sphere.

Ackerman (1938) noted that the common clinical tendency and technical mistake of the period was a concentration on the maladaptive behavior of either the child or the parent (usually the mother). His early work at Menninger Child Guidance Clinic, influenced by the work of Bowlby at the Tavistock Clinic, broadened the practice of child psychotherapy by looking at the family as the unit of diagnosis and treatment. Ackerman particularly favored visiting families at home to observe spontaneous family interactions without interference from nonhousehold surroundings. His work continued as a driving force in psychodynamic family therapy, particularly with regard to the relationship between the intrapsychic and interpersonal psychopathology. Another of his additions to family theory was the formulation of the rigidly structured symbiotic relationship between the mother and child, particularly in families with schizophrenic children.

Bowen, a towering early figure in family therapy, has contributed as much to the psychodynamic school of family therapy as to intergenerational family therapy. In 1951, he housed client parents in cottages at the Menninger Clinic to live with their disturbed offspring. His project of hospitalization of children and their entire families simultaneously was carried out between 1954 and 1959. The detailed examination of the family interactions in both inpatient and outpatient settings allowed Bowen to formulate the concept of "family projection process," wherein parents and children played active parts in the transmission of the parental problems to the child. He used the model of mother-child relationship to arrive at the concept of "undifferentiation."

Whitaker, as early as 1943, developed the practice of bringing spouses and children into sessions together. This resulted in the elaboration of three concepts: the use of *cotherapy*, *play*, and *affect* in family therapy. Whitaker's close working relationship with Warkentin and T. Malone led to the elaboration of the cotherapy technique and process in family therapy (Gurman and Kniskern 1981b). Whitaker's emphasis on the role of affects that are defended against is a key emphasis of psychodynamic psychotherapy. The use of play in therapy is particularly consonant with the ego psychology school of psychoanalysis, where conflict-free functions of the ego become an important aspect of an individual's personality, complementing the symptomatic and conflicting aspects of the individual.

J.L. Moreno used therapeutic group processes and psychodrama in 1925 to shift emphasis from the individual to the context of the individual's life. He assigned special significance to the nonverbal aspect of communication, in addition to the verbal dimension (Kaplan and Sadock 1971).

Theoreticians were clearly conceptualizing the family as a unit as early as the 1930s when they were studying the quality of the relationship between parents, the selective traits of children, the relationship between siblings, and the dyadic relationship of the marital couple. This culminated in the investigation of the family as a continuous functional whole.

The period between 1952 and 1961 saw a rise of interest in studying the transmission of schizophrenia in the family. The work of Lidz, Bowen, Wynne, Jackson, and Ackerman made significant contributions to this area. It is noteworthy that all of the above major contributors were psychoanalysts. Theodore Lidz (1963) introduced a significant shift from individual psychoanalytic concepts to one of an interpersonal and social perspective. He began looking at the family as a social unit in itself, with its own dynamic characteristic. Lidz described the role of shared family defenses in cases of conflict or arrested development in the oedipal phase. He attempted to examine the effect of the parents' relationship to each other on their offspring. He described how the child's ego development was affected by the "parental coalition" and the marital relationship; both the coalition and the relationship figured in the redirection of oedipal fantasies and identification with the parents. Lidz clearly recognized the systemic aspects of the family and emphasized that the actions of any component affected all members. The need for relationship assumed a fundamental position in the intrapsychic life of individuals and achieved parity with the dual drives of sexuality and aggression.

The work of Lyman Wynne and his multiple co-workers at NIMH (Wynne et al. 1958) moved psychodynamic family therapy to a new phase, in which the focus was on the ongoing transactions among family members and with the therapists. Family interactions became the locus of exploration in the determination of psychopathology. Wynne focused on directly observable interactional data to discover the motives and links between the past and present. His work in this area resulted in the delineation of psychodynamic defense mechanisms such as projective identification but most importantly the concept of *pseudomutuality*. In addition to recognition of the basic drives of relatedness, sexuality, and aggression, he recognized a basic need for an identity within a relationship. Wynne's concepts moved psychodynamic family therapy toward a truly interactional model. As a result, the term "exploratory family therapy" was coined.

More recent developments in psychoanalytic family therapy include the application of object relations theory to families and couples (Scharff and Scharff 1987; Zinner and Shapiro 1974); separation and individuation of adolescents from their families (Stierlin 1974); marital contract theory (Sager 1976); family images (Sonne 1981); and triadic and dyadic family transference (Sonne 1981). These developments will be described in detail in the section below on theoretical concepts.

Theoretical Concepts

A number of key theoretical concepts from psychoanalysis have been applied in the field of psychodynamic family and marital therapy. These key concepts include transference, countertransference, resistance, socially shared psychopathology, projective identification, family myths, family image, represented and practicing family perspectives, holding environment, bonding/attachment, true self/false self, self pathology, unconscious assumptions, and continuity-discontinuity.

Transference

The concept of transference was first described by Freud (1912/1958) and has been applied to family therapy in terms of transference reactions among family members as well as between the family members and the therapist. Transference is a regressive phenomenon by which unconscious infantile and childhood conflicts are gradually and progressively mobilized and reexperienced in current life situations inside and outside of therapy. Transference is formed with all people in all places and at all times. However, it achieves its greatest intensity among family members and in intensive psychoanalytic treatment, where such attitudes are thoroughly mobilized and reexperienced in current relationships. In psychoanalytic situations, the intensification of the transference reaction results in transference neurosis, and its exploration in the treatment situation can result in the resolution of the neurotic conflicts. Transference reactions among family members represent the natural outgrowth of the earliest dynamic interactions within the family. Ackerman (1962, p. 41) emphasized intrafamilial transferential experiences as being mutual and a true social experience—that is, an interaction between two or more minds as compared with the patient and analyst's regressive transference experiences. This historically based phenomenon is therefore *transgenerational* in nature. Interactions involve displacement of transference residues from earlier levels of experiences with the extended family, and a complex pattern of interlocking projections and introjections based on internalizations from previous generations. The term "interlocking transferences" (Meissner 1978, p. 82) implies the complex and multidimensional nature of this phenomenon. Treatment of interlocking transferences requires the identification, clarification, and interpretation of the family's own projection process toward each other and the therapist.

In addition to the transference reaction toward the therapist by each family member, the family or the couple as a whole can develop certain transference distortions toward the therapist. Families with more severe disturbances form stronger and more apparent transference distortions toward the therapist, while the more highly functioning families react to the therapist in a more integrated and less distorted way.

Transference reactions in family and couples therapy provide important information on each partner's (and the joint dyad's) feelings, perceptions, misperceptions, attributions of each other's (and the therapist's) intent, motivation, and loyalties about specific actions (Gurman 1978). Family and marital therapy provides an exceptional opportunity for the therapist to recognize the transference reactions based on the repetition of historical attitudes, and to use such ready-made reactions and attitudes as the basis for interpretation and insight. This makes the therapist less dependent on the emergence of transference reactions in the therapeutic situation, which requires time-consuming regression not usually available in an active, brief therapeutic encounter. The study of transference reactions obviates the need for extensive interpretations in order to yield meaningful and enduring change in the individual partners or in the marital relationship itself (Gurman 1978, pp. 469–470).

The transference reaction toward the therapist can be a valuable tool to provide empathic clues on the transferential nature of interactions between the couple. Transference in family therapy does not refer to a reaction toward the therapist stemming solely from the past and unrelated to what the therapist "really" does or what he or she is like. Transference here is understood as the patient's idiosyncratic way of construing and reacting to what the therapist is doing (Wachtel 1978, p. 111). Interpretation of transference reactions toward the therapist or toward other family members is "integrative" in nature. It attempts to clarify and sort out the feelings of the family members in the current family or therapeutic situations, rather than to try to recreate regressively the family's childhood feelings. Interpretation of transference toward the therapist is consistent with the interpretation of intrafamilial transferences. Such interventions can take place in the process of family and marital therapy, which tends to be shorter in duration. These interpretations can be made in the initial phase of family treatment rather than waiting to use them only when they have become more fixed in the therapeutic situation.

The various transference reactions of patients in family and marital therapy have been described by object relation therapists as 1) contextual transference, 2) focused transference, and 3) shared contextual transference (Scharff and Scharff 1987). *Contextual transference* refers to the therapeutic situation, management of the therapeutic situation, and the patient's expectations about the therapy. Great attention is given to the details of the therapeutic setting, handling the arrangements for sessions, conveying concern for family safety, the therapist's competence in interviewing, and seeing the whole family. Such care is necessary to provide for effective handling of contextual transference. This expectation of safe and sensitive provision of care is based on internal models of "holding" functions provided by primary figures for the family. The mother's "contextual holding" function is to provide a safe and responsive environment for the infant. In contextual transference, the therapist likewise provides a "container" for anxieties and fantasies that are unmanageable for the patient (Scharff and Scharff 1987, p. 62). Contextual transference occurs in the early stages of treatment when the family tells the therapist about their life and problems; contextual transference leads later to focused transference.

The second form of transference, *focused transference*, consists of the patient's focused projections onto the therapist based on the early experiences. The third type of transference, *shared contextual transference*, reveals the couple's difficulties with the holding situation. The therapist's holding of the couple in treatment can help show the family or couple how to provide holding for each other (Scharff and Scharff 1987).

Several prominent family and marital therapists have developed a view of transference as it applies to family therapy. Sonne (1991) emphasized the importance of recognizing the triadic transferences that are the partial recreation and replication of pathological family images constructed in father-mother-child triads during childhood.

Sager (1967, 1976) emphasized the many unconsciously determined transferential factors involved in mate selection. He describes this in his definition of marital contracts.

Lansky (1986) emphasized that transference interpretations are not always a primary vehicle for cure. However, transference can be used to help understand the couple's deep anxieties about the therapist and, hence, the transference between the spouses. An example would be when the mode of defense is *preoccupation* with outside obligations, blaming, provoking blame, or exclusive focus on the actions of one person. This phenomenon points to anxiety about the therapist or therapeutic situation; it is particularly applicable to addressing the transference reaction between the spouses, especially in treatment of narcissistic disorders.

Dicks (1967) utilized the concept of *transitional* objects to understand the transference reaction toward the therapist. One task of the therapist is to accept the patient's projections and unreal expectations but to respond to these communications in such ways that it will increase the patient's insight. Interpreting and working through negative transference is a significant source of insight.

Countertransference

Countertransference refers to the phenomenon of unconscious feelings in the therapist in reaction to the patient's verbal and/or nonverbal communications in treatment. Countertransference can become a potent impediment to the progress of treatment if it influences the interventions of the therapist. However, the therapist's relatively early recognition of his or her feelings toward the patient can become a valuable tool for understanding the nature of the patient's transferential projections onto the therapist in the treatment situation.

There are superficial and fleeting reactions on the part of the therapist toward the patient, based to a large degree on objective reality and under good control of the therapist. In superficial types of countertransference reactions, the therapist is aware that he is concealing his own responses to the patient and that his responses may be the projection of his own fantasies rather than the reality. More serious types of countertransference reactions are relatively stable, fixed, focused, and *unconscious* reactions of the therapist to the patient, based on some infantile aspects of the therapist's personality provoked by the patient's behavior or material. The countertransference feelings in the therapist are usually the result of the therapist's defensive behavior, based on his early life experiences or current circumstances. Countertransference arises out of the therapist's identification of himself with the patient's internal objects (Racker 1981). Behaviors such as distancing, unempathic interpretation, taking sides and reversal, reverting to dyadic or individual therapy, simplification of the issues, preoccupation and rationalized emotional withdrawal, shaming the patient, or impulsive attempts to control one of the spouses are some of the ways countertransference is exhibited. Termination of treatment is likely to occur at this point because of the unresolved transference.

Countertransference in family therapy is often the result of several factors, some of which are listed below:

1. The presence of multiple persons in family and couples therapy is likely to give rise to oedipal transferential configurations because of alliances, coalitions, rivalries, jealousies, boundary disturbances, and triangulations (Dare 1986). Interpersonal expression of intrapsychic defenses is a common phenomenon with the more disturbed, boundary-lacking families.
2. The active and self-revealing nature of family therapy promotes expression of countertransferential reactions in the sessions. The therapist's task is to remain outside the conflict and not take sides.
3. It may be technically more difficult to completely avoid collusion with a family member in family therapy, particularly when the painful issues involved may be similar or mirror those encountered by the therapist in the course of his or her own past or current intimate relationships.

Sager cautioned therapists that countertransference often occurs in the triangular relationship of the therapist and two patients, as in marital treatment. Such countertransference reactions take the form of becoming competitive or resorting to "male chauvinistic," "feminist," or "anti-male" thinking. He cautions to "check one's value system constantly so that it is not imposed upon the couple" (Sager 1976, p. 207).

Resistance

The concept of resistance describes all oppositional forces within the therapeutic situation that hinder progress in treatment (Greenson 1965). Resistance may be conscious, preconscious, or unconscious. Any human behavior can be used as a resistance in treatment; such behaviors include emotional expressions, attitudes, ideas, impulses, thoughts, fantasies, or actions. Object relations psychotherapists see the motive for resistance as reluctance on the part of the patient to allow a painful relationship into awareness. The patient therefore avoids the return of the repressed bad object relations and the attendant pain of the earlier experiences with the bad object (Guntrip 1969; Scharff and Scharff 1987). In family and marital therapy, resistance exhibits itself by the collusive behavior of the family. The common forms of resistance in family therapy include avoiding conflictual topics, scapegoating, becoming depressed to avoid expression of anger, refusing to consider one's own role in dysfunctional interactions, seeking individual sessions or individual treatment, keeping secrets, threatening to leave treatment or changing therapists, and acting-out. All of these forms of resistance allow the patient to avoid pain, including the anxiety about remembering previous painful experiences.

Sonne, Speck, and Jungress (1962) described one form of resistance to family therapy called the "absent member maneuver in family therapy."

Family members representing one side of the family conflict can absent themselves from family sessions as a collusive behavior to conceal and avoid family conflicts. This resistance can only be successfully overcome once all family members are encouraged to attend the sessions and express their viewpoints.

Socially Shared Psychopathology

The concept of "socially shared psychopathology" is the end result of a number of interpersonal psychological mechanisms such as projective identification and delineation. Through these mechanisms, a person delineates part of his psychopathological tendencies and imparts it to another intimate member of his social group, particularly his family. The other person invites and receives this psychopathology and claims ownership of the projected part.

Projective Identification

Projective identification is an interpersonal defense mechanism shared by two or more people based on a shared fantasized object relationship. Here, the parts of the self and internal objects are split off and projected onto an external object. The object then becomes "identified" with the split-off part as well as possessed and controlled by it. In family and marital treatment, a therapist can easily become involved in projective identification; he or she subsequently gets pulled toward one partner's side of the battle and begins to act out against the other partner, thereby disrupting treatment.

Projective identification occurs extensively and frequently between the spouses as well as between parents and children. The mechanism of projective identification between marital partners is facilitated by choosing a partner that shares one's neurotic conflict and then accusing the partner for the problem. A parent's continued use of accusations (i.e., "You'll become just like your father") can initiate projective identification. This is the colloquial "self-fulfilling prophecy." In parent-child relationships, projective identification can occur readily and extensively because the child may view the parent's projections as reality. Children often base their developing identities on these projections.

Family Image

The concept of family image described by Sonne (1981, p. 82) refers to a developing child's recognition of the existence of a marital dyadic relationship between the parents and his internalization of such an image. The child learns to relate to the parental dyadic relationship in a fashion similar to how he or she relates to individual parental figures. This family image expands the child's possibilities for identification with the roles assumed by both parents. The development of triadic family image is influential in the issue of mate selection as well as transference distortions outside of the marital relationship.

Holding Environment

The concept of holding environment developed by Winnicott refers to a quality and characteristic of interaction between the mother and infant. This concept has been further utilized to describe a certain aspect of the therapeutic situation. The function of "holding" refers to those facilitative aspects of the environment that provide the infant with the feeling of safety, constancy, and "containment." The holding environment produced by the mother provides safety, constancy, and protection for the infant. It also would provide a precise reflection of the infant's experience and gestures to him or her that can facilitate growth as well as allowing temporary regressions. Winnicott (1958) refers to this holding environment provided by the mother as "good enough mothering," through which the infant experiences an omnipotence that is essential for the child's healthy development. This holding provides sufficient security for the infant to ultimately tolerate the inevitable failures of empathy.

The concept of the holding environment can also be applied to the nonspecific and supportive continuity provided by the therapist and the therapeutic situation. The regularity of visits, the steadiness of the therapeutic environment, and the very continuity of the care by the therapists all contribute to a metaphorical holding that can help contain the disruptions that occur during meaningful treatment (Moore and Fine 1990, p. 206). The provision of therapeutic holding is particularly important for patients who have not experienced a satisfactory "holding" experience in their early childhood. An important aspect of therapeutic holding is to accept the total range of expressions by the patient, to contain such expressions, and to help the person to integrate his or her experiences in a growth-promoting fashion. Kohut's (1971a) concepts of idealizing and mirroring functions in self psychology are very similar to the concept of holding environment.

Bonding/Attachment

The concept of bonding or attachment is based on Bowlby's ethologically based observations on the child's tie to his mother. Bowlby (1988, p. 27) defined attachment as any form of behavior that results in a person's attaining or maintaining proximity to some other clearly identified individual who is conceived as better able to cope with the world. The presence of an available and responsive attachment figure gives a person a pervasive feeling of security and encourages him or her to value and continue the relationship. This definition addresses both the protective aspects of attachment as well as the relational nature of this type of behavior. The need for personal relationships is the basis for bonding and attachment rather than the need for food or some other sustenance necessary for life. Proximity to the attachment figure and the security therein is a crucial aspect of the therapeutic situation. The environment for the patient must be safe and secure. Bowlby labeled this protective environment a *secure base*. The concept is related to the concept of holding or containment described by Winnicott (1958) and Bion (1962), respectively, and incorporated into the theory of object relations in family therapy.

True Self/False Self

The concepts of true and false self proposed by Winnicott (1958) are rooted in his view of early development. The "true self" is based on the child's experience of nurture by a "good enough mother" who appreciates the importance of need satisfaction in the infant.

The disorder of the "false self" can indicate the absence of this experience: as an infant, this individual had a caretaker (usually a mother) who was unable to meet his or her instinctual needs. Instead, the caretaker deprived the infant through her own self-involvement. As a result, the child often withdrew from spontaneity and authenticity. Intellectualization is often associated with the false self. The concepts of true and false self have central relevance to family pathology and family therapy because the predominance of false self and intellectualization can significantly reduce a married couple's ability to satisfy one another in the relationship. Since marital choice or love object choice is a matter of idealization and looking only at the best in the loved one to complement oneself, persons with a false self will hide their own unpleasant feelings but seek the needed love from the partner.

Separation-Individuation Theory

The separation-individuation theory of Margaret Mahler (1975) has become an increasingly dominant theory for the explanation of childhood development, particularly in the first three years of life. Mahler's theory is based on her observation of the developmental process in infancy and early childhood. It proposes that the infant enters a symbiotic relationship with his or her caregiver after a brief phase of being primarily preoccupied with the establishment of internal homeostasis. In the first three years of life, the child goes through a succession of phases by which he or she attempts to arrive at a differentiated sense of self and the mother (object). By the end of the third year, the child is "on the way to individuation," a process which would take many evolutionary years. However, at the third year of life, the child is expected to have achieved the minimum level of individuation and separation from the caregiver and be able to function with relative autonomy, for a period of time, in the physical absence of the caregiver. This capacity is related to the achievement of "object constancy"—the establishment of an internalized and relatively stable sense of self and object that can withstand the anxiety of the separation.

A decisive period in the separation-individuation process is the "rapprochement" phase, in which the infant is pulled between two forces: the need to stay close to the caretaker while being pushed to function autonomously. This results in the "rapprochement crisis" that reaches its height in the second half of the second year of life. The failure to negotiate the rapprochement phase successfully can result in the inability to establish a satisfactory distance and harmonious relationship with the caregiver or other people in the future.

Self Psychology Theory and Self Pathology

The model of "self" proposed by the school of self psychology of Kohut (1977) has clear application to family therapy, because the disturbances of self can readily result in the projection of a person's inner experience onto intimate relations in family. "Self" or "self organization" refers to three phenomena: the cohesive self, the fragmented self, and the self-regulatory structure. The person with a cohesive self exhibits a high level of well-being, self-esteem, vitality, and productivity. The "fragmentation" of self occurs when there is a failure to establish the cohesive self. The person with a fragmented self exhibits a lack of vitality, low self-esteem, unstable mood, and depression. "Self-regulatory structure" refers to the psychic capacity to maintain self-esteem, cohesiveness, and vitality and to regulate tension or mood.

The disorder of the self, or narcissistic personality disorder, can be the result of an unempathic parent who deprives the child of a needed "selfobject." Selfobject refers to an object, similar to a "transitional object" in Winnicott's terms or a "symbiotic object" in Mahler's language, that is cognitively *perceived* as external to the self but is *experienced* as part of the self.

A person functioning as a selfobject for another is perceived as performing some essential psychological function for the subject. Without available external selfobject support, the individual is liable to feel helpless, ineffective, overwhelmed, unworthy, unreal, incomplete, or empty.

Unconscious Assumptions

Wilfred Bion (1962) described three "basic assumption groups" and processes: dependency, fight/flight, and pairing. The basic assumption groups are regressive in nature in contrast to "working groups." The basic assumption groups can support or subvert tasks. Bion has described unconscious assumptions with their characteristic "valency" as the individual's readiness to join a group that acts on the regressive basic assumptions. The valencies are similar to the transference phenomenon described in broader psychoanalytic literature. The end result of this type of functioning is the phenomenon of merging or fusion (in contrast to fission) that can occur as a defense against the threat of personal identity dislocation and alienation (Scharff and Scharff 1987).

Fusion basic assumption group functioning supports harmony, empathic identification, and togetherness appropriate to the early infant-mother bonding. The domination of the group by fusion is generally an attempt to deny difference, conflict, and loss; Bowen and Minuchin describe this phenomenon as "undifferentiation" and "enmeshment." *Fission basic assumption group functioning* promotes conflict, difference of opinions, and divergent goals. Fusion-fission basic assumptions are the two poles in group dynamics.

Continuity/Discontinuity

Belief in the importance of "traumatic" experiences in the formative years of early childhood and an interest in identifying individuals at risk for later psychiatric disorders have led researchers to look intensively for significant continuities in development (Zeanah et al. 1989). The continuity/discontinuity model of psychopathology led early psychoanalytic theorists to predict that psychological traumas and biological propensities lead to predictable sequelae and consequences. Contrary to expectations, one of the major results of the search for continuities in behavior has been the recognition that discontinuities in early development are far more readily apparent than continuities (Emde and Harmon 1984; Zeanah et al. 1989). This recognition, coupled with evidence of adequate coping in some resilient children and adults despite adverse early experiences, has led some investigators to ascribe little if any significance to experiences in the early years (Kagan 1984).

The contemporary psychodynamic model incorporates the models of both continuous and discontinuous development. As Mitchell (1988) proposed, early experiences result in patterns of interaction that will be repeated in different forms at different times over the years. Present family interactions merely maintain patterns of behavior initiated in the past.

Emotionally Focused Therapy

The expression of affect in family and marital therapy can be loud, excessive, and defensive and can often conceal rather than reveal the significant issues. Emotionally focused therapy (EFT) (Johnson 1996) has proposed an intelligent framework to concentrate on affects to enhance the treatment process and reduce the disruptive impact of *defensive affects*. The therapist focuses early in therapy on the expression of affects that are usually defensive, self-protective, and accusatory toward other family members. The exploration of such affects in a manner similar to defense analysis can lead the therapist to the discovery of soft *attachment affects* that are the roots of relational dissatisfaction. Emotionally focused therapy is based on the application of attachment theory in family therapy.

Goals

The primary goal of psychodynamic family therapy is similar to those of other family therapy approaches that attempt to create a more highly functioning family unit, free from enduring conflicts and inhibitions. As such, the family can enhance the maturation of all family members, particularly children. Psychodynamic family therapists subscribe to the principles of resolution of presenting problems, enhanced self-esteem in family members, flexibility and adaptability of family roles, tolerance of difference among family members, clear boundaries and lines of authority, and a balanced sharing of the power in the family. However, these therapists also place a very strong emphasis on personal maturity and individuation in family members. This reduces the likelihood of projection of inner perceptions based on past experiences on other family members, or responding to distorted projections of other family members in a shared pathological way. From this point of enhancement of maturity and individuation, psychodynamic family therapists and practitioners of Bowen's family systems theory are closely tied. Both schools of thought agree that family members need to take the following steps in family therapy:

1. Develop a sense of self that is both differentiated and internally integrated (Meissner 1978)

2. Resolve conflicts over the differences between the partners and failures of complementarity, thereby interrupting the collusive processes in the relationship (Ackerman 1958)
3. Resolve transference projections among family members that represent the split-off part of the self, which is projected onto and experienced as a part of other family members

Applicability and Methodology

Therapeutic Situation

The psychodynamic therapeutic situation is a modification of the concept of the analytic situation that is a central point of psychotherapeutic methodology. In response to the attentive, responsive, relatively nondirective, and neutral position of the therapist, family members express their wishes, fantasies, and memories in regard to current and past ideas and events. This enables the therapist to uncover transference reactions among family members. Transference reactions are a "new edition" of residual infantile experiences and traumas with early objects in patient's lives that have remained beyond consciousness but that affect current relationships of family members with each other. The recognition, clarification, interpretation, and working through of such residual experience and traumas can help family members integrate their past with the present, nullifying to varying degrees the pathological effects of previously unconscious and unrecognized conflicts.

The psychotherapeutic situation is the vehicle for the actualization of the psychodynamic therapeutic process. The psychotherapeutic situation enables the family or couple to examine the reactivated pathogenic or potentially pathogenic elements from their early development. Such pathogenic elements rooted in the early development of the family members are usually embedded in their personality structure and traits and are also externalized in their current relationships and interactions. The rigid interactional pattern in the family has a syntonic quality by which each family member feels confident about the accuracy of his or her actions, impressions, and judgment and blames other family members for the negative consequences of events and interactions. The psychotherapeutic situation enables the family or couple to identify with the observing and accepting function of the therapist in a neutral environment and to gain objectivity and a heightened perception and sense of reality. As a result, there will be a weakening of shared defenses, such as projective identification, and expansion of the self-observation function and other autonomous ego functions of family members. Furthermore, family members will be able to gradually and incrementally recognize the impingement of their pathogenic pasts, as well as the shared and complementary conflicts and defenses that impinge on the adaptation of the family and its members to the current reality.

The psychotherapeutic situation in many ways is an operational definition of the psychodynamic method itself. Its purpose is to create a field that is dynamically unstable so that the therapist, from the position of neutrality, may observe the conflicting components as they shift in their unstable equilibrium. Triggered by the property of the psychodynamic situation, various mental phenomena begin to emerge in a flow of affect and ideation—or rather affectively tinged ideation. The psychotherapist listens to the statements of the patients and observes their behavior as "metaphorical" enterprise that ambiguously relates in a distorted and disguised way to what the patient and family members unconsciously fantasize (Lansky 1986; Scharff and Scharff 1987).

Object relations family therapists use the term *frame* instead of "psychoanalytic situation" to describe the provision of safety and security in treatment, which allows for the exploration of problems and provision of interpretations. The establishment of boundaries and guidelines, as well as the regularity and predictability of the time, space, arrangements, and structure of the family sessions is an important element for the achievement of the therapeutic frame (Scharff and Scharff 1987).

Therapeutic or Working Alliance

Therapeutic alliance and *working alliance* are somewhat equivalent terms that characterize realistic cooperation and collaboration in the therapeutic process. It is assumed that the therapist is capable of such an effort but that the patient's ability and willingness to respond similarly is in question (Moore and Fine 1990, p. 175).

The therapeutic alliance is based on both the positive transference relationship of the patient with the therapist and the "real" relationship between the two people. Transference involves the repetition in the therapeutic situation of childhood attitudes of trust, reliance, and cooperativeness in the therapeutic collaboration. The "real" relationship implies that the therapist is also perceived and reacted to simultaneously as a "real person," a dynamism somewhat free of transference contaminations. The "real" relationship is based on socially valuable character traits, capacities, and areas of functioning in patients that are relatively autonomous from problems of infantile or conflictual origin. "Real" relationships describe the patient's collaboration and involvement in the joint therapeutic enterprise as reasonable and realistic (Moore and Fine 1990).

In family and marital therapy, the formation and maintenance of the therapeutic alliance is more difficult because such collaborative attitudes need to be developed with each family member as well as the family or couple as a unit. The therapeutic alliance can be disrupted rapidly if one or more family members perceive the therapist as biased or aligned with the wishes of other family members. Therefore, the therapist should keep an exceptionally watchful eye on the conscious and unconscious wishes of each family member and strive to position himself or herself in a balanced way among such opposing and contradictory forces. The existence of a therapeutic or working alliance between the therapist and family members is based on positive trust and confidence in mutually shared goals and helps the family continue working in the face of strong resistances. In the advanced stage of treatment, the family or couple will experience a dramatic decrease in shared defensive activities and the heightening of their ego capacity of self observing function toward their own activities and those of other family members. The enhanced observational function in family members is generally a result of a mature identification with the therapist and his or her therapeutic goals in the psychotherapeutic situation. Therefore, through therapy there is a shared and complementary self-observational field, composed of integrated self-observational capacities of family members, replacing to some degree the previously shared pathogenic defenses.

Use of History and History Taking

The developmental history of family members is a significant tool in the hands of psychodynamic family therapists. The history alerts the therapist to the parallel interactional patterns in the patient's past and present functioning. The therapist is then in the enlightened position of recognizing how current interactional patterns that are impinging on the patient's current reality are, in effect, the continuation of past pathogenic events. An example would be a father who has lost his own father in early childhood; has resented having to grow up without the support, love, and guidance of a father; and, in spite of his great love for his son, continues to absent himself from the son's activities. This same process is evident on relational and interactional levels in the mother who was raised in a family with a father prone to explosive and frightening outbursts. Her father usually absented himself from the family scene after explosive and frightening scenes and left the patient almost exclusively dependent on her mother. This early pattern of upbringing is reproduced in the current family situation being addressed in therapy by the mother accepting, welcoming, and even encouraging the father's lack of involvement with their son. The mother is consequently allowed excessive closeness with the son, reproducing the mother's own family experience.

In the initial course of treatment, the history serves as a roadmap for the therapist. The history's utilization with family members may have little more than an intellectual impact. However, with the progress of treatment, the family members should arrive at the point where they can recognize the troublesome and restricting effects of early developmental events and conflicts on their current functioning.

Empathy

Greenson (1965) defined empathy as an "emotional knowing." It is an experience of the feelings of another person without the subject having expressed the feelings verbally. It requires a type of partial, temporary identification of the therapist with the patient that permits participation in the patient's experiences. The use of empathy as a tool for psychodynamic psychotherapy requires that the therapist remain both detached and involved—both observer and participant (Langes 1981, p. 244). Empathy may require the therapist to tolerate intense feelings that are beyond the capacity of the patient's tolerance.

Empathy has also been described as a mode of perceiving by vicariously experiencing the psychological state of another person. Literally, it means "feeling into" another person, as contrasted with sympathy, which means "feeling with." The capacity for empathy is thought to be developmentally related to preverbal mother-infant interactions in which there is a concordance of wish, need, and response. It is an essential prerequisite for the practice of psychodynamic psychotherapy. In the therapeutic situation, empathy derives in part from the therapist's evenly suspended attention that is part of his or her work ego. From an object relations perspective, projective identification *into* the therapist is the basis of empathy. The therapist's self-perceptions or introspections then become a source of information about the patient. Empathy is therefore a partial ego regression in the service of the therapeutic process, permitting an easy, reversible, and trial identification with the patient. It may occur during a loss of verbal communication and understanding and is a preconscious, silent, and automatic process (Moore and Fine 1990).

From the perspective of psychoanalytic self psychology (Kohut 1959), empathy signifies a fitting and appropriate perception of and response to the patient's feelings and needs.

Within treatment generally, empathy implies a consistent focus on the patient's inner experience. Thus, we speak of empathic aspects of understanding, interpretation, and intervention, without giving empathy a subordinate position in psychoanalytic technique. Empathy is a nonjudgmental phenomenon and should be differentiated from sympathy, which lacks objectivity and encourages overidentification and can lead to enactment of rescue fantasies by the therapist.

Nichols (1987, p. 121) discusses listening, understanding, and empathy as part of the interpretive process in family therapy. Empathy requires "actively imagining what things look like from inside someone else's lifeworld" and implies active participation on the therapist's part.

Boszormenyi-Nagy (1972) also refers to the active role of the therapist. He says that the therapist must be able to side with one member and then in turn with other members, instead of refusing to commit himself or herself to anyone's claim for merit or justice. Boszormenyi-Nagy calls this "multidirectional partiality" (refer to Chapter 6, "Contextual Therapy," of this text for a more comprehensive discussion of this contextual term).

Empathy may be more difficult to achieve in family therapy because it requires consideration of different family members' viewpoints. Also, families themselves find it hard to empathize. They rarely understand each other's point of view and are unlikely to be receptive to interpretations. A statement by the therapist such as, "No one understands what you mean, do they?" creates an honest empathic intervention, but it also creates a tension that challenges the family to try to understand each other's point of view.

Intersubjectivity refers to the therapist's capacity to understand what the patient is experiencing through one's own attunement and empathic stance (Lachkar 1992; Stolorow et al. 1983; Trevarthan 1980; Trevarthan and Hubley 1978). This capacity allows the therapist to understand the patient's partially undifferentiated and archaic feelings and helps the patient to do the same. It is based on Daniel Stern's concept of "intersubjective relatedness," which begins in the second half of the first year of the infant's life (Stern 1985). Intersubjective relatedness serves as the foundation for reading and sharing the affective state of the other person, in degrees ranging from attunement to the more complex phenomenon of empathy. The application of such capacities in treatment can be an effective therapeutic tool.

Interpretation

Interpretation is the ultimate therapeutic activity in psychoanalytic treatment. It is a process whereby the therapist expresses what he or she comes to understand about the patient's mental life. This understanding is based on the patient's description of memories, fantasies, wishes, fears, and other elements of psychic conflict that were formerly unconscious or known to the patient only in incomplete, inaccurate, or otherwise distorted forms. Interpretation is also based on observation of the way the patient distorts the relationship with the analyst to meet unconscious needs and to relive old experiences (Moore and Fine 1990, p. 103).

Two forms of interpretations are common. The first is *genetic interpretation*, which connects present feelings, thoughts, conflicts, and behaviors with historical antecedents, often dating back to early childhood. The second form is *reconstruction*, which is part of the process of genetic interpretation, consisting of "piecing together information about psychologically significant early experiences" (Moore and Fine 1990, p. 103).

Interpretations in individual therapy are usually sparse and succinctly stated, utilizing everyday language suitable to the patient. Most of the therapeutic work involves clarification of already conscious material that is stored in a disintegrated and isolated manner in the mind of the patient. Before interpretation can take place, very extensive clarification of the conscious material is needed to find connections among feelings, thoughts, and behavior. However, in family therapy, the process of interpretation becomes more complex and somewhat richer, because family members can more readily recognize each other's unconscious feelings and thoughts. For example, a father's harsh and sadistic treatment of his child based on his reliving a similar relationship with his own father may be beyond consciousness in the patient but readily observable by his wife or children. However, the family generally does not make use of such observations and stores them away as part of their shared defensive functions. Within the therapeutic situation and with the accepting attitude of the therapist, family members can allow shared defensive mechanisms to relax or breakdown, paving the way for the emergence of unconscious material into awareness of the family members. Appropriate therapeutic handling can allow the family to incorporate such information as part of their everyday knowledge of one another and therefore expand the family awareness.

Working Through

Working through refers to the process of repeated interpretation of the conflictual expressions of the patient, formed through traumatic experiences, in different forms and circumstances. The goal of working through is to make insight more effective and bring about significant and lasting changes in the patient by altering the conflictual modes. The strong force of unconscious conflict attempts to override the temporary ability of the ego to recognize the nature of the conflict in light of interpretations. Working through is necessary because it is unlikely that the patient's active conflictual processes will yield immediately to interpretation, or that theses processes take a new path simply because it has been opened. Therefore, the patient must be allowed time and repeated exposure to multiple expressions of conflictual material in different situations so that he or she can become conversant with his or her own resistance. In family therapy, the process of working through may be easier, because different family members can keep alive the interpretations made during the sessions. This makes it more difficult for any family member to continue producing new resistances to maintain past conflicts.

Termination

Termination has more importance in psychodynamic family therapy than in other approaches for a variety of reasons. One reason is the relatively longer course of psychodynamic family therapy in comparison to behavioral family therapy approaches. An even more important reason is that the termination phase enhances the regressive tendencies in families: family members may attempt to revert to earlier modes of symptomatic and dysfunctional interaction under the threat of losing the therapist and the breakdown of the therapeutic alliance. The effective interpretations of such elements and tendencies can enhance and consolidate the identification of the family members with the therapeutic goals of the therapist. This would enable the family to continue its corrective interactional course after the termination point.

Conclusion

Psychodynamic family theory provides comprehensive integration of the most valuable traditional concepts in psychiatry with more recent behavioral methodologies and their application to the field of interpersonal psychology. Theoretical concepts of psychoanalysis that have endured over decades can be combined with some of the newer concepts of social learning theory and applied within a systemic perspective. General systems theory has proved to be a valuable overall perspective through which to integrate the interactional aspects of family functioning, while exploring the individual's conscious and intrapsychic characteristics. In psychodynamic family therapy, behavior change can occur by the reduction of pathological defenses exchanged among family members, and by gaining insight into family members' unconscious needs that have been expressed in a destructive way.

A major application of psychodynamic family therapy has emerged recently through the work of Susan Johnson and her colleagues in Ottawa, Canada. *Emotionally focused family therapy* (Johnson 1996; Johnson et al. 1999, 2001) applies attachment theory in order to understand the nature of marital conflicts and helps couples resolve their arguments and move toward a more intimate relationship. The distinction between defensive affect and attachment affect is the basis for this intervention.

Chapters on Related Topics

The following chapters describe concepts related to psychodynamic family therapy:

- Chapter 5, "Multigenerational Family Systems Theory of Bowen and Its Application"
- Chapter 6, "Contextual Therapy"
- Chapter 14, "The Family Life Cycle: A Framework for Understanding Family Development"
- Chapter 20, "Couples Therapy: An Overview"
- Chapter 21, "Psychodynamic Couples Therapy"
- Chapter 33, "Family Therapy With Personality Disorders"

5

Multigenerational Family Systems Theory of Bowen and Its Application

Michael Kerr, M.D.

Introduction

In the early 1950s, psychiatrist Murray Bowen developed a new theory of human emotional functioning and behavior called *family systems theory* or *Bowen theory*. The theory not only describes the human family and provides a basis for family psychotherapy but also applies to nonfamily groups (including society as a whole) and may apply to other species.

Family psychotherapy can result in change within individuals as well as change in relationships. Psychotherapy based on Freudian theory occurs in the context of the therapist-patient relationship, but psychotherapy based on Bowen theory occurs largely in the context of an individual's family relationships. Family theory incorporates Freud's observations from two-person therapy relationships, but it also conceptualizes the multiperson system of the family. As a result, it is possible for a person to work directly on unresolved emotional attachments to her or his family. Since it is unnecessary to replicate the unresolved attachment with a therapist via transference, family therapy requires much less frequent sessions.

Change in individuals resulting from family psychotherapy can affect biological functioning as well as psychological processes and behavior, and change in one family member's functioning affects the behavior and internal functioning of other family members. This interrelationship between biological, psychological, and social functioning means that clinical problems that have a biological component can be treated with family psychotherapy. Moreover, by providing a broader framework for evaluating clinical problems than a patient-focused one, family theory is useful for making clinical assessments about if, when, and how to use biological treatments.

History

Bowen's formal psychiatric training began in 1946 at the Menninger Clinic in Topeka, Kansas. There he became an avid student of Freudian theory and underwent personal psychoanalysis. In time, he concluded that Freud had developed an elegant and useful theory, but because it included considerable subjectivity, Freud had foreclosed the possibility of his theory ever becoming an accepted science. Besides this problem, Bowen and others recognized that psychoanalysis was effective for neurotic problems but largely ineffective for more severe problems such as schizophrenia. The ineffectiveness of Freudian therapy in many situations motivated a few pioneers to broaden their focus from the patient to the family.

Bowen was unusual among these early pioneers because of assumptions he made about human nature and his efforts to develop a science of human behavior. Extensive background reading in the natural sciences and other fields convinced him that science could accept a theory of human behavior that was based on the ways humans are similar to all life, but could not accept one based on the ways humankind is unique and different. Emphasis must be on what humankind is, not on what humans say they are. Psychology and culture are important influences on human behavior, but they do not liberate humankind from natural forces that govern the behavior of all life.

Bowen attempted to develop a theory based on proven and provable facts, not on subjectivity. Proven facts are generally accepted, but provable facts require more substantiation. Many of the provable facts on which Bowen's theory rests concern functioning that is observable in all families and all cultures. Observing facts of functioning requires distinguishing between content and process. Content is often subjective and unverifiable, but process is factual and provable. For example, a husband may feel neglected by his wife and accuse her of not "caring" about him. She may respond to the content of his accusation by saying and doing things to prove to him that she does "care." As a consequence, his accusations of "not caring" cease. What "caring" is and whether the wife "cares" are totally subjective, but the pattern of how each spouse predictably functions in reaction to the other spouse's words and actions is factual. It is easy to observe facts of functioning, but not easy to measure them.

At the Menninger Clinic, Bowen studied and treated a wide range of severe clinical problems. He also had considerable contact with relatives of hospitalized patients. His library research and clinical observations led to a hypothesis about the forces that create and maintain a symbiotic relationship between a mother and her schizophrenic child. Others had explained the intense attachment using psychoanalytic ideas, but Bowen held that the forces creating and maintaining the process are deeper than human psychology. The forces are biological, rooted in our mammalian ancestry. The human mammal is not the only mammal in which the young sometimes fail to separate from the parents.

In 1954, Bowen moved to the National Institute of Mental Health (NIMH) in Rockville, Maryland. There he directed a project in which families with a schizophrenic member lived with a research unit for long periods. Bowen's group observed that the family as a whole strongly governed each member's functioning, including the schizophrenic member. By observing the whole family at once, the researchers saw that an individual's words and actions function to perpetuate a process in the group, and the process in the group functions to foster behaviors in individuals, even "sick" behaviors. This explanation of individual behavior differs radically from theories based on individual psychopathology. In other words, descriptions of each member's psychopathology do not adequately explain family process.

The research of Bowen's group showed that the relationship between a mother and her adult schizophrenic child was more intense than originally thought. It also showed that the father and other family members helped create and maintain this intensity. The family functions as an "organism," as if its members are living under the same skin. Change in the emotional functioning of one member is automatically compensated for by changes in the emotional functioning of others. The overfunctioning of the parents compensates for the underfunctioning of the schizophrenic child, but the underfunctioning of the schizophrenic child also compensates for the overfunctioning of the parents. The parents *feel* their child's "sickness" forces them to overfunction and to make decisions for the child, but parents and child form a mutually reinforcing system.

The NIMH project ended in 1959. Bowen then moved to the Department of Psychiatry at Georgetown University School of Medicine in Washington, DC. His family research continued on an outpatient basis. By the early 1960s, the new theory had come together into a coherent whole. Patterns of emotional functioning in schizophrenic families are not unique to them but are more intense versions of patterns occurring in all families. Furthermore, the low level of functioning of people with schizophrenia and similar impairments represents one end of a continuum of human emotional functioning. Bowen's theory addresses the full range of human functioning, not just "pathological" functioning.

Bowen instituted a form of therapy for the family (family group therapy) in 1954, the first year of the NIMH project. His therapeutic approaches changed dramatically in the ensuing years. By 1960, he no longer recommended a personal analysis for therapists in training. He regarded family psychotherapy with one's spouse as the most efficient and productive way to increase emotional maturity. By 1967, he had worked out a method by which therapists and patients alike could change themselves in relationship to the family of origin. After experience with this approach, he concluded that it had the most therapeutic potential.

The family programs at Georgetown grew to include teaching, training, clinical services, sponsorship of symposia, and research in numerous specialized areas. Bowen developed a faculty of multidisciplinary mental health professionals. In 1975, the family programs were consolidated in an off-campus facility, the Georgetown University Family Center. Bowen was the center's director until his death on October 9, 1990. The center became administratively separate from the University in July 1990. It is now a nonprofit organization with a continuing academic orientation. Michael E. Kerr, M.D., a psychiatrist who worked with Bowen for many years, is now director of the Georgetown Family Center.

Theoretical Concepts

Bowen theory consists of eight interlocking concepts (Bowen 1978; Kerr and Bowen 1988; Papero 1990). Rather than focus on each concept in detail, the discussion that follows emphasizes the interrelatedness of the concepts and their underlying assumptions. The discussion begins with a brief synopsis of systems thinking.

Systems thinking contrasts with cause-and-effect thinking. The following are two examples of cause-and-effect thinking as applied to human behavior: 1) the husband of an alcoholic wife claims that he tells her not to drink because she drinks too much, and 2) the alcoholic wife claims she drinks because her husband nags her about it. In contrast, systems thinking holds that the more the husband tells his wife not to drink, the more she drinks and that the more she drinks, the more he tells her not to drink.

Each spouse triggers certain behaviors in the other, but because each operates in reaction to the other, neither spouse "causes" the other's behavior.

Systems thinking easily encompasses multiperson systems and interactions on many levels. For example, a wife interprets her husband's facial expression to mean that he is angry with her, and she consequently withdraws from him. The husband feels angry in reaction to her withdrawal and it shows in his face. Reacting to the husband's more intense expression, the wife starts nagging their son. The son yells back at his mother, which not only increases her nagging but also makes the husband feel more critical of his wife. The husband's intense reactions aggravate his ulcer, the pain of which puts a different look on his face. The wife responds sympathetically to his new facial expression. The father feels less angry with his wife, and she in response moves closer to him. Her shifted focus to her husband allows the son to calm down.

Systems thinking addresses the how, what, when, and where of life processes, but not the *why*. Focussing on *why* someone thinks, feels, or acts in a certain way inevitably leads to cause-and-effect thinking. Implicit in a "why" question is the assumption that what someone thinks or feels "causes" his or her behavior. Seeking a "cause" for behavior *within* a person automatically obscures a view of the relationship forces governing that person. Processes within people are important for understanding what transpires between them, but from the standpoint of systems thinking internal processes do not "cause" behavior.

Systems thinking permeates the natural sciences. A number of systems theories exist; two examples are general systems theory (von Bertalanffy 1968) and cybernetics (Wiener 1961). Both of these theories attempt to deal with nonliving as well as living systems. Bowen theory is a "natural systems theory" in that it derives from the direct study of living systems, not from an extension of principles that apply to nonliving systems. The core concepts in Bowen theory do not exist in other systems theories.

The Emotional System

The emotional system is a central concept of family theory not present in other theories. The emotional system is an attribute that humans share with nonhuman species. Simple life forms have emotional systems that govern their behavior. The emotional systems of complex organisms are a product of their phylogenetic history. The human emotional system probably retains fundamental characteristics of the emotional systems of primitive organisms; it no doubt retains most characteristics of the emotional systems of recent evolutionary ancestors. The emotional system compels human beings to act like human beings. Emotional behaviors are naturally occurring, but in complex organisms developmental experiences can shape and the nervous system can modulate many of these behaviors. Emotional reactivity is necessary for life; a cornered rat reacts emotionally to survive. Plants and animals are always reactive to some extent, adjusting to and affecting the environment.

The emotional system is not equivalent to feelings. People only *feel* the more conspicuous or superficial aspects of their emotional system functioning. They do not feel emotional reactivity such as cell division or DNA repair, but people do feel the emotional system working when they react to the death of close kin or the physical injury of others. Feeling systems, as opposed to emotional systems, have evolved in species with fairly complex brains (MacLean 1989).

The intellectual system is a recently evolved function of the human brain, a product of the cerebral cortex. Humans appear to have a far more advanced capacity to think, reason, and reflect than other species. In addition, the human intellectual system can distinguish between thoughts and feelings, objectivity and subjectivity. The ability to be factual about emotional functioning is referred to as "emotional objectivity." A person can use factual knowledge about his or her emotional and feeling reactions, and about what others say and do that trigger those reactions, to increase emotional self-control.

Heightened anxiety tends to increase emotional reactivity and to "fuse" the emotional, feeling, and intellectual systems. The higher the level of anxiety, the more reactive people tend to be and the more that reactivity tends to dictate their functioning and behavior. When anxious, a person may "want" to act one way (intellectually determined) but acts in another way (emotionally determined). For example, when people prone to compulsive eating get anxious, they eat what they earlier resolved not to eat. They watch themselves buying and preparing the food, feeling calmer as they do so, but thinking of themselves as "crazy" for doing it. A mother may want her son to lose weight but will give him extra food when she is anxious about his health. Another example of fusion of systems is a person ignoring the facts about something to cling to a subjective impression of it that makes him feel good. Insofar as anxiety is "bound" or linked to compensating but irrational actions in these and many other types of emotional functioning and behavior, an individual may actually feel less anxious.

If the intellectual system is functioning separately from the emotional system, people can be more aware of their anxiety and of their propensities for binding it. Consequently, through an intellectual process, people can exert some control over emotional functioning; they can tolerate anxiety rather than bind it internally or act it out. If aware of anxiety, they can also choose to manage it in various ways. For example, they may have a drink or a sexual encounter to relax.

Symptom Development

Symptom development may erupt as a result of increased emotional reactivity coupled with other necessary variables. The symptom may be psychiatric, medical, or social in nature. In other words, all clinical dysfunctions are linked to the emotional system: the same basic emotional forces govern all the dysfunctions. Depression, agoraphobia, shoplifting, homicide, cancer (Kerr 1981), and psoriasis (Kerr 1992) all reflect a disturbance in the balance of the emotional system.

The intensity of the anxiety and emotional reactivity significantly affects the degree of dysfunction. The degree of functional impairment is considered more important than a specific diagnosis. Illnesses are conceptualized on a continuum of functioning. In other words, a disease can impair functioning, but the more impaired the emotional functioning, the more severe a disease tends to be. In psychiatric illnesses, for example, people with the most impaired functioning are the most vulnerable to chronic psychosis and people with less impaired functioning are more likely to manifest the impairment as a mild depression. Bowen theory substitutes the term "emotional illness" or "emotional dysfunction" for "mental illness." This is because the emotional system creates the aberrations of mental processes associated with psychiatric illnesses. Mental functioning reflects emotional system functioning, but it also reinforces emotional system functioning. Medical and social illnesses exist on similar continuums of functioning. Individuals with more impaired medical functioning are likely to have more severe cases of diabetes; people with more impaired social functioning are likely to show more extreme degrees of antisocial behavior.

Family systems theory considers most illnesses to be functional dysfunctions. This implies that a chronic illness can improve if one of the following occurs: 1) a family becomes less anxious, 2) a family shifts the focus of its anxiety off the dysfunctional person, or 3) the dysfunctional person reduces the degree to which he or she absorbs family anxiety. The forces that create and maintain illness, in other words, are not confined to the disease process itself or to the dysfunctional person.

Defective genes, pathogenic organisms, and other such factors are important in disease development, but people may adapt successfully (no illness occurs) or unsuccessfully to the presence of such factors. The emotional system is a fundamental influence on adaptation. Genes, the immune system, the endocrine system, and other physiological systems are all part of the emotional system. Therefore, an excessive or inadequate immune system response to invading bacteria may reflect a dysfunction of the emotional system.

Life Forces for Fusion and Differentiation

"Life forces" akin to those that make bacteria divide, grasses grow, insects swarm, birds migrate, elephants mate, and whales sing govern the human emotional system. These forces regulate the activity of family relationship systems. Families function as if two counterbalancing forces were governing them. One force is for fusion, which is manifest in people overtly and covertly pressuring each other to think, feel, and act in certain ways. They press for oneness, sameness, and agreement. Everyone exerts this pressure on others and everyone responds to it; our needs for approval and acceptance reflect this responsiveness. The opposing force is for differentiation, which is manifest in people thinking, feeling, and acting for themselves. They are individuals in their own right. Capable of maintaining emotional separateness while in emotional contact with others, their interactions do not determine who they are. They do not force others to be a certain way; nor do they capitulate to such pressure from others.

Anxiety disturbs the fusion-differentiation balance. Anxiety is the reaction of an organism to a threat, real or imagined. Real threats (what is) usually seem solvable and time-limited, and therefore tend to generate acute anxiety. Imagined threats (what might be) usually seem to have neither an obvious solution nor a foreseeable end, and therefore tend to generate chronic anxiety. Chronic anxiety most disturbs the balance of family emotional forces.

Increased chronic anxiety intensifies the pressure for relationship fusion (as well as for fusion of the emotional and intellectual systems) and intensified relationship fusion increases chronic anxiety. As the process escalates, people increasingly act as if they feel both more dependent on one another and unpleasantly crowded together. On the one hand they need more from one another, demand more from one another, and worry more about one another; on the other hand they are more reactive to one another's needs, expectations, and anxieties. The process erodes people's ability to think, feel, and act for themselves as well as their ability to permit others to do the same.

As anxiety increases in a family system, each family member automatically tries to reduce his or her own anxiety. Efforts by individuals to reduce anxiety in themselves fuel predictable patterns of interaction among family members. The interactions have the effect of shifting anxiety around the family system such that certain relationships and certain individuals temporarily or chronically absorb a disproportionate share of family anxiety. The concept of the triangle describes the predictable interactions that occur in all families (and in other groups) that direct the flow of anxiety in the system.

The Triangle

A triangle is an emotionally fused three-person system. The characteristics of a triangle vary depending on the level of anxiety. If anxiety is low, triangles are largely inactive. If anxiety is moderate, two people maintain a comfortable fusion in their relationship (and in themselves) by excluding a third person. The preference of the two "insiders" for each other rather than for the "outsider" calms both "insiders." The outsider reacts to the exclusion by attempting to break into the twosome and form a comfortable fusion with one of them. If anxiety is high, exclusion of a third person may not sufficiently reduce the anxiety between the insiders. Hence, one of the insiders will try to escape the intensity of that relationship either by getting more involved with the outsider (thereby forming a new comfortable fusion) or by maneuvering the outsider into more involvement with the other insider (thereby escaping the uncomfortable fusion).

Triangles are the smallest stable emotional units, since two-person systems tolerate little anxiety before involving a third person. A triangle can contain much more anxiety than a two-person system, but one triangle may get sufficiently "saturated" with anxiety that the anxiety spreads to other triangles. This creates "interlocking triangles" that allow the anxiety both to diffuse among many people and to shift back and forth between triangles. The capacity to shift anxiety enhances the stability of the overall system. Interlocking triangles can extend beyond a nuclear family to the extended family and community.

The process of triangling can reduce anxiety in one family relationship at the expense of raising it in other relationships. Anxiety activates mechanisms or "patterns of emotional functioning" in a relationship to manage the anxiety. Each pattern manages anxiety in a different way, as described below.

Patterns of Emotional Functioning

Four basic patterns of emotional functioning exist in relationship systems. Each pattern has psychological components but is anchored in the emotional system. All four patterns are present in every family, but one or two patterns may predominate in certain families. The activity of the patterns intensifies as anxiety increases. Both members of a given relationship contribute equally to the patterns of emotional functioning in that relationship. The four patterns are as follows:

1. *Emotional distance.* This pattern is active to some degree in all relationships. If made anxious by contact, people reduce anxiety by reducing contact. The distance binds the anxiety. People establish distance through

physical avoidance or various forms of internal withdrawal. Distance reduces anxiety generated by contact, but it also precludes the calming effects of emotional contact. Consequently, people automatically monitor the balance between contact and distance. Too much distance triggers behavior that functions to promote contact and too much contact triggers behavior that functions to promote distance. Automatic avoidance of aversive stimuli appears to be characteristic of all life forms.

2. *Emotional conflict.* This pattern is fueled by people's reactions to differences rather than by the differences themselves. Each person fights to "hold his own" in the fusion. Each is unsure of himself or herself, which manifests in overreactions to agreeing with or giving in to the other person. Each criticizes the other for such things as not meeting needs, not listening, being critical, being controlling, or being dependent. In a conflicted marriage, brief periods of fairly harmonious contact usually interrupt longer periods of conflict and distance. Conflict functions to provide both emotional contact and emotional distance, making it another way to balance the two. People externalize their anxious responses to each other into the relationship. The conflict binds anxiety. The relationship is tumultuous, but up to a point, the people are calmer.

3. *Dominant-submissive.* In this pattern one person gives in to the other to avoid conflict. The pattern preserves harmony but over time can impair the subordinate person's functioning. Either spouse may dominate, since the forces at work are unrelated to sexual differences. Every marriage requires giving in on both sides based on the realities of a situation. In this pattern, however, emotional forces result in one spouse giving in more than the other. Each tries to reduce his or her own anxiety by keeping the relationship smooth and by relating to the other in a way that is most comfortable for himself or herself. Each spouse exerts overt and covert pressure on the other, aggressively or passively, to accomplish this. The emotional postures they have to each other bind anxiety.

A discrepancy in the emotional functioning of the two spouses can occur over time; the higher the anxiety, the greater the discrepancy. In reciprocal fashion, one spouse "overfunctions" and the other "underfunctions." Depending on the intensity of the process, the discrepancy may occur in most areas of the marriage or in just a few areas. The overfunctioner usually seems dominant and the underfunctioner usually seems submissive, but that can be deceiving. Either one can be the one making the most adjustments in his or her internal functioning and behavior to preserve harmony. The spouse who gives in the most absorbs a disproportionate share of family anxiety.

Overfunctioners, driven by their own makeup as well as by the real expectations of others, get "done in" by trying to do more than they can do. They feel overwhelmed and overloaded. They work to make things "right" for others. In making and being relied on for most decisions, they appear dominant, but the family system governs their functioning more than they govern it. Underfunctioners get "done in" by doing less than they can do. Their self-confidence gets eroded to the point of feeling unable to make decisions or to take initiatives on their own behalf. They feel excessively dependent on others for their direction. They too are just reactors to the system.

Anxiety absorbed by "done in" spouses is bound up in their emotional functioning and behavior. Sufficient anxiety coupled with the presence of other necessary variables may surface as a psychiatric, physical, or social illness. The higher an individual's level of anxiety is, the more severe the illness tends to be. If symptoms develop, they may stabilize a relationship. Spouses assume "caretaker" and "patient" positions, a process that fosters chronic illness. It is easier for both to live with the symptom than to change the relationship. The emergence of symptoms can also increase family anxiety, fueling more severe symptoms.

4. *Overinvolvement with a child.* In this pattern a family binds its anxiety in one or more children. A simplified example can illustrate the basics of the process. Two people marry and initially have a calm relationship. Then they have a child. The transition from a two- to a three-person system triggers anxiety, disturbing the balance of family emotional forces. The parents manage this fusion-generated anxiety with emotional distance. The mother gets more involved with the child than with her husband. Parental anxiety rather than the child's reality needs dictates the mother's involvement with the child. The father fosters the process by investing more of himself in work. A second child is born, again intensifying anxiety, but the triangle with the older child primarily absorbs it. As the children grow, the first child reciprocates the mother's focus with a focus on her. The parents have an easier relationship with the second child, who is less of a worry. This child's reality needs, rather than the parents' anxieties, dictate their involvement with him.

Overinvolvement with a child can have varying degrees of intensity and either a positive or negative tone. The father may be most overinvolved, but usually it is the mother. He generally reinforces the process through withdrawal and/or anxious inputs of his own. The result is that a child absorbs a disproportionate share of family anxiety. A clinical vignette can illustrate how parental anxiety transfers to a child. A husband's long hours at work increases his wife's anxiety. She worries that the husband's absence is making their child feel insecure. She treats the child as if her fear is a fact. Reactive to her worry, the child accentuates behaviors that most worry her. Gradually, what began as a feeling in the mother becomes a fact in the child. The more the child appears insecure, the more the mother tries to correct the problem, which makes it worse. The child is a worry to the parents, but it is easier for the parents to focus on his immaturity than their own.

Anxiety can impair a child's emotional functioning. The impairment may surface at any age and manifest as psychiatric, physical, or social illness. It might surface as hyperactivity in a young child or as rebellion in a teenager. The acting-out adolescent often has a harmonious relationship with the mother as a preadolescent, but then distances from her to the degree he or she was overinvolved with her. The mother reacts to the distance by worrying about what might be wrong and by pressuring the child to talk. The father often sides with the mother, which intensifies the process. Poor academic performance and behavioral problems reflect the child's anxiety. An impairment may not surface until a child leaves home, perhaps a psychotic episode or serious physical illness. Less involved siblings separate more easily and are less vulnerable to symptom development. Emergence of a dysfunction can increase parental focus on a child, which creates a vicious circle that further escalates anxiety.

In summary, four basic patterns of emotional functioning manage anxiety in a family system. The more anxiety one pattern binds, the less anxiety other patterns must bind. For example, in a family with intense marital conflict, the children may be quite functional. In a family with a severely alcoholic father, his drinking and impaired functioning are a source of anxiety for the family, but his dysfunction also absorbs family anxiety. If anxiety is sufficiently high, a family may require several patterns to bind it. For example, the parents may be fighting, the mother may have a chronic physical illness, and two of the children may be in legal trouble.

Some situation-related fluctuations in emotional functioning occur in all individuals and families over time, but individuals and families differ in their ability to adapt to stressors that can affect functioning. The scale of differentiation conceptualizes both the possible range of human emotional functioning and the range of human adaptiveness.

The Scale of Differentiation

The scale of differentiation distinguishes between functional and basic levels. Anxiety-related shifts in emotional functioning in the same individual or family over time are termed changes in functional level of differentiation. The different abilities of individuals and families to adapt to potentially anxiety-generating stressors reflect differences in basic levels of differentiation. Adaptiveness is the ability to adjust to real or anticipated changes, particularly in important relationships, without a prolonged escalation of anxiety that can impair the physical, mental, or social functioning of oneself or others.

The higher individuals' basic levels of differentiation, the greater their capacity to be in emotional contact with others without fusing with them, even if anxiety is high. The ability to maintain differentiation makes it possible for one family member to be anxious without its triggering an infectious spread of anxiety in the group. If family members neither focus anxiously on one another nor distance reactively from one another, the family is more adaptive to stressors on its members. Because of the low probability that a relationship process will create an escalating spiral of anxiety, families whose members are fairly high on the differentiation scale tend to have low levels of chronic anxiety. The preservation of comfortable emotional connections among family members also makes it easier for each person to manage his or her own anxiety. One way the low level of chronic anxiety in well-differentiated families is manifested is in the low incidence of serious clinical dysfunctions; if serious dysfunction does occur, recovery is usually rapid and complete.

Well-differentiated people can think for themselves and make decisions without being impulsive. They are not emotionally invested in convincing others of their viewpoint and they can respect a viewpoint different from their own without attacking or dismissing it. Their beliefs and values can change, but they change based on a thoughtful process rather than an emotional one. They have an unusual tolerance for feelings and anxiety in themselves and others, which permits free expression of feelings and thoughts in their relationships. Excessive need for approval and affirmation and undue aversion to the dependency of others do not destabilize their relationships.

The lower individuals' basic differentiation levels, the smaller their capacity to be in emotional contact with others without fusing with them, especially if anxiety is high. When people are fused, one person's heightened anxiety easily triggers an infectious spread of anxiety in the group. Because family members focus anxiously on one another or reactively distance from one another, the family is less adaptive to stressors on its members. Because of the strong tendency for a relationship process to create an escalating spiral of anxiety, families whose members are fairly low on the scale tend to have a high level of chronic anxiety. The inability to maintain comfortable emotional connections among family members also undermines each person's ability to manage his or her own anxiety. One way the high level of chronic anxiety in poorly differentiated families is manifested is in the high incidence of serious clinical dysfunctions, which often develop early in life and become chronic.

Poorly differentiated people live their lives with a mixture of compliance with and rebellion against the relationship system. Emotional and feeling reactions so govern and inundate them that they may become numb to feelings. They yearn for love and acceptance, but their intense need for others combined with their aversion to too much contact with others all but precludes comfortable and stable relationships. Less able to stay in emotional contact with others, they are vulnerable to lapsing into chronic psychosis, chronic alcoholism, major physical illness, or other chronic disability. They may live out their lives in a penal institution.

The differentiation scale is not an instrument that provides exact assessments, but it does describe many gradations of emotional functioning between two extremes. Midpoint on the scale marks where people begin to use intellectual principles to override emotional, feeling, and subjective reactions when it is important to do so. At each increment above the midpoint, people have more capacity to keep the intellectual system in charge; at each increment below the midpoint, feelings and the automatic urge to relieve anxiety govern more of an individual's functioning. People in the lowest quarter of the scale have such ill-defined beliefs and values that changing them is not an issue.

Although the differentiation and fusion forces are anchored in biology, individuals' family experiences during the developmental years largely determine the relative influence the two forces come to have on their functioning. In other words, the particular balance of the two forces determines the basic level of differentiation. The experiences of the total spectrum of children of the nuclear family in society are widely different, which results in the wide range of basic levels of differentiation developed by the children. The wide range of nuclear family experiences results from a multigenerational emotional process.

Multigenerational Emotional Process

The multigenerational emotional process results in two parents, over the course of many generations, having descendants that register at almost all points on the scale of differentiation. It takes many generations to create large differences in basic levels among family members, because the basic levels of the members of a succeeding generation are only slightly higher or lower than the basic levels of members of the preceding generation. The following three factors largely determine the basic levels members of each generation develop:

1. *Basic levels of their parents.* People marry spouses with basic levels of differentiation identical to their own. The mates fuse to a degree commensurate with those levels. This sets a basic differentiation-fusion balance for the family. The balance creates an emotional climate that affects the differentiation of their children such that the children develop basic levels close to, but not necessarily identical to, their parents' levels.
2. *Level of anxiety in their nuclear family while growing up.* The level of chronic anxiety fuels the patterns of emotional functioning that promote or retard emotional separation of children from their families. Three factors determine a nuclear family's average level of chronic anxiety. The first factor is the parents' basic levels of differentiation: the greater the fusion between parents, the less adaptive a family is to stressors. The second factor is the number and frequency of stressors encountered by the family, such as deaths, geographical relocations, births, and occupational setbacks: the more numerous and frequent the stressors, the more strain on a family's adaptive capacity. The third factor is the degree of emotional contact with extended family and social systems: the better the emotional contact with extended family and social systems, the more potential for tempering and diffusing nuclear family anxiety.
3. *Dominant patterns of emotional functioning in their nuclear family while growing up.* Children absorb less family anxiety when the patterns of emotional functioning most active in a nuclear family bind anxiety in the parental generation. The binding of anxiety in the parental generation fosters children's developing basic differentiation levels somewhat higher than their parents. Children absorb more family anxiety when the pattern of emotional functioning most active in a nuclear family binds anxiety in the children. The binding of anxiety in the children fosters their developing basic differentiation levels somewhat lower than in their parents. If there is marked overinvolvement with one child, it may result in less overinvolvement with another child. In that case, one child develops a basic level lower than his parents, and the other develops a level equal to or higher than his parents.

These three interrelated factors explain how every multigenerational family produces people at most points on the differentiation scale. A simplified hypothetical example illustrates the process. Two people marry who are at the midpoint on the scale. They have two children. The children have basic levels similar to those of their parents, but depending on the level of family anxiety and dominant patterns of emotional functioning, one child's basic level may be slightly higher than his parents' and the other's slightly lower. Each child marries, but because their basic levels are different, one's marriage is a little more fused than his parents' marriage and the other's marriage is a little less fused than his parents' marriage. Depending on the anxiety level and dominant patterns of emotional functioning in each of the children's families, each child may have children with basic differentiation levels slightly higher and slightly lower than his own. So in one multigenerational line, there may be a successive decrease in basic levels (least differentiated child of the least differentiated child), and in another line there may be a successive increase (most differentiated child of the most differentiated child).

Because these processes repeat down the generations, with basic levels changing at a rate dependent on the mix of relevant variables, nuclear families are produced that range from highly fused to highly differentiated. Unstable relationships, less productive life courses, and a high incidence of severe clinical problems characterize the most fused families. Some individuals in these families function better than others. Stable relationships, more productive life courses, and a low incidence of severe clinical problems characterize the least fused families. Some individuals in these families function worse than others. Well-differentiated people can have psychotic episodes or cancers during the prime of life, but such events are more likely to occur in people lower on the scale. The functioning characteristics of families vary at each increment between the extremes.

An estimate of a person's basic level of differentiation requires an assessment of the functioning of that person over his or her entire lifetime and an assessment of the functioning of those connected to him or her emotionally such as parents, siblings, spouse, and children. Consideration of all these factors is necessary because significant shifts in an individual's functioning can occur based on changing life circumstances, and because of the interdependence of emotional functioning that exists among family members.

Methodology

The methodology based on Bowen theory rests on three primary assumptions:

1. Reduction of family anxiety automatically reduces symptoms.
2. One family member's raising his or her basic level of differentiation increases family adaptiveness.
3. Whether the presenting symptom is marital conflict, illness in a spouse, or illness in a child, the fundamental problem is in the functioning of the family system. The technical approach based on the three assumptions attempts to facilitate a) reduction of family anxiety, and b) a family member's raising his or her basic level of differentiation. Anxiety can subside quickly, but basic levels change slowly.

People can raise basic levels by learning to function with more emotional separateness in their most fused relationships. Everyone has some degree of unresolved attachment or fusion to their parents and extended family: the lower a person's basic differentiation level, the greater the unresolved attachment to family. Rebelling against the family or leaving home physically does not resolve the attachment. Maintaining distance from the family may appear to resolve an attachment, but it is only dormant. The degree of unresolved attachment with the family of origin matches the degrees of fusion people have with a spouse and children. People may fuse into work and other relationships with an intensity approaching the original attachment to family.

Therapeutic techniques vary because individuals can raise basic levels through efforts in any or all of their most fused relationships. Conjoint treatment of spouses emphasizes each one developing more of a self in relationship to the other. If seen conjointly, spouses need not restrict their focus to the marriage. Treatment works best if people are trying to raise basic levels in many relationships. Multiple family therapy involves the treatment of several couples together: a therapist treats one couple at a time while the others observe. Individual sessions are particularly valuable if the family of origin is a principal focus.

Even if the presenting problem is a child's, treatment is usually not directed at the child. Not treating a child directly is based on three assumptions:

1. A child's problem reflects a family problem.
2. If one family member raises his or her basic level, the entire family will improve its functioning and the child's symptoms will resolve.
3. The parents, as heads of the family, are the only ones capable of changing the family.

If a family situation is volatile, it may be useful to see children individually as well as seeing their parents. However, treating a child after things have calmed down usually results in the parents waiting for the therapist to make the child better. Outside forces affect families, but a persistent family problem reflects a family's inability to adapt to the impact of those forces.

The effectiveness of any technical approach depends on the therapist's emotional functioning. People must deal with their own problems before they can think through systems consistently and foster differentiation in others. By trying to improve their own emotional functioning, therapists learn they cannot "make" a family less anxious or more differentiated. If therapists have not learned this lesson, when faced with an anxious family they will do the family's thinking for them and tell them what to do. Anxious families benefit most from contact with therapists who know theory fairly well and who can maintain differentiation from the family. Families do not need someone telling them what to do. If therapists manage themselves adequately, someone in the family will begin to calm down, which helps others, and someone may work on differentiation, which is also a stimulus to others. Not everybody wants to attempt to raise their basic level of differentiation, particularly if anxiety decreases and symptoms resolve.

When mental health professionals observe family psychotherapy based on Bowen theory, they commonly say that the family seems to be making progress, but the therapist does not appear to be doing any therapy. In fact, it looks as if the family is doing therapy on itself. The family looks as if it is doing its own therapy because family members are often talking about theory and their attempts to apply it in their lives. If observers at least tentatively accept that a family could do therapy on itself, they then ask, "How did you (the therapist) get the family to do this?" This question is unanswerable without some understanding of differentiation of self.

All children go through a process of differentiation from their parents and family. No one differentiates completely because of the counteracting force for fusion in the child and in the parents. Children do not differentiate at a specific age; differentiation begins in infancy and continues. A poorly differentiated adolescent was generally a poorly differentiated toddler. Differentiation is evident in young children, but they add new elements as they grow. Individuals probably reach the limit of their differentiation by adolescence. The basic differentiation level usually does not change after adolescence, but levels of functioning can vary. By describing the natural process of differentiation, Bowen theory also provides guidelines for resuming the differentiation process as an adult. Strong biological, psychological, and relationship forces tend to keep basic level fixed, but people can raise it some though a structured, long-term effort.

There are two fundamental components of attempting to increase a basic differentiation level as an adult: 1) using the intellectual system to become more factual about the family emotional system and one's participation in it, and 2) using the factual knowledge as a basis for actions that increase one's emotional separateness from others. Actions that increase separateness automatically trigger emotional reactivity in oneself and others that functions to sustain fusion. A factual understanding of the emotional process is critical for maintaining differentiation in the face of such reactivity. If one family member can function with a little more differentiation despite this reactivity to it, other family members will eventually function with more differentiation as well. Consequently, the family will be slightly less fused and slightly more adaptive.

The intellectual system is essential to resuming the process of differentiation. The intellectual system's capacity to distinguish thoughts and feelings, objectivity and subjectivity, permits a choice about whether to act based on thoughts or on feelings. Human beings tend to focus strongly on feelings and to be mesmerized by subjectivity. Awareness of feelings and subjectivity is important, but such awareness alone is inadequate for guiding an effort toward differentiation. Differentiation depends on viewing feelings in the context of facts.

A simplified example can illustrate the importance for differentiation of understanding feelings in the context of facts. One way a woman's unresolved attachment to her mother is manifested is in her continual anger with her mother. The anger is a function of the following processes:

1. Interconnected emotional reactivity, feelings, and subjectivity in the woman that affect her functioning in relation to her mother
2. Interconnected emotional reactivity, feelings, and subjectivity in the mother that affect her functioning in relation to her daughter
3. A relationship process between mother and daughter that is both produced by and reinforced by each other's functioning

Both women play equal parts, but it usually does not feel that way to either one. The three processes and their interrelationship can be described factually. The overall process generates the anger in the daughter and the anger reflects and helps perpetuate the overall process. If one person can be more factual, she then has a choice between acting on feelings or on facts. Acting on a more factual view of a relationship process—without cutting off from the other person—increases differentiation in the relationship.

Another component of attempting to raise the basic differentiation level is overcoming the automatic tendency to diagnose oneself and others; that is, to attribute unwelcome behavior to a flawed character. By describing how emotional positions in a family shape and maintain much of people's thoughts, feelings, and actions, systems theory provides a rationale for not diagnosing people. The theory replaces diagnoses such as "cold" parent or "warm" parent, "good" child or "bad" child, and "giving" person or "ungiving" person with a view of how such characteristics reflect the functioning of a family relationship system. In other words, "good" and "bad" children are created and maintained more by interlocking triangles than by the children's inherent qualities. Replacing idealized and denigrative notions of oneself and others with a comprehension of emotional positions makes possible a remarkable degree of emotional neutrality about people. The neutrality is not feigned or forced but emanates automatically from a systems view. More neutrality coupled with actions that increase emotional separateness in one's most fused relationships can resolve feelings and attitudes linked to the past.

Efforts to increase the basic differentiation level also depend on knowledge of triangles. It is essential to be able to think in terms of triangles rather than dyadic relationships. A simplified example can illustrate this. A mother habitually gets quiet and withdrawn when she feels her husband treats her unfairly. Their daughter, sympathetic to her mother, reacts to her mother's mood by blaming and confronting her father. Confrontations over the years have left the daughter feeling that her father does not respect her opinion. The daughter has viewed the problem as being in the relationship with her father rather than in the parental triangle. To address the triangle, the daughter picks an issue that reflects the process between her parents. For example, the father criticizes the daughter for being "too critical." Instead of defending herself, she says, "Why do you criticize me when you know it upsets mother?" The effort is to move the problem out of the relationship with her father and back to where it came from, namely, the marital relationship. Similar efforts with both parents repeated over time can slightly increase the daughter's differentiation from her parents.

People learn best about differentiation by attempting to live it rather than by someone explaining it. Consequently, the description of some aspects of the process has probably not answered the question about how a therapist could get a family to do therapy on itself. Suffice it to say, therapists who are somewhat successful at functioning with more differentiation in their own lives are then able to facilitate a similar process in others. Besides therapists' efforts on themselves, some teaching of theory during therapy is also useful. The purpose is not to tell a family what to think, but to communicate a way of thinking. Families learn not only from what therapists says but from the way they attempt to live the theory in relationship to the family. This occurs provided what therapists do is consistent with what they say. People also benefit from studying the theory through reading and lectures. Those who accomplish the most with differentiation not only work on themselves in key relationships but systematically study their multigenerational family. The study provides objectivity about the past that can bestow greater flexibility on the future.

Applicability

Medicine has long been steeped in a biological paradigm. Psychiatry, after a half-century of domination by Freudian theory, has courted the biological paradigm in recent decades. However, psychiatry has traditionally been unique within medicine in its commitment to integrating psychological and social variables with biological ones. Given that Bowen theory addresses the full range of human emotional functioning, including all types of clinical dysfunction, the theory, if it proves to be accurate, could provide psychiatry with the broad conceptual framework it has been seeking. Since Bowen theory conceptualizes most clinical problems the various medical specialties address, the theory could guide clinical assessment and treatment decisions in every specialty.

Besides its applications in psychiatry and medicine, Bowen theory helps explain the functioning of nonfamily groups. Concepts such as the emotional system, differentiation, chronic anxiety, and triangles apply to churches, small businesses, civic groups, and large organizations (Comella 1995, 1997; Sagar and Wiseman 1982). The emotional functioning of the director of an organization plays a central role, through interlocking triangles, in problems existing anywhere in the organization. Communication breakdowns and irresponsibility by members of an organization are more the symptoms of an organizational problem than its cause. If the leader can change his or her functioning, most organizational problems correct themselves automatically. Using Bowen theory, an organizational consultant deals primarily with the leader. Someone down the organizational ladder is responsible for himself or herself and affects the functioning of subordinates, but this person cannot change a company. A consultant does not presume to tell a leader what to think or what to do, but provides a way of thinking about the nature of the organizational problem.

About 1970 Bowen began to extend his theory to society as a whole. Like families, society undergoes periods of anxiety-driven regression in emotional functioning. Following World War II, societal functioning began a decline that accelerated during the 1960s. Fluctuations occurred over the next two decades, but the overall trend was down. A hallmark of the regression is the trend of individuals and institutions making more decisions to relieve the anxiety of the moment, decisions that complicate the long-term future. More focus is on "rights" than on "responsibilities." Greater polarization exists among factions in society, and each faction acts more out of self-interest than community interest.

The functional level of differentiation in society has now declined over several generations, so the percentage of poorly functioning people in society is much higher. The dramatic increase in serious drug abuse probably reflects this increased percentage of poorly functioning people. High divorce and crime rates, a proliferation of lawsuits, an accentuation of bigotry, a decline in academic performance, an increase in white-collar crime, and a large homeless population are symptoms of a less functional society.

A regression will reverse in a family if one member functions with a little more differentiation. One or a few individuals have less impact on large systems such as society. However, the distress associated with opting for short-term solutions, with taking the easy way out, will eventually exceed the distress associated with acting based on a long-term view. This will turn the tide by forcing enough people to act more unselfishly. Societal anxiety will begin to decrease and the regression will reverse. Until then, those who blame everyone but themselves for the morass in which they are mired will drown out the more thoughtful and principled voices in society.

Research

Theory leads science, provided facts are the basis of the theory and provided allegiance to theory never exceeds allegiance to facts. Theory guides the discovery of new facts and the rediscovery of old facts. It gives clues for what to look for and where to look for it. It takes a long time to prove a theory. Enough proven or provable facts exist to support the development of Bowen theory, but not enough facts yet exist to prove or disprove it. This is the nature of theory. Researchers attempting to prove an aspect of the theory generally exclude so many variables to "measure" something that the results are inconclusive.

Bowen theory has been the basis for numerous descriptive studies. Researchers have compiled many multigenerational family studies, which are all consistent with what the concept of multigenerational emotional process predicts (Baker and Gippenreiter 1996). Families can generate a wide range of functioning in as few as four or five generations, but changes are usually gradual from one generation to the next. The research is difficult because of the difference between basic and functional levels of differentiation.

Several clinical projects have examined the interplay between family process and health problems such as cancer (Kerr 1981) or social dilemmas such as divorce (Kuhn et al. 1979). Similarly, the physical or mental health problems that can accompany aging were studied in the context of family process (Bowen et al. 1977). Each study found parallels between the severity of the problem or dilemma and levels of differentiation. One study examined the relationship of biofeedback to family theory (Kerr 1977a). Biofeedback involves control of autonomic functioning by higher brain functioning. Unpublished work with AIDS, infertility, family violence, incest, chronic illness, and alcoholism all describes links between these clinical problems and family emotional process. Several studies have examined the link between relationship systems and physiological functioning (Crews 1998; Papero 1996; Rauseo 1995). A study of Bowen theory–based psychotherapy with juvenile delinquents showing a low recidivism rate after 1 year will be published soon.

Aspects of Bowen theory appear to apply to other species (de Waal and Embree 1997; Kerr 1998). Concepts such as differentiation, fusion, anxiety, triangles, and patterns of emotional functioning are part of humans' evolutionary heritage. Given that the human family is an emotional unit, these concepts have implications for understanding other species. If a family of elephants, a troop of baboons, a colony of insects, a pride of lions, a school of fish, a gaggle of geese, and a cluster of trees are "emotional units," another dimension is added to our understanding of how emotional functioning and behavior evolve. The theory may enrich the study of subhuman species as much as the study of those species enriches Bowen theory.

Several studies demonstrate a consistency between Bowen theory and evolutionary theory (Berman 1996; Comella 1995; Gubernick 1996). Knowledge about mammalian evolution can help explain mother-child symbioses that persist into adult life (Noone 1988). An unpublished study applied the concept of differentiation to monkeys and primates. The study included observation of monkey social groups and a review of Goodall's (1986) work with chimpanzees. Variation in emotional functioning exists among members of these species that is similar to that of human beings. Another unpublished study included observation of colonies of overcrowded mice and a review of Calhoun's (1962) research on the effects of overpopulation on mice and rats. Density-induced regression in rodent colonies has similarities to anxiety-induced regression in human colonies.

Bowen conducted a videotape clinical research project for over 20 years, first at the Medical College of Virginia in Richmond and later at Georgetown (Kerr 1977b). Entire courses of family psychotherapy with several families were recorded on tape. The tapes are stored at the Georgetown Family Center and the National Library of Medicine, both located in the Washington, DC, area. Among other things, the tapes demonstrate the relationship between theory and therapy, and the process of differentiation.

Research in all the life sciences is important for supporting or refuting Bowen theory. Sociobiologists attempt to use evolutionary theory to explain social behavior in all species, including *Homo sapiens* (E.O. Wilson 1975). Research by ethologists such as Lorenz (1981) argues compellingly for understanding human behavior in the context of all life. MacLean's (1989) brain research is consistent with family theory. Comparative neuroanatomical studies show that brains of higher mammals are triune brains; that is, three brains in one. Besides the neocortex, the human brain has components that are structurally and functionally similar to reptilian (R-complex) and lower mammalian (limbic system) brains. Naturally occurring human behaviors are anchored in the older brains; for example, ritualized and imitative behaviors in the R-complex and the triad of family behaviors (nurturance of the young, isolation call, and play behavior) in the limbic system.

Conclusion and Future Directions

Amplifications and extensions should characterize the future of Bowen theory. Each concept requires amplification. Further research, for example, can better define the biological, psychological, and relationship functioning of people at each point on the scale of differentiation. Extensions of the theory will require more than analogies between human and nonhuman relationship systems. The regressions in mouse and human societies are analogous, but it is necessary to demonstrate common emotional processes for this observation to be an extension of theory. Differentiation in man is analogous to cellular differentiation, but the actual relationship between the phenomena is unknown. Fusion in *Homo sapiens* is tantalizingly similar to the "togetherness" in prides of lions, troops of baboons, and pods of killer whales, but it is not proven that common emotional forces create the similarity.

If facts about natural systems prove consistent with Bowen theory, two factors will still probably slow the theory's acceptance. The first is the emotional reactivity generated by linking the forces that govern all life with the forces that govern human behavior. Many people want humankind to be a special case in nature; to suggest otherwise is to strip humankind of meaning and purpose. These people try to retain two viewpoints: they endorse the pursuit of "what is" (science) but suggest that what they imagine about human nature (nonscience) is also part of "what is." Inevitably, students of human nature confront making a choice between fact and a belief that makes them feel good. I think this is a more difficult choice than most people realize. A second factor that will probably delay the theory's acceptance is the emotional reactivity generated by describing emotional connections between people that profoundly link their functioning. People may say they accept this but will not live their lives as if they really believe it.

Human beings do have a unique adaptation: the elaborately developed cerebral cortex and prefrontal lobes. The more they use this adaptation to create an image of themselves that separates human nature from the rest of nature, the more the forces that govern all life will blindly govern mankind. The more human beings use this adaptation to understand their connection to all life, the more potential they have for controlling their destiny.

Chapters on Related Topics

The following chapters describe concepts related to this chapter:

- Chapter 4, "Psychodynamic Family Therapy"
- Chapter 6, "Contextual Therapy"

6

Contextual Therapy

Catherine Ducommun-Nagy, M.D.
Linda D. Schwoeri, Ph.D.

Introduction

Contextual therapy is the product of more than 40 years of research and clinical work by its founder, Ivan Boszormenyi-Nagy, M.D. (hereinafter referred to as Nagy). His main goal over the years has been to reach a definition of what constitutes the healing moment in therapy and to use his finding to develop a unique approach that bridges the gap between individual and family therapy. In his work, Nagy demonstrates that relationships are determined by four clusters of elements—four dimensions of relational reality—that cannot be reduced to one another and that coexist at any time: facts, psychology, transactions, and relational ethics. The dimension of relational ethics accounts for a universal characteristic of relationships: our striving for trustworthiness and fairness in close relationships (Boszormenyi-Nagy 1966/1987a; Boszormenyi-Nagy and Spark 1984).

Contextual therapy allows for the development of specific treatment strategies and offers a motivational theory that informs several aspects of relationships that are not explained by individual psychology, or systemic laws. Nagy believes that it is not just the internal drives and needs described by classical psychoanalysis that determine people's actions. Nor does he believe that transactions between family members are the sole product of supra-individual, systemic, regulatory forces. He shows that ultimately any action between two individuals amounts to either giving or receiving, and he describes the two persons as being in a relational balance of entitlement or indebtedness. The sum of all the interpersonal balances constitutes the relational context in which future relationships will be anchored and by which they will be influenced.

Contextual therapy has, from its beginning, made room for biological components in the etiology of mental illness. It also has refrained from relying on a naive transactional explanation to account for either psychosis or the complexity of human relationships. To this extent, contextual therapy is in a good position to resist the serious challenges posed by biological psychiatry to any kind of psychotherapy.

In contextual therapy, the therapeutic contract must include all persons who could be affected by the consequences of the therapeutic interventions. By successively exploring relationships from the vantage point of each of the participants involved, the therapist is able to take into account the individuals' respective vulnerabilities and interests. This design is referred to as *multidirected partiality* and forms one of the core strategies of contextual therapy. Multidirected partiality has been recently rediscovered by many therapists as an answer to the challenge posed to the family therapist who needs to establish a therapeutic contract with more than one client. In seeking to understand the position of each of the family members who could be affected by their interventions, whether present or absent, contextual therapists are less likely to blame their clients' relatives at a time when more and more family members, believing that their needs and rights have been ignored, sue therapists for compensation.

At present, contextual therapy influences therapists worldwide, and many family therapy training programs in the United States, Europe, and South America include contextual therapy in their curriculum.

Background of the Contextual Approach

The Path of the Founder

Nagy's path to becoming a psychiatrist was determined by his striving to find ways to help psychotic patients. Starting his clinical work as a psychiatrist in Budapest in the late 1940s, he became interested in the relational implications of individual psychotherapy. His mentor and friend Kalman Gyarfas was a relationally oriented psychiatrist who eventually moved to Chicago, where he became an influential educator of many, including Virginia Satir.

Nagy also had a strong background in philosophy and was familiar with the writings of Hegel, Heidegger, Jaspers, Bergson, Sartre, and others. His knowledge of Hegelian dialectics was a formative base of his early integration of existential thought with object relations theory (Boszormenyi-Nagy 1965/1985, 1966/1987a). Later, he found in Martin Buber's writings the philosophical parallel to his own clinical discoveries and a model for his formulation of the dialogical aspects of relationships.

After he immigrated to the United States in 1950, Nagy attempted to develop a biochemical research approach in order to establish correlates between observed clinical symptoms and biochemical abnormalities in schizophrenic patients (Boszormenyi-Nagy 1958/1987b). Although he gained the respect of the scientific community for the sophistication of the methodology he used for studying cellular metabolism, he soon returned to his original interest in psychotherapy.

In Chicago, Nagy became familiar with the work of the psychoanalyst Franz Alexander and met Thomas Szasz, who introduced him to the British school of object relations theory.

In 1957, he became director of an inpatient research therapeutic department at Eastern Pennsylvania Psychiatric Institute in Philadelphia, which later became the Department of Family Psychiatry. He maintained this position until the research institute closed in 1980. As a researcher, Nagy initiated many groundbreaking changes in the management of clients hospitalized for schizophrenia, and he later developed innovative outpatient programs.

The discovery of family therapy stemmed from early experiences that Nagy had with his research inpatient unit. One of the first innovative steps in caring for clients with schizophrenia was the establishment of community meetings under the personal inspiration of Maxwell Jones of London, the founder of the *therapeutic community* approach. Soon, Nagy and his team took the step of inviting family members to participate in the community meetings that had already brought together staff members and patients. The research team discovered that patients who seemed lost in senseless talking when dealing with staff members would suddenly engage in meaningful discussions when they talked with their relatives. This finding motivated Nagy to invite families for joint sessions attended by the patient, the available family members, the patient's individual therapist, and Nagy himself, while other team members functioned as observers behind a one-way mirror (Boszormenyi-Nagy 1958/1987c). Over time, an enormous amount of clinical material accumulated. In drawing parallels between family dynamics and some aspects of individual pathology, it became possible to establish hypotheses that led to innovative treatment strategies. One of the first steps was to stop providing individual sessions that still emphasized the role of the individual therapist and to shift to a clear family therapy design. This period of rapid discovery led to the first formulation of what by the early 1960s had became known as intensive family psychotherapy. By then, Nagy and some of his co-workers had already established contacts with other pioneers in the field, such as Ackerman, Bowen, Wynne, and Whitaker, and started to visit other early family therapy centers. They also had contacts with therapists such as Searles, Burnham, and Will, who were involved at Chestnut Lodge near Washington, DC, in the intensive individual psychotherapy of patients with psychosis.

Soon, Nagy formulated a complex model of relationships that was informed by the integration of Hegelian and existential philosophy, systemic knowledge, and object relations theory (Boszormenyi-Nagy 1965/1985, p. 65). Multidirected partiality was established both as a core theoretical concept and as a methodological tool for conducting therapy (Boszormenyi-Nagy 1966/1987a).

As Nagy's understanding of intergenerational dynamics progressed during the 1970s, he began to define his approach as intergenerational family therapy (Boszormenyi-Nagy and Spark 1984). The key element of this shift was the diminished role of psychodynamic psychology and the discovery of the importance of justice dynamics for relationships, based on Martin Buber's writings (Buber 1957). Seeking to understand what was helpful to his psychotic patients and to determine the elements of effective therapy, Nagy had come to the conclusion that trust and guilt were the fundamental elements needed to understand health and pathology. Nagy's observations paralleled those of many individual therapists before him. However, his contribution was to demonstrate that it was not the psychological aspects of trust and guilt that counted, but their existential, relational component. Ultimately an individual's psychological capacity to trust is anchored in his or her early experiences of not only reliable but also equitable ways of relating as exhibited by his or her caretakers. If trust is anchored in the trustworthiness of the relationship, there must be a connection between trust and justice. Conversely, the experience of actual injustices can eventually damage a person's capacity to trust: Nagy believed that children are less damaged by objective deprivations than by any form of exploitation that damages their capacity to trust.

Nagy found in Buber the needed language to describe the phenomenon that he had discovered in the therapy room. He demonstrated that the existential guilt rooted in actual harm done to others is what matters in relationships.

Following Buber, Nagy underlined the difference between the guilt stemming from actual harm done to others and guilt that originates in the ego as a response to internal conflicts between the instinctual drives and the superego.

As Nagy became aware of the importance of justice dynamics in close relationships, he found in the term *loyalty* a good description for the dynamics that were holding families together. Family members are linked by the obligation to offer their commitment to one another as a repayment for care received. He described how a transgenerational web of expectations and obligations keeps family members connected regardless of possible psychological or transactional cutoffs.

About the same time, Nagy coined the term *parentification* to describe situations in which parents try to find in their children the caring adult they missed while growing up, and children try to live up to this expectation at the sacrifice of their own needs.

Later, Nagy established the term *contextual family therapy*. It was created to allow for a clear emphasis on the ethical dimension of relationships. By then, the notion of justice based on equitable returns and injustices as a source for destructive entitlement was well established. The reestablishment of some measure of fair giving and receiving between family members became the focus of the contextual therapist's interventions.

More recently, Nagy shifted his attention to the fact that there is a reward for giving, regardless of the actual returns by the recipient. Nagy uses the term *constructive entitlement* to describe the experience in which one gets a reward for the act of giving, regardless of the recipient's ability to reestablish an equitable balance of giving and receiving. The therapist's focus of interventions, therefore, had to shift from an exploration of avenues for fair receiving to a dialogue of fair giving, where chances for every participant in a relationship to give appropriately are explored. The concept of loyalty was revised to encompass these newer ideas. Nagy emphasized the broader implications of his approach for any form of therapy for individuals and couples as well as families. To underscore the fact that his principles apply to any of these treatment modalities (Boszormenyi-Nagy 1958/1987c), he chose to rename his approach *contextual therapy*.

Besides its implications for psychotherapy in general, contextual therapy also has applicability for the exploration of cases that involve relationships between conflicting groups, whether in business situations, interethnic conflicts, or other situations. The expansion of reproductive technologies also posed new challenges to the field of family therapy, that contextual therapy is well prepared to address since it involves people with conflicting interests (the infertile couple, the potential donors, and the yet unborn child).

In recent years, Nagy has taken a very strong stand: He believes that without serious consideration of the implications of the ethical dimension of relationships for any kind of therapy, psychotherapy as a field may not survive long into the 21st century. He believes that the concerted efforts of all therapists are needed to address family and societal issues, restore responsible parenting, and help prevent social disintegration. He sees social disintegration as a threat to human survival that parallels the irresponsible handling of our planet's natural resources (Boszormenyi-Nagy 1966/1987d).

Basis of Contextual Therapy

A Dialectic View of Relationships

Nagy's original work integrates psychoanalytic theories, especially object relations theory and systems theory, with existential philosophy (Heidegger, Bergson, and mostly Buber) and Hegelian dialectic.

Nagy starts by examining Freud's contribution to the understanding of the functioning of the psyche. According to Freud's structural view of the individual's internal world, the ego is the locus of a compromise between the instinctual drives (libido, aggression) and the forces of the superego (internalized parental image and societal taboos). To that extent, psychoanalytic theory is essentially a theory of internal conflicts and defense mechanisms vis-à-vis these conflicts. In Freud's theory, the object is understood as the person, a part of a person's body, or the actual object that is the source of gratification of internal drives. In *object relations theory*, the object is understood as an internal image of the other, based on the early experience of actual relationships, to which the individual is relating in accordance with various internal needs. Nagy specifically stresses Fairbairn's contribution in emphasizing the object—the seeking rather than pleasure-seeking nature of the mind's dynamic forces (Fairbairn 1952). Nagy, following Hartmann's (1964) definition, sees the self as the part of the person that is in contradistinction to the object and the ego as in contradistinction to other intrapsychic structures. Nonetheless, Nagy stresses that all psychoanalytical theories remain psychological theories, based on an individual perspective: The individual mind is regarded mostly as a closed system determined by its own dynamic laws. Object relations theories are individually rather than relationally based. They do not take into account the fact that the other person is also a subject in need of an object. Boszormenyi-Nagy (1965/1985) demonstrates that the self can be both a subject-agent of an action and an object-target of the action; the same is true of the other, who can be either the subject or the object of an action involving the self. The self can be the subject of the action, when for instance a client shouts back at the voices that he hears, or the object of the action, when the voices are commanding him to act.

Self-Delineation

The self-delineating aspect of the self-other relationship was another fundamental element of relationships underlined by Boszormenyi-Nagy (1965/

1985). For him the real struggle of each person is to possess a secure ground for one's own sense of self, and this ground is the *other*. The *other* is not in dichotomous relation with the self but serves as an antithesis to the self and to that extent becomes an indirect constituent of this self. Boszormenyi-Nagy's vision of the self-other relationship is dialectic in the sense that the self (thesis) that emerges in contraposition with the *other* is also transformed by this other, which therefore becomes a constituent of the self (synthesis). Individuals depend on the availability of a partner to assert and fulfill their own need of self-delineation.

Furthermore, as individuals enter a relationship, both partners will try to assign a role to the other and use the other in accordance with individual "need-templates." "I am what I make of the other" (Boszormenyi-Nagy 1965/1985). If both partners have need-templates that complement each other, the relationship can remain stable (homeostasis) or both partners may engage in a power battle for the use of the other (escalation). The form and outcome of such confrontation will be determined both by the nature of the needs involved and by systemic laws of interaction. This can lead to the collapse of the relationship unless both partners can move toward fairness and reciprocity instead of exploiting each other.

Self-Validation

Each person needs someone to give to as a ground for self-validation and for the earning of entitlement; thus, partners serve yet another function. At any time when I have someone to give to, my merits augment. I also gain freedom from the guilt that I would have accumulated if I had not tried to meet the other's needs. By giving, I validate myself and my self-worth increases. In this sense, the justice that underlies the relational ethic is based on the alternation of benefits issuing from giving and receiving. "The contextual principle of receiving through giving is another example of a dialectical synthesis that resolves the antithesis between selfishness and altruism" (I. Boszormenyi-Nagy, personal communication, 1992).

Relational Ethics

Relational ethics, for Nagy, can be translated as an ethic of fair consideration for both self and others. It includes the capacity to take responsibility for the consequences of one's action, the capacity to care for the vulnerabilities of children and helpless people, the acknowledgment of burdens and advantages, and the courage to claim one's own dues.

The self's dependence on an *other* to exist as a self has not only existential and power implications but ethical ones. What do I do to *the other* when

I use him or her for my own needs? Without a measure of reciprocity, the relationship is doomed to fail. Each person involved in a close relationship is entitled to expect fair consideration of his or her needs in return for having been available to the needs of the partner. Nagy's clinical experience converges with Martin Buber's writings about the dialogue that enriches the language used in the further development of contextual therapy (Friedman 1989).

Transgenerational Dynamics

Constructive Entitlement

The contribution of the contextual approach to the understanding of transgenerational dynamics lies both in the dialectical description of self-object relationships and in the way the parents' entitlement (constructive or destructive) affects the next generation.

One of the most common avenues for adults to earn constructive entitlement and to increase their self-worth is to give to their children. This giving also benefits the next generations, since children who have received are also more likely to give when they become parents. One should remember, however, that overgiving can amount to the unilateral exploitation of the child, if the child is cut off from chances of repaying or giving in general, which blocks him or her from earning entitlement in turn.

Destructive Entitlement

Conversely, having been wronged or exploited leads to the accumulation of destructive entitlement. Each person who has been wronged has a legitimate claim to compensation for the damage inflicted on him or her. If the one who caused the damage is not available to make up for the damages incurred, the injured party may seek redress from an innocent third party, such as a spouse or a child. The victim's entitlement becomes destructive if it places an unfair demand on others. This could lead in turn to a cascade of transgenerational exploitation, if parents who have been wronged start to excessively tap into their children's generous availability to get compensation for past injustices. The child will tend to adjust to the parent's needs and to remain available to the parent even if not acknowledged. Nonetheless, children who have not been protected from unfair expectations can in turn become depleted and prone to misusing their own offspring. Winnicott's description of the early *stage of concern* in the child (Winnicott 1958) parallels Nagy's observations.

Loyalties

The term *loyalty* has been used by Nagy to describe a relational constellation that includes at least three parties: the party who deserves the commitment, the party who offers the commitment, and a third party who could also expect commitment from the second. To that extent, loyalty is anchored in the ethical dimension of the relationship and cannot be separated from the notion of loyalty conflicts. Having received care from parents, the child is obligated to them and must repay them by later trying to meet their needs (availability) or by supporting them when they are challenged by others (display of loyalty). If loyalty were based only on the merits of the parents, one would not expect children to remain loyal to their nondeserving parents. According to Nagy's newest definition, loyalty to family members is also based on a need to give to the ones who are close to us, even if they have exploited us. If *earning of entitlement* by giving to others in close relationships becomes a right for each of the persons involved, they all can increase their self-worth by displaying availability to their parents in the form of a loyal commitment. Loyalty as a form of giving benefits the self as much as the parent toward whom this loyalty is manifested, and being loyal to parents becomes, therefore, a right of any child.

Invisible Loyalties

Invisible loyalties are expressions of loyalty that take an *indirect form*. They are potentially destructive for both the individual and others, including the one toward whom the person is indirectly loyal. In general, invisible loyalties can be considered the result of a complicated compromise between contradictory forces (resentment toward the parent and guilt over one's lack of availability to that parent). As one starts to resent a parent, one is blocked from giving to this parent, and this can become a new source of destructive entitlement if being able to give is a right of any human being. Instead of being free to loyally commit to the parent, one starts instead to establish other relationships. A very common example is the situation in which an adult child rejects his parents and at the same time vehemently criticize his in-laws. Neither the parents nor the in-laws benefit from this criticism, but the result is the same: the criticism amounts to an *indirect* display of loyalty to his parents. The child who has been wronged is often blocked from the possibility of giving to the parents in a direct, visible way and is more likely to give in an indirect manner by sabotaging other relationships. People occasionally can become aware of indirect loyalties. For example, an individual may realize that each time she becomes angry with her parents and cancels a visit with them, she ends up fighting with her spouse. She might not understand the deep dynamics underlying this sequence of interactions but still realizes that there is a connection between her cancellation of the visit to the parents and bad treatment of her husband. Often the ways in which a person remains indirectly loyal to a parent are difficult to see. For example, a patient may enter individual therapy to deal with the bad relationship he had with his parents and spend a lot of time blaming them for his difficulties. He does not realize that in choosing individual therapy rather than family therapy to deal with these issues, he shields his parents from the direct complaints that they would have heard in a family therapy session.

The goal for the contextual therapist is to help each individual find terms of giving that are compatible with the interests of both the giver and the receiver. Many can be helped to find constructive ways of direct giving that are not destructive, rather than refusing to consider the realistic needs of parents and continuing to give to them in an indirect and costly manner.

Contextual Strategies

Assessment: The Four Dimensions of Relational Realities

Nagy postulated that one has to take into account four dimensions, four aspects, of four clusters of elements to account for all the elements that determine relationship (Boszormenyi-Nagy and Spark 1984). These have to be assessed in order to get a full perspective on both pathology and resources. Each dimension of relational reality is governed by motivational forces that need to be understood by the therapist.

Facts

The first dimension describes the givens in a person's life—biological endowment, including health and illness; gender; nationality; religion; and country of residence—as well as the factual elements of one's personal history (e.g., being an orphan, an only child, the last of many children). Physical assets and conversely genetic diseases or illness will contribute to success or failure in relationships with others. For instance, a person who is weakened by an illness and whose long-term survival is threatened will enter relationships with a more limited set of options than a healthy person. The early loss of one's parents will forever change a person's life, whether or not the person was provided with good parental substitutes.

Therapists should carefully assess the factual elements of an individual's life and design interventions to alleviate the detrimental impact of certain conditions.

Nagy also reminds us that despite the pretenses of many biologically oriented psychiatrists, no scientifically acceptable or irrefutable correlates have been demonstrated between any well-defined biological characteristics (or qualities) and a specific mental illness. The biological treatment of mental illness is not based on specific etiological knowledge, as it may be in the case of internal medicine, for instance. Nagy nonetheless recognizes the helpfulness of psychotropic medications for some patients. Other factual elements can also be modified by external interventions. For instance, a social worker can mobilize financial aid to relocate a family or a psychologist can recommend a school transfer for a child with special needs.

On the other hand, recognizing the inescapable nature of some of these facts can be therapeutic. The therapist can explore the consequences of a distributive injustice (or injustices of life) as a source of destructive entitlement for the person whose life is marked by an unusual hardship. As the recipient of such injustices seeks redress by expecting special consideration from others, he or she creates a new injustice by making unfair demands of others and becoming, in turn, the source of a retributive injustice (unfairness in the relationship). For example, the person who is affected by diabetes cannot change this predicament, and nobody can be held responsible for this person's fate as a sick one (distributive injustice). However, a person who expects others to be responsible for reminding him or her to follow a prescribed diet has unfair expectations (retributive injustice) of others. (People can be sympathetic to the sick person, but they should not be held responsible for his or her treatment.)

The articulation between distributive and retributive justice forms the link between the dimension of facts and the dimension of relational ethics.

Individual Psychology

The second cluster of determinants is formed by the uniqueness of each individual psyche that encompasses the person' emotional functioning and cognitive abilities.

Here we can list the psychological determinants that have been described in psychoanalytic theories. Relevant to this dimension is Freud's theory of instincts with its description of instinctual drives and internal conflicts, as well as the concepts of object relations theory: internalization of the object, externalization, displacement, and projective identification. In this category also belongs any theory that accounts for intellectual functioning and learning processes, including Piaget's description of stages of intellectual and moral development.

The contextual therapist working with the family group observes the ego strength or weakness of the various family members, their capacity to endure frustrations or cope with anxiety, and the nature of their defense mechanisms such as projection, denial, or displacement. The therapist may also become aware of some of the transference phenomena that begin to occur as family members become more engaged in the therapy process.

Contextual therapists do not interpret what they observe and do not see the increase of insight for those they treat as the goal of their interventions. To this extent, contextual therapy is clearly separated from individual treatment modalities that are inspired by psychoanalysis.

Of course, any kind of individual psychotherapy based on insight or cognitive awareness and any remedial therapies (e.g., speech therapy, special education) use tools that can provide new options for improving individual functioning. Rather, they seek to help individuals free themselves from psychological bondage through coming to terms with the justice dynamics of their situation rather than simply rejecting others, which is itself a sign that they are still deeply affected by some adverse psychological phenomena. These tools can be helpful to clients during the course of a contextual treatment as long as the therapist does not betray the principles of an ethics of fair consideration for all persons affected by the treatment and as long as the therapist understands that autonomy as a goal of therapy cannot be gained by a simple rejection of others.

Transactions

Transactions form the third cluster that regroups all the aspects of systems theories that apply to families and have served as a theoretical backbone for ordering the discoveries and observations made by family therapists. "All family therapies share the ideal goal of affecting a superordinate gestalt of relationships which is more than the sum of the dynamics of individual family members" (Boszormenyi-Nagy 1966/1987a), and to that extent contextual therapy is fundamentally "systemic."

Phenomena such as power alignment, alliances, and collusions belong to this dimension. Contextual therapists observe the various transactions involved while proceeding with their interventions. The therapist will register the communication patterns established in a given family and relate them to motivational elements found in the other dimensions of relationships. On the other hand, Nagy's major contribution to the field of family therapy, in addition to being one of the inventors of this treatment modality, has been to postulate that systems theories alone cannot account for all of the supra-individual forces that determine the sequence of transactions between family members.

Relational Ethics (Context of Fairness)

Relational ethics, composing the fourth cluster of elements, describe a characteristic of human relationships understood by all of us but not usually discussed by therapists. At any moment in a close relationship, we know the status of the balance between what we have given to the other and what we have ourselves received, and this balance determines our next actions. As described earlier, each transaction between two closely relating partners amounts to either giving or receiving. Each individual is involved in a multitude of such balances, to which each individual has to respond by new actions. Nagy defined this aspect of relationships as the dimension of relational ethics. One has to realize that this dimension does not represent a remote intellectual or moralizing principle but a reality of our daily life with others.

In a symmetrical relationship—that is, when both partners have similar options to give and receive from each other—the partners will find a measure of fairness in their relationship; if they do not, the mistreated one can choose eventually to leave the unfair one. In comparison, children and their parents are in an asymmetrical situation: The child does not have the option of leaving the unfair parent. Instead, the child accumulates an entitlement that is based on his or her right to fair treatment. As described earlier, this entitlement can become destructive if the child later uses his or her own children as a source for compensation for the past lack of attention.

The capacity of a parent to tend to a young child's needs and to give generously to a child is based on a balance of giving and receiving. "As I have been given to generously while growing up, I will be free to give to my offspring and meet their needs." Conversely, "If I have been exploited myself, I will expect compensations for what I suffered and will rely on the unrealistic hopes that my child could be available to meet my needs."

The therapist's task is to help each family member take a position and examine the balance of giving and receiving from the vantage point of both the giver and the receiver. Each person is expected to gain both from claiming due consideration and from offering care to others. Earning of entitlement through giving to others in close relationships becomes a right for any of the persons involved because each of them will benefit from increased self-worth. The contextual therapist who is informed by the recent developments of the contextual approach will aim at helping each family member to earn constructive entitlement. Elements of destructive entitlement will be explored and its sources tracked. One of the characteristics of the destructively entitled person is his or her blindness to the perpetration of new injustices. Moreover, the person who has been wronged may end up being blocked in his or her capacity to give to others and consequently be further cut off from options to earn constructive entitlement. The therapist's optimism is based on the notion that each person can come to experience that generosity does not require altruism in as much as it also benefits the giver (Boszormenyi-Nagy 1995; Ducommun-Nagy and Schwoeri 1990).

The Therapeutic Contract

In the individual contract, the client is the patient whose goals and needs the therapist tries to respond to. When a therapist invites more than one person into the therapy room, he or she is faced with some major questions:

- Who is the client?
- Who is to be the beneficiary of the changes?
- Is there a difference between client and patient?
- Can I be at the same time the therapist to the abused person and the therapist to the one who harmed the other? How can I address the conflicting needs of two adults seeking marriage therapy. (More recently, this question has gone beyond a theoretical consideration to finally reach the courtroom, where family members attack therapists who they allege have alienated them from each other.)

As Nagy pointed out early in his writings, bringing more than one person into the therapy room does not resolve the issue of the therapeutic contract. Nagy has demonstrated that the therapist who sees families will soon face a dilemma: Does the therapist continue to serve the goals and interests of one specific member, often the identified patient, or can he or she respond to the needs of more than one person?

The therapist who believes that family members should change their behaviors so that his or her client can get better implicitly endorses a *unilateral view* of a therapeutic contract, even if the family is asked to participate in many treatment sessions. In this sense, there is not much difference between the individual therapist and a family therapist who retains an individual perspective of his therapeutic contract. The systemic therapists who do not want to fall into this trap seek a haven in neutrality. "I am neutral vis-à-vis the family members" and "The family is my client" are statements often made by such therapists, as if the so called *family* could be an entity with a mind to make decisions and assume responsibility for them. Nagy opposes this personification of the family as a living creature because he believes that each family member is uniquely responsible for the consequences of his or her own acts and decisions. Nagy proposes that the therapeutic contract should include the interests of any person affected by the interventions of the therapist, whether present or absent, yet unborn or deceased.

Multidirected Partiality

Several schools of family therapy have begun to appreciate and utilize what Nagy defined in the late sixties as *multidirected partiality*. Every therapist must define a strategy to address the conflicts of interest that eventually emerge from the confrontations of family members' diverging needs in the establishment of the therapeutic contract and later in the course of therapy. Nagy proposes that multidirected partiality as an offer of fair consideration for the respective position of each of the persons involved allows for both self-delineation and self-validation of each family member in turn. This strategy helps the therapist to hear each family member's side in full, paying attention not only to his or her expressed goals but especially to his or her expressed or unexpressed existential vulnerabilities. By maintaining a multidirected stance, contextual therapists do not take sides; they do not remain neutral. Instead, they listen with concern for *all* members present as well as absent.

Contextual therapists tend to structure their interviews according to the guidelines offered by multidirected partiality. They address people in an order that is determined by their respective vulnerabilities without letting themselves be distracted by the interventions of other family members who try to seek the therapist's attention, unless the interaction becomes clearly destructive or dangerous. Soon people learn that the best way to capture the therapist's attention is by making positive contributions to the discussion: this provides a tremendous leverage for maintaining order in the therapy room. Each person is offered an opportunity to describe his or her position and to give concrete examples to illustrate his or her points: in offering an example, one person clarifies his or her position and allows for the response of others based on their personal perspective of a shared event. This is a powerful tool to increase self-delineation between family members. Contextual therapists extend their concern to absent members of the family and to anyone who could be affected by the impact of the therapeutic process. If a couple seeks therapy because they are struggling, after discovering that they are both carriers of a recessive gene that could affect their children, with the decision to continue with their marriage or separate, the therapist will address the two young people as parents and focus his or her attention on the interest of the child to be born or not, as much as on the distress of the couple.

Young children are welcomed in sessions and encouraged to express their concerns. Indeed, in allowing children to express their realistic worries about their parents, for instance, the therapist does not increase the child's parentification. Instead, it will be easier for the therapist to support the child if he or she understands the child's predicament. If the child were to be simply scolded for undermining the parents' role by reporting his or her concerns to a stranger (the therapist), the child would be left alone with his or her worries, which increases parentification.

Applicability

Contextual therapy can have applicability to many societal problems and situations. From a clinical perspective, it has important applications for the treatment of psychosis, more specifically, schizophrenia. Therapeutic resources can be mobilized by the discovery and acknowledgment of the deep forms of giving and of availability of the patient to his family members. From that standpoint, an exploration of giving and receiving between family members is not contradictory with any individually diagnosed condition, nor is an exploration of burdens resulting from this condition included for the identified patient. Any attempt to motivate people to be responsible in responding to others can be helpful and is never contraindicated. In fact, depressed patients, in spite of their condition, may benefit from being helped to give to others. They may find an opportunity for self-validation instead of having to to ask for more support for themselves, which could further decrease their self-esteem. The whole range of neurosis, personality disorders, and behavioral problems of the child and the adolescent can be explored in terms of contextual therapy. The implications of handicaps, physical or mental, and of genetic diseases for the individual and for his or her family are a known focus of contextual therapy interventions. The therapist will usually focus on an exploration of the handicapped person's right to get help from other family members to design situations in which the vulnerable family member can find ways of becoming a meaningful contributor to family relationships. Contextual therapists are also concerned with the rights of yet unborn children and potential (unconceived) offspring to not be conceived if they will be born into detrimental circumstances.

As much as systemic theories offer an invaluable core of knowledge and a valid instrument to account for actual interactions, they cannot account for all aspects of relationships. Nagy likes the image of a spiral to encompass both the circularity of phenomena that contribute to the homeostasis of the system and the linearity of the passing of time with its cascade of cause and consequences engendering irreversible changes.

Case Example

The vignette below illustrates some of the elements discussed in this chapter. The client's identifying data have been changed for the sake of confidentiality.

Identifying Information

John was 4 years old when he was diagnosed with severe developmental delays in the areas of speech and socialization. He was otherwise a healthy boy, and his mother's pregnancy and his delivery had been uneventful. Since no clear explanation was found for his presentation, it was initially assumed that his delay was of psychogenic origin, and possibly rooted in his mother's depression and lack of availability when he was a baby. His parents were advised to send him to a special kindergarten program that offered individual and family therapy. With time, John made good progress and was able to attend a specialized school, although he remained very slow in verbal expression and in math. He was eventually diagnosed with severe learning disabilities. As he grew older, his behavior started to deteriorate and he was referred to a residential treatment facility that offered intensive individual psychotherapy several times a week in addition to other treatment modalities.

Background

John's parents came from a similar social and ethnic background and married young. John was their first child. Their second son, Jimmy, 4 years younger, was doing well. The parents had uneventful contacts with their relatives, and the children appeared to like visits with the extended family. The only noticeable point was that the father had little time for his family while he was taking evening classes to become an accountant. His wife was responsible for managing the children and was often at a loss over John's oppositional behaviors and occasional rage outbursts.

During John's long stay in the residential program, the parents started to attend family therapy sessions led by the team social worker and one of John's counselors. John's father became more available after he graduated and learned, with the help of the family therapist, to support his wife in disciplining the children. He also became more involved in family activities. John's mother received a lot of reassurance from the therapists and learned to be firm with John and to set limits without feeling guilty. However, John's temper tantrums continued during home visits, and the mother was still very distressed by some of his odd behaviors. One day John smashed a mirror in the family dining room just before the arrival of his parents' guests. Another time, he threw away all the flowers that his mother had bought for a sick neighbor. On several occasions, he slipped out of the home in the middle of the night to play outside, which scared his parents.

At the same time, John was doing so well in the residential program that the team suggested he be allowed to return home and attend public school in a special class for children with leaning disabilities. The family was very disturbed by this recommendation and asked for a new evaluation and recommendation, which is the point at which the consultant (Catherine Ducommun-Nagy) assessed the family.

Assessment

The factual elements at hand were John's scholastic limitations and the fact that his younger brother had already surpassed him in many school activities.

Psychologically, John was clearly exhibiting low self-esteem, poor impulse control, and possibly faulty reality testing. As described above, his cognitive abilities were significantly limited.

The family transaction patterns were noticeable in the parents' making John the scapegoat and the mother's over-involvement with him.

Having heard a list of complaints about John and realizing that the parents had great difficulty in being attentive to his positive contributions, the consultant began the therapy by asking the following question: "Does father notice when John is worried or discouraged?" John interrupted, saying, "Daddy only plays with Jimmy, he does not want to play with me because I am dumb!"

The father answered that that was not true, that John was invited to participate in the games but did not seem interested. As more questions were asked about the kind of games they played, it became obvious that John felt left out because either he did not understand the rules of the game or he could not count his points. Engaging him in a game that was too difficult for him was unfair, given his condition.

The consultant then turned to John and asked bluntly, "John, are you hurt to see that you are not as smart as your brother?" John responded immediately, "Yes, it is not fair." John was then asked, "What is unfair? Do you blame anyone for what is happening to you?" John's immediate answer, surprising for a boy suffering from difficulties in communication, was, "My mother, she did not make me right!" John became agitated, and his mother became speechless and then defensive: "How can you say that? First, I did not make you alone, and second don't you think I am hurt too?!" She was clearly responding as a parent who had been hurt by John's failures and nasty behaviors. The father came to the mother's rescue, "Neither your mom nor I could choose anything about the way you were made, and it would have been nicer for us too if you did not have difficulties." Jimmy interrupted to say that winning at games did not make him happy because he knew that his brother was not able to challenge him. John appeared surprised by all these comments. For the first time he realized that others, not just him, had been hurt by his limitations and that his parents did not intend to favor his little brother. His was also visibly surprised that his own handicap was a burden for his little brother.

The end of the session was used to explore how to help John in turning family activities into times when he too could succeed. Mother was encouraged to express her own needs and tell John what she expected from him rather than letting herself be hurt and later snapping at John in an unexpected way. Father was asked if he could spend time explaining soccer to John, who was a fantastic goal keeper but could not play with his team because he did not understand the rules.

Besides the systemic dynamics already explored by the therapist, the consultations underscored the importance of understanding the balance of giving and receiving between family members to approach John's behavior and remotivate him as a positive contributor to family life. John experienced his limitations as an injustice for which he had secretly blamed his mother. He acted toward her in a vengeful way when he destroyed things that she had bought. He also expected his family to make up for his unhappiness by meeting some unrealistic demands, but his overentitled behaviors were only a reflection of a real distributive injustice: nobody could be blamed for a condition that affected his entire life and had placed him at a real disadvantage vis-à-vis others, such as his little brother, who had not experienced any difficulties in learning. Nonetheless, by acting unfairly towards others, he was committing new injustices for which he was in turn punished: he was not allowed to return home despite his good behavior in the residential program.

As the consultant showed interest in John and helped his parents to credit him for the unfairness of his condition despite their own hurt, John became less destructive and more able to cooperate with others, which helped him feel good about himself. As his reliance on his destructive entitlement decreased, his behavior improved rapidly and he started to get rewards for his improvement. His parents agreed to a trial discharge, and he eventually returned successfully to his parents' home and made a good adjustment to a new specialized school.

Chapters on Related Topics

The following chapters describe concepts related to contextual therapy:

- Chapter 4, "Psychodynamic Family Therapy"
- Chapter 5, "Multigenerational Family Systems Theory of Bowen and Its Application"

7

Behavioral Family Therapy

Ian R. H. Falloon, M.D.

Behavioral family therapy (BFT) encompasses a broad range of therapeutic strategies with a primary focus of enhancing the efficiency of family functioning. The common thread that binds these strategies is the manner in which they have been subjected to empirical studies to examine their efficacy. This empirical focus has led to a convergence of strategies that have been demonstrated as having consistent benefits when applied in a clearly specified manner across a wide range of problems, family groups, cultural settings, and clinical disorders. This chapter introduces these approaches and the manner in which they are implemented in clinical settings.

Historical Development

Some 30 years ago behavioral approaches to family therapy emerged in the form of a series of case reports describing specific strategies that were shown to benefit specific problems in childhood disorders, such as nocturnal enuresis, aggressive behavior, tantrums, autism, and learning deficits. These case reports focused on training parents to apply specific strategies to reduce the disturbed behavior of young children. The family members were co-opted as members of the clinical team. Prior to training, their best efforts to resolve the disturbed behavior patterns were carefully assessed from a social learning theory perspective, and patterns of family behavior that were thought to promote and sustain the specific disturbances in the child were observed. These early formulations were derived mainly from operant conditioning paradigms and in retrospect appear overly simplistic. Nevertheless, they gave rise to straightforward interventions that involved relatively minor changes in the responses of key family members, interventions that were often dramatically effective. Most interventions involved training family members to eliminate those responses that were observed to increase the frequency of the disturbed behavior, and to increase those responses that appeared to promote desirable behavior. The training involved active learning through guided practice, therapist demonstration, and direct coaching of skills in the home setting. Benefits were measured by counting the frequency of disturbed responses, both during the training sessions and between sessions.

This early approach was further developed by Gerald Patterson and John Reid and their colleagues in Eugene, Oregon (Patterson et al. 1975). They recognized the limitations of the basic operant approaches, particularly when dealing with multiproblem families and with children who showed disturbances in multiple settings such as home and school. They demonstrated that the behavior of disturbed children was often the culmination of coercive patterns of parent-child interaction, and thereby validated the reciprocity concepts that were emerging from the theoretical constructs of the early systems theorists.

The reciprocity construct was given further support by Richard Stuart (1969), a social worker who was developing strategies for reducing marital distress. He devised a strategy known as *contingency contracting*, in which the aim was to increase pleasurable exchanges between marriage partners in a noncoercive manner. The partners agreed to exchange specific responses that each found pleasing, rather than to make demands for such responses from an unmotivated spouse. Stuart described this more rewarding interaction pattern as the "give-to-get" principle. To get the responses that you desire from other persons, it might be more efficient to give them what they want so that they will be motivated to reciprocate by meeting your needs.

A third major figure in the development of behavioral family therapy was the psychiatrist Robert Liberman. Liberman trained in social learning principles, which he applied to his work with adult patients with mental disorders (Liberman 1970). In addition to applying an operant conditioning framework to family interaction, he introduced the imitative learning principles of Bandura and Walters (1963). This included the use of modeling and role rehearsal to assist family members in acquiring more effective interpersonal communication patterns. Liberman emphasized the need for developing a collaborative therapeutic alliance with all family members and encouraged therapists to use their own expression of positive reinforcement, usually praise, to support the efforts of all participants. A final contribution involved the provision of straightforward education about mental disorders and their clinical management to all patients and their informal caregivers. This education was often provided in multifamily seminars and became the forerunner of the psychoeducational approach to family intervention (Falloon and Liberman 1984).

More recent developments encompassed the efforts of a broad range of scientist practitioners. Major innovations included the refinement of methods for assessing the strengths and weaknesses of family interaction, the introduction of structured training in problem-solving strategies, and the inclusion of the entire range of research-validated cognitive-behavioral strategies whenever they are specifically indicated. These innovations will be covered in greater depth later in this chapter.

Core Theoretical Assumptions

A core theoretical assumption of behavioral family therapists is that the family in its many guises constitutes the greatest natural resource for both the management of the stresses associated with personal development and the maintenance of a productive, satisfying life in our communities. It is all too easy to criticize the family when its breakdown appears to contribute to major health or psychosocial problems even though those problems are due to poor physical and emotional nurturance or to a lack of skills in dealing with major life crises such as bereavement, childbirth, or the breakup of a relationship. In contrast to these dramatic events, the everyday efforts that families contribute to the quality of life of their members may be readily overlooked. However, recent developments in research on the way people cope with stress suggest that the role of the family is crucial in helping people resolve major stresses in their lives. Furthermore, a series of studies has shown that the way in which a family helps its members cope with stress may be an important factor in their recovery from major physical and mental illnesses (Falloon and McGill 1985).

The stress-vulnerability model underpins most applications of BFT in the health field and can be readily adapted to provide a theoretical construct for psychosocial disturbance. Stress may be defined as an individual's response to threat. This response may be psychological, such as a recognition and emotional response; behavioral, such as an escape or avoidance response; physiological, such as an autonomic arousal, hormonal, or biochemical response; or a combination involving all three systems. In everyday terms, a person may realize that a situation is likely to be stressful, feel apprehensive about it, try to find ways to avoid dealing with it, and find that his or her blood pressure, heart rate, and adrenal hormone level are all higher than usual.

However, no two people react in exactly the same way to the same stress (Cooper et al. 1985). There is substantial variation in the patterns of stress responses, even when the stresses are of a similar nature, such as the death of a parent. It is likely that each person's response to stress is multidetermined, with biogenetic factors determining physiological response patterns, and psychological factors, such as personality, conditioning to past experiences, coping skills, and being prepared for an expected occurrence all determining the individual's actions in response to the specific stress. Thus, one person may react to a stressor by producing excess stomach acid leading to heartburn, another may react to the identical stressor by becoming quiet and socially withdrawn, another may react with feelings of frustration, and yet another may have no reaction at all.

Although patterns of stress responses vary widely from person to person, individuals tend to develop their own characteristic patterns. When that response is excessive, it may lead to a physical or mental disorder, such as a peptic ulcer or a depressive disorder, or a maladaptive psychosocial response, such as an aggressive outburst or self-destructive action (Kety 1984). Health problems are more likely to be triggered when a person is highly vulnerable to a specific disorder. This may be due to an inherited weakness, previous episodes of a major illness, or current poor health.

It is postulated that the risk of stress-related episodes of impairment is increased when stress exceeds an individual's vulnerability threshold. The level of this threshold is determined by a person's overall vulnerability at any point in time. Exceeding this threshold is associated with a high risk of impaired health or social functioning. Two types of stressors have been extensively researched: ambient stress and life events.

Ambient stress is the stress experienced in dealing with the day-to-day hassles of life in the community. It is an accumulation of stresses in the household, in social and leisure pursuits, and in the work environment (DeLongis et al. 1982). Such a wide range of stresses is extremely difficult to quantify (Cooper et al. 1985). However, household stress has been measured by indices such as expressed emotion (Vaughn and Leff 1976) and "family burden" (Grad and Sainsbury 1963). Work-related stress and stress in social relationships, including the stresses associated with homemaking, child care, unemployment, and interpersonal relationships, are less readily measured, yet undoubtedly are as important as family relationships as sources of ambient stress. Indices of ambient stress have been shown to predict the risk of recurrent episodes of major mental disorders (Brown and

Harris 1978; Leff and Vaughn 1985; Miklowitz et al. 1988), as well as many physical disorders (Cobb and Rose 1973; Friedman and Rosenman 1959).

Life events such as the loss of a job, the death of a close associate, or the breakup of an intimate relationship are more discrete stresses. Life events that lead to long-term increases in ambient stress have been associated with the onset of major health problems (Ambelas 1987; Brown and Birley 1968; Brown and Harris 1978; Edwards and Cooper 1988; Holmes and Masuda 1973; Tennant and Andrews 1978). It seems likely that regardless of the specific origins of stress, the longer a person's overall stress level remains above his stress threshold, the greater his chance of succumbing to the major health problems to which he is most vulnerable.

The coping behavior of an individual will modify the level of stress experienced from any stressor. This behavior includes all efforts to resolve the problems associated with the stressor and the individual's immediate responses to it. It encompasses the problem-solving capacity of the person's intimate social network, particularly the family unit (Billings and Moos 1981; Pearlin and Schooler 1978). If a person is able to communicate readily with other people in his or her social habitat, together they are able to assist in developing efficient strategies for handling the key problems, and the risk of a detrimental outcome is likely to be minimized (Falloon and McGill 1985). This process is summarized in Figure 7–1. It should be noted that all members of the household may experience increases in their stress levels as a result of shared concern for a major stress that impinges most directly on one member of the living group (e.g., one member losing a job, another having a baby, or another sitting important exams), and that the everyday tensions in the household may themselves exceed some persons' stress thresholds at times. Therefore, as well as dealing with the more dramatic life events, effective family management of stress involves dealing with everyday hassles and tensions and the problems of all members of the household, not merely those most vulnerable to health or psychosocial disorders.

It is concluded that the family, or alternative intimate living group, is the basic care unit in industrialized societies. It is the natural setting where members share their stresses with one another and seek assistance in its effective and efficient management. Considerable skill is required among all members of the living group to facilitate this process. Those skills are seldom taught in a systematic way in modern family development, which probably accounts for the high rate of family breakdown and family violence. It may even contribute to the higher rates of morbidity associated with mental and physical disorders found in industrialized societies when compared with tribal settings, where stress management is a highly structured part of everyday life (Falloon and McGill 1985). Certainly, when one

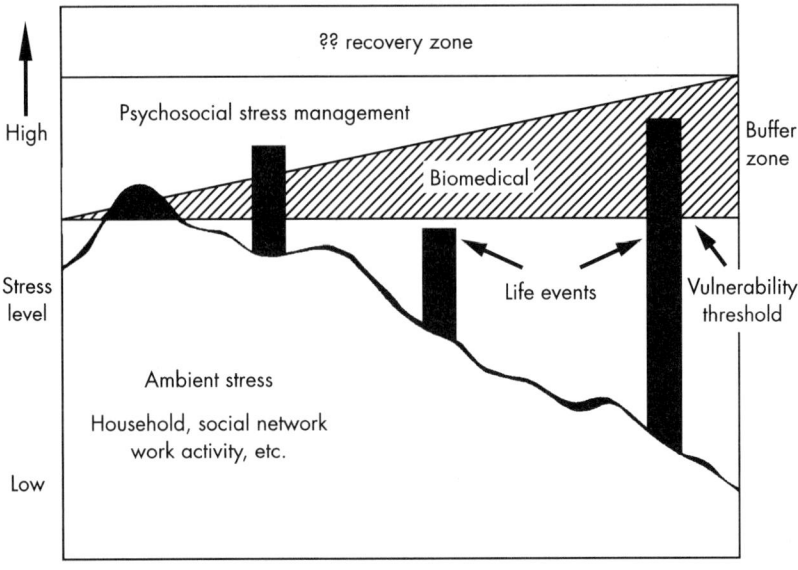

Figure 7–1. Stress, vulnerability, and clinical management in the determination of outcome of major health problems.

member of a household develops a disabling disorder of any kind, exceptionally efficient stress management is essential, not merely in assisting with that person's rehabilitation but also in enabling the other household members to sustain their efforts toward their own personal goals (McCubbin et al. 1980).

The Family as a Behavioral System

Although BFT is rooted in empirical concepts derived from social learning theory, it has also incorporated many aspects of systemic thinking. The concept of reciprocity in the exchange of reinforcing responses is one of the basic assumptions that underlies many strategies. Thibaut and Kelley (1959, p. 12) postulated that

> [t]he exact pattern of interaction that takes place between [family members] is never accidental; it represents the most rewarding of all the available alternatives…it represents the best balance which each can achieve between individual and mutual rewards and costs.

Family members are considered to always select the responses to specific situations that at each point in time represent their best efforts to resolve the problems that they confront. This is considered to apply even when the chosen responses appear destructive rather than constructive to harmonious relationships. Thus, behavioral family therapists have always acknowledged the problem-solving efforts of all family members rather than their achievements and attempt to build on the strengths of individuals, rather than focus on their all too obvious defects. Any attempts to change the response patterns of individuals must aim either to

- Increase the "rewards" or pleasant consequences an individual gains from the response
- Reduce the "costs" in terms of effort and unpleasant consequences
- Alter the contingencies that trigger that specific response pattern

Early social learning theory considered rewards in terms of basic reinforcement by primary reinforcers such as food, drink, and sex. However, a much broader view is considered in BFT. Tharp and Wetzel (1969, p. 3) summarized this as follows:

> Reinforcers lie within the environment of the individual, and are imbedded within this social nexus: whether the reinforcer is a smile or a candy, a bicycle or a slap, reinforcement is frequently displaced by people articulated into the individual's social environment. If the environment is the hospital, these people are the nurses, doctors or other patients; if the environment is the school, they are the principal, teachers or other pupils; if it is the family they are the siblings, the spouse or the parents.

What Is a Family?

Most family therapies address the needs of the typical, Western middle-class family of Mom, Dad, and two children, preferably one boy and one girl. However, households consisting of such stereotyped family arrangements are found less and less frequently. There are numerous other combinations of families, such as multigenerational, single parent, multiparent, multifamily, adopted parental, sibling, or avuncular households. There are in addition many people who live in family-style households who are not legally related. These include young adults sharing households and gay couples. Family-style households with unrelated members can also be found in residential schools and training centers, hostels, boarding homes, and lodgings.

Furthermore, family care extends well beyond the confines of the family home, with continued and extensive support being provided for family members when they are residing in households other than the family home. Vast improvements in telecommunications and modern transportation enable people to remain in close contact while at different ends of the earth.

The concept of the intimate social network that provides both emotional and physical support for an individual on an everyday basis probably encompasses the notion of a "family" much better than that tied solely to people sharing a living space, or those related by birth. Even the homeless person sleeping on the streets may have a close support network of fellow itinerants who are deeply concerned for his or her day-to-day welfare. It is a sad reflection that sometimes people in such situations may receive greater supportive human contact than those living in mansions with relatives or those in the splendid social isolation of modern housing estates.

The definition of family as used in BFT is a broad one that requires one of two features to be present. A family can consist of either

- Those people who live in one household unit, sharing the everyday responsibility for the organization and maintenance of that unit; or
- Those people who are the key providers of emotional support for an individual on an everyday basis, regardless of the location of their residence.

Methodology

Behavioral Analysis of Mental Disorder in the Family

The baseline assessment of family functioning and the continual review that is conducted as part of every session is the framework on which behavioral intervention strategies are constructed. The initial behavioral analysis may involve several hours of painstaking individual and conjoint interviews as well as systematic observation. When one member is vulnerable to a major disorder, a range of stressful problems is often evident. Each of these problems is explored in the assessment process. The therapist attempts to obtain the following:

- *A therapeutic alliance with all family members.* The presenting problems are used as a starting point for the analysis of the functioning of the family as a problem-solving unit. Each component of the system (individual, dyad, triad, etc.) is explored in order to discover its strengths and weaknesses in relationship to those specific issues. At its most straightforward level this step consists of defining the specific contingencies that surround a specific problem behavior. For example, what precedes a family argument, or increases agitated behavior, and what are the usual consequences of that behavior? By interviewing each family member individually rather than obtaining the consensus view provided by a family

group, the therapist gains a broader picture of the setting of the presenting problems. Generalizations tend to be avoided. However, reports of problem behavior are often distorted by the search for simple causal relationships, so that at this stage the therapist can derive only a series of hypotheses to be confirmed in subsequent observation of the actual behavioral sequences.
- *Detailed information about each family member's observations, thoughts, and feelings about the presenting problems.* This includes the level of understanding of the nature and treatment of the index patient's disorder, when this is a relevant aspect of family stress.
- *Information about each family member's interaction within the family system.* This includes the family member's attitudes, feelings, and behavior toward the other family members and his or her support for efforts to resolve presenting problems.
- *Information about each family member's functioning in settings outside the family unit.* This includes his or her personal assets and deficits that might be relevant to problem-resolution processes.

Ideally, observations of family functioning are conducted in the circumstances in which the presenting problems arise, usually at home. Although such naturalistic observations are invaluable, they may be too costly for routine practice. Alternatives include the family's tape-recording interactions at targeted times, time sampling of recordings with automated time switches, reenactment of problem situations by family members, or family discussions about "hot issues." Nevertheless, at least one home visit is an essential part of the behavioral assessment and usually provides the therapist with an abundance of valuable information seldom accessible in clinic-based assessments.

The behavioral family therapist is interested not merely in pinpointing the setting in which problem behavior is most likely to arise, but also in ascertaining the family's past and current efforts to cope with the behavior. It usually emerges that any problem is present only a small proportion of the time and arises only on a proportion of occasions when it might be expected. Even a severely depressed person has extensive periods when his or her main symptoms are not observed, and episodes of violence or criminal misdemeanors tend to be episodic. From another viewpoint, most behavior observed in families is positive or neutral (i.e., nonproblematic), and for the most part families have already learned some strategies to cope with the major problems. Thus, the therapist is interested in uncovering those contingencies that exist when the targeted problem is quiescent, as well as those that exist when the problem is present but results in minimal distress. It is assumed that although the family may have developed responses to cope with the problem, these coping behaviors are only partially effective, often because family members apply them in an inconsistent manner or do not persist to derive benefit from these coping efforts. When such effective strategies can be pinpointed, the therapist is left with the relatively straightforward task of assisting the family to enhance the efficacy of their preexisting interaction patterns. Such a targeted intervention may take a mere session or two, but the behavioral analysis that precedes it may be a much longer process.

Major health and psychosocial problems play havoc with the everyday routine of family living. A survey of the current activities of all family members is contrasted with their desired activity patterns. Each family member is invited to describe his or her most frequent activities, as well as the people, places, and objects that he or she spends most time in contact with. Discrepancies between current and expected activity levels help the therapist pinpoint key areas of dissatisfaction that may assist in defining specific goals related to each family member's quality of life.

In addition to listing activities that induce pleasing responses, the family is asked to discuss aversive situations. Unpleasant situations that tend to be avoided may vary from simple phobias to various family interactions, such as arguments, discussions about finances, or sexual concerns. Feelings of rejection, isolation, frustration, coercion, lack of support, mistrust, and intrusiveness may be discussed in this context. Family members are asked to provide clear examples of interactions in which they experience these negative feelings.

This survey of reinforcing and aversive situations often provides a fascinating picture of the manner in which families' everyday activities intertwine in patterns of mutual reinforcement, positively in happy families and negatively in distressed families in which marked avoidance of intimacy, confrontation, or coercion may predominate. Interviews of daily activities are notoriously unreliable, particularly when the family members are interviewed at times of high stress. In obtaining a more precise assessment of family activity, it may be necessary to invite family members to complete daily activity schedules.

A final use of the reinforcement survey involves the selection of positive reinforcers that may be employed in the promotion of specific behavior change during the intervention phase. Activities, places, people, and objects that are deemed highly desirable can be employed to mediate change when used as specific rewards for performance of targeted behaviors.

At the completion of the behavioral analysis, the therapist will be able to specify the short-term personal goals of each family member and the conflicts and problems that may need to be resolved to achieve these goals. These may include symptoms of the mental disorder, as well as relationship difficulties that appear to impede problem resolution within the family unit.

Functional Analysis: A Behavioral System

The behavioral analysis provides a clear basis for identifying a list of potential intervention targets. However, such a list does not tell us where to begin. The behavioral family therapist aims to pinpoint the key deficits within the family group whose resolution will lead to maximal change. As mentioned earlier, it is assumed that the patterns of family behavior that are observed at any point in time represent the optimal response of every family member to the resolution of the existing problem. Even when chaotic, distressing responses are observed, every family member is attempting to resolve the problem (or achieve the goal) in the manner he or she considers most rewarding (or least distressing), given all the constraints imposed by the biopsychosocial system at that time.

Rather than attempt to impose his or her own optimal solutions to the problem, the behavioral family therapist aims to employ minimal intervention that will build on existing family assets. For example, when one family member is observed to be able to get a disturbed adolescent to assist with household chores, the therapist examines that person's behavior closely and pinpoints the specific effective strategies that person employs. A note is made that effective strategies are already present within the family unit and that the skilled member may be co-opted to train others in the intervention plan.

The functional analysis involves the exploration of the family system from a behavioral perspective so that a long list of potential targets for intervention can be reduced to one or two key deficits that often can be addressed in a straightforward manner. These issues are not restricted to purely psychosocial parameters, but may include biological variables such as changes in hormonal systems that may trigger or maintain mood disturbance, or the specific benefits of drug therapies. If the latter are observed to produce significant relief of specific symptoms of a medical condition in an efficient manner, they are strongly advocated, despite evidence that family patterns of behavior may appear to have contributed to the onset or maintenance of the disorder.

Thus, a purely pragmatic approach is employed that endeavors to facilitate effective problem resolution and goal achievement for every family member in the most efficient manner. Of course, this includes efforts to ensure that similar problems do not recur in the future. In most cases of major disorders, interventions are targeted to multiple systems. Drugs are used to correct biological deficiencies, psychological interventions to correct cognitive-behavioral disabilities, family interventions to enhance family problem-solving functions, and social interventions to deal with financial, work, and friendship stresses.

These varied biomedical and psychosocial strategies can be subsumed under a problem-solving paradigm. Maximizing the efficiency of the mutual problem-solving functions of patients and their family members enables them to become actively involved in all aspects of clinical management. The final assessment of family functioning involves observation of the family group attempting to resolve a problem that is a current hot issue for them. Behavioral observation focuses on the strengths and weaknesses of interpersonal communication, such as clear expression of unpleasant feelings and active listening, as well as specific components of problem solving such as problem definition, choosing solutions, and planning.

At the completion of the functional analysis, the behavioral family therapist is able to draw up an initial intervention program with one or two clearly defined therapy goals and a systematic treatment plan targeted to these goals. A time frame is defined and a contract of a specific number of sessions is agreed on with the family. Continuous measures of progress toward the goals are defined to guide the therapist from session to session, and a date is set for a detailed review at the end of the contracted sessions. After this review, goals and intervention plans may be modified or changed and a further contract for therapy may be developed.

The key intervention strategies employed in BFT include

1. Education about specific disorders and their clinical management
2. Communication skills training
3. Problem-solving training
4. Specific cognitive-behavioral strategies
5. Crisis intervention
6. Managing therapist concerns

Education About Specific Disorders and Their Clinical Management

The initial sessions are usually devoted to providing the patient and family with a straightforward explanation of the nature of the disorder and its treatment. Handouts are provided and the index patient is invited to describe his or her experiences of the disorder and its treatment. The vulnerability-stress theory is outlined as a framework for integrating the benefits of combining biomedical and psychosocial interventions to reduce morbidity. Throughout treatment, revision of this education is conducted whenever indicated; for example, when patients display reluctance to continuing with the recommended diet or to apply a reinforcement program in the appropriate manner, or on occasions when major stresses threaten to overwhelm the coping resources of the family. The early warning signs of imminent episodes of an index patient's disorder are clearly delineated so that the patients and family members can take immediate action to avert major episodes.

Communication Skills Training

The goal of communication skills training in BFT is to facilitate family problem-solving discussions. The ability to define problems or goals in a highly specific fashion, to reinforce progress toward objectives in small steps, to prompt behavior change without coercion, and to listen with empathy enables problems and goals of all kinds to be dealt with in an optimal fashion. Most families can improve their interpersonal communication substantially and benefit from several sessions of communication training. The skills are trained through repeated practice among family members, with instructions, coaching, and reinforcement of progress in a manner identical to that employed in social skills training. Homework practice is a key component to ensure that the skills are not restricted to practice within the therapy sessions but can be generalized to everyday interaction.

Problem-Solving Training

Enhancing the efficiency of the problem solving of the family unit is the key goal of BFT approaches (D'Zurilla and Goldfried 1976). In BFT, unlike most family interventions, the therapist aims to teach families to convene their own structured sessions of problem solving, rather than to assist them in their problem solving during therapist-led sessions. The therapy sessions resemble training workshops in which the families learn the skills that they apply later in their own problem-solving discussions. Only at times when stresses threaten to overwhelm the family problem-solving capacity, or when the early signs of an impending major episode of a mental disorder are detected, does the therapist consider becoming an active participant in the family problem-solving effort.

The steps employed include

1. *Definition of the problem or goal.* Pinpointing the exact issue that is to be addressed.
2. *Listing alternative solutions.* Brainstorming to produce a list of five or six possible solutions.
3. *Evaluating the consequences of proposed solutions.* Making a brief review to highlight the main strengths and weaknesses of each alternative solution.
4. *Choosing the optimal solution.* Asking the participants to choose the solution that best suits the current resources and skills of the family.

5. *Planning.* Drawing up a detailed plan to define the specific steps to ensure efficient implementation of the optimal solution.
6. *Review of implementation.* Reviewing the efforts of the participants in their attempts to implement the agreed-on plan in a constructive manner that facilitates continued efforts until resolution has been achieved.

The family assigns one of their members as the chairperson and secretary to assist in convening a regular family meeting at least weekly, in administering the meeting, and in reporting back on their efforts during each therapy session. A guide sheet that outlines the six-step method is used to record family discussions and assist the therapist in his or her review. Social skills training is provided whenever family members are deficient in their use of one or more steps of the method. The therapist avoids getting personally involved in suggesting or choosing solutions, leaving that to the family.

Specific Cognitive-Behavioral Strategies

Once participants learn to use the problem-solving approach there are relatively few occasions on which families are unable to devise effective strategies to resolve their problems or achieve their goals. However, when a family appears to be struggling to come up with an effective strategy and there is a well-validated procedure for the management of that particular issue, the therapist may offer that procedure to the family as one possible solution. Common examples of this include

1. The use of operant reinforcement procedures to enhance motivation to perform tasks that are not inherently reinforcing, such as household chores and work activities
2. Desensitization procedures for specific anxiety-provoking situations
3. Cognitive strategies for persistent negative or unwanted thoughts
4. Social skills training for coping with difficult interpersonal situations
5. Coping strategies for persistent hallucinations or delusions; strategies for sexual dysfunction
6. Relaxation strategies for muscle tension and insomnia

Although this six-step method is preserved, the therapist outlines the strategy in detail for the family and assists them in its implementation.

Drug treatment can be targeted in a similar fashion to specific problems, including tranquilizers for overactivity and psychotic perceptual distortions; lithium for mood swings, especially elation; and tricyclics for generalized anxiety, retardation, appetite reduction, and late insomnia.

Crisis Intervention

A second occasion when the therapist may become involved directly in the problem solving is when a major crisis impedes family ability to conduct its own problem solving in a calm, constructive manner. On these occasions the therapist may choose to chair the problem-solving discussion in order to facilitate rapid stress reduction and thereby prevent symptomatic exacerbation.

Managing Therapist Concerns

Finally, when family members fail to adhere to the recommended treatment program, thereby producing strong negative feelings in the therapist, the therapist may choose to express his or her feelings directly to the family and to chair a problem-solving discussion that aims to relieve his or her personal distress. Issues such as failure to complete homework tasks, missing sessions, and not adhering to prescribed drug regimens are among the issues that engender high levels of therapist distress.

Wherever possible the specific effects of each intervention are assessed by introducing them one at a time and by measuring specific change on the targeted problem behavior in a multiple-baseline design. This process assists in the continuing functional analysis of the disorder. For example, when generalized improvement occurs from the introduction of an antidepressant drug directed primarily at severe anorexia, it may be postulated that a primary disorder of biological systems existed. When a cognitive-behavioral strategy produced similar changes, it would tend to support a predominantly psychosocial deficit. However, the conclusions of such speculation should be viewed with caution in the light of our very limited understanding of the origins of mental disorders.

The severity of the disorder in the index patient and the management skills of the family members will determine the level of input from the therapy team. This will vary from once-a-week sessions to working with the patient and family two or three times a day. Whenever possible, these sessions are conducted in the family home so that generalization of skills is maximized. Each session involves practical training in specific skills with instructions, demonstrations, guided practice, and supportive coaching. Emphasis is placed on shaping the preexisting skills of family members and self-help strategies for patients. Session-by-session review is conducted to evaluate patients' and family members' progress toward their personal goals, acquisition of efficient problem-solving functions, and reduction in specified problem behaviors.

The range of problems that are likely to benefit from the application of BFT is summarized in Table 7–1.

Table 7–1. Problems likely to benefit from behavioral family therapy strategies

Psychosocial	Biomedical
Conduct disorders in children	Depression
Mental handicap and autism	Bipolar disorders
Adolescent behavioral disturbance	Schizophrenia
Marriage and family conflict	Anxiety disorders
Sexual dysfunction	Relapse prevention
Drug and alcohol misuse	Chronic physical health problems
Family violence and child abuse	Dementias
Premarital counseling	Stress-related disorders in high-risk groups (prevention)
Divorce mediation	
Eating disorders	
Suicide prevention	
Residential care: homes, hostels, etc.	
Criminal offending problems	

Summary

Behavioral family therapy provides a structure for assisting people living together in small, shared living groups to enhance the quality of their efforts to help each other in coping with the multitude of stresses that they encounter in their everyday lives, as well as those less frequent major life crises. This is achieved mainly through improving the efficiency of the problem-solving functions of the group through enhancement of interpersonal communication skills combined with clearer structuring of regular problem-solving discussions. The overall aim is to minimize periods of high stress that threaten to overwhelm the coping capacity of members of the household, particularly those members who may be highly vulnerable to stress-related health or psychosocial problems. Additional strategies, including the full range of cognitive and behavioral strategies, psychoeducation, and targeted pharmacotherapy may all be combined with this approach to provide a comprehensive plan of care for serious psychosocial and health problems.

Research

Efficacy of BFT in Major Mental Disorders

The first question for the behavior therapist is whether the specific goals of the therapy were achieved in a specific manner. The main goal of BFT in treating major mental disorders is to enhance problem-solving efficiency of the family unit. In a controlled study that compared BFT with individual supportive therapy (IST) of similar intensity in the long-term management of schizophrenia, measures of family problem-solving indicated that after the intensive first 3-month phase the quantity of problem-solving statements in the BFT condition had trebled, whereas no significant change in the numbers of family problem-solving statements was noted after 3 months of IST (Doane et al. 1986). Perhaps more significantly, the quality of family problem solving that was observed by independent assessors who interviewed the families about everyday stressful events showed a significant linear improvement over the first 9 months of treatment in families receiving BFT. No benefits were noted for IST families. Similar levels of stress were encountered by families in each condition. Thus, it is reasonable to conclude that BFT may be associated with specific improvements in family problem-solving functions and consequent stress management.

It was hypothesized that specific changes in the ability of families to cope with a wide range of stressful life situations would be associated with clinical benefits. The evidence for this is impressive. First, BFT patients experienced fewer major episodes of schizophrenia during the 2-year period. Three BFT patients (17%) experienced a total of seven major episodes, while 83% of IST patients experienced 41 major episodes of schizophrenia and in addition 11 major depressive episodes (compared with 5 major depressive episodes in the BFT patients). These clinicians' observations were supported by blind ratings of psychopathology that indicated that not only were the florid symptoms of schizophrenia more stable in BFT patients, but there was a sustained improvement from baseline levels, suggesting that BFT may have promoted further symptom remission (Falloon et al.1985). A trend (almost reaching statistical significance at the 5% level) was noted on the Brief Psychiatric Rating Scale (BPRS) withdrawal factor that suggested that the BFT was associated with reduction in negative symptoms of schizophrenia. At the end of 2 years, one-half of the BFT patients showed no evidence of any mental disorder on blind Present State Examination interviews. By contrast, 83% of IST patients still showed evidence of schizophrenic symptoms at 2 years, although they too showed a trend toward remission, albeit on a much slower trajectory. Thus, the benefits for BFT appear genuine and not attributable to a comparative deterioration of the IST group. Nor were these benefits associated with differences in the drug treatment received by patients in the two conditions. Indeed, BFT patients tended to have lower doses of neuroleptics than IST patients, and although the latter had more difficulty maintaining adequate compliance, this was remedied through the use of intramuscular preparations and other compliance strategies.

The achievement of clinical stability and remission is an important goal in the rehabilitation of a chronic disorder. However, a more crucial goal from the patient's perspective is the restoration of social functioning. We should never forget that clinical stability is readily achieved by removing persons with schizophrenia from community living and placing them into less stressful settings (Lamb and Goertzel 1971). BFT, with its emphasis on achieving functional goals for patients, was associated with social benefits. BFT patients doubled the time they spent in constructive work activities compared with the 2 years before the study. Blind ratings of measures of social performance showed significant improvements over the 2-year study period as well as significantly greater benefits than those achieved by IST patients. The greatest comparative benefits for BFT were in the areas of work activity, household tasks, and friendships outside the family (Falloon et al. 1987).

The family members of persons with chronic disorders tend to lead impoverished lives and experience considerable distress themselves (Hatfield 1981). An effective management approach would be expected to reduce levels of burdens on caregivers. BFT was associated with increased satisfaction for relatives as well as patients, even when the benefits to individual patients were limited. The burden associated with the care of the patients was reduced over the 2 years so that 17% of family members reported moderate or severe levels of burden at that point. On the other hand almost two-thirds of families who received IST continued to complain of moderate or severe burden at 2 years. Together with the earlier evidence of enhanced management of a wide range of family stresses, this finding suggests that the benefits of BFT extended beyond those for the index patients and were experienced by the family as a whole.

Although the number of subjects in this study was too small to allow detailed multivariate analysis, the data supported the conclusion that the specific changes in family problem-solving behavior that were induced by BFT were associated with the clinical and social benefits (Doane et al. 1986; Falloon 1985).

Furthermore, increasingly efficient family problem-solving behavior was shown to generalize to a wide range of family stresses and appeared to have an impact on major life events. BFT families appeared to use their problem-solving behavior to reduce the stressful impact of life events (Hardesty et al. 1985). During the first 12 months of the study, the 18 families experienced only three life events that were associated with high levels of long-term threat, as defined by Brown and Harris (1978). Thus, the benefits of BFT appeared to derive from a reduction in both the stress of everyday household difficulties and the stress associated with major life events. This combined effect appeared to be sustained throughout the less intensive second year of the study, although the data were incomplete and a comprehensive analysis was not conducted. It is probable that the continued benefits in both clinical and social morbidity were achieved as a result of continued use of the structured problem-solving approach in the management of stress and the promotion of social functioning.

Studies With Schizophrenia and Depression

The third generation of BFT studies, including studies of the effects of BFT on schizophrenia and depression, are now well under way. These studies are of two types. The first type attempts to employ the BFT methods with different clinical and social populations. The second type attempts to analyze the relative contributions of the major components of the approach. Studies are in progress in Munich, Los Angeles (three studies, one with Hispanic families), Providence, Naples, Athens, Manchester, Birmingham, Southampton, Sydney, and Bonn. There is also a multicenter collaborative study now in progress in five U.S. cities. Publication of the results of these studies is awaited. Preliminary results suggest that most will replicate the major findings of the University of Southern California (USC) project. One major study completed in Salford, England, found similar benefits for a behavioral problem-solving approach that was applied with families (Tarrier et al. 1988b). Unfortunately, no specific benefits for social functioning appeared to be associated with this rather less intensive approach in the more chronically disabled population studied. Additional field trials showed that similar results can be obtained when the approach is applied within everyday clinical practice (Brooker et al. 1992; Curran 1988; Whitfield et al. 1988).

The large number of controlled and uncontrolled studies of BFT with schizophrenic disorders is contrasted with the few attempts to evaluate its effectiveness with affective disorders. Apart from the Seattle study with depressive disorders (Jacobson 1988), the only other study in progress is comparing the effects of adding BFT to lithium in the long-term management of bipolar disorders (Miklowitz and Goldstein 1990).

The NIMH Treatment Strategies in Schizophrenia Collaborative Study is attempting to examine the interaction between neuroleptic drugs and family interventions in the aftercare of schizophrenia. Five centers—Payne Whitney Clinic; Hillside Hospital (Long Island); Emery/Grady University; San Francisco General Hospital; and Medical College of Pennsylvania (EPPI)—have been selected for the study. Therapists at each center have been trained to stabilize patients who have experienced a recent episode of schizophrenia with optimal doses of neuroleptic drugs before randomly allocating them to double-blind fluphenazine decanoate in one of three doses:

1. Continued optimal dose
2. One-fifth the optimal dose
3. Targeted doses of fluphenazine associated with periods when early warning signs of an impending episode are detected

Random allocation to BFT or a supportive family intervention is made independently. All families are invited to participate in an educational workshop and a monthly educational support group and receive crisis support when needed. The BFT is similar to that employed in the USC study, with one significant modification: the therapists are not behavior therapists and have not been trained to apply sophisticated behavioral programs, such as depression or anxiety management, social skills training, or token economies, within the family problem-solving framework. Thus, the method concentrates almost entirely on enhancing the general problem-solving functions of the family units.

BFT is provided for at least 12 months after stabilization and continues throughout episodes of florid schizophrenia or hospital admissions, in a manner similar to the USC study. The main hypothesis being tested in this study is that BFT, with its effectiveness in enhancing stress management, may reduce the need for higher doses of neuroleptic medication and hence the detrimental effects associated with these drugs. However, the large number of cases entering the study will enable a wide range of secondary issues to be explored. These include the association between therapist competency and therapeutic outcome; the association between problem-solving skills and outcome; the specific benefits of more intensive, targeted family therapy; the cost-effectiveness of these approaches; and predictors of therapeutic efficacy.

The Buckingham Early Intervention Project was based on the assumption that if BFT is effective in reducing the frequency of major schizophrenic and depressive episodes in established cases of schizophrenia, a similar approach might reduce the morbidity associated with initial episodes of schizophrenic and major affective disorders. An attempt was made to detect cases during the prodromal phases of these disorders, when major episodes appeared imminent. The current absence of clear biological measures of vulnerability limited early detection strategies to recognition of the clinical features through screening by primary care physicians, who worked in close collaboration with highly trained mental health professionals. The detection of a suspected prodromal state led to immediate intervention with BFT and targeted low-dose neuroleptics or antidepressants when appropriate. BFT focused on stress management and educating the index patient and caregivers to recognize the main symptoms of these mental disorders. The drugs were discontinued as soon as the prodromal features remitted.

Early results support the feasibility of this approach, with more than 100 cases being successfully managed in this way. A tenfold reduction in the expected incidence of schizophrenic and major affective disorders has been observed. Further efforts are being made to conduct a controlled evaluation of this approach.

The increasing sophistication of intervention strategies has been accompanied by similar advances in the assessment process. Rather than merely counting the numbers of positive and negative responses observed during problem-related discussions, methods of examining sequences of family interaction have been developed. The methods developed by Hahlweg and his colleagues (Hahlweg et al. 1984a, 1984b) allowed heated arguments to be mapped and contrasted with constructive expressions of unpleasant feelings that contribute to effective conflict resolution. It was established that the expression of unpleasant feelings in a manner that assisted in the clear definition of a specific problem, rather than through coercive nagging or hostile comments, was a crucial first step in conflict resolution.

Efficacy of Behavioral Family Therapy in Other Disorders

The effectiveness of BFT interventions has been demonstrated in a wide range of client group concerns, including marital distress (Jacobson and Margolin 1979; Weiss 1980), premarital counseling (Markman and Floyd 1980), childhood conduct disorders (Griest and Wells 1983), adolescent conflict (Alexander and Parsons 1982; Foster et al. 1983), developmental disability (Harris 1983), and dementias (J. M. Zarit and Zarit 1982; S. H. Zarit and Zarit 1982).

Controlled-outcome studies of BFT approaches for major affective disorders have been conducted in Los Angeles and Colorado (Miklowitz and Goldstein 1997). These studies showed that benefits similar to those found in studies of schizophrenic disorders can be derived from BFT for bipolar disorders. The adjunctive use of BFT strategies in a range of other disorders, such as anxiety, anorexia and bulimia, depression, and substance abuse, showed added benefits from this integration (Falloon 1988).

Recent Developments

In the past 10 years further outcome research led to the conclusion that family therapies based on the BFT model are among the prime treatments of choice for psychotic disorders. More than 20 high-quality studies have been conducted. The studies vary considerably in the specific BFT intervention strategies examined. The most basic merely provided several sessions giving information about drug treatments (Hornung et al. 1995). Others extended for several years, with continued education, stress management strategies, social skills training, vocational training, specific cognitive-behavioral strategies, and home-based crisis management when necessary (Hahlweg et al. 1995; Hogarty et al. 1986; McFarlane et al. 1995a, 1995b, 1996; Tarrier et al. 1988b; Veltro et al. 1996).

Since 1980, 14 random, controlled trials have compared individualized case management and maintenance medication with or without the addition of a BFT-based family approach. Of these, 11 showed a significant advantage for the stress management approach (Falloon et al. 1984, 1985; Hogarty et al. 1986; Hornung et al. 1995; Leff et al. 1982; McFarlane et al. 1996; Randolph et al. 1994; Tarrier et al. 1988b; Veltro et al. 1996; Xiong et al. 1994; Zhang and Yan 1993; Zhang et al. 1994); two showed no significant difference (Buchkremer et al. 1995; Linszen et al. 1996); and one showed a significant advantage for individual case management (Telles et al. 1995). An analysis of the benefits in terms of the proportion of cases maintained in treatment for 1 year without any form of major psychopathological exacerbations showed a 26% advantage for the stress management strategies (relative risk of exacerbation $RR=0.61$; CI $0.57<RR<0.65$; chi-square=222.49; $P<0.00000001$). During the 12-month period, 62% of cases had a successful outcome, compared with 37% of cases not receiving family-based stress management.

But the absence of major exacerbations is not the only goal of long-term treatment. Most patients experience continuing psychotic and deficit psychopathology for some time after a major psychotic episode. The benefits of stress management strategies in reducing this residual psychopathology, and thereby enhancing the trend toward full remission of schizophrenia, were assessed in 11 studies (Buchkremer et al. 1995; Falloon et al. 1985; Hahlweg et al. 1995; McFarlane et al. 1996; Montero and Asencio 1996; Randolph et al. 1994; Telles et al. 1995; Veltro et al. 1996; Xiong et al. 1994; Zastowny et al. 1992; Zhang et al. 1994). These studies compared rating scales of psychopathology at the time of random assignment, when patients entered the comparative phase of the studies, with the ratings obtained a year later. In all but one of these studies (Zhang et al. 1994), an overall trend toward recovery was observed, both with experimental and control treatments. Zhang and his colleagues (1994) noted this trend only in patients receiving the family management, who remained free of exacerbation. The benefit of adding a BFT-based approach was again evident, with the finding of a mean reduction of psychopathology of 32% from the stabilized baseline levels, compared with a 14% reduction for case management and drug treatment.

Perhaps the most important goal of BFT is to enhance people's abilities to function in a full range of social roles. The social benefits of 11 methodologically adequate studies showed a mean gain of 18% for family management and 2% for control conditions. Four studies showed significantly greater benefits for BFT strategies (Falloon et al. 1985; Veltro et al. 1996; Xiong et al. 1994; Zhang and Yan 1993), one showed a clear trend (McFarlane et al. 1996), and three showed no significant benefits when compared with drug treatment and case management (Buchkremer et al. 1995; Hornung et al. 1995, Randolph et al. 1994).

BFT strategies also aim to enhance family functioning and reduce stress, particularly that associated with caregiving roles. A mean reduction in the stress of caregiving of 34% was reported in four studies using family interventions (Falloon et al. 1985; Hahlweg et al. 1995; McFarlane et al. 1996; Zhang and Yan 1993). This was contrasted with a stress reduction of 9% in the drug and case management conditions. Four of the five studies that compared standardized family stress ratings associated with stress management and drugs and case management showed significant advantages for the stress management approach (Falloon et al. 1985; Veltro et al. 1996; Xiong et al. 1994; Zhang and Yan 1993). In one study (Buchkremer et al. 1995), no change was noted in family problems associated with the patients' illness, but the relatives showed increased warmth and reduced hostility toward the patients.

The studies included in this review varied in the duration for which BFT strategies were applied from 6 months to 4 years, with most of the studies providing this treatment for 9–12 months. It was apparent that benefits endured, and trends toward clinical and social recovery continued, when the treatment approach was continued without major modifications throughout the study period (Falloon et al. 1985, 1996; Hogarty et al. 1991; McFarlane et al. 1995a, 1995b, 1996). In cases in which treatment was not continuous, it was noted that the stress of impending termination of a successful treatment program might have contributed to an excess of episodes during this period (Hogarty et al. 1991). However, withdrawal of BFT was not usually associated with an immediate cessation of apparent clinical benefits. The studies that examined clinical benefits over at least 2 years showed a 23% advantage for BFT in minimizing major clinical episodes (Falloon et al. 1985, 1996; Hogarty et al. 1991; Hornung et al. 1995; Leff et al. 1988; McFarlane et al. 1995a, 1995b, 1996; Tarrier et al. 1989).

Field Trials

One major concern raised by previous reviews (Lam 1992; Lehman et al. 1995; Pharoah et al. 2000) has been the ability to apply BFT methods in routine clinical practice or field trials. There has been a tendency to dilute the methods, using only part of the intervention program, usually education about mental disorders (Atkinson et al. 1996; Bäuml et al. 1996; Ehlert 1989; Goldman and Quinn 1988; Greenberg et al. 1988; Hill and Black 1987; Kelly and Scott 1990; Lebrun et al. 1991; Leung et al. 1989; MacCarthy et al. 1989; McCreadie et al. 1991; Pilsecker 1981; Seltzer et al. 1980; Smith et al. 1990; Vaughan et al. 1992; Williams 1989; Xiong et al. 1994). Although some of these studies showed limited benefits, particularly improved adherence to medication and better relationships with professionals (Bäuml et al. 1996; Cozolino and Goldstein 1986; Kelly and Scott 1990; Xiong et al. 1994), more substantial clinical and social benefits are generally less than those associated with more comprehensive programs applied over longer periods. A series of comprehensive field trials have been completed, with almost all reporting successful replication of the controlled trial results (Berglund 1996; Bertrando et al. 1992; Brooker et al. 1992, 1994; Curran 1988; Falloon and Fadden 1993; Held 1995; Kavanagh et al. 1993; McGorry et al. 1996; Rund et al. 1994).

Multifamily Versus Single Family BFT

A series of seven studies that compared BFT in multifamily groups with that provided in individual family sessions showed a mean advantage of 2% greater clinical success (37% versus 34%) in the first year of treatment (Falloon et al. 1996; Hornung et al. 1995; Leff et al. 1989; McFarlane et al. 1995a, 1995b, 1996; Montero and Asencio 1996; Schooler et al. 1997). Only one study compared a multiple family group with a medication and case management control (Buchkremer et al. 1995). This study of relatives' groups, which did not involve the patients and which was not strictly a BFT approach, showed a higher rate of hospital admissions than the control condition. High attrition from multifamily groups reduces the effectiveness of this approach, which nevertheless may be delivered at a lower direct cost (McFarlane et al. 1995a). However, adequate economic analysis that includes all costs and benefits is not yet available to support this preliminary conclusion. A well-controlled multicentered study in Italy may provide clearer information about the advantages and disadvantages of multi- and unifamily strategies.

The addition of social skills training strategies to help patients cope more effectively with stresses in community settings outside the family orbit appears to confer an added benefit to those methods that focus more on stresses within the patient's immediate social network. Five studies that combined social skills training strategies with family-based stress management appeared to have had the best clinical outcomes (Falloon et al. 1985; Hogarty et al. 1986; Tarrier et al. 1988b; Veltro et al. 1996; Wallace and

Liberman 1985). Only 19% of patients receiving this integrated approach had poor outcomes during the first year of treatment.

Attempts to substantially lower dosages of drugs below those deemed to be clinically optimal proved relatively unsuccessful (Hahlweg et al. 1995; Schooler et al. 1997). However, in both these studies the dose of drugs was rapidly and substantially lowered, rather than gradually reduced in the manner recommended in optimal clinical practice. Hahlweg et al. (1995) showed a relatively low rate of major episodes with a targeted dose strategy while regular stress management sessions were conducted.

Conclusions and Future Directions

Behavioral family therapy is a highly effective treatment approach for a wide range of mental health disorders. Future clinical and research efforts should focus on refining the strategies and improving the effectiveness and efficiency of the approach. To do this, improved methods of assessing the needs of patients and their relatives that can target specific stresses and strategies in an individualized manner may prove helpful. To this end, the type and amount of different strategies can be tailored to need and phase of illness, as well as to the life goals of the individual (American Psychiatric Association 1997). This may mean applying these strategies in residential care settings, which are alternatives to family care (H. Katschnig, personal communication, 1994). There is a need to develop strategies to maintain the use of the specific skills after the intensive training has been completed so that the prophylactic benefits continue and the potential for full and lasting clinical and social recovery is facilitated.

The high rates of successful application of these methods somewhat obscure the problems associated with the approach, including failure to derive any benefits. Although it has been accepted that some families are slower learners than others, it has been assumed that given sufficient time, all families can acquire the skills and utilize them to manage their stresses. However, in recent years greater emphasis has been placed on those people who have major problems incorporating these communication and problem-solving strategies into their everyday lives (Birchler 1988). At the moment, there is little research to support the use of any particular strategies for enhancing adherence to the relatively small, but highly significant, changes in lifestyle that these methods seek to achieve. However, there is evidence that the training methods employed by therapists may play an important role (Patterson 1988; Patterson et al. 1975). This has led to the development of methods of assessing the competence of therapists in the application of behavioral interventions with families (Laporta et al. 1989).

Behavioral family therapy has made a major contribution to clinical practice, supported strongly by controlled research trials. It has proven highly adaptable to a wide range of problems, including major mental disorders. Therapists can deliver this form of family therapy in a competent manner after relatively brief training. However, these benefits have yet to be fully realized in clinical practice, where BFT remains a relatively rare commodity.

There is an urgent need to ensure that all clinicians are trained to employ these methods in a competent manner (Lehman et al. 1995). This requires a major international training effort with considerable resources. One such effort is currently under way to provide training in these and other effective strategies for schizophrenia in several countries and to examine the benefits when they are maintained throughout a 5-year follow-up period (Falloon et al. 1996). This effort, the Optimal Treatment Project (OTP), has led to the development of a series of workbooks for therapists, as well as guidebooks for families, that facilitate the training process and help ensure the fidelity of the treatment strategies (Falloon et al. 1998).

Chapters on Related Topics

The following chapter describes concepts related to behavioral family therapy:

- Chapter 22, "Behavioral Couples Therapy"

8

Psychoeducational Family Intervention

Linda D. Schwoeri, Ph.D.
G. Pirooz Sholevar, M.D.

Introduction

Psychoeducational family intervention is a therapeutic and secondary prevention approach to the treatment of serious mental disorders. It focuses on educating the family about the nature and characteristics of the illness, and how they can best cope and intervene by providing the most positive and functional environment for the patient. The psychoeducational approach is based on the view that there is interaction between biological, social, family, and individual variables on mental disorders. This approach is sensitive to the stress of caregiving roles as well as the day-to-day stress created by the medical or psychiatric condition itself and experienced by both patient and family. Families encounter a wide range of psychological, social, and financial problems when a member has a serious mental illness. Many times they are unjustly blamed for making the patient's problems even worse. These families are dealing with the enormous burden of chronic and severe mental illness (Beels and McFarlane 1982). The mere fact that the patient needs hospitalization makes families feel guilty and in subtle competition with the hospital staff. Each relapse further heightens the family's sense of inadequacy.

Psychoeducational family intervention emphasizes the family—its stresses, needs, and strengths. It is not family "therapy" in a classical sense, but clearly it reflects a family system orientation. It provides families with an adequate and accurate knowledge base about the illness in order to help them develop reasonable expectations for the patient and to enable them to understand the many limitations imposed by the illness. The psychoeducational approach attempts to transfer knowledge and skills needed to help the patient and the family members become agents of their own healthy adaptation. Thus, the patient and family themselves, not the therapists, effect growth and change.

The psychoeducational approach is rooted in the understanding of three basic principles: 1) the *biological* and *genetic* factors that make individuals vulnerable to illness; 2) the *interpersonal* context that can either increase or decrease vulnerability; and 3) the *psychological* makeup of the patient. This model of intervention was born out of the complex study of schizophrenia as an illness that requires an optimal emotional climate for the patient to prevent relapse and enhance the quality of the patient's and family's life. Relapse prevention, enhancement of recovery, and mitigation of the impact of the illness on family members are the major goals. The psychoeducational model originated in the search for a more effective way to treat schizophrenia. However, it can be applied to any mental illness that has a complex etiology, especially when the goal is the enhancement of the rehabilitative capacity of the family.

This chapter describes the psychoeducational approach as it developed through the combined research goals of finding both a more effective treatment for schizophrenia and a solution to the problem of a high relapse rate in schizophrenic patients once they returned to their home environment. We review the psychoeducational model developed by C. M. Anderson et al. (1980), who originally applied the approach to the treatment of schizophrenia and subsequently adapted it to treat a range of affective disorders. We also describe McFarlane's multifamily approach with schizophrenic patients and families (McFarlane 1991, 1997) and discuss briefly the preventive intervention model for children of parents with affective disorders developed by Beardslee et al. (1988). An extensive discussion of the preventive model for families with depression can be found in Beardslee and Schwoeri (1994).

This chapter further shows the application of the psychoeducational approach to families facing emotional manifestations of physical trauma. Psychological manifestations of traumatic events predispose families to a comparable range of stresses as does the traumatic event itself. Furthermore, the aftermath of the trauma can also dramatically alter the family's adaptive coping skills, weaken family members' ability to manage ordinary family crises, and leave them without appropriate models of functioning. Brief family-based interventions can impart basic information that the family can use during the crisis and rehabilitative phases of crisis treatment.

At the turn of the twentieth century, the psychoeducational model has been applied effectively to a variety of new situations. These applications include extensive application to bipolar disorders (Miklowitz 1997; Miklowitz and Hooley 1998; Simoneau et al. 1999). Psychoeducational therapy has been used preventively with children of depressed patients (Beardslee et al. 1997, 1998), and suicidal children and adolescents (Goldman and Beardslee 1999), and in the contexts of death and dying (Pettle 1998), pediatric cancer (Koocher et al.1996), and maltreatment and substance abuse (McCreary et al. 1998).

History

The historical context of the research-generated psychoeducational approach is in part the atmosphere of the 1950s and 1960s, decades during which research underscored the genetic predisposition and vulnerability to schizophrenia. Antipsychotic medication was found to be effective in reducing or eliminating symptoms of schizophrenia. Psychosocial factors of the illness were also studied. However, despite the widespread use of antipsychotic medication, progress in family treatment, and expanded residential and rehabilitative services that lessened institutionalization, only 25% of first-episode patients recovered. The remainder of patients lived their lives in social isolation and rejection (Yolles and Kramer 1969). Even with medication, schizophrenic patients were estimated to have a 40% chance of relapse in their first year after any given episode (Schooler et al. 1988).

With the advent of antipsychotic pharmacotherapy and the insights of biological research (including in vivo observation of cerebral blood flow and brain metabolism), multiple, interrelated factors for schizophrenia came to be considered, included inherited and acquired vulnerability and environmental stress. Focus shifted from etiology to multiple determinants occurring over the course of the illness, and in light of this change, new clinical approaches were considered that combined antipsychotic medication with a family-based program to educate and support members. The role of antipsychotic medication was central to the psychoeducational approach to schizophrenia and mood disorders (McFarlane 1991, 1997; Miklowitz 1996). Therefore families, psychiatrists, and family clinicians were required to work together with patients to ensure compliance with medication regimens.

Antipsychotic pharmacotherapy and biological research created new goals for psychoeducational research. The role of the family in the etiology and maintenance of schizophrenia was studied, as well as the family's long- and short-term reactions to the disturbed behavior of a member. If a patient's disturbed behavior *preceded* the family's individual or collective emotional reactivity, was the future relapse of the patient inevitable, regardless of family input? In other words, did the cause of the disturbed behavior reside primarily in the individual? Or could family members *cause* the relapse, regardless of the patient's former functioning, by reacting to disturbed behavior? These questions broadened the scope of work with these families; environment was now considered as a factor associated with greater patient relapse. Eventually the vulnerability-stress model of Zubin and Spring (1977) emerged, suggesting the existence of a biological predisposition in at-risk individuals that was kindled by environmental (family) stress. In this model, the way in which families communicated and interacted with patients would have an impact on the future course of the illness.

To help families cope with the stress and social alienation that caring for a schizophrenic member can cause, and to help families understand this illness, Laqueur et al. (1964) designed *the multiple family groups* program. The original group structure called for two or three therapists to meet with four to eight families for about an hour weekly. The social support focus of the group enhanced the families' resources. Social functioning was significantly improved, and patients and families felt protected and safer knowing that other families were struggling with the burdens created by this illness. By the late 1960s the program had caught on, and multiple family groups were formed with patients and families from both inpatient settings and aftercare services such as day hospitals. The experience was both supportive and educational. Group process was encouraged, and in time families began to develop a sense of their own competence in dealing with the patient and his or her illness. These multiple family therapy groups had the ambience of self-help groups; the therapists acted as advisors and also provided structure and agendas for the meetings.

Despite the observed efficacy of antipsychotic medication, as well as the increased family treatment and expanded residential and rehabilitative services that lessened institutionalization, only 25% of first-episode patients recovered. Many patients lived in social isolation and rejection (Yolles and Kramer 1969). Schizophrenic patients were estimated to have a 40% chance of relapse in their first year after any given episode (Schooler et al. 1988).

Although antipsychotic medication proved central to the psychoeducational approach to schizophrenia and mood disorders (McFarlane 1991, 1997), McFarlane and his colleagues were also aware of the shortcomings of a simple pharmacological approach. Their response was *multiple family therapy*, an expansion of the single-family format of Hogarty and Anderson (C. M. Anderson et al. 1980, 1986). Multiple family therapy provided a valuable avenue of support for families in the management of illness-related behavior. Schizophrenic patients themselves attempted to promote new rehabilitative efforts that would benefit both patients and their families and lessen the burden and stigma of severe mental illness.

Contemporary Research on Families With Mentally Ill Members

In this section, we discuss contemporary research on families with mentally ill members. We first note that the psychoeducational model is rooted in the research of George Brown and his colleagues (Brown and Birley 1968; Brown and Harris 1978; Brown et al. 1962, 1972). Their studies revealed a significantly elevated rate of relapse in schizophrenic patients returning home after discharge, compared with patients going to boarding homes. The studies suggested that critical attitudes, familial overinvolvement, and high expressed emotion (EE) were the reasons for the increased relapse rate. The studies of Brown and his colleagues were replicated by Falloon and colleagues (1985), Vaughn and Leff (1976), and others. They indicated the need for family education about the nature of the illness, treatment, and outcomes (see Chapter 27, "Family Variables and Interventions in Schizophrenia," for a detailed description).

Psychoeducational Model Applied to Depression

Description

The original psychoeducational model was designed as a single-family approach to the treatment of schizophrenia. The model's application to the treatment of depression by C. M. Anderson et al. (1980) represents a comprehensive reworking of the structured, goal-directed approach of the original method. In treatment of depression, psychoeducational principles help families recognize the systemic nature of their involvement in a member's illness. The overarching goals of psychoeducational intervention in depression include resolution of the presenting problem, removal of the symptom, utilization of the family's existing resources, and development of coping skills to handle future as well as present difficulties. Psychoeducational interventions also attempt to increase patient and family skills for dealing with the complexity of depression. The emotional stability of the family environment is enhanced by the following guidelines (Anderson 1976; C. M. Anderson et al. 1980, 1986):

1. Provide the family with information about the illness, and help increase the family's ability to manage the patient's behavior without becoming reactive, overprotective, or overfunctioning.
2. Reduce the family's stress, guilt, and worry.
3. Offer the family alternatives to negative and possibly destructive interactions with the patient.

4. Provide the family with hope for change by mobilizing the resources of the family and its social network.

This use of psychoeducation is guided by social learning principles such as imitation, reward, and the fundamentals of social support through social networks, as well as research data on the illness involved. It is sensitive to the many family and interactional factors that contribute to the etiology, maintenance, and relapse of a serious mental illness. Although originally designed as an *aftercare research project* to compare medication management and psychosocial family intervention for serious psychiatric disturbances (C. M. Anderson et al. 1980, 1986), the psychoeducational treatment of depression has been adapted and applied in many inpatient and day treatment settings for a variety of illnesses.

Principles and Application to Depression and Other Disorders

The psychoeducational approach is considered most valuable when the family as a whole is involved in the intervention program. The program for depression was based on the assumption that a biological/genetic vulnerability *interacts* with the family's environmental stress to produce depressive symptoms. Biological and genetic contributors to onset and maintenance of depression include genetic history, history of previous episodes and life stressors, and current interactional patterns in close relationships. Family environmental contributors to onset and maintenance of depression include marital and family discord, the interactional stress of living with a depressed person, dysfunctional problem solving, and impaired communication. The intervention of family members can actually make the patient's problems worse. The depressed person can appear demanding, coercive, and controlling, which drives people away, leaving him or her feeling angry and unwanted. This mutual exchange of negative interactions can exacerbate the depression as well as increase family stress and conflict. Information can alter beliefs about depression and the depressed person's behaviors, which can modify negative family attitudes. Psychoeducational interventions were designed to address the family's need to learn appropriate strategies that will mitigate symptoms. The strategies are tailored to the individual family's situation and presented in a supportive manner with support offered in ongoing family sessions.

Phases

Holder and Anderson (1990, p. 160) outlined three phases in a program for depression:

1. Engaging the family
2. Providing information and enhancing coping skills
3. Facilitating the application and retention of this information in everyday life

Engaging the family. Phase 1 involves *engaging the family* and enlisting their cooperation in the program. The family is seen as a vital resource, and as such the clinician attempts to join the family by a) adapting to their style of relating; lowering their anxiety by providing concrete, practical information; and positioning himself or herself as a family ombudsman being available for emergency calls and contact. This is particularly important in the initial phase, because the family's stress level is very high. The family often feels that the mental health professional will not be sensitive to their feelings of guilt, blame, and so forth. The clinician also tries to emphasize family strengths through positive *reframing* of problems.

An important aspect of this opening phase is the treatment contract, which is a mutual agreement about the goals, content, number of sessions, rules, and methods of treatment (C. M. Anderson et al. 1980, 1986). This occurs within seven days of the admission. Information about the family's reactions to the particular illness, their coping styles, and the reactions of other family members and friends to the patients is elicited. Knowledge of the family's strengths and the availability of other resources can diminish the family's anger and self-criticism. The family can be mobilized by reorganizing what it already has and what is needed.

Education and enhancing coping skills. Phase 2 includes education on the particular illness (depression, schizophrenia, etc.) This stage of intervention is referred to as the *workshop phase*. The workshops can run one-half to a full day. During this phase, details about the course and nature of the illness are emphasized, as well as the limits, purpose, and side effects of different medications. Guidelines for setting limits and what behavior to expect from the patient are discussed, as well as how to manage the behavioral and interactional complications of the illness. Families are encouraged to maintain their own activities and not become isolated. Unlike the workshops with schizophrenic patients, workshops for depressed patients *include* the patient for both educational and interactional purposes. Families react differently when the patient is present, and this presents an opportunity for open discussion. Families are encouraged to keep discussions from becoming too wordy, detailed, or vague; to speak in terms of what happened rather than how one feels; to accept responsibility for what one says; and to express positive and supportive comments rather than critical ones.

Other aspects of work with depressed families include sessions on defining depression; describing the interactional ambience of a depressed person; explaining the different types of treatment available; helping family members learn to cope with and avoid problems created by overinvolvement, over- and underresponsibility, and reactivity; encouraging family members to care for themselves; and helping them cope with threats and attempts at suicide. The program looks at the impact of depression on family life while providing strategies and suggestions for coping. The work of Coyne (1976) on the interactional nature of depression and Beck et al. (1979) on the role of cognition in depression and depressive symptoms is emphasized. Table 8–1 presents an outline, based on Holder and Anderson's (1990) discussion, for the psychoeducational sessions for depression.

Facilitating application and retention of information in everyday life. Phase 3 is concerned with the application of the principles learned during the workshops. With schizophrenic patients, careful attention is paid to the patient's needs in order to move him or her gradually toward independence. Families with schizophrenic members need help with boundary formation. Families must learn to understand patients' signs of emotional overload and allow them to retreat from interaction; conversely, families need to know when patients can begin to resume responsibility for themselves without precipitation of a relapse. For depressed patients, the focus is on discussion of basic problems manifested by patients in depression: poor sense of self-worth, lack of energy for activity and productivity, and lack of coping skills. Families and/or spouses are instructed and encouraged in taking steps to reduce stressful interactions. The educational component in this approach addresses what families need to know about etiology, the interactional context, and effective coping skills, while the program's direction and support help families integrate and use information learned in the program.

Multifamily Psychoeducational Model

Description

McFarlane (1991, 1997) developed a psychoeducational model that can be applied in both single and multifamily contexts. His family approach remains simplistic, giving families easy access to information and advice while building a collaborative alliance with significant relatives in the patient's life. Many aspects of the approach are similar to network therapy in terms of the role taken by the therapist and the goal of utilizing the family network (see Chapter 9, "Social Network Intervention").

The model directs the clinician to offer methods for handling the patient, provide guidance regarding medication and other management issues, and discuss the nature of the illness. The family, on the other hand, is

Table 8–1. Outline of topics for patient-family psychoeducational sessions on depression

I. Defining depression
  A. Definitions and descriptions of depression and mania
  B. How depression differs from "the blues" we all experience (length of time it lasts, impact on mood, functioning, self-esteem, responsiveness to the environment)
  C. Possible causes: the stress-vulnerability model
    1. Genetic factors
    2. Biochemical factors
    3. Life events, stresses, and family problems

II. Depression and the interpersonal environment
  A. What depression looks like: interpersonal difficulties
    1. Oversensitivity and self-preoccupation
    2. Unresponsiveness (to reassurance, support, feedback, sympathy)
    3. Behaviors that appear willful
    4. Apparent lack of caring for others, unrealistic expectations
    5. Apparent increased need to control relationships
    6. Inability to function at normal roles, tasks
  B. Negative interactional sequences
    1. Family attempts to help by: coaxing, reassuring, and protecting; the potential for overinvolvement is always present
    2. The patient is unresponsive; the family escalates attempts to help or it withdraws
    3. The patient feels alienated; the family becomes withdrawn, angry, or both
    4. The family feels guilty and returns to overprotective stance
    5. The patient feels unworthy, hopeless, infantilized
    6. Families burn out over time but remain caught in guilt/anger dilemma

III. Treatments
  A. Psychotropic medication
  B. Psychotherapies
  C. Other treatments

IV. Coping with depression
  A. What to avoid
    1. Too rapid reassurance
    2. Taking comments literally
    3. Attempting to be constantly available and positive
    4. Allowing the disorder to dominate family life

Table 8–1.	Outline of topics for patient-family psychoeducational sessions on depression *(continued)*

IV. Coping with depression *(continued)*
    B. Creating a balance (neither over- nor underresponsive)
        1. Recognition of multiple realities
        2. Distinguishing between the patient and the disorder
        3. Decreasing expectations temporarily
        4. Providing realistic support and reinforcement
        5. Avoiding unnecessary criticism (but providing feedback when necessary)
    C. Taking care of self and family members other than the patient; skills for self-preservation
        1. Time out (away from patient)
        2. Avoiding martyrdom
        3. Accepting own negative feelings
        4. Minimizing the impact of the disorder
    D. Coping with special problems
        1. Suicide threats and attempts
        2. Medication
        3. Hospitalization
        4. Atypical responses

Source. Adapted from Holder and Anderson 1970.

most knowledgeable of what is effective with the patient based on their ongoing experience with solving problems. The added self-help dimension is the inclusion of other families and patients for support and new ideas, as well as emphasis on the family's strengths by reinforcing tolerance and efforts to cooperate in meeting goals for the patients. The clinician maintains a much less traditional role in this approach and one that changes depending on the particular phase of therapy. For example, during the engagement or *joining* phase, the clinician will listen nonjudgmentally, allowing families to mourn the patient's loss of healthy functioning during the course of the mental illness. The clinician will also encourage families to recall happier memories that predate the onset of the illness. The validation of these memories and the facilitating of grieving for losses allow the family to move forward in treatment.

Structure

A typical session for both multiple and single family intervention involves socialization, family information, problem solving, communication, skill building, and practice.

Phases

Similar to Anderson's model with schizophrenic families, McFarlane's program consists of four phases:

1. Engagement of the family at the time of crisis
2. An educational workshop
3. A reentry period of biweekly group sessions that focus on stabilizing the patient
4. A rehabilitation phase that emphasizes raising of the patient's functional level

A clinician meets with the family during the engagement phase. Schizophrenic patients are present only during the reentry and rehabilitation phases.

Engagement and joining. The joining phase occurs during an acute episode and *excludes* the patient initially. Its purpose is first to help form an alliance with the family members and lessen their worry about the patient. The second purpose of this phase is to assess the crisis and the family's way of handling it. During the crisis, observations and assessments are made of the family's coping style and coincidental events that might create more stress. More extensive information is then gathered, including facts about the family's interactional style, alliances, splits, communication style, and coping strategies. The available family and social resources are evaluated, usually through the use of a genogram. The clinician attempts to learn details about the family's sources of enjoyment, recent life events, changes in the family membership, and its strengths and limitations.

Educational workshop. Once a few families are engaged, the clinicians conduct an educational workshop with them. This multifamily meeting takes place one day on a weekend. The workshop is designed to interrupt the emotional process in the family that contributes to the schizophrenic patient's difficulty with emotional interaction. Families are essentially taught the following principles:

- *Go slow.* Reduce the family expectation for rapid return of the patient's former level of functioning.
- *Keep it cool!* Families are encouraged to take a more relaxed approach with the patient and to be less critical of the patient's need to sleep and withdraw.
- *Give the patient space!* The family is encouraged to keep the environment calm, offer joint activity to the patient, but not become upset if it is refused.

- *Ignore what you can't change!* The patient's symptoms often elicit family curiosity. The family is told to avoid discussion of delusional material or lecturing the patient.
- *Keep it simple!* Be aware of the patient's cognitive difficulties in the area of attention and keep all requests simple. Conversation should not be arousing or confrontational.
- *Carry on business as usual!*
- *No street drugs or alcohol!* Drugs must not become a part of the patient's life.
- *Pick-up on early signs to avert a relapse!* The family is encouraged to use the information it has gained about signs of relapse.

Community reentry. The community reentry phase refers to the time when patients are starting to show an interest in seeing a friend, attending a social event, and so forth. It is a reengagement with their environment. This process usually takes 2 to 18 months depending on the severity of the illness and the family's ability to follow guidelines set forth to prevent relapse. They must

- Be alert to the early signs of relapse
- Strengthen the interpersonal boundaries
- Set limits on behavior
- Help adherence to the medication regimen
- Encourage taking responsibility in and out of the home
- Judiciously handle suicidal or dangerous activity

McFarlane (1997) demonstrated the value of combining assertiveness training with community reentry initiatives to help patients deal effectively with obstacles they may encounter.

Rehabilitative phase. The rehabilitative phase follows 1 year of slow, gradual recovery. The family's task is to encourage the patient to engage in social activities and to show initiative in looking for part-time work. Care is taken to encourage the patient to talk with other patients who have been able to get back into a more functional way of living.

In multiple family therapy, McFarlane encourages therapists to engage in small talk with families, thereby modeling a relaxed interactional posture that they can use with each other. Group process is very much a part of this initial phase. The group is only as productive as the network of families it encompasses and the effective communication that occurs within that network. As the group becomes more cohesive and supportive, it exerts collective pressure on the families to help patients become more responsible.

Leadership in the group is provided by the emergence of an "optimal leader" (see Chapter 9, "Social Network Intervention"). By now the group has developed its own objective and direction. With the emergence of leadership in the group, problem solving occurs more easily, and at times patients themselves contribute to solutions. Group acceptance and membership become strong motivators and serve as a healthy substitute for the families' overinvolvement with the patient. A viable social network develops among families, and they begin to socialize outside of the therapy. The clinicians encourage this process, especially on holidays and social occasions, and suggest that families further expand their social network and become advocates for change by joining national self-help organizations and local branches of such organizations as the National Alliance for the Mentally Ill (NAMI).

The effectiveness of the multifamily psychoeducational model with depressed patients and their families has been consistently confirmed in the past decade (Miklowitz and Hooley 1998; Simoneau et al. 1999). The application methodology has since been further refined.

Intervention With Children of Depressed Parents

Description

William Beardslee and his colleagues (Beardslee and Schwoeri 1994; Beardslee et al. 1988, 1997, 1998b; Goldman and Beardslee 1999) developed a preventive intervention model designed to be used by a broad cross section of practitioners, including psychiatrists, family therapists, psychologists, social workers, pediatricians, school guidance counselors, and pastoral counselors. This model is family-based and addresses the primary and secondary prevention levels and to some extent the tertiary level. *Primary prevention* aims to prevent or undermine the future transmission of the disorder, whereas *secondary prevention* aims to identify early signs of the disorder and initiate treatment before the onset of symptoms. *Tertiary prevention* reduces further dysfunction in patients through effective treatment of the disorder. Beardslee's approach is based on extensive empirical findings concerning children who grow up in a family in which a parent has an affective disorder.

This psychoeducational model involves the whole family and is geared toward informing members about the illness, helping them discuss the problem and arrive at solutions, and better preparing them for the task of coping with the illness. The model also emphasizes the recognition of individual characteristics of a patient, including their vulnerability or resiliency, and attempts to help all family members understand and utilize their own resources and strengths. The favorable outcome of this intervention model has been recently reviewed by Beardslee et al. (1997, 1988, 1998b).

Structure and Phases

The number of sessions is variable. Usually there are at least 6 but no more than 10. There is a combination of sessions involving parents alone, child (or children) alone, and parent and child (or children) together.

Assessment of Family Members

Assessment of family members is accomplished through family sessions. One or two parent-history sessions are held either with each spouse alone or with spouses together. The focus is on the parent's recent illness and past disorder and each spouse's experience and understanding of it. Parents are asked to describe not only their histories but also how they think the children have experienced those historical events. This helps the parent to take in the child's perspective and elicits descriptive and useful information about everyday events.

The Beardslee model focuses heavily on family discussion. During the discussion, children can gain a different perspective on the issues and can learn to understand that the depressed behavior is really discontinuous from normal behavior. Adolescents learn that their parents do not want to be the way they are and that there is an alternative course in the future. It is essential that the clinician demystify what has been a complex and confusing experience for the children. Children need to know that this event does not have to overwhelm them; they can understand it both cognitively and emotionally. This intervention model builds on family and individual strengths, identifies risk factors, and helps the family plan for the future. It requires that the clinician be flexible in approach, as well as honest and open in discussing whatever the family feels is relevant. In sessions with the children, their experiences in school, with friends, in the family, and in outside activities are explored, as well as the parent's major symptoms if any.

Cognitive Teaching

Cognitive teaching refers to passing on factual knowledge and developing logical conclusions about disorders. In sessions with the parents alone, the clinician reviews what is known about the etiology of depression, its psychosocial manifestations, and the risks to children growing up in families with serious affective illness. The adaptive capacities of youngsters who function well in this and related risk situations are described.

Children's Experiences and Development of Plans for the Future

Sessions with both parents specifically explore strategies that the family can use in discussing the patient's illness and plan for the future. The major areas of discussion are as follows:

1. Clarify for children what has happened to the parent and to the family.
2. Ensure that children do not feel guilty or responsible.
3. Encourage children's understanding of the nature of the illness, and stress that the parent's unavailability and incapacity need not limit the children.
4. Encourage exploration of networks of support for children, particularly reestablishment of any that may have been disrupted by parental illness.
5. Discuss difficulties that the children may face.
6. Anticipate possible illnesses in the children in the future and seek prompt treatment.
7. Work on the ongoing process of understanding in the family. At the end of the sessions, the parents define what they hope to accomplish in the family sessions with the children.

Family Discussion

Two family sessions are held to present the material listed above to the children. Special care is taken to explain to children that they are not to blame. During these sessions, there is discussion of aspects of the depression that may have been confusing or frightening to children. For example, children may ask how someone becomes depressed and if they too will become depressed. A depressed mother may explain that when she was acting irritated, she was not angry with her family. She could not do anything about her irritability because it was part of her illness. Plans for the future are discussed in terms of continued exploration of the best course to take in helping the family adjust to the illness.

Family Intervention With Children

Family intervention with children may be efficacious with at-risk individuals. The psychoeducational model has been applied to child and adolescent populations therapeutically and preventively. Brent and his colleagues applied the model in the aftercare of the children with self-harm and suicidal behavior (Brent et al. 1997). They compared three types of psychosocial interventions: psychoeducational, cognitive, and supportive psychotherapy with depressed adolescents (Brent et al. 1997). Psychoeducation proved an effective therapeutic approach for children at risk for self-harm and suicide. The effectiveness of psychoeducation with suicidal adolescents was also confirmed by Goldman and Beardslee (1999).

Psychoeducational intervention also has proven effective with children with pediatric cancer (Koocher et al. 1996) or in cases of impending death of the children or parents (Pettle 1998). It has been particularly effective in treatment and prevention of childhood maltreatment by helping the families of chronically ill children identify immediate stressors and their long-standing vulnerabilities (McCreary et al. 1998).

Family Intervention With Trauma Patients

Psychoeducational intervention can be applied to families facing the devastation of massive physical trauma. The lives of many trauma patients have been saved due to effective on-site administration of emergency medical treatment and rapid transportation with helicopters. With the general advancement of technology however, trauma patients who survive may experience a prolonged and uncertain period of slow recovery while their families are struggling with the issues of life and death without any preparation. Families and patients alike are generally unaware of the impact of the trauma, the short-term and long-term losses involved, and are uncertain about the differential outcome according to the course of illness. Family interventions should include provision of support to the family in the *initial, acute phase* when the family is highly apprehensive and overwhelmed. Information about the impact of trauma and the differential outcome should be provided to the family according to their ability to receive and utilize such information. Clinicians should refrain from overloading the family with too much information but also should not withhold information that the family may need to make appropriate decisions.

Phases

Intervention with families is focused on understanding the importance of the trauma on family life and behavior and adopting new ways of handling the crisis both immediately and in the long term. Families experience different reactions to the trauma. The intervention format used by C. M. Anderson et al. (1980, 1986) can be followed with some variation:

1. Involve the family at the time of crisis.
2. Hold an information session that includes the patient and family.

3. Hold individual sessions with the patient.
4. Hold biweekly family sessions that focus on stabilization.
5. Conduct family sessions and multifamily group sessions involving patients and families whenever possible. These sessions can be conducted with one family until it becomes possible to expand the intervention by providing a group structure and inviting several families.

In the first phase of the intervention following the trauma, clinicians should collaborate closely with the medical or surgical trauma team to keep abreast of the condition of the patient. During this phase, the family is extremely preoccupied with the physical condition of the patient and will ask questions requiring the full attention of physicians and surgeons. Clinicians can function as the communicator, translator, or integrator of the information exchanged between the family and the trauma team. They can supply information about the patient, and describe the nature of the trauma, such as the impact of head injury or loss of consciousness, in an accurate manner. They may need to be available as a sounding board as the family repeatedly attempts to mentally process different scenarios. It is essential to allow the family to maintain control of the initial phase, to define the nature of the clinical interaction, and to ask questions repeatedly to reduce their anxiety. Generally, the family prefers clinicians to be responsive but passive, letting the family control the sessions. It is essential to answer the questions of family members while acknowledging the vast areas of uncertainty predominating in this stage. Clinicians should refrain from dashing the hopes of the family and should allow them to wish and pray for miraculous recoveries, even if this seems totally unrealistic. The family should be allowed to maintain their denial, which may be their way of titrating the level of reality tolerable to them. Denial should be dealt with only if it interferes with necessary medical interventions such as amputation of a limb. If a connection between preexisting conditions and current traumas can be made readily, the family would make such connections and interpretations on their own. Clinicians should make gentle attempts at reduction of family guilt only if guilt weighs heavily on families, especially when they are the survivors of the trauma.

In the second phase following the trauma, patients are stabilized and the degree of functional losses becomes apparent to the family and health care providers. Families utilize different mechanisms for dealing with losses, ranging from extensive denial to accepting the losses too readily and completely. During this phase clinicians should remain available to the family and provide them with sensitive and warm support until the family is ready to accept the bitter reality on their own. There are many alterations in family roles and lifestyles during this phase. Many functions of the patient, such as being the primary income provider, may have to be taken over by other family members. Intervention becomes more task-focused in response to these needs. Families who lose a member enter the grieving process during this phase.

In the third phase, the extent of functional losses is more or less accepted by the family and patient and the family becomes involved in the long road to recovery. The complete acceptance of functional losses motivates whole-hearted participation in the recovery process. This acceptance varies depending on the nature of the trauma. Denial and the projection of blame on others, including the health care providers, can significantly interfere with motivation for recovery. In particular, with open and closed head injury the family needs specific education on expectations and ways to interact with the patient.

Preexisting conditions or new psychopathological developments have to be addressed during this phase. Preexisting conditions would include a high prevalence of alcohol and substance abuse; these are significant preexisting conditions in as many as 40% to 50% of severe trauma cases. Equally disabling are severe personality disorders, family conflicts, or underemployment. All could have been contributory factors to the accident. The severe changes in social and family roles and loss of function may also result in the development of new psychopathological states such as substance and alcohol abuse and depression. Family, group, and individual psychotherapies, as well as rehabilitative programs for substance abuse, are most beneficial to these families.

Trauma patients and their families are generally totally unprepared for catastrophic losses brought about by trauma. Broad-based educational programs through media and other educational vehicles may be necessary to prepare the general population to seek adequate measures for dealing with trauma. An additional educational goal is extensive public education on how to prevent severe traumas by such simple measures as wearing seat belts and helmets.

Structure of Approach

The treatment structure and approach for both the single family group (SFG) and multiple family group (MFG) were the same. However what seems to have made the difference is the multiple families involved in MFG.

The cost effectiveness of this approach deserves mention. The psychoeducational MFGs require exactly one-half the staff time per patient per month compared with SFGs. MFGs helped reduce the isolation experienced by patients and family members through the creation of a social network that served both. Therapeutic tasks of MFGs include the following:

1. Engage key members within seven days of admission of the patient.
2. Provide information on the biological aspects of the disease to the family through the use of video, lectures, and written guidelines.
3. Expand the family's social network and resources.
4. Provide ongoing support for at least 2 years after the end of therapy to help prevent relapse.
5. Intervene early in cases of relapse.

Outcome Data

Outcome data show that family psychoeducation has proven more effective in the prevention of relapse than individual treatment or medication alone for schizophrenia (Falloon et al. 1985; Hogarty et al. 1986, 1991; Leff et al. 1985; McFarlane 1991, 1997; McFarlane et al. 1995a). Earlier studies have detailed psychoeducational multiple family groups as more effective in the prevention of relapse than single family treatment (Beels 1975; Detre et al. 1961; Laqueur 1972; Levin 1966). The multiple family group has been a well-known approach in the treatment of schizophrenia for three decades. It was designed to replicate methodology set forth in the SFG model, except that instead of one family, the treatment was directed at several families and utilized two clinicians. In their 4-year study, McFarlane et al. (1995a) found MFGs to be more effective in extending remission and enhancing the overall functioning of the patients than the same techniques conducted in a single-family format or in traditional MFG therapy without psychoeducation.

Furthermore, psychoeducational MFGs offered social network interventions as well as training in coping skills and problem solving, which enhanced the effectiveness of the intervention. The main benefits were supported in the study by McFarlane et al. (1995a). Psychoeducational MFGs, compared with SFG, yielded the lowest relapse rate—50% versus 12.5% per year. At the end of the 4-year study, 78% of patients in the SFG cohort had at least one relapse. There were few relapses in cases with treatment longer than 4 years. McFarlane et al.'s (1995a) study supports the findings of Hogarty et al. (1991) that family intervention, combined with standard-dose medication, may delay but not completely prevent relapse in at-risk patients.

Conclusion

Psychoeducational family intervention is a family-based intervention that operates within the framework of family theory, yet is different from traditional family therapy. The psychoeducational model of intervention is an effective and eloquent model of collaboration between families and the mental health system that effectively meets the challenge posed by emotional illness. The model addresses the significant issue of preventing the recurrence of emotional illness and enhancing the family's successful adjustment to emotional disorders. Clinicians provide the family with extensive information with which to understand the nature, course, outcome, and treatment of mental illness. This information empowers the family to better cope with adjusting to the illness and supporting the patient. The patient benefits from a better family environmental adaptation and experiences increased community involvement and better adjustment.

Extensive research supports the effectiveness of psychoeducational family intervention with a number of affective illnesses, particularly schizophrenia and depression. Its methodology focuses on provision of information about multiple aspects of mental illness to the family using the full range of the clinician's clinical and communication skills. The provision of information in a group setting allows families to support one another in their common struggle against the plight of emotional illness.

Psychoeducational family interventions began with chronic and severe mental illness in adult patients, particularly schizophrenia and biopolar disorders. Its application has gradually expanded to the treatment of children with depression and suicidality and, more recently, to situations such as death and dying and pediatric cancer.

Chapters on Related Topics

The following chapters describe concepts related to psychoeducational family interventions:

- Chapter 19, "Parent Management Training"
- Chapter 27, "Family Variables and Interventions in Schizophrenia"
- Chapter 28, "Depression and the Family: Interpersonal Context and Family Functioning"
- Chapter 29, "Family Intervention and Psychiatric Hospitalization"
- Chapter 30, "National Alliance for the Mentally Ill (NAMI) and Family Psychiatry: Working Toward a Collaborative Model"

9

Social Network Intervention

Ross V. Speck, M.D.

Introduction to Network Therapy: Editor's Note

Social network therapy was a bold attempt to place family therapy within the larger social context in the heyday of family therapy. When early family therapists were placing the family unit above and beyond other entities, social network therapy introduced a note of caution and maturity by placing the family unit within a hierarchical paradigm. The rationale for including social network therapy as a contemporary theoretical system is based on a number of reasons. Most importantly, the field of therapy is now recognizing the disintegration in some family units who are cut off from larger social support for economic, geographical, cultural, and psychological reasons. The recent emphasis on family preservation, family-based services, home-based services, wraparound services, and therapeutic and temporary foster homes underlines the phenomenon of progressive family deterioration and disintegration when the family receives insufficient support from its social context. The school of family therapy emphasizes that the external support for the family is essential in order to maintain or restore the internal family unity and cohesiveness. The introduction of therapeutic staff support in wraparound and other services recognizes the importance of support for the families if they are to carry on with their responsibilities and functions such as child rearing.

The social network model can also provide a sensible way of aligning the therapeutic foster family or temporary foster family with the biological family; one of the former groups can provide the additional support and reduce stress in order to help the biological family to reintegrate. Additional data on family disintegration have emerged through the work of family therapists with hospitalized and institutionalized patients (Glick et al. 1993; Sholevar 1988), the work of multisystemic therapists (Henggeler et al. 1998a, 1998b), and the work of multidimensional family therapists (Liddle et al. 1995a, 1995b).

Social network therapy presents a clear perspective on the disintegration within the family unit due to the lack of sufficient external and internal resources and describes a methodology for reconstructing the family unit, which is significantly and chronically decompensated. The application of this methodology to the new social initiatives such as family preservation services can enable the family therapist to search for, recognize, and utilize the sources of support available to the family.

G. Pirooz Sholevar, M.D.

Introduction

Barnes (1954) was the first to introduce the idea of a social network to describe the order of social relationships that were important in understanding social behavior, as opposed to structural concepts such as groups defined by occupation or territory. He used the term "network" to describe a set of social relationships for which there is no common boundary. Bott's (1957) book *Family and Social Network* describes a theoretical framework for understanding the surrounds or next layer mediating between the family and the larger social system. The social network concept was translated into clinical terms (Speck and Attneave 1971, 1973) by assembling the entire social network of a given family together at one time—as in a family reunion, a wedding celebration, a funeral feast, or a cousins' club. The clinical techniques of a large assembly social network intervention have evolved by trial-and-error, pragmatic, and heuristic methods. These methods were used when simpler methods of treatment failed to produce results with families in extremely difficult circumstances. The assembly of family, friends, neighbors, and other helpful network persons brought a large psychosocial field into operation for innovation, repair, and option finding in human relationships.

Theory of Social Network Intervention

There are at least *four kinds of healing:* psychotherapeutic, organic-biologic, mystical-faith, and social action. For our purposes, the concepts of "healing" and "change" are regarded as similar. All four levels of healing may be involved in varying degrees in social network interventions. The network intervention team (usually three to five persons, but the team can be larger in special situations) has the task of catalyzing the network and getting its members to define goals for the problem family as well as a few options or solutions. In large-group psychology it is relatively easy to get the network to cooperate in helping the family to change. When 40 or more persons begin to exert an influence on an individual, it doesn't take long before that person becomes overwhelmed with information processing and new options appear.

When large network assembly occurs—40 to 100 or more friends, family members, neighbors, and acquaintances—the whole social fabric of the family is present. Networks have both a time and space representative. The time or *vertical element* consists of family members from several generations and helpers, friends, and others who have had long-standing involvement with the individual family members. The space or *horizontal dimension* includes all who assemble and who are currently involved in the life of the family.

It is the network and the assembly of the network members that produces healing or change. The professional's job is to keep the network process moving, to deal with resistance, and to facilitate or catalyze and choreograph the group. The network intervention is selected when earlier, simpler methods, such as individual, group, or family therapy, have not been effective. The professional who leads the network team is called the *interviewer*. He or she orchestrates the network intervention and encourages the helpers and innovators in the network to become active agents of change.

There are many routes to change. In some networks it appears that shame is a factor in getting a person to change his or her behavior. The group exerts social control. In other networks, a mystical-faith effect, in some ways akin to hypnosis, occurs. In these networks, the professionals are cast in the role of shaman, and there are many similarities to tribal healing. Frequently, the enactment of family problems stirs up latent conflicts in other network members, who then seek their own marital, family, or individual therapy. Network intervention has been called *backdoor entry* into psychotherapy.

It is usually impossible to predict who or what will be instrumental in producing the network effect. Sometimes it happens by reframing the meaning of behavior. In one case, the labeled patient, a 19-year-old, marched up and down the sidewalk of his parent's home between sessions. The network members feared this meant psychosis and hospitalization. When the interviewer labeled this behavior as "picketing," the network treated this boy in a totally different way and went on to help him get free of the symbiosis with his parents.

However, networks of 40 or more members are capable of producing extended families and networks. The loosening of secret bonds and binds is a frequent element in attaining the goals of a social network intervention.

Techniques of a Social Network Intervention

Assembling the Network

Referrals for a social network intervention are usually made by family therapists who are dealing with a difficult family situation in which the family is often in chronic crisis, a crisis that has not responded to the usual family therapy methods. Common indications for network assembly include the family's wish to avoid hospitalization of one of its members, suicidal threats and behaviors, and emotional exhaustion of the immediate family.

An experienced network intervention team is assembled and a home visit is scheduled in order to meet with the family, assess the problem, and answer questions about what the family can expect. The family is told that they are to invite at least 40 persons who might be willing to help solve the family's presenting problems, including friends, relatives, neighbors, and service and professional persons. It is the family's task to contact as many people as possible who can form support systems for each and every family member. We have repeatedly estimated that 400 to 800 telephone calls and other contacts occur, in the 7 to 10 days before the first scheduled meeting. The "network effect" (Speck and Attneave 1973) is already in progress before the big meeting. There is great curiosity, excitement, anticipation, and even some anxiety about this large tribal-like meeting. Second- and thirdhand rumors flow from person to person. Bateson (1979) has described the *ho-ho-pani-pa* ritual in Hawaii in which the network convener may take up to a year making the rounds of persons who will be talking and thinking up innovative solutions before the big feast and assembly that solves family problems.

The family picks the date and time for the network assembly. We insist on a minimum of 40 persons, as smaller networks have less energy and fewer natural leaders (who we call "activists"). We have also found empirically that this is about average network size, even in cases of schizophrenia as long as the person has not been hospitalized for years at a time.

A team of 3 to 5 members is usually adequate to handle most network assemblies, although we once had a team of 10 in a particularly difficult situation. The team has a leader called the *convener*, and the others are his *consultants*. Usually one consultant handles brief encounter techniques in the event of a stalemate or blockage of the network process. All team members huddle occasionally and move about the assembled network of people who are seated as in a theater-in-the-round. Decisions are made on how to facilitate the network activists who are making decisions, options, or plans for resolving the family problems.

Network meetings last for 2 to 3 hours with the team in attendance. For most meetings we meet with the network only once. Some networks continue to meet without the presence of the team for months after the initial meeting.

A typical large assembly begins with the team arriving half an hour before the scheduled time. This allows us to move furniture if necessary, set up tape recorders or video cameras, and then observe and meet the members of the network as they arrive. Large groups of people never all arrive on time. People who travel long distances, such as from Europe, South America, or the opposite coast, usually arrive early and visit the family prior to the meeting. We wait until the house is full of anxious, talking persons (as at a noisy cocktail party) to begin the meeting. The serving of drinks or food is avoided because it trivializes the process.

Beginning the Process

The convener starts the meeting by signaling (usually loud hand-clapping) everyone to be seated. A short talk is given about social networks, tribal healing, and the purpose of the assembly. People are told that secrets may be revealed by network members and that confidentiality is impossible in a network. The family is expected to tell the assembly what the problem is and what kind of help they would like to get.

At this point the intervener (convener) asks everyone to stand, hold hands, and sway silently with eyes closed. They are to remain silent. After a minute or so he or she asks members of the group to say what they are feeling in one word. This gives the team an opportunity to gauge how cooperative or resistant this particular network is going to be. Some ethnic networks do well with humming and then singing a song that has special solidarity and meaning for them. War whooping sometimes loosens up timid groups. The purpose for these and other warming-up exercises is to transform a group without process (e.g., a bus queue) into an interactive group with a purpose and a goal and also to get them ready to act as activists, smaller support groups, and problem-solvers.

The next step in the program or process is to get the family with the problem into the center of the room and seated and to have each family member tell in his or her own words what the problems are and to ask the network for help. As this happens, various network members are asked to address the family with questions or comments that evolve into clarifying what is needed for the index family. We thus have an inner group (the family) and an outer group (the network) interacting with each other. In many networks, polarizations occur between network members. This is usually determined by the individual innate network structure, such as elders versus young, male versus female, city versus rural, religious versus not so religious, ad infinitum. This polarization often makes two groups within the network, and thus the whole assembly has an inner and two outer groups. Polarization is very useful in raising energy in the assembly and defining political power, side-taking, and the eventual setting up of support groups for all family members.

Phases in the Intervention Process

Network intervention process goes through six cyclical spiral phases that may also temporarily reverse at times. From repeated experience they have been labeled

- Retribalization
- Polarization
- Mobilization
- Depression-resistance
- Breakthrough
- Exhaustion-elation-termination

Retribalization begins when the assembly is given its task by the family and the intervention team. The opening ceremonial ritual attests to the uniqueness of the network and the awareness that this network-tribe assembly is united as a group with a special purpose. The team gives the stamp of approval to the assembly by supporting and encouraging them to bring about changes in the index family. *Polarization* begins when differing opinions are expressed about what is taking place. This can get quite emotional and leads to splits and coalitions in the assembly. The team intervenes if the polarization becomes sidetracked or repetitive or leads in the direction of violence. In over 25 years, I have seen two men square off only once, and they were easily separated.

Polarization is an important phase in that it reveals who the innate group leaders are, and it pushes them to begin to make suggestions that may reframe the family's problems. We call these innate leaders *network activists*.

The next phase is the *mobilization* of activities. In this phase the assembly acknowledges the wisdom, energy, and action of five or six members who lead the group in exploring innovative solutions. At this point the network may split up into half a dozen or more support groups, each meeting in a separate room of the house. The task is for each group to map out an agenda and plan for the family member they are to support (who is a member of that group).

After a few hours of intense interaction it is not unusual for fatigue, defeat, and sadness to overtake the network. This phase is called *depression-resistance*. It is not difficult to recognize this phase in large groups, as it will induce similar feelings in the team. We have found that we can best break through this phase by brief-encounter techniques such as those in Rueveni's *Networking Families in Crisis* (1979). We usually have a team member who can get the group into an exercise or two for a few minutes. Then we are ready to resume work in the mobilization phase.

When the assembly realizes that their efforts have produced a clear-cut plan, the mood changes into a high that we call the *breakthrough* phase. This is rapidly followed by a feeling of *exhaustion and elation* and the task for that evening is done.

At this point the team links up solitary network members with subgroups and then leaves *(termination)*. We have routinely found that after the team leaves, our departure is scarcely noticed. Coffee and cake are usually served, and the subgroups are so tightly locked that the network often continues for another 3 hours. Networks are so asymptotic that we continue to get news or feedback for many years, often from great distances.

Clinical Example

The Nelson family consisted of a 55-year-old mother and her 19-year-old son. The father had died mysteriously in another city where he worked prior to the son's birth. The mother said there was poor mother-child bonding right from the start because of her son's abnormal behavior. He made no friends and attended school only sporadically until he was 17, when he began to refuse to leave his lower-middle-class home. At about age 5 he became and remained interested and obsessed with the local traffic routes and memorized most of the local bus routes. He learned to tie his shoes at about 12 and his tie at about 17.

A careful family and network history was taken and I suggested that we assemble the network the following Thursday evening. The extended family was small, consisting of only three cousins and five other distant relatives. I insisted that we needed a minimum of 40 persons, and it was agreed that friends, friends of friends, neighbors, and any other helpful persons should be invited. The meeting was to be held in the Nelson's small two-story row house.

At the first meeting about 40 people showed up, many of whom did not know each other. I later learned that this is a loose-knit network and as such has the potential to reach outside of the family network. Tight-knit networks are less open to outside influence and thus may be more rigid and resistant to change. Also very few persons had any notion of what the family problem was that they would be getting involved in. Peculiar to this network was the role of Jack, the wealthy uncle who was anxious to establish himself as the leader of the network. Over the next few weeks, it became obvious that the basic problem to be solved was the symbiosis between mother and son, and that Jack was using the network instead for his own aggrandizement. After one stormy session in which he attacked several younger network members by disparagement, the network asked him to leave, which he did in a huff (polarization).

This prepared the way for a subgroup of younger members to propose a plan (mobilization of activists). This plan consisted of renting a small apartment for Harold, packing his belongings, moving him, and then setting up a schedule for visits, movies, phone calls, etc. Harold look bewildered but did not object. Mrs. Nelson however, had an immediate panic attack. She looked like a cornered animal, then rushed about, arms flailing, crying, and saying, "He'll starve, he can't open a can." Another subgroup of the network, closer to her age, began to organize a support system for her also.

The plan to physically separate the two worked, and Harold continued to attend the network meetings. Now the topic switched to future plans for Harold and his mother. The network went through several weeks of mobilization, resistance, and depression. Then one night a younger cousin proposed that Harold get a job. This seemed preposterous, as Harold did unusual things such as turn somersaults when he saw a pretty girl. However, the network pursued the plans.

A few weeks later a woman who was about 35 years old arrived at the family home requesting permission to join the network. She had heard about it in a mental hospital from which she had been discharged that day. She offered him a badge and placed it on his shirt. Harold blushed deeply and looked scared. Five minutes later he moved the badge to over his heart. Nothing further was said.

Two months later a networker member gave Harold a job in a household item repair shop. He functioned quite well in this job. The network continued social support of both Harold and his mother. By this time the network members had labeled themselves a "Family of Families" and held several informal meetings and picnics at sporadic intervals.

Two years later Harold became a cabdriver. Although eccentric and isolated, he supported himself and lived on his own. After 20 years and his mother's death, he decided to go on Social Security disability. During the course of this network intervention 11 people changed jobs, 3 experienced temporary marital separations, and 4 requested referrals for psychotherapy.

Research Directions

Research on social network intervention has exhibited its impact on many areas of therapy. The interventions are now used frequently in the field of drug and alcohol rehabilitation. Pattison et al. (1975) devised the Pattison Psychosocial Kinship Inventory, and Carolyn Attneave (Speck and Attneave 1973) pioneered a sophisticated network-mapping inventory for use in the research of both social networks and mental health. Sholevar (1983) has applied the social network concept to the treatment of hospitalized and institutionalized adolescents.

The Mount Tom Institute in Holyoke, Massachusetts, has had a network intervention team for more than 10 years. Schoenfeld et al. (1985) have shown that the cost of network therapy in mental health centers is about 25%

of the cost of individual care. David Trimble and Jodi Kliman have had numerous network projects in the Boston area, including some involving adolescents, some involving patients with chronic schizophrenia, and one involving a large "network of networks" composed of the assembled networks of each person in a halfway house. There have also been network therapy projects in Minneapolis, but in general, funding for network research in the United States is minimal. Although there are lively pockets of activity with social networks in the United States, growth of this approach to social problems has been limited largely due to its political bent. On the other hand, the spread of social network research outside of the United States is very impressive. Countries that are more socialized medically and politically tend to give much more support to social network research.

The Canadian Occupational Therapy Association Social Network Therapy Program has six social network therapists working in the metropolitan Toronto area. They are funded by the Ontario government to work with the chronically mentally ill, with patients who have Alzheimer's disease, and with adolescents who have psychiatric problems. In Winnipeg, research projects are under way to study neighborhood networks where child abuse is prevalent.

Mauro Croce in Verbania, Italy, has been working for years with Gruppo Abele, a network of therapists dealing with networks of drug-abusing adolescents. Stockholm has an Emergency Network Center dealing with child abuse and other family problems. Gunnar Forsberg and other team members have written a book on social network intervention teams throughout Europe. In Belgrade, Yugoslavia, Branko Gacic has run a highly successful network intervention project for patients with alcohol or drug addictions.

Chapters on Related Topics

The following chapters describe concepts related to social network intervention:

- Chapter 17, "Family Therapy With Children and Adolescents: An Overview"
- Chapter 34, "Impact of Culture and Ethnicity on Family Interventions"

10

Gender-Sensitive Family Therapy

Linda D. Schwoeri, Ph.D.
G. Pirooz Sholevar, M.D.
George S. Villarose, M.A.

Introduction

The emergence of family therapy in the late 1940s provided a focus on the multiple sources of stress and support within the family and for all family members. In the social and political climate following World War II, families were reuniting, gaining stability, and providing a needed respite. There was a return to a Parsonian scheme of social values and its typical division of family gender roles. This postwar social equilibrium was clearly upset in the mid- to late 1960s, partially by much political upheaval and most dramatically by the events surrounding protest to the Vietnam War, the civil rights movements, and the assassinations of political and religious leaders. The 1960s and 1970s also gave a new voice to women in the form of feminist values and principles.

New changes emerged in families: Women were postponing motherhood or planning smaller families; fewer women opted to remain home with their children. Although marriage was still seen as the best option for women, divorce statistics reached the highest rate ever in the 1970s. Women began to explore their choices and options concerning conception, pregnancy, and childbirth. Accompanying the new options and choices for women was the economic fact that women who worked outside the home were, in relation to men, in lower-paying jobs, had fewer opportunities for advancement, and had less access to the experience or credentialing required for career advancement (Goldner 1985b; Hare-Mustin 1978). Women had entered the workplace, but men maintained control over women's roles both at home and in society. Women were given reproductive choices but still had to face the choice of forgoing or postponing pregnancy to pursue career opportunities. The 1970s ushered in a rise in the age at first pregnancies and fewer pregnancies among women of childbearing age (Notman and Nadelson 1993). Women with children worked not simply because it was an option but because it was a necessity in both a financial and psychological sense. In light of these changes in women's lives, gender issues became a topic for heated discussion and debate. Feminists voiced criticism of family theory for its inadequacy to promote a gender and family role structure congruent with the social changes.

Our purpose in this chapter is to summarize the central gender issues in families and family therapy and to explore the conceptual and technical implications of these issues in clinical practice.

Challenging the Traditional View of Women in Families

Challenges to traditional views of women's role in families and established family structures in general began to arise due to divorce, the more frequent occurrence of second and third marriages, and women's decisions to raise children on their own. Single parents (both heterosexual and homosexual) were raising children; these children joined others in reconstituted families or were adopted into single-parent homes. Questions about family history became more complex in view of changing family structures and parental configurations.

More recent models of family structure and organization are presenting a diverse view of family life that requires changes in ideology and clinical orientation. For example, in "The Saturated Family," Gergen (1991) presented a view of today's family with its ambiguities and formlessness. The family of the 1990s is described as the "floating family," resembling foam drifting on the ocean waves. Gergen's symbol evokes the loose ties and weakened emotional bonds existing in our postmodern society—that is, after the 1960s. He noted that it is possible to live within a family group in which no one is related by blood. Divorce and remarriages separate the lines and ties that once held families together. Ministers, therapists, and physicians, rather than the biological entity, became the family support system.

Family theory and therapy developed in a period when the mother's place was clearly in the home and with her children (Goldner 1985a). The theory and rules of behavior behind family interventions are therefore best interpreted as part of a historical context. The female gender role is a culturally constructed concept that refers to attitudes, behaviors, and expectations. Although the range of roles is considerable across cultures, raising children is a role consistently assigned to women (Levine and Padilla 1991). Fathers continue to take a less active role in child rearing (Seeman 1995). Family theory and therapy appear to have accepted these enduring gender roles and have long addressed a narrow view of women's development in which early gender-based experiences influence later interactions between the sexes. The pioneers of family therapy were primarily charismatic male physicians who created strategies to get fathers involved in "helping" mothers with children or chores. The gender bias in these well-intended strategies resulted in an even more lopsided view of the power differential in families. Women and men had their assigned roles, and now it was clearly upfront and obvious!

As noted by Goldner (1985b), developmental differences play a significant role in family interaction patterns. Female development builds on the importance of maintaining attachments and relationships (Gilligan 1982; Jordan et al. 1991). Gilligan (1982) noted that it is difficult for females to maintain attachments while struggling to become autonomous. The female child learns to control anger and aggression, and this makes it difficult for her to behave in assertive ways. The threat of loss of relationships and aggressive conflicts may motivate behavior that puts her at risk for depression or abuse.

A large part of the criticism of early family theories underlined the need to address power inequities in women's roles both in the family and in the workplace. The most often cited criticism was that family therapists, while claiming a nonjudgmental position as systemic theorists, were blaming mothers and absolving fathers for their actions in the sessions. General systems theory was criticized for *presuming* equality among subsystems. The cybernetic model of family interaction presumed *no blame*, only circular responsibility. Viewed in isolation from the larger context, this appeared to be a generous egalitarian perspective on families. However, in reality, certain aspects of systems theory work against women. For example, the concept of circularity implies mutual responsibility and mutual reinforcement. It is not uncommon for family members to renounce all responsibility for actions. Fathers who were out of the home providing a living and too tired to bother with the disciplining of children remained shielded from blame for family problems. Mothers on the other hand were usually singled out for children's problems.

Feminist family literature began to raise questions about gender roles and to define power by such elements as money, job status, and credentials (Chodorow 1978; Goldner 1985a, 1985b). Traditionally, gender roles assigned to women (housekeeping and childcare) have had a lower status and less influence in terms of day-to-day decision making. Therefore, the use of the term "overly involved mother" in relation to the interaction between mothers and their children came to be viewed as a derogatory and sexist criticism of the parental style. The term confused the mother's role as caregiver or authority figure. A major focus of gender-sensitive and feminist family therapy is to assist women in obtaining power and having an equal say in the decision-making process, rather than simply following established family routines.

The early work of Dinnerstein (1976), Chodorow (1978), Hare-Mustin (1978, 1988), and Brodsky and Hare-Mustin (1980) posed some related arguments about gender roles to the field of family therapy and psychotherapy as a whole. Dinnerstein (1976) discussed the different ways male and female power is exhibited in parenting and noted how the domination of childcare by women actually creates a lopsided view of women's power, making them appear more powerful than men. Historically, men have been portrayed as playing a less direct and therefore a less threatening role in regard to discipline. Chodorow (1978) argued that women from early childhood are more involved in interpersonal relationships, whereas men have learned to suppress such attachment. The claim was that girls were taught to value attachments that would prepare them for family life and connectedness. Women's role as a caregiver implied that they should serve others first.

Carol Gilligan's (1982) classic work on women's style of conflict resolution in moral dilemmas is pivotal in discussing gender differences. Gilligan's thesis is that women's morality is based on caring, whereas men's morality is based on individual "rights" (Prozan 1997). Women assess the needs and vulnerability of the people involved in conflicts and seek solutions involving the least damage to those individuals and to the relationship itself (Gilligan 1982). As a result, women's individual needs suffer. This is commonly referred to as the "fear of selfishness": "The inflicting of hurt is considered selfish and immoral in its reflection of unconcern, while the expression of care is seen as the fulfillment of moral responsibility" (Gilligan 1982, p. 73). This applies to major decisions regarding women's responsibility to their families, to their careers, and others. The dichotomy of men being prone to autonomy and women being prone to relatedness created a framework for blaming mothers for their children's problems.

Hare-Mustin and Mareck (Hare-Mustin 1978; Mareck and Hare-Mustin 1991) maintained that psychotherapy is based on a history of insensitivity to gender issues. They argued that most psychodynamically based psychotherapy sets the stage for blaming mothers when there are deficiencies in the socially and psychologically driven system of caregiving and nurturing relationships. Women tend to stretch the rules to preserve relationships, whereas men subscribe to certain standards of truth and justice. These differences can be seen in how women are taught to not question or oppose power or challenge inequities in salary, position, and leadership.

Misapplication of Basic Concepts in Gender Roles

A number of basic gender-role concepts described by the different schools of family therapy have been criticized strongly by feminist and gender-sensitive family therapists. The following concepts can undermine the position of women in the family, impede their development, and reduce their potential contribution to the family. The most alarming issue is the clinical mismanagement of spouse abuse and violence in the family.

Circularity

Circularity is a significant and foundational concept in family therapy. It is very helpful in examining the interrelatedness of behaviors and interactions among different family members; it allows the examination of problematic interactions without blaming one or more family members. However, the concept is hardly applicable to a situation when violent and potentially disabling or fatal actions are perpetrated on one family member by another, as in cases of spouse or child abuse. Abusive and potentially disabling acts can be better understood and handled by holding the perpetrator responsible for his or her actions according to legal principles and consequences. Examination of "circular" facilitating or triggering roles of different family members is helpful only after the potential for violence in the family is eliminated through the appropriate use of legal and social systems.

Being the perpetrator of or a victim of violence does not necessarily coincide with gender. In cases of physical violence against children, both genders make their unfortunate contributions. In cases of spouse abuse and spouse murder, men perpetrate a higher rate of physically and psychologically damaging violence, but women exhibit a sizable level of violence too. In terms of violence against the elderly, the bidirectional nature of violence is skewed, because women's "violent" acts are more neglectful than physically abusive. In terms of sexual violence in the family, men are decidedly overrepresented, although women also commit some of the sexual abuses. For example, it is estimated that 10% of incest cases involve mothers and sons but remain unreported due to a variety of factors (see Chapter 32, "Family Intervention With Incest").

Complementarity of Roles

Complementarity of roles is a concept that has been in use since the early days of family and marital therapy. It allows for the recognition of how family members can function as a team, enhancing one another's functioning and roles along the lines of their mutual and collective strength. Due to ignorance of inequity in gender role assignments, as well as prejudicial societal attributes, women are burdened with laborious and less rewarding roles, while men received more rewarding roles and functions.

Family therapists are rightfully criticized for their ignorance of traditional family role assignments, the detrimental impact of these roles on women and daughters, and the field's inadequate efforts to remedy the situation. The goal of *gender-sensitive family therapy* is to equalize the level of reward and burden in the family while allowing intelligent assignments of family roles to members based on their talents, ability, and productivity, rather than gender. Essential issues to address in reaching this goal are finances, working hours, and equal power to make crucial decisions. The most detrimental inequality is the assignment of childcare solely to women. It deprives men of optimal contributions to the development of their children of both genders, reduces the pleasure of men's relationship and the amount of time spent with their children, and reduces women's opportunities to pursue their interests in careers, the workplace, and other activities.

Role Rigidity

The rigidity in role assignments increases generally and is proportional to the level of family dysfunction. Each spouse has a variety of marital and family roles. Many of the roles assigned to women are tedious, unending, and undervalued and carry low levels of concrete and financial rewards. For instance, the wife may do bookkeeping for her husband's business without pay, while sacrificing her own job that could provide reasonable financial compensation. In contrast, the functions carried out by men outside of the family can be more rewarding financially and in terms of career progression.

The symptoms and syndromes women suffer, such as depression and their lack of adequate response to treatment, may be the product of women's feeling hopelessly "stuck" or "trapped" in unrewarding, burdensome, and degrading family roles and positions. Family therapy can be an effective tool in increasing role flexibility to allow women to search and pursue more rewarding tasks and careers that are in line with their talents and the available opportunities. Some remedies can be found in applying new ways of raising children according to nonprejudicial gender roles, but more important is the intelligent and equitable modification of gender roles within the family.

Closeness and Distance in Relationships

The different socialization goals and process of men and women complicate closeness and distance in relationships. Because men and women are socialized to value different interpersonal qualities, tension, conflict, and potential family dysfunction can result. Women's socialization places a high premium on relationships and taking care of others, whereas men's socialization emphasizes achievement and independence (Gilligan 1982). Prevailing family theories, reflecting cultural biases, tend to undervalue relatedness and pathologize intense relatedness or involvement in terms such as "enmeshment," "overinvolvement," "symbiosis," "fusion," and "undifferentiation." The high prevalence of such labels in clinical reports suggests that some of the normative but intense relationships of women are labeled as pathological.

While downgrading the value of relationships, the field has overvalued and glamorized qualities attributed to men's socialization model and relational distance by concepts such as "differentiation" and "clear boundaries." Only the most extreme levels of relational distance are recognized as pathological; examples of terms applied to these extremes are "isolation," "disengagement," and "cut-off phenomenon." This observation is supported by clinical reports, which find this extreme group of dysfunctions much less prevalent than the pathologized types of intense involvement.

Technical Application

Prejudicial views of gender roles affect women in families. Common family issues include

- Power, money, and finances
- Sharing childcare responsibilities
- Childcare after divorce
- Mother blaming
- Empowerment and disempowerment
- Culturally defined gender roles

The specific culture and the cultural context of women have a marked influence on role definition and enactment. Different individuals view the world around them, especially the world of their family and family relationships, in special and diverse ways. This knowledge is essential to the clinician in today's multicultural and multiethnic societies. Motherhood is a valued role in all cultures, but the responsibilities and privileges vary according to the culture.

Power, Money, and Finances in the Family

Power, money, and finances in the family form an interconnected system. Poor earning capacity can have a decisive effect on the power structure and leverage in families. Frequently men are left in control of financial resources, which can be used as a means of exerting power over the wife and children. The "rewarding" of the wife financially can place her in a dependent and demeaning position. It is common to overvalue the man's financial contributions to the family while devaluing or minimizing that of the woman. Financial inequities in the family are significantly increased when the wife has the responsibility for childcare; this allows the husband to work and possibly earn a higher level of income, which unfortunately can be wielded as power over the wife.

The following case summary demonstrates the exploration of money and jobs in a gender-sensitive approach.

> The husband works as a mason and the wife as a part-time receptionist in a dentist's office. He is frustrated with his job, undecided about long-term career plans, and wants to do trucking in the interim; this is a job he had quit a few years ago so that he could spend more time with his wife. The interim plans require buying a truck for $100,000. The wife doesn't want their home and savings to be used as collateral for the loan. Two gender-related aspects of the case come to light: 1) the wife reveals that the husband denies the job-related physical pain that is driving him to change his job; and 2) he also denies his strong wish to be with his wife rather than on the road. In response to the therapist's inquiry the wife states that she makes 10% and the husband makes 90% of their total income. Simple calculations reveal that the wife brings in at least one-third of their joint income through her direct income and bookkeeping for her husband. The career aspirations of the wife are completely ignored by the couple. She wishes to become an accountant and is well positioned, interested, and has proven ability. Becoming a dental hygienist was her backup career plan. However, her promising and practical plans are put on the back burner in deference to the husband's questionable interim plans. The couple is encouraged to invest in the wife's career plans, which seem very promising, and the husband is encouraged to explore less risky interim job possibilities.

Sharing Childcare Responsibilities

Childcare should be a mutual responsibility of the couple rather than the predominant obligation of the mother. The childcare tasks of the mother can be excessive and exhausting. Her basic responsibilities may include driving children to their multiple social activities, supervising their homework, and tutoring them in areas of educational weakness. The responsibility for waking up with the babies and young children at night may be totally assigned to the mothers in some families rather than shared by the parents. This arrangement weakens the relationship of the children with the father. In some families, the father's work is considered to be finished when he arrives home, whereas the mother's work is unending. The mother may be held back from obtaining further education or employment because she has to stay home and take care of the children: such restrictions often do not apply to the father. The father may be able to take multiple days off without criticism to attend an out-of-town meeting, whereas the exercise of the same option by the mother can portray her as disinterested and neglectful. Family therapy strategies are well suited to bring about equality in responsibility for childcare by assignment of this duty to both parents. The traditional bias toward women as the nurturers in families implies that caregiving is a gender-related responsibility. Tied into this is the idealization of motherhood, which may also create conflict for women who choose to not be mothers or choose to combine motherhood and a career.

Childcare and Child Support After Divorce

Childcare and child support following a divorce can be very difficult financially for women, due in large part to contemporary no-fault divorcee laws. In the majority of divorced families, the mothers are responsible for all aspects of childcare, including health care. In many cases, reduced financial resources and inadequate or unreliable child support complicate the mother's responsibilities. Statistics indicate that more than 60% of biological fathers provide no financial support (Furstenberg et al. 1987). Further complicating matters is the fact that women workers in the United States continue to make about 74 cents for every dollar made by male workers (U.S. Department of Labor 1996).

Financial contribution toward a child's future, including plans for a college education and financial protection in case of death, is often omitted from divorce settlements. The lack of attention to children's future wellbeing and the custodial parent's resources is an indication of the difficult position in which women are often placed; they become the sole caregivers, while being blamed for their extensive involvement in the child's upbringing. Gender bias ignores the majority of fathers who are capable of developing necessary childcare skills and who are interested in their children's economic security. Too often children develop the view that dad is the good guy since he is not stressed-out on visits or vacations, whereas mom is always tired and nags about cleaning up or doing homework.

Mother Blaming

Mothers are often held accountable for the emotional difficulties of the children. Blaming one or both parents is generally counterproductive. Very often, errors of omission due to the emotional absence of the father are mislabeled as the mother's errors of commission. Vulnerability to biological factors such as attention-deficit/hyperactivity disorder (ADHD), depression, or separation anxiety can hardly be blamed on one of the parents. A comprehensive evaluation of the individual, family, and biological contributions to maladjustment is generally more conducive to a successful outcome.

Empowerment and Disempowerment

The empowerment and disempowerment of women have a number of remedies and causes. For example, women entering the workforce can help reverse the disempowering impact of the prejudicial treatment of women in the society and the family that limits their options and withholds adequate resources and rewards from them. The lack of appropriate rewards in society and family stifles women's true creativity and productivity and generates self-doubt and withdrawal from challenging and potentially rewarding activities. A young woman consulted one of the authors of this chapter about depression and anxiety. She expressed severe doubts about her ability to go to graduate school to obtain a meaningful job, although she graduated with high honors from a highly competitive Ivy League school. Her self-confidence had significantly diminished during several years of caring for a child with pervasive developmental disorder. The therapist uncovered her impressive educational history, succeeded in helping her to enter a graduate school, and shared the pleasure of the woman and her husband when she graduated and began a rewarding career. The son's emotional disorder improved moderately during this period.

The empowerment of women includes making them aware of their options. Most importantly, it helps women to speak up, find their own voice, become aware of their talents, and actively search for fulfillment without fear of failure or feeling guilty ("self-guilt"). It is a premise of family theory that the fulfillment of women enhances the status of all family members. Conversely, stifling women's development and growth produces stagnation in other family members.

The case study below describes a wife who was "stuck" in an unrewarding situation in her family. She had a master's degree, came from a very achievement-oriented family, and was married to a well-trained but non-achievement-oriented husband.

> The wife initiated treatment for anxiety and agoraphobia. Her role was that of a housewife. The husband did not make enough money to comfortably support the family of five, didn't want to work harder, and enjoyed relaxing with the children. The mother was not needed on a full-time basis because the three children were teenagers. A well-positioned friend asked for her help with his consulting business, an opportunity that was exciting and possibly lucrative. The husband felt very comfortable with his wife's wish to change her role in the family, that is, from a housewife to a working woman. She actually had functioned well in her career prior to the birth of their children. In addition, this change would have allowed the husband to work less. Within a few years, the wife's income increased sevenfold in comparison to the husband's income. She felt as accomplished as her male siblings and father and became a positive role model for her children, and her husband enjoyed the reduction in his financial responsibility as well as his increased time with the children. Subsequently, he asked several times to work for his wife, a request that she declined. Continued but sporadic clinical work with the family over a period of 10 years exhibited her positive impact as an exceptional role model for her son and daughters. In summary, the family therapist uncovered the women's many talents, the opportunities open to her, and the husband's flexible view of gender roles. The therapeutic plans to empower the woman thus bore fruit, which further empowered the whole family.

Spouse Abuse

The subject of spouse abuse (also called wife abuse) has been studied more seriously over the past 15 years and has gained visibility in the media, particularly after the O.J. Simpson trial. Violence toward the spouse can originate from either gender. It is generally underreported due to fear or shame, particularly in cases of abused husbands. Spouse murder can occur frequently within the context of domestic violence. Wives and husbands are victims in 60% and 40% of reported abuse cases, respectively (Coleman and Straus 1986). Violence and cruelty toward women and children as two vulnerable groups are part of American social history. The right to *not* be beaten or battered is more recent than one would expect (Gordon 1988; Straus and Sweet 1992). The first known women's shelter was started in

England only in 1971; the first U.S. shelter opened in St. Paul, Minnesota, during the mid-1970s (Fleming 1979).

One of the major difficulties of studying violence in intimate relationships has been the sanctioning of different forms of abusive behavior within the framework of cultural, religious, and kinship groups. Victims of domestic violence often hide their shame to protect the spouse's position or status, or most commonly because of embarrassment and fear brought about by the sequence of events. The middle class often chooses the anonymity of a private physician instead of reporting to an emergency room. More frequently reported are the abuse cases of less affluent families brought to an emergency room by the police. A National Institute of Mental Health (NIMH) project on violence found that 21% of all women who use emergency surgical services are battered; 50% of all injuries occur as the result of partner abuse; and 50% of all rapes of women over 30 years of age are part of this battering syndrome (Straus and Gelles 1990).

Violence in the marriage or in an intimate relationship is not determined by culture or social class. It is part of the pattern of destructive and aggressive behaviors associated with other forms of abuse, emotional as well as sexual, toward both women and children in families. Recent explanatory theories of abuse relate it to the status and psychological and social power of men; inequalities in the provision of economic resources to women; the politics of the discussion of motherhood versus career or employment; and, more fundamentally, issues related to the marital contract (C. Sager 1976) that may be ill-fated from the start. Coleman and Straus (1986) found that when family relationships were either female-dominant or male-dominant, there was the highest likelihood of violence, whereas with shared responsibility in decision making, there was little violence. The conflict over control and the limitation of both psychological and economic resources intensified the expression of family violence.

Alcohol is closely associated with violent behavior. As Gelles (1972) has noted, intoxication provides an excuse and a justification for the violence because it leads to arguments (usually over the alcohol) and serves as a trigger for long-standing, repetitive disputes that may culminate in violence. A study by L. Walker (1989) found that in cases of battered women who were killed by their abusers, the abuser's drinking had increased over time as had his unpredictability and violence. A national drug use survey by the National Institute on Drug Abuse (NIDA), reported in Gelles and Straus (1990), found that 53% of respondents who reported being drunk more than twice a month became aggressive and angry when they drank. Serious arguments as a result of the drinking were reported by 41% of respondents. Of the men in the 1,600 cases studied, 80% were drunk every time they were violent.

In the intimacy of a marital relationship, violence can easily escalate and become reciprocal. Although women are more likely to cry or yell or run from the room, a significant number of women can and do hit back, as witnessed by incidents of victims killing their abusers.

Treatment of spouse abuse should initially concentrate on the protection of victims using all measures, including police involvement and temporary shelter. Psychological issues such as helplessness, victimization, substance abuse, stress management, and gender role considerations should be addressed within a comprehensive framework and *after* the safety of the potential victims is established.

Prevalence

A 1990 survey estimated that 2 million wives are severely beaten by their husbands each year (Straus and Gelles 1990). Other researchers have estimate that 4 million women are severely assaulted each year (Browne 1993). Despite the presence of domestic violence throughout American history, the first nationally representative survey reporting prevalence data of marital violence was not conducted until 1975 (Straus et al. 1980). In some samples 80% of the battered women were injured by their partners so badly that they needed medical attention. Of the batters, 20% had been arrested for domestic violence. Sociodemographic correlates of domestic assault reveal higher rates of violence among couples who are younger, poorer, less educated, unmarried, African American, Hispanic, and urban. The higher reported prevalence rate for domestic abuse of a nonwhite population in comparison with a white population has not been a consistent finding in the literature (Lupri et al. 1994; Rosenberg and Fenely 1991).

National survey results indicated that women are as likely as men to report engaging in assault against spouses or partners (see Straus et al. 1980); these results fueled theoretical and methodological debates. Feminist scholars have offered a methodological critique of the use of large-scale surveys to research domestic violence. Although most therapists acknowledge that in heterosexual relationships, men have a greater capacity to injure women, controversy remains about whether there is a fundamental asymmetry between men and women who are violent. For example, men are more likely to use severely violent tactics, less likely to be injured, and less likely to be intimidated by their partner's violence (Cantos et al. 1994; Cascardi et al. 1992; Dobash et al. 1992; Langhinrichsen-Rohling et al. 1995). While men and women alike employ violence to express anger, release tension, or force communication, women tend to use violence for self-defense, escape, and retaliation (Straus and Gelles 1990). In working toward an integrated sociological theory of domestic violence, it is important to analyze theories of domestic violence in relation to violence perpetuated by women and men. Examining victims of husband abuse and wife abuse, Christian et al. (1994) found that victimized wives reported more negative impact and more frequent and severe injuries than did victimized husbands, and female perpetrators experienced more depression than male perpetrators (Vivian and Malone 1996). A husband's violence produces fear in the partner. In couples in which the man has been quite violent, wives are verbally aggressive in reactions to husbands' violent behaviors, whereas husbands are violent in response to a variety of nonviolent wife behaviors. Because men report becoming more violent when their partners attempt to use force (Mederos 1995), it can be helpful to discuss with women how they can balance their need for retaliation or self-defense with efforts to enhance their safety.

Clinical innovations developed by experts on domestic violence have failed to reach the field of family therapy (Jacobson and Gottman 1998). It is still the exception rather than the norm for a family therapist to receive state-of-the-art training in detecting violence in couples, assessing lethality of batterers, and knowing when to refer the batterers to a specialist in domestic violence rather than keeping the batterer in couples therapy. Due to the pervasive minimization, denial, and distortion in batterer's self-reports and the subjectivity in retrospective accounts of violent incidents (Jacobson and Gottman 1998), some researchers have looked toward a more comprehensive battery of assessments.

Assessment

Domestic violence is not a new social phenomena, but it has been steadily rising or increasingly recognized in the American culture. Initial prevalence estimates suggest that one adult woman in five is physically abused by a partner. Of the injured women who enter emergency rooms, 22%–35% are abused by their partners. Violent relationships are all too often the result of the changing roles of women and rising expectations for marital satisfaction and personal growth. Violence toward women occurs in the context of male dominance and women's subordination. It encourages timidity, passivity, and a sense of powerlessness in women (Gordon 1988). Domestic violence is not merely another women's health issue; it is part of a complex web of women's health problems including birth control, pregnancy, AIDS, and mental illness. Women today are more encouraged to take action in reaching their potential and making choices in life. This includes making good choices in relationships. Women *continue* to be defined in relation to marriage and their relationship with men. When these relationships become violent, women often get caught up in what has been called a "cycle of violence" (Walker 1989). Abused women often feel trapped and helpless but remain in abusive relationships because they fear reprisal or are seduced into believing that the abuser will change. They remain dependent and unable to fight back, and worst of all, they "no longer feel the pain" (Walker 1989).

Walker (1989) describes three phases of domestic violence:

Phase one: Tension builds during which minor incidents occur. During this phase the *victim* tries to calm the abuser by using whatever tactics work. She denies feeling angry, helpless, and terrified, yet the anger and the terror increase. The abuser becomes fearful that the victim will leave him, yet becomes more possessive and often jealous of her interactions with others. As the victim withdraws more, the minor incidents increase and the tension becomes unbearable.

Phase two: An acute battering incident occurs as a result of the mounting tension. The abuser loses control and wants to "teach the woman a lesson, not to hurt her." He tries to justify his behavior by accusing her of something. Men usually do not remember much during this incident; however, women do. The victim waits for the incident to end, fearing more harm if she retaliates, but the anticipation causes severe psychological stress, including headaches, appetite changes, and constant fatigue. Shock, denial, and disbelief occur. Women typically do not seek help during phase two unless badly hurt and then return to the abuser after treatment in the emergency room.

Phase three: Kindness and contrite loving behavior are demonstrated by the abuser. This is part of the denial but welcomed by both parties. He knows he went too far and "tries to make it up to her." This completes the victimization of the woman. Finally, a calm returns; he begs forgiveness and promises to stop. The victim unfortunately wants to believe him as he "reminds" her how much he loves her. The many roadblocks to leaving the abusive relationship include lack of job skills, threats of loss of custody of children, fear of loneliness, fear of escalating violence or death, and, worst of all, the psychological stripping of her self-respect and esteem. The victimization leaves her exhausted and more vulnerable to the kindness the abuser provides after the assault. Women in abusive relationships demonstrate how difficult it is to break out of the cycle of violence. Violence in relationships is transmitted over generations and becomes part of a family's way of interacting. In addition to the culpability of traditional cultural norms of femininity and masculinity, Prozan (1997, p. 236) writes, "It takes two times two to produce the phenomenon of the battered woman—the parents of the victim and the parents of the abusive, battering male."

A related issue in the abuse of power is the *misuse of a professional relationship* through patient-therapist or student-teacher sex. Rutter (1979) describes how men by virtue of their professional status and power can control women's access to jobs, careers, and education. The potential for misuse of the power by the men always exists. Rutter also distinguishes between sexual harassment on the job and the violation of trust, which occurs in professional relationships, and is especially harmful in a therapeutic relationship. Rutter's position is that the person in the position of power has a clear responsibility to assure that sexual behavior does not occur in the therapeutic relationship.

Treatment Issues With Family Violence

Assessment of the potential for violence or the observation of violence and abuse in the family requires action on the part of the therapist. Frequently, battering is inaccurately assessed and remains undetected, allowing the abusive behavior to escalate. Attention should be paid to the potential for abuse from the initial referral phone call to the therapist. Hare-Mustin (1978, 1988) lists the following guidelines for determining the level of abuse:

- *Mild abuse:* yelling, pushing, slapping, shoving, verbal abuse, or name calling
- *Moderate abuse:* punching with fists, hitting in the face or head, pulling, dragging by the hair, or kicking
- *Severe abuse:* use of a weapon (gun or knife), choking, or running down with a car

Once the therapist assesses the nature of the abuse, he or she may decide to see the woman alone, especially in cases of mild to moderate abuse. The patient may find it easier to describe the situation without the domestic partner present. During the session, the therapist will elicit descriptions of the three most recent episodes and of the worst episode. The therapist questions what was happening prior to the incident, what happened after the battering stopped, who else might have been involved, and the impact of the battering on the woman. In the course of the session the therapist should consider the following issues:

1. Inquire if police assistance has been called for, a legal complaint made, and restraining orders obtained. The legal steps will make the abuser aware that his actions are judged by criminal standards rather than as family disagreement. Involvement of the police also ensures the protection of the victim from the abuser.

2. Ensure the woman's safety by either finding a way to stop the violence, enlisting the help of police, or helping her to find a shelter or safe home with a friend or relative (Walker 1989).
3. Review backup plans and a hold a rehearsal of safety plans.
4. Listen to and believe what the woman says. Take the story seriously and gather the essential information on the history of the relationship and the abusive acts to help her understand her situation.
5. Identify the woman's feelings. For example, she may experience numbness or helplessness much like the response of a trauma victim. The therapist may need to label the feelings for her, especially the right to be angry.
6. Identify the impact of the violence on the woman's behavior. She may help understand how she has adapted to the violence as a way of protecting herself. She may also have "contributed" to the abuser's behavior.
7. Foster self-empowerment. The therapist should point out how the woman's patience and tolerance may have contributed to maintaining the abusive relationship (Goodrich 1991).
8. Assist in the development of problem-solving skills. Once the woman's safety is assured, the therapist can help her focus on how to get help from different agencies, help her make a list of problems, and assist her in taking small steps toward solutions.
9. Advocate social agency support.
10. Encourage the woman's participation in support groups to move beyond isolation and guilt about the situation.
11. Encourage the continuation of a therapeutic relationship until the violence is no longer a threat and the woman may return to the relationship.

The relationship issues involved with violence are complex and based on both conscious and unconscious defenses and needs. One of the primary considerations is attention to the social context of the couple and the safety of the patients. Understanding the nature of the relationship can only come once the threat of violence is removed. The goals of treatment would be to eliminate the violence, help the couple recognize their behavior, and ultimately to assist them to recognize the maladaptive reasons which brought them together. The decision to separate is the last, not the initial, step in treating these relationships.

The advanced stage of intervention and treatment for family violence focuses on shared responsibility for the battering. This stage is part of the systemic view of causality. Theories differ regarding how to treat the abuser and victim as a couple. Some clinicians question the need to involve the victim in couples therapy since it implies blame and responsibility. Other clinicians maintain that the victim should learn strategies to protect himself or herself, including learning about a victim's own subtle contribution to the abuse. This does not mitigate the role of the batterer, but looks at the dynamics in the relationship. Many strategies and interventions used in strategic, structural, and psychodynamic approaches can be viewed as enhancing the victimization of women in both direct and indirect ways. In an effort to unravel unconscious motivations for violence in the relationship, it is conceivable to discuss coresponsibility; however, the therapist should be *very aware* of how easily the victim can be blamed. Mental health professionals can easily and unwittingly blame the victim when exploring the subtleties of the relationship.

As with all psychotherapies, personal values and philosophies enter into treatment in quite subtle ways and can become part of the therapeutic process for both male and female clinicians. There are many possibilities for countertransference in treating these cases. It is incumbent on both male and female clinicians to become familiar with gender-related issues, which include the legal aspects of domestic violence, the clinical signs of abuse, knowing where to refer a patient for help and protection, and in general how to intervene when a patient presents with a problem with the potential for spouse abuse.

The goals in conjoint therapy are to eliminate the violence and preserve the adaptive qualities in the relationship. Therapy should focus on the positive aspects of the relationship in addition to exploring the damaging aspects of the couple's interactions. The assessment of the couple's ability to engage in treatment, to communicate feelings, and to observe their own behavior and work toward problem solving is important.

An additional goal is to reduce the overwhelming emotional experiences of rage by the abuser and fear on the part of the victim. The intensity of the emotions exhibited in the interactions may impair the couple's ability to accurately perceive their intentions and behaviors. The therapist should monitor emotions to prevent the couple from becoming overwhelmed.

Helpful family therapy techniques include asking the couple to speak to the therapist, not to each other. This breaks the cycle of mutual blaming and criticism and gives the couple a "time out." Reframing of statements is useful to prevent blaming and negative escalation. It can also help to suggest that the couple seems to be "very close and involved" in cases of enmeshment. The therapist should emphasize the strength of the relationship before pointing out mutual projections of blame, particularly in the beginning stage of therapy. Furthermore, allowing old battles and issues to reemerge in therapy sessions without a specific purpose is counterproductive, especially with couples who have demonstrated violence in their relationship (Bagarozzi and Giddings 1983).

Another important goal is to increase both partners' awareness of choices: violence and submission are not the only paths. The basic feelings behind violent outbursts are hidden. The therapist can help identify the fear, powerlessness, and sense of loss behind the couple's interactions as well as the sources of stress.

The most important therapeutic goal is to establish that *violence is unacceptable*, and the couple should commit themselves to a contract of nonviolence. If necessary, the legal process should be called on to ensure this requirement is met before the therapist attempts to identify and rehabilitate the interactional problems between the couple.

Comprehensive Intervention in Family Violence

Training of Healthcare and Law Enforcement Personnel

Careful training of healthcare and law enforcement personnel in gender-based issues is essential to the mental and physical well-being of women. Women's mental and physical health issues have become a matter of great concern and urgency, especially in light of the rise in violence toward women in society today. At Massachusetts General Hospital, for example, considerable attention is paid to the role of domestic violence in today's culture. The hospital's Law and Psychiatry Program calls attention to the need for physicians, especially psychiatrists, to become aware of manifestations of violence toward both women and children. Knowing the law and what can be done is part of responsive and responsible medical practice.

It is not only psychiatrists or mental health professionals who need to become more aware of gender-based issues, but also primary care physicians and especially OB-GYN specialists. Considering the trend in healthcare delivery that emphasizes brief intervention, it is incumbent on *all* physicians to become more sensitized to the impact of economic, social, and family contexts on a woman's mental health. Recognizing the struggle to keep a family together can benefit a patient enormously. A good working relationship between psychiatry and primary care is a definite asset in furthering the mental and physical health of women. Physicians must know how to listen to a woman's problems and look beyond physical complaints. Very often an empathic physician's response and the safety and confidentiality of the physician's office will allow a woman to reveal her need for psychological intervention due to symptoms of abusive relationships, posttraumatic stress disorder, eating disorders, serious depression, and/or severe anxiety. These signs could easily go undetected and untreated without the assistance of a physician trained in gender-based issues.

Different educational programs are available to improve the physician's approach to violence and sexual abuse. Medical schools and residencies now teach students and residents to *ask* all or almost all patients about domestic violence. This awareness is vitally important for all primary care physicians, but especially for emergency room physicians and OB-GYN specialists. Very often these specialists' observation of the patient's demeanor and presentation during an examination could make the difference in averting or prolonging violence and abuse. A psychiatric referral for medication and treatment, including the treatment of anxiety and depression, can be made based on the observation and history of the patient.

Feminist readings that present and clarify ideology, readings in the sociology of the family, and courses in women's psychology and development are recommended as part of the physician's curriculum. Familiarity with specific family approaches to treating depression, eating disorders, and sexual abuse can also sensitize the clinician to gender issues. Continuing medical education courses in violence and sexual harassment can further educate physicians on how changes in role structure, power, and position affect women and families today.

Training in Gender Issues

Piercy and Sprenkle (1986) advocate several principles for training family therapists in gender-related issues:

- Make gender issues part of the ideology of treatment. This may necessitate a shift in thinking to counter old attitudes regarding women's abilities and the standards for judging their behavior, their successes, and their need to compete.
- Ensure that the conceptual framework for evaluating families addresses changes in the structure of families as well as power differences in families. Family structure need not be hierarchical; it can and should be reciprocal, mutual, and democratic in nature.
- Strive to empower women to value their skills and assert their feelings and needs in the following ways:
  1. Build self-confidence by pointing out their contributions to the family.
  2. Support them in building social supports.
  3. Prepare them to handle any backlash from family when they do assert themselves.
  4. Affirm women's rights to pursue careers beyond the home.
- Recognize the prevalence of violence in families and review the extensive research in this crucial area.

Conclusion

The promise of family theory to create a conceptual model to enhance the development of all family members has been compromised by lack of attention to the importance of gender roles. Societal prejudices against women have penetrated deeply the practice of family therapy through the misapplication of basic family theory concepts. The potential for clinical mismanagement is particularly significant when an intervention for spouse abuse and family violence is necessary.

Feminist family therapists were the pioneers of gender sensitivity in psychiatry. They focused attention on the serious inequities in gender roles and the partial blindness of some of the leading family therapists to these problems. Gender-sensitive family therapists further defined household inequities in the distribution of power, money, and household responsibilities, including childcare. The position of women in families is thus undermined, and they are denied the power to achieving personal fulfillment. Gender-sensitive family therapists have provided guidelines for the examination of biased views of gender roles and the detrimental effect of such biases on the welfare and development of women. These therapists have also proposed the remedy: women should have equal access to opportunities and rewards to help them fulfil their potential. Just as important as counteracting bias is to address ways of preventing spousal abuse and family violence through therapeutic and preventive measures. Educating healthcare and law enforcement personnel in gender-related issues is an essential step in the prevention of family violence.

Chapters on Related Topics

The following chapters describe concepts related to gender issues:

- Chapter 2, "Structural Family Therapy"
- Chapter 3, "Constructing Therapy: From Strategic, to Systemic, to Narrative Models"
- Chapter 4, "Psychodynamic Family Therapy"

11

Techniques of Family Therapy

G. Pirooz Sholevar, M.D.
Linda D. Schwoeri, Ph.D.

Introduction

The interventions directed at change in family relationships fall into two broad categories: strategies and techniques. These interventions are guided by multiple principles, prominent among which are the following:

- The theoretical model employed by the therapist to evaluate, diagnose, and alter family relationships
- The therapist's understanding of a particular family and its responsiveness to therapeutic interventions
- The style, personality, and values of the therapist

The field of family therapy is moving toward a stage wherein multiple theoretical paradigms can be combined into a preliminary comprehensive model of evaluation, diagnosis, and intervention with families. Practitioners are noticing that multiple theoretical systems often address and present the same dimensions of family life as novel findings. For example, *boundary diffusion* between family members is referred to as diffuse boundaries, lack of differentiation, enmeshment, and other terms, but it refers primarily to the same dimension. The breaching of family boundaries is referred to as *triangulation, coalition formation, or collusion;* basically these terms describe the same phenomenon.

Family therapy is also moving away from a variety of relatively dramatic technical interventions that are primarily rooted in the therapist's personality and style but not effective with multiple family types of therapy. More commonly accepted is the belief that effective therapists have a broad repertoire of techniques and styles that are applied, when appropriate, to different families. At the same time, there is a movement away from a chameleon type of stylistic performance that imitates the pioneers in the field. The more current practice for therapists is to adapt their strategies and styles to the contextual needs of families rather than adhere to rigid therapeutic techniques.

The *theoretical orientation* of individual therapists affects their data collection methods and interventions. *Behaviorally oriented family therapists* are particularly interested in systematic evaluations of reinforcement practices in a family. These clinicians attempt to enhance positive reinforcement and undermine punitive, coercive, and avoidant interactions. *Structural family therapists* focus on family boundaries and attempt to alter boundaries, thereby providing healthy and flexible support for different family members and family subsystems while countering enmeshment and isolation. *Psychodynamic family therapists* search for unexpressed and conflictual feelings that, although hidden, can produce rigidity in the family system.

Psychodynamic and object relations family therapists often view the current relationship dysfunctions of patients as reflecting the unsatisfied basic needs in the mother-child dyad. *Experiential family therapists* attempt to improve families' tolerance of intense affect and to produce more adaptive behaviors through enhanced self-awareness and the expansion of the domain of the self. Such expansion of self will also include the dimensions of communication and problem solving emphasized by behavioral family therapists.

Protection of the family unit from external forces is an important goal of all family therapists, but *intergenerational family therapists* and *network therapists* address it in particular. Intergenerational family therapists address the transmission of undifferentiation, anxiety, and conflict from prior generations by exploring the triangulation, loyalty conflicts, indebtedness, and entitlement issues that can transcend multiple generations. Network therapists address constrictions and dysfunctionality in the family network that obstruct the normative feedback needed for maintenance and progression of family development.

Therapist Styles

Therapists' styles of relating to families can be intimate, distant, technical, or almost manipulative (Beels and Ferber 1972). Although they practice a combination of these styles, most therapists can be grouped into two major types: *conductors* and *reactors*.

Conductor Type

The *conductor type* refers to active, assertive therapists who place themselves in the center of the family as experts or teachers. They initiate interactions rather than waiting for the family to start. Conductors are often described as vigorous personalities who hold their audiences' attention through strategic moves and eclectic techniques; Ackerman (1955) and Satir (1964, 1972) represent this style. Ackerman's style was to watch for nonverbal gestures and interactional clues to themes, and Satir's communication exercises enhanced the capacity of the families to listen and attend to one another's expressions. Bowen (1978) and Minuchin (1974a, 1974d) are also conductor types because they take charge of and control interactions in sessions. Bowen de-emphasizes his role as a therapist because he feels that it only fosters dependency on the therapist. Minuchin uses himself as an agent for change through his mimetic unbalancing and reframing maneuvers. Both Bowen and Minuchin emphasize differentiation but do so using different tactics and strategies.

Reactor Type

The *reactor* type refers to therapists who are more indirect than the conductor type. Boszormenyi-Nagy (1976), David and Jill Scharff (1987), Sonne (1981), and Whitaker (1953, 1976a, 1976b) represent the *analyst* type of reactor by conceptualizing interactions in psychoanalytic terms, attending to the projections and internalizations, and actively exploring transference and countertransference issues. Haley (1962, 1967, 1976), Jackson (1965), Madanes (1980), and Zuk (1971) represent a second reactor type, *system purists*, so called because they attend to the family's power to maneuver to exclude and control the therapist. System purists use directive, problem solving, and strategic approaches with the families.

Intensified Family Interactional Technique

The *intensified family interactional technique* calls for therapists to encourage family members to interact with each other on a certain issue to make the covert family interactional pattern more visible and subsequently demonstrable to the family. The therapist remains in the room but does not respond to the family's overt or covert maneuvers to involve him or her in the discussions. Once the family interactional pattern becomes clear, therapists may make suggestions with the goal of altering particular patterns. For example, the therapist may prompt a silent *member in a family* dispute to take a more active part in the resolution of conflict.

Funneling Through the Therapist Technique

In the *funneling through the therapist* technique each family member is encouraged to converse *only* with the therapist while the other members listen. This allows the therapist to get each family member to describe his or her ideas, feelings, and perspectives while minimizing collusive and defensive maneuvers by other family members that can diffuse issues, create collusion, and prevent problem solving. The technique allows each family member to describe his or her experiences fully; family members are thereby helped to see each other objectively, rather than through the mutual projection of distorted expectations. Funneling through the therapist helps reduce fusion, undifferentiation, collusion, and triangulation. Bowen is considered the strongest proponent of the funneling technique.

Structural Therapy Techniques

Structural therapy techniques attempt to alter structural and boundary deviations in the family and are particularly effective with families in crisis.

Boundary-Making

Boundary-making is a structural technique that creates both the psychological and physical distance in a family system necessary for the differentiation process. The goal is to decrease *enmeshment* or *overinvolvement* within the family system by constructing a new, functional boundary between subsystems. Boundaries are defined, respected, and maintained. There is no "mind reading" or talking for someone else (Minuchin and Fishman 1981). The therapist can symbolically create boundaries by rearranging the seating or by using hand gestures to stop or cut off comments. Boundaries are likewise created by having one subsystem interact while excluding another.

Joining

Joining is a set of techniques whereby the therapist attempts to enter a family system and form a type of partnership with the family. Being positioned within the family allows the therapist to change dysfunctional family transactions, minimize symptoms, and reduce conflict and stress (Minuchin and Fishman 1981). Joining allows the family to accept the therapist as a helper and reassures the family that it is supported, understood, and confirmed.

Tracking

Tracking refers to the therapist's careful, attentive listening to family dialogue and to the observance of family behavior and communication. It provides information about family interaction, structure, roles, process, and content. By attending to his or her own reactions, the therapist comes to appreciate how the family includes and excludes members and how they allow alliances and coalitions to form. This observation helps the therapist avoid being inducted into the system.

Mimesis

Mimesis is the adoption of the family's style of communicating—its affect, humor, speech patterns, tempo, and the extent of communication—in an effort to accommodate or join with the family.

Family Mapping

Family mapping visually depicts the structure of dysfunctional families. Systems and subsystems are drawn and labeled for clarification.

Actualization

Actualization refers to the process of enacting or replaying a particular transactional family pattern within the session. Minuchin and Fishman (1981) discuss three types of enactment:

1. Enactment may take the form of spontaneously occurring sequences that the therapist observes and earmarks for later replaying.
2. A therapist may ask the family to enact a usual manner of interacting and then intervenes to change the script, requiring the family to find a new solution. This type of enactment is used for diagnostic and restructuring purposes.
3. The most change-producing type of enactment happens when a new, successful interaction occurs. The individual then experiences himself or herself as competent and capable of organizing and creating a totally different interaction.

Intensity

The *intensity* technique attempts to highlight a family theme or emphasis with the expectation of eventually modifying family interactions. For example, a therapist may allow a child to have a temper tantrum in the session and then encourage the parents to take charge and get control of the situation. Another approach to the intensity technique is to immediately highlight successful sequences of behavior.

Unbalancing

The *unbalancing* technique attempts to change stalemated conflicts and hierarchical dysfunctions among members of the family subsystem. To be effective, the therapist must first join with the family as a leader and maintain affiliation with all members of the system. The therapist can create unbalance by ignoring family members, affiliating with certain ones, or entering into a coalition with some family members against others. The therapist can create hierarchical unbalancing by supporting joint parental decisions, while also supporting an adolescent's right to question changes in the parents' approach to decision making.

Reframing or Relabeling

The *reframing* or *relabeling* technique is used by structural, strategic, and behavioral family therapists. In reframing, the therapist alters information presented by the family to give a new and more helpful meaning. For example, a jealous spouse can be told, "You really care about your husband and don't want to lose him."

Use of Cognitive Constructions

Cognitive construction refers to providing the family with an alternative view of what they are experiencing. The altered cognition provides additional options for enhanced interaction. For example, the therapist asks a child "How old are you?" and then states "Oh, I thought you were younger because 7-year-olds do not need their mothers' help to tie their shoes."

Strategic, Systemic, and Triadic-Based Techniques

Strategic techniques provide the therapist with specific and powerful tools to counter the rigid, homeostasis-maintaining posture of the family. The specific techniques are very similar to those of behavioral and structural family therapists but are mainly focused on the therapist's strategy as a way of undermining the potent resistance of highly rigid families.

Therapeutic Strategies

Therapeutic strategies refer to the overall plan and intervention strategy designed by the therapist to promote change in highly change-resistant families. Therapeutic strategies are closely related to the strategies used by the family to maintain family dysfunctional patterns. These strategies focus directly on the family interactions, usually by incorporating symptomatic interactions, and do not include collaboration with the family.

Directives

The assignment of *directives* is the cornerstone of strategic and systemic family therapies. The therapist assigns therapeutic tasks to the family to practice between sessions with the goal of breaking inappropriate sequences of behavior and realigning the family relationships. The goal of the directives can be straightforward or paradoxical.

Circular Questioning

Circular questioning refers to interview questions directed by the therapist to family members in an effort to learn more about differences between the family members or changes in family relationships. Circular questioning is also referred to as a *triadic questionnaire*, because a third party is asked to describe the behavior and interactions of the first and second parties. The answers provide the therapist with clues to how one party thinks the other would answer a question or how a family member would behave in certain circumstances. The therapist can then proceed to generate interventions and help the family to view themselves systematically in the context of their interactions with each other (Penn 1985; Selvini Palazzoli et al. 1978). Circular questioning attempts to bypass the defensiveness caused by direct questions.

Therapeutic Paradox

Therapeutic paradox refers to the seemingly illogical instructions used to change family relationships. Interventions appear illogical because they represent apparent contradictions to the goals of therapy (Haley 1976). The therapist needs to forge seemingly powerful arguments to persuade the family to follow the contradictory instructions. Major classes of therapeutic paradox include symptom prescription, restraining, and positioning.

Symptom Prescription

Symptom prescription or prescribing refers to strategies whereby the therapist uses powerful rationales and arguments to encourage or instruct the patients to perform their symptoms. For example, a couple requesting treatment for the reduction of marital fighting may be instructed to continue the fight in order to resolve the underlying issues and eventually have a more harmonious family life.

Restraining

Restraining is a paradoxical instruction that discourages patients from the achievement of their therapeutic goals. Restraining usually entails informing patients of a range of dangers implicit in improvement. For example, a couple may be told that improvement in the symptoms of their child may result in increased marital alienation or fighting.

Positioning

Positioning is a paradoxical intervention that refers to the enthusiastic acceptance of the family's statements by the therapist. This can eventually reveal the absurdity of the situation and force the family to change its relationship. At times, the accusatory party may move to defend the accused family member following the positioning of the therapist. For example, a mother reluctant to visit her sisters gives the excuse that her husband would drink in her absence, get their 12-year-old son drunk, and murder him. She is encouraged by the therapist to visit her sisters and pursue her own plans instead of acting as a guardian for the alleged "dangerous and irresponsible father." The visitation between the mother and her sisters results in the mother's increased closeness with her family of origin as well as increased closeness between the son and the father.

Pretending

Pretending involves the therapist's instructing a family member *to feign* his or her symptom. The expectation is that gradually the symptom will appear as voluntary behavior, rather than behavior outside of the patient's control.

Relabeling or Reframing

In *relabeling*, or *reframing*, the therapist assigns a new and usually positive meaning to a situation in order to alter its negative effects or consequences. For example, the runaway behavior of an adolescent may be relabeled as an attempt to gain autonomy.

Positive Connotation

Positive connotation refers to the relabeling of family behavior in a positive light. For example, a nagging mother could be relabeled as a *concerned parent*.

Family Rituals

Family rituals refers to the design and assignment of a well-planned, individualized prescription of one or more actions designed to alter family relationships. The family is instructed to practice the ritual multiple times every day. For example, the family of an anorexic teenage girl is instructed to kneel around her bed on a daily basis and thank her for sacrificing her life in order to allow the mother to maintain daily contact with her own mother over the objections of the father (Selvini Palazzoli et al. 1978).

History

Taking a *family history* can be a sensitive tool for therapists to track the developmental course of a dysfunctional relationship and arrive at corrective interventions.

Triadic-Based Go-Between Technique

Pathogenic relating manifests itself by a range of collusive and destructive interactional processes that include silencing and scapegoating. It is based on the covert role of a family member who is involved in a struggle with another family member, denies his or her own role, and provokes fights in the family by getting someone else to fight another member as his or her proxy. The technique proposed by Zuk (1971), which he called *go-between*, will succeed in forcing the person to reveal his or her intention and to fight openly rather than acting as an impartial observer.

As a *go-between* in the family, the therapist identifies the pathogenic process, refrains from being drawn into a role assigned by the family, and helps to break the collusive, repetitive, and destructive patterns of interaction in order to help create more productive forms of interpersonal relating. For example, the therapist can select a covert family problem to work on, make the covert problem overt, take a mediator role, and then switch roles.

Narrative Techniques

Narrative techniques focus on the narrative or the dominant story that constitutes the meaning patients assign to their problems. The patient's dominant story may result in an *internalizing* process that constructs a negative view of others and an intractable, negative view of oneself. As a result of this intractable position, patients revisit the same problem again and again and cannot try new solutions (Eron and Lund 1996; White 1989, 1995; Zimmerman and Dickerson 1996).

Narrative therapy attempts to empower patients to rewrite their dominant stories and arrive at an alternative narrative. The therapist searches for exceptions to past problems to use as liberating gateways that empower patients to try alternative narratives and new solutions (see Chapter 3, "Constructing Therapy" for a full description of narrative techniques). In couples therapy, spouses are helped to enter *collaborative conversations* by which to coauthor their dominant narratives. Another intervention pathway focuses on the better or *preferred* view of spouses and their partners (Eron and Lund 1996).

Narrative techniques (Nichols and Schwartz 1998) include

- Reading between the lines for a *problem story*
- Rewriting the whole story through collaborative work
- Reinforcing the new story
- Deconstructing dominant cultural discourses

Behavioral Family Therapy Techniques

The techniques of behavioral family therapy can be utilized beneficially with all types of family treatment. These techniques focus on enhancing the family reinforcement system, promoting high levels of rewards for positive interaction, and encouraging pleasing interactions between members to undermine the avoidance and punishing behavior within the family. Rewarding positive interaction encourages the family to become involved with one another. The introduction of affectionate exchanges, caring days, and loving days are highly effective in reducing the persistent negative affect that is the hallmark of families with depressed members.

The basic concepts and techniques of behavioral family therapy derive from behavioral exchange theory; costly behaviors that provoke aversive reactions from family members are replaced with more beneficial behaviors.

Behavioral Exchange Interventions

Behavioral exchange interventions aim to increase behaviorally and emotionally rewarding behaviors and reduce costly behaviors that bring about aversive reactions from the partner.

Establishment of a Baseline

To establish a *baseline*, the frequency of the target behaviors is recorded initially in order to determine the subsequent response to therapeutic interventions.

Positive Reinforcement

Positive reinforcement refers to family members rewarding one another for certain behaviors such as making *appreciative statements*.

Negative Reinforcement

Negative reinforcement is similar to positive reinforcement, but instead of a direct reward, an aversive condition is removed following a behavior that is pleasing to the first party.

Coercion and Punishment

Coercion and *punishment* refer to the type of interaction, common in dysfunctional families, in which a person uses aversive behavior to control other family members.

Contracting

Contracting refers to a procedure that institutes a contract between family members with the goal of producing the desired interaction. In a *good faith* or *parallel* contract, the person will produce certain behavior independently of other family members. In a *quid pro quo contract*, the behavior of one family member is contingent on certain behaviors of other members.

Coaching

Coaching refers to the provision of verbal instructions by the therapist on how to achieve the desired result in interactions. For example, the therapist can coach a spouse to gently ask his or her partner for a desired behavior instead of nagging.

Modeling

Modeling refers to acquiring new behavior by observing another person exhibiting behaviors that produce rewards. Modeling can strengthen desirable behavior or weaken undesired learned responses.

Caring Days

In the *caring days* approach, spouses identify various desirable behaviors in their partners; each spouse then commits to increasing the frequency of those behaviors and thus the emotional rewards of the relationship.

Loving Days

In the *loving days* approach, the spouses are asked to increase behaviors that are pleasurable to partners on specified days, regardless of the spouse's reaction—for example, bringing flowers or giving kisses (Jacobson and Margolin 1979).

Reciprocating

Reciprocating refers to an interaction between two people in which rewards to the two parties are equitable over time and therefore self-reinforcing.

Token Economy

A *token economy* uses secondary reinforcers, such as points or stars, to reward the performance of appropriate tasks. Fines are given for undesirable behaviors.

Functional Analysis

Functional analysis techniques study the functions of symptoms in a family system. Symptomatic behaviors in family members typically arise from unmet needs for self-expression and/or closeness (Alexander and Parsons 1982). Symptoms can be reduced once the functions they serve in the family are discovered and the family has found healthy ways to perform those functions.

Shaping (Successive Approximation)

Shaping rewards small steps and gradual changes in behavior leading toward the accomplishment of a final goal.

Time-Out

A *time-out* helps reduce inappropriate behavior by removing patients from situations in which their behavior is rewarded with attention. Thus, the negative consequences of inappropriate behavior are emphasized. For example, children may be immediately removed from a classroom to avoid reinforcing negative behavior with the attention of their peers.

Counterconditioning (Reciprocal Inhibition)

Counterconditioning weakens an undesirable behavior by reinforcing its desirable counterpart. For example, anxiety can be reduced by assertiveness. In systematic desensitization, relaxation techniques are combined with imagining progressively anxiety-provoking situations.

Extinction

Extinction helps remove the undesirable behavior by eliminating its reinforcement. For example, the family will ignore the irritating and disruptive behavior of a family member, thereby bringing about the extinction of that behavior through lack of reinforcing attention.

Discriminating Stimulus Cue

The *discriminating stimulus cue* is a signal that indicates an upcoming event; the signal directs a person to fulfill a task and receive rewards. For example, a person may be given advance notice of an upcoming event such as getting ready for dinner or leaving home and be rewarded for timely preparation and departure.

Psychodynamic and Object Relations Techniques

Psychodynamic psychotherapy views dysfunctional structures as the end products of developmental deviations produced by shared family defenses. The techniques used are tools for the exploration and resolution of unexpressed feelings and conflicts.

Some of the goals of the psychodynamic psychotherapy approach are listed below:

- Establish therapeutic relationships with each family member, or key family members in particular if appropriate
- Promote empathic listening within the family
- Broaden self-expression and self-observation in each member and collectively in the family
- Reduce collective family defensiveness
- Enhance supportiveness
- Broaden functional family relationships and structures to replace dysfunctional ones

The provision of a supportive environment for child development is a significant aid in ensuring the resumption and continuation of a healthy developmental course for children. Furthermore, the healthy development of children interrupts the transmission of dysfunctional relationships and behavior across generations.

Psychodynamic psychotherapy helps couples recognize their distant and covertly punitive interactions and move toward the establishment of an empathic relationship in which listening, understanding, and satisfying the partner's needs are of paramount importance. The delineation and reconstruction of early patterns of relationships help couples recognize the powerful hold of the early interactions on their contemporary marital and parental interactions. Mutually provocative interactions between the couple need frequent delineation and the institution of corrective measures. The empathic response of the therapist to the couple helps establish a therapeutic framework and encourages the couple to change their relationship into one that is rewarding and nondepressive. However, it is important that the therapist does not become a rewarding alternative to the nonrewarding and distant spouse; such a development could further undermine family relationships.

Therapeutic Frame

The *therapeutic frame* refers to the time, space, and structure for the therapy. The therapist creates the frame by observing the family mood, how they create it, when they accept therapeutic tasks, and so forth; these observations help define the therapeutic frame.

Provision of the Holding Environment

Therapists provide and communicate a *holding environment* for families by listening, following family themes, and addressing anxieties, thereby increasing the family's *holding capacity*. The provision and enhancement of the family members' holding capacity is a major focus of all therapeutic interventions, including interpretation (Scharff and Scharff 1987). Family holding capacity is analogous to the mother's holding of her baby and the father's support of maternal holding through paternal support and the marital alliance.

Interpretation

Interpretation is a central technique by which therapists join with families and share their understanding of family problems while mirroring back to family members what they have said. The language of interpretation is kept clear, direct, simple, and short (Scharff and Scharff 1987). Interpretation may include information learned from observing the family members' transference reactions to one another and to the therapist.

Enlarging the Field of Participation

Enlarging the field of participation refers to the engagement and communication of each family member's point of view to reveal the family's dynamics. *Enhancement* of the family's capacity for self-observation counters shared family defenses and heightens the family's sense of their actual, contemporaneous emotional experiences. These "core affective exchanges" (Scharff and Scharff 1987) and the living family history (Ackerman 1958) provide the intrapsychic and interactional evidence for transference interpretations.

Use of Play

The *use of play* by the child and the parents' ability to participate in the elements of play can both be therapeutic tools. The therapist uses the following methods in play therapy (Scharff and Scharff 1987):

1. Observes the play but does not directly comment
2. May ask the child to elaborate on the theme of the play or the story behind a drawing
3. Observes if a drawing is related to the parents
4. Often uses the play as a metaphor for the content of the session
5. May use clarification and interpretation after observation—for example, by saying that the child is trying to use drawings of animals to explain what he or she sees happening in the family

This technique is most useful once families have a beginning awareness of their conflict and behavior.

Family History

The developmental *history* of family members is obtained through a genogram that reveals both dysfunctional and functional interactional patterns across generations. Acknowledgment of defensive and conflictual patterns in families allows interpretations to enhance both the current reality in the family and recognition of how the past influences the present. Exploration of family history is best conducted in a spontaneous and dynamic manner.

Empathy

Empathy refers to the ability of a therapist to perceive and vicariously experience the emotional state of a patient. Partial ego regression on the part of the therapist enables him or her to experience the projective identifications from the patient. Empathy develops as the therapist joins the family, listens intently and actively, and explores the family dynamics.

Therapeutic Alliance

A *therapeutic alliance* is the collaborative and cooperative efforts of the therapist and family members in the therapeutic process following the joining of the therapist with the family at both unconscious and conscious levels. This alliance with the family as a whole and with individual members must be impartial and balanced because countertransference easily occurs when so many personalities are involved.

Working With Affect

The expression of *affect* in family and marital therapy can be loud, excessive, and defensive. Feelings expressed in the sessions often conceal, rather than reveal, the significant issues due to their defensive nature.

Emotionally focused therapy (Johnson et al. 1999) utilizes an intelligent framework that concentrates on affect to enhance the treatment process, and in particular aims to reduce the disruptive impact of defensive affects. The therapist focuses early on the expression of hard and defensive affects that are usually self-protective and accusatory toward other family members. The exploration of such affects in a manner similar to defense analysis can lead the therapist to the discovery of soft attachment affects that are the roots of relational dissatisfaction. Emotionally focused therapy is based on the application of attachment theory in family therapy.

Multigenerational Family Systems Theory of Bowen

Key concepts of Bowen's influential multigenerational family systems theory include differentiation of self, emotional cutoff, emotional divorce, family projection process, and the use of therapeutic family voyages. Details of these and other concepts are given below.

Enhancement of Differentiation

The enhancement of differentiation involves establishing a one-to-one relationship between individual family members, usually each of the spouses, and the therapist. The goal of these relationships is to enhance family members' self-differentiation and self-definition and to encourage a cognitive way of viewing relationships rather than an emotional one. Differentiation and growth occur through relationships without triangulation; that is, without involving a third family member in the relationship between the spouses. Triangulation serves to relieve anxiety by allowing a partner to invest emotionally in a person outside the couple for defensive reasons (see Chapter 5, "Multigenerational Family Systems Theory of Bowen and Its Application," for more discussion of triangulation).

Coaching

Coaching (Bowen 1978) refers to the process of instructing and supervising patients in the process of differentiation.

Reversal of Emotional Cutoff

Reverse of emotional cutoff refers to the encouragement of family members to reverse their isolation, withdrawal, and denial. The reestablishment of relationships with families of origin is encouraged. Family members are coached to reverse emotional cutoff while preventing triangulation. In addition, detriangulation takes place after the person has been triangulated but frees self up. The fear of triangulation makes family members reluctant to reverse the cutoff phenomenon.

Reversal of Emotional Divorce

Emotional divorce occurs due to the fear of fusion and loss of individual identity and autonomy in the relationship. The therapist helps to reverse this process and increase intimacy in the couple.

Detriangulation

In *detriangulation*, the family members keep themselves rational and outside of the emotional field of other family members who attempt to triangulate them. The therapist also resists being triangulated by family members during sessions, which helps family members to detriangulate themselves within their nuclear and extended families.

Therapeutic Voyages

Couples are encouraged to make *therapeutic voyages* to the family of origin, once they have succeeded in resisting triangulation within the nuclear family. They are encouraged to establish one-to-one relationships with one parent at a time and resist attempts by that parent to triangulate them against the other parent. Obtaining a family history is helpful in weakening triangulation initiatives by one parent.

Cognitive and Emotional Modes of Relationships

There is a *cognitive* and *emotional* basis to relationships. The therapist first encourages each family member to describe his or her relationship from a *cognitive* point of view. The *emotional* basis of the relationship is de-emphasized because it leads readily to fusion and triangulation.

When cognition and emotion are not in balance, an individual's behavior can appear compulsive, rigid, and intellectually driven, or global, hysterical, anxious, and emotionally driven. However, when the dichotomous systems of cognition and emotion operate separately and harmoniously, individuals can function rationally and not be swayed only by emotions. In general, the cognitive mode represents a higher level of functioning and counters emotional fusion.

Countering the Family Projection Process

When *countering the family projection process*, parents are helped to define themselves and their anxiety rather than projecting it onto their children. Projection and triangulation are the building blocks of undifferentiation.

Person-to-Person Relationship

Person-to-person relationships are fostered by instructing two family members to relate personally to each other and to talk only about each other. Their conversation should include details of their therapeutic voyages to families of origin. To avoid triangulation, conversation should not include a third person.

Assumption of an "I Stand" Position

The evolutionary assumption of "I stand" positions (i.e., "I stand for…") results from the gradual differentiation of the couple. In this process, the individuals define clearly for themselves and others their thoughts, interests, actions, and beliefs that will discourage others from triangulation attempts.

Boundary Formation

Boundaries can be effectively formed both by the enhancement of differentiation and the assumption of *I stand* positions.

Contextual Family Therapy Techniques

Contextual family therapy explores the contributions from families of origin of pathogenic conflicts over loyalty, indebtedness, and lack of normal feelings of entitlement.

Multidirected Partiality

Multidirected partiality refers to the therapist's open, impartial listening to each family member's accounting of their needs, expectations, and entitlements, as well as what family members have to say about each other's needs. Multidirected partiality is a vital part of the contextual approach because it addresses the dimension of relational ethics and the context of fairness (Boszormenyi-Nagy 1972).

According to the contextual approach, family members have the right to express their respective positions concerning the balance of giving and receiving in the family relationship. The therapist's task is to help each family member take a position and then address and examine the existing balance of give and take. Each family member is thus helped to gain constructive entitlement (Boszormenyi-Nagy 1986). Constructive entitlement refers to the right to receive fairly from others in return for giving to them.

Therapeutic Contract

The *therapeutic contract* refers to the therapist's commitment to equitably treating individuals in relation to their families. *Fairness* is ensured through multidirected partiality.

Invisible Loyalty Commitments in the Family

Invisible loyalty commitments hold and bind a family together. These commitments are unwritten but shared patterns of expectation that inform such attributes as trust, faithfulness, and devotion in relationships. By ascertaining each family member's ability to give as well as receive in the family relationship, the therapist draws up an account of family obligations and merits. The more a member is able to give and take, the higher his or her merits with the family; and the less a member gives and takes, the greater his or her obligations to the family. The goal is the recognition and resolution of pathological loyalty commitments to the parents.

Exploring the Loyalty Context

The therapist explores the loyalties and disloyalties in the family by first listening carefully to complaints voiced by family members and then exploring the *opposite* position. The goal is not the removal of negative feelings, but a form of exoneration that releases family members from unresolved and lingering resentment toward a sibling or parent. Without exoneration, resentment only repeats itself multigenerationally (see Chapter 6, "Contextual Therapy") and creates an imbalance in family relational justice.

Genograms

Genograms are diagrams of a three-generational family relationship system (McGoldrick and Gerson 1985). Symbols are used to indicate systems, subsystems, and their characteristics, thereby providing a type of blueprint of the family's character. Important events such as illnesses, deaths, and marriages are also highlighted.

Experiential Family Therapy Techniques

Experiential family therapists use interventions familiar to Gestalt and other psychodynamic therapists. Experiential therapists aim to intensify relationships in order to expand the experiential self, so as to counter personality and relational constrictions.

Self-Confrontation

Self-confrontation refers to the use of audio and videotape playback, documents, diaries, family photographs, and sculpting as methods to help individuals reevaluate, reexamine, and face their behavior and its effect on others. Self-confrontation techniques attempt to inculcate awareness and responsibility for behavior by making individuals compare their idealized, subjective self-concepts with the image they present to others. This makes family members aware of and responsible for their alliances and defensive coalitions, as well as individual development and change.

Family Choreography

Family choreography is a nonverbal, action-oriented technique in which the family is sculpted and visually depicted. Family choreography attempts to reenact the parts played by different family members in a dysfunctional family. It was developed by Duhl, Kantor, and Duhl (1973) and used widely by Satir (1964, 1972) and Papp (1981) to illustrate dyadic and triadic relationships, alliances, triangles, and different transactional patterns. With the use of a multigenerational genogram to identify patterns across generations, the family roles are acted out and observed by other family members.

Role-Playing

Role-playing is an elaboration of the concept of enactment within a session. The players either represent themselves in a hypothetical situation or assume the role of a partner. Often the players swap roles. The role of each person in the family is identified and made available for self-exploration by the individual and the family. Parents can be asked to role-play conflictual family scenes from childhood in session and then find alternative solutions to the scenes (Rubinstein et al. 1976).

Videotaping

Recording behavior on videotape and showing it to a patient is a self-confrontational technique that helps develop the ability to observe, compare, judge, discriminate, and subsequently generate new and more adaptive behaviors. Repetitive, destructive, and collusive patterns of behavior can be identified, discussed, and interpreted. Video playback is a method of integrating old and new learning in therapy.

Family Drawing

Through the Kinetie *family drawing* and family scribble, members can symbolically express conflicts and anxieties and possibly disclose secrets and produce new insights.

Being "With the Family"

Being with the family refers to Carl Whitaker's view that techniques are the product of the therapist's personality and the co-therapy relationship (Keith 1986; Whitaker 1976a, 1976b). Whitaker symbolizes the family's conflict and style of interaction by modeling, parenting, and disciplining children.

Stories, Fantasies, and Dreams

Patients' stories about how they successfully solved their problems offer hope to others (Bodin and Ferber 1971).

Family Albums and Pictures

Family albums and pictures refers to an evocative exercise that can stimulate discussion about relationships, losses, and changes.

Use of Films and Arts in Therapy

The *use of films or film segments* draws on the emotional processes portrayed and explores conflicts, triangles, problem resolution, and the general relational atmosphere.

Psychoeducational Techniques

Psychoeducational techniques offer clinicians psychotherapeutic knowledge and teaching skills needed to enhance problem management and problem solving and to capitalize on the resources and skills of the family. The approach is particularly effective in the treatment of schizophrenia and depression (see Chapter 8, "Psychoeducational Family Intervention"). The intervention package includes preplanned and phase-specific techniques that help prevent relapse and enhance the family's ability to cope. Techniques include systematic instruction to the family about such issues as the

- Nature and symptomatology of the illness
- Nature of stress precipitating the illness or its relapse
- Vulnerability of the patient
- Course of illness with or without treatment
- Role of medication and treatment
- Ways of reducing stressful family interactions such as high expressed emotion

Conclusion

The multiple therapeutic intervention techniques available to family therapists are largely drawn from the more established theory and practices of individual, group, psychodynamic, and behavioral psychotherapies. The significant element added here is the focus on the the cooperative and collaborative efforts among resourceful family members. The synergistic collaboration of family members can significantly improve their creative problem-solving skills and remedy dysfunctional and symptomatic interactions that result from overt and covert power maneuvers among members. More skilled and effective family therapists are deeply confident about the family's power in resolving problems. Their interventions are primarily geared toward realignment of family forces to enhance cooperation and reciprocity, diminish power plays, and control punitive maneuvers.

Families in crisis situations are particularly susceptible to the loss of structure, specifically in terms of boundaries between both the generations and between family members. Such families are therefore highly responsive to restructuring techniques that strengthen boundaries among members and different subsystems. The establishment of better functioning boundaries generally results in the development of cooperation and effective problem solving based on the emergence of family members as distinct components of the larger family systems. Prognosis can be determined readily by assessing the integrity of boundaries and family structure prior to the present crisis, and the nature and impact of the critical event on the family structure. Families with young children are particularly prone to excessive reaction and disorganization following an acute or prolonged crisis. The forces of recovery may be strong here, and quick therapeutic gains can undermine any resistances on the part of the family. Therefore, the therapist may not need to work systematically with resistances that are present in cases with long-standing developmental problems in the family.

The presence of multiple and poorly defined symptoms in a number of family members is a characteristic of families with *midrange family dysfunction* (Lewis et al. 1976). The symptoms fluidly shift in one family member or among multiple family members, indicating the significant underlying developmental conflicts and deficits. Such families generally have maintained a high level of functioning in educational, financial, and social areas. They should play an active and collaborative role in the establishment of a treatment plan that addresses family deficiencies and utilizes family assets. A *collaborative* relationship with the therapist may depend on a deepening level of trust and can enhance therapeutic effectiveness. Conversely, such families may become either indignant or resistant to therapeutic intervention if they perceive that they are excluded from a meaningful contribution to the treatment plan or view the treatment strategy as emanating primarily from the therapist. The principles of psychodynamic psychotherapy based on delineation and progressive resolution of collective family defenses, shared family conflicts, and intrafamilial transference reactions can be helpful with such families.

Assessment of the therapeutic outcome becomes more complicated if the family chooses to leave treatment through quick symptomatic recovery, known as a *flight to health*. This escape from treatment can reflect a family's wish to maintain their deep developmental failures. The family may also perceive the therapist as an unwelcome intruder into their value system.

Families with *symmetrical midrange dysfunctions* (Lewis et al. 1976) that exhibit overt behavioral problems may initially require a combination of behavioral, psychodynamic, and strategic approaches. Families with *complementary midrange disorders* that exhibit covert or *neurotic* behavioral difficulties can be more responsive to a treatment strategy based on psychodynamic psychotherapeutic principles.

Families with severe and chronic dysfunctions produce severe and chronic symptomatology based on multiple intergenerational failures along different developmental lines. Symptomatic behavior in the offspring of such families, which may be grown children (adults), is usually coupled with developmental arrests and ego restrictions in the parents, who are excessively dominated by the grandparents. The domination by grandparents usually produces a lack of differentiation in their children and grandchildren. These families can be most responsive to multigenerational family therapy according to the theoretical model proposed by Bowen (see Chapter 5, "Multigenerational Family Systems Theory of Bowen and Its Application"). If the families are not motivated or capable of utilizing this theoretical model, multigenerational family therapy coupled with individual therapy for the younger generations may be a satisfactory substitute. At times, the excessive and dysfunctional ties between the parental and the grandparental generations are based on pathological loyalty, indebtedness, or destructive entitlement within the family system that can produce severe psychopathology in the grandchildren. Contextual therapy with the family as proposed by Boszormenyi-Nagy and his colleagues (see Chapter 6, "Contextual Therapy") can be effective with such families, particularly if it is coupled with individual therapy for the younger generations.

Families at an advanced and prolonged stage of disintegration usually have disturbances in their social network (see Chapter 9, "Social Network Intervention"). Such families often require interventions based on the social network of the family and combinations of family therapy with other modes of treatment, including individual and group therapy, medication, and hospitalization (see Chapter 19, "Parent Management Training"). Family interventions addressing social network disturbances should be eclectic and flexible and utilize a combination of different psychotherapeutic strategies.

Medication is considered a significant ally of family therapy, particularly when a family member is suffering from depression, psychosis, panic attacks, or attention-deficit/hyperactivity disorder (ADHD). Medication can improve the psychobiological functioning of individual family members resulting in stable mood, decreased anxiety, enhanced reality testing, or, in cases of ADHD, diminished distractibility. Together these interventions form the all-important armamentarium available to family therapists in the treatment of mental illness. No theory or technique alone should be regarded as self-sufficient.

Chapters on Related Topics

The following chapters describe various family therapy models and their applications:

- Chapter 2, "Structural Family Therapy"
- Chapter 3, "Constructing Therapy: From Strategic, to Systemic, to Narrative Models"
- Chapter 4, "Psychodynamic Family Therapy"
- Chapter 5, "Multigenerational Family Systems Theory of Bowen and Its Application"
- Chapter 6, "Contextual Therapy"
- Chapter 7, "Behavioral Family Therapy"

- Chapter 8, "Psychoeducational Family Intervention"
- Chapter 9, "Social Network Intervention"
- Chapter 10, "Gender-Sensitive Family Therapy"

Family Theories: Conclusion

G. Pirooz Sholevar, M.D.

Despite the apparent contradictions among different schools of family therapy, their unique contributions can be understood from a developmental-hierarchical perspective. *Structural family therapy* can enhance family organization through the restructuring of family relationships. The effectiveness of this approach is undisputed in crisis situations in which boundaries are obliterated, creating extreme forms of enmeshment or disengagement. The approach is also highly effective if the family has young children with behavior problems. Restructuring maneuvers can reestablish adequate boundaries among family members and family subsystems and bring about rapid improvement. The effectiveness of structural methods is reduced if the family has inadequate precrisis adjustment or insufficient differentiation from the families of origin. We believe that the structural approach can be applied effectively by experienced therapists to some of the long-standing family problems that undermine or interfere with structural development. However, other family therapists have questioned its utility in this area.

Strategic family therapies are closely related to structural family therapy and behavioral approaches. The initiation of strategies for change through avoidance of power plays and negative labeling of family behavior can reduce opposition and enhance cooperation of the family. Theorists of the strategic approach have developed a well-articulated conceptualization of the "resistance" phenomenon within families. The work of these theorists parallels recent changes in the concept of resistance in psychoanalytic psychology.

Strategic approaches evolved significantly in the 1990s. At the turn of the twenty-first century, some of the dominant approaches have adopted a collaborative working relationship with the family, focusing on the inner experiences of the family and its members and emphasizing the inner resources of the family to empower them to deal with their "problems."

The departure from early strategic approaches is particularly striking in *narrative therapy*. This approach still acknowledges its debt to Gregory Bateson but has distanced itself from the cybernetic model and strategic techniques. Narrative therapy highlights the impact of cultural pressures and contradictions on the family, which result in noncollaborative and oppressive interactions. Family members internalize cultural and interactional discourse, which results in a negative and disempowering internal narrative. The reauthored narrative, developed collaboratively between the therapist and the family, can help the family to move forward (Nichols and Schwartz 1998; White 1993, 1995; Zimmerman and Dickerson 1996).

Families that lack sufficient "behavioral organization" (Greenspan et al. 1987) are particularly unaware of the continuity between one member's behavior and behaviors exhibited by other family members. Members of these families are inclined to feel punished by other people and employ punitive countermeasures. *Behavioral and strategic family therapies* are particularly effective in making such family members aware of the contextual contingencies of their behavior and helping them learn principles of positive and negative reinforcement, thus reducing reliance on punishment, avoidance, and power play.

Behavioral family therapists have consistently enlarged their approach to treatment and have incorporated principles once considered characteristic of other family therapy approaches. The new "integrative" behavioral models emphasize 1) the importance of *accepting* symptoms before attempting to change them and 2) the significance of collaboration with the patients. These two principles tend to reduce resistance to treatment and make the patients full partners in their own treatment.

Psychodynamic family therapy is most applicable to families exhibiting a wide range of mild or moderate inhibitions that restrict the personalities of their members, limiting their full enjoyment of and success in life. These patients, defined as individuals with neuroses, have achieved a measure of behavioral organization in their development. They are also aware of the contextual contingencies of their behavior and the principles of reinforcement that account for their social and vocational success. However, these patients' restrictive and conflicted conceptual and fantasy systems limit their adaptation to life events, particularly if they choose a partner with "neurotic tendencies." The couple can have areas of shared conflict, develop a shared unconscious conflictual fantasy life, and employ shared defenses to contain their fantasies and underlying implied dangers. Interlocking neurotic mechanisms in such marriages are so subtle that detection is difficult, particularly if the family suffers from narcissistic disorders that are difficult to delineate, and require an especially strong alliance between the family and the therapist. Psychodynamic family therapy can be combined concurrently or serially with individual therapy because of its theoretical and technical continuity; the combination of these therapies produces an optimal outcome.

The psychodynamic approach received significant boosts in the 1990s. Emotionally focused therapy (Johnson 1996; Johnson et al. 1999) demonstrated empirically the significance of dealing with strong affects in the couple and family relationships. Defensive affects should be differentiated from attachment affects, and relational changes can be brought about on the basis of this differentiation. Other principles of psychodynamic family therapy have gained broad acceptance: examples are the importance of a collaborative rather than an asymmetrical relationship between the therapist and the family; the need to accept symptoms before attempting to change them; and patients' unique contributions to solving their own problems (see Chapter 20, "Couples Therapy: An Overview"). More importantly, psychodynamic practitioners have become more cognizant of the helpfulness of a comprehensive theoretical system by which to understand the nature of intimate relationships and guide interventions.

In some families, the dysfunction is passed down through the extended family to the parental generation, which remains highly involved with its own *family of origin* through fusion, triangulation, pathological entitlement, and invisible loyalties. Such involvement deprives succeeding generations of the progressive, creative energies necessary for continued individual and family development. Resolving conflicts between two or more senior generations helps resume individuation and development in the families. This is especially apparent if senior family members are still living and available and can be engaged in a new style of multigenerational relationship based on detriangulation techniques learned in therapeutic situations. Bowen's multigenerational family systems theory and Nagy's *contextual therapy* are effective approaches with such families.

Psychoeducational family intervention is most applicable to chronic mental disorders in which genetic and biological factors play an important role. The family is considered a major resource in the treatment and management of the illness; they are provided with significant information about the illness, treatment, and available community resources.

The extreme levels of pathology apparent in chronic and severely disturbed people and their families are generally the result of debilitated and constricted social networks that cannot foster good personal relationships. *Social network therapy* is an effective way to expand and rehabilitate such social networks.

The field of family therapy is rapidly reaching maturity. Field cohesion can be immeasurably enhanced by the clarification and definition of conceptual elements and dichotomies common to all theoretical systems, such as boundaries-differentiation, undifferentiation-enmeshment, and so forth. The field should further attempt to describe the unique concepts of family therapy (e.g., interactional restructuring, shared unconscious fantasies, narratives in the family) and demonstrate their possible therapeutic utility with different types of disorders and families.

III

Family Assessment

12

Initial and Diagnostic Family Interviews

G. Pirooz Sholevar, M.D.

Introduction

The diagnostic family interview is an invaluable tool to assist the psychiatrist in the development of diagnostic and therapeutic goals. The multiple goals of the family interview may vary depending on the clinician's theoretical orientation or the nature of the problem and can shape the structure, form, and content of the session. The diagnostic interview can take place as the initial contact with the family, regardless of the nature of the *presenting problem*; it can be part of the comprehensive assessment of a symptomatic child or adult; or it can occur when therapeutic efforts of any type are partially or totally ineffective. It can occur in an outpatient or an inpatient unit.

The assessment of the total family is important because a person is part of the family as an emotional unit rather than an autonomous psychological entity. In treating a patient, a psychiatrist may fail to recognize how the problematic relationship between child and parents, or between parents and grandparents, contributes to the disorder and may therefore prescribe a prolonged and relatively ineffective course of individual or conjoint family therapy. A broader evaluation of the problems addressing multiple sets of variables can result in more successful treatment choices.

The family diagnostic interview is guided by the theoretical orientation of the clinician. A psychodynamic family therapist would pay special attention to traumatic events, developmental failures, and intrafamilial transference reactions that may shape the contemporary interactions and identity of the family members in a decisive manner. The behavioral family therapist focuses on the antecedents and consequences of the problematic behavior and collect extensive data in this area. A communications orientation leads to an interest in the homeostatic mechanisms and rules maintaining the family transactions. A multigenerational family therapist would be most interested in the level of differentiation and the pathologic loyalty and indebtedness between the parents and their families of origin.

The goals of clinicians vary and may include 1) identifying family and individual variables that may play the decisive role in shaping the behavior of a problematic family member; 2) assessing the adequacy of family functioning, structure, and development according to the family life cycle; and 3) conducting an initial family treatment session, when the necessity of such a course has been recognized by the family or by the referral source.

The multiple goals stated above can influence the strategy of the clinician. In the first category, the clinician pays equal attention to the interpersonal, individual, and intrapsychic data. In the second category, the systematic exploration of the family structure is complemented by some interventions aimed at testing the flexibility of the family system and by rules to determine if the most leverage and the least defensiveness can be gained in the individual or family treatment. In the third category, raising the positive expectancies of the family as a group may assume the first priority.

Stages of the Initial Family Interview

The diagnostic family interview is commonly divided into the three segments of *social stage*, *multidimensional inquiry* into the presenting problem, and *exploration of the structure and developmental phase* of the family (Haley 1976, pp. 9–47; Minuchin 1974b).

Social Stage

In the *social stage* of the interview, the clinician acts as a host to the family according to the prevailing customs. The family is put at ease by engaging in mutual introductions, asking the family to introduce themselves by name, matching the names with family members, and inviting them to make themselves comfortable in the office. The family should be provided with adequate seating, preferably in a conversational living room arrangement, and with play material, table, and chairs for young children. Zilbach (1986) recommends that the clinician crouch down to establish eye-to-eye contact with young children when they enter the office and be alert to the possibility that some young children may be afraid of handshakes or physical touching. A few minutes may be spent in small talk, inquiring, for example, if the family had any difficulty finding the office or problems with transportation.

Multidimensional Inquiry

In the stage of *multidimensional inquiry*, the clinician asks the family to describe the problem that has prompted the clinical contact. The clinician can share his or her prior information about the family with them, which may exhibit the therapist's interest and style. Such information can include what the psychiatrist learned in the initial phone call about the presenting problem and recent events involving the family. The family members generally feel very comfortable with the initial part of this stage of evaluation because their statements are largely prerehearsed and allow them to present their *official* image to the clinician. The initial inquiry may be directed to the father, in recognition of the often tenuous motivation of many fathers to attend the therapeutic setting, or to the mother, as the person who may be most knowledgeable about the family life and problems. After hearing the views of one parent, the clinician should ask the other parent to express an account of the problem. The therapist should then inquire about the views of different family members on problematic areas in the family. It is preferable to elicit the views of the siblings of the troubled family member (the *identified* or *index patient*) about the problematic areas in the family before moving to that individual, because an early solicitation of his or her views may increase defensiveness and further polarize the family.

The clinician should be prepared to encounter resistance from the family members to broadening the focus of the explorations and establishing a true multidirectional partiality (Boszormenyi-Nagy 1972). Such resistance will become apparent if one or both parents demand a solution to the presenting problem from the therapist, or instruct the therapist about what to do (i.e., prescribe medication for a child's hyperactivity). Understanding such attempts as signs of a high level of family tension, the clinician should avoid confrontation with the parents and gently underline the importance of understanding everyone's viewpoint on family life as a necessary step for establishing a corrective course of action for the problems.

The family's manner of negotiating boundaries with the clinician as a member of the outside world may be exhibited by a readiness to include the therapist immediately in their conflicts, projections, and blaming. The emergence of an intense, negative transference to the therapist can give rise to countertransferential feelings, which should be used as a clue to the level of family health and pathology.

While listening to the family's presentation of the problem, the therapist should observe carefully the family's relatively unconstrained nonverbal behavior. The observation of any restless behavior in the children following a look at one of the parents and interruption, qualification, and negation of messages by one or more multiple family members are the signals used to regulate family transactions and should provide the interviewer with useful clues on family structure to be tested in the next stage of the family interview. By the end of the second stage, each family member should have experienced a sense of participation in the interview and the opportunity for input in the evaluation. However, an excessive accommodation to some family members, particularly the autocratic and tyrannical ones, may undermine the potential trust of the *scapegoated* and peacemaking members because the family members may assume the therapist and the alleged *victimizers* have formed an alliance.

Exploration of Structure and Development

The *exploration of family structure* through observation of family interactions provides the clinician with valuable clues, including the level of differentiation, boundary formation, and boundary flexibility of different family subsystems and family members. The clinician is particularly interested in the functional adequacy of different family subsystems. The common family subsystems include the 1) marital-parental, 2) parent-child, and 3) sibling subsystems. Grandparental involvement, very common in certain ethnic and socioeconomic groups, would provide additional subsystems of grandparent-parent and grandparent-grandchild.

Assessment and Diagnosis

In the advanced phase of the family interview, the clinician devises active interventions or interpretations to test the flexibility and adequacy of different family subsystems, such as the marital or parental subsystems. Some family therapists may ask some family members to discuss in the session a potentially conflictual subject, which will reveal their hidden disagreements, as well as their flexibility in family negotiation and compromise formation.

Generally, most clinically referred families reveal observable deficiencies in at least one of the family subsystems, such as the parent-child one, while proving adequate and resourceful in other ones, such as marital or sibling subsystems.

The strategy of broadening the focus of exploration extends the reach of the clinician beyond the problems of the identified patient to other functional and dysfunctional aspects of the family life. Depending on the level of tension in the family and the skill of the family therapist, the session may oscillate between two competing forces: 1) the family's drive to focus the discussion on the identified patient when the tension mounts and 2) the therapist's attempting to guide the discussion toward other family issues involving different family subsystems.

While attempting to broaden the focus on a problem, the psychiatrist may uncover hidden or apparent marital problems. Generally, an early focus on marital difficulties is correlated with a high rate of dropout from treatment and negative therapeutic outcome due to heightened family tension. Additionally, the family may present the marital problems in an attempt to diffuse the therapeutic efforts directed at the identified child, without genuine motivation to deal with marital issues (Montalvo and Haley 1973).

Maintaining the family's motivation to return for treatment is an important therapeutic goal. Therefore, at the time of heightened tension during the sessions, the therapist may choose to retreat from uncomfortable family topics until the tension is reduced.

In the first session, siding with or confronting family members in a family with a rigid structure may result in the interruption of the family evaluation. The clinician should always be aware of the unity of the family system as a natural group with strong ties of loyalty, common history, and rigid homeostatic rules dictating the behavior of each family member. A close and intricately functioning family can close ranks readily and extrude the therapist if the family's tolerance is exceeded, based on an incorrect assessment of the family's power or the therapist's status.

Specific Procedural Considerations

The benefits of the family diagnostic interview include the recognition of subtle parental pathology, different aspects of individual and family dysfunction, and, most important, the presence of powerful dysfunctional interlocking relationships and loyalties. Such dysfunctional relationships can play a decisive role in the ability of the family to adapt and also may produce symptoms in one or multiple family members.

For the initial family session, all members of the household and significant others should be invited; these include young children, toddlers, and infants, who are an important source of diagnostic data about the family. The invitation should be extended in a matter-of-fact manner, emphasizing the importance of all family members' views for a full understanding of the problem. Simple statements such as "I'd like to meet you all, including the little ones" can readily communicate the clinician's goal. The success of the invitation is dependent on the conviction of the clinician about the importance of family interactional data. The clinician should avoid any lengthy phone discussion to justify the participation of all family members because a prolonged explanation based on general assumptions may make the therapist appear as if he or she lacks confidence. Once the family members recognize the importance of the family interview to the diagnostic process, they usually comply. The common parental fear about the *contamination* of younger children and *well siblings* by their exposure to the problems of the identified patient can yield readily to the clinician's reassurance. Other sources of fear in the family include the parents' fear of blame for the child's problems and the fear that the entire family may be pronounced "ill." The clinician can reduce the fears of the family by emphasizing the consultative nature of the family diagnostic interview, which does not imply any commitment to treatment on the part of the family. The refusal of an adolescent to attend a family diagnostic interview usually indicates parental apprehension about the session or the weakness of parental authority.

The family assessment can occur during one or multiple family sessions. The diagnostic interview preferably should be scheduled for 90 minutes to allow a systematic evaluation of the family in an unhurried fashion. One should be prepared for a high rate of cancellation for the initial family interview with little hope of receiving remuneration for the canceled session.

The assessment of family structure should include the determination of the characteristic constellations of family conflicts, patterns of control, clarity of parental authority and generational boundaries, expression of feelings, and family rigidity, including the brittleness of family defenses. Structural flexibility of the family includes the accessibility of alternative action patterns.

The assessment of family functioning should include the exploration of instrumental-adaptive functions of the family, geared toward enhanced adaptation and problem resolution, as well as their expressive-integrative function, addressing the expression of affect and provision of comfort. The lack of balance between these two sets of functions can result in an unbalanced family system with reduced adaptability. The elucidation of multigenerational dynamic and relational patterns may be an important factor, particularly with chronically and severely dysfunctional families.

The diagnostic family interview can be extended into interviews with family subgroups, such as parents or children, or with one child for exploration of other important information that may not be readily shared in a conjoint session. The intimate aspects of the parental relationship, such as their sexual functioning, can be explored in such an interview. When the children are seen alone, they may reveal phobias, food fads, or eating and elimination problems that may be too embarrassing for revelation in a diagnostic family session.

In the advanced stage of the initial interview, the impact of the clinician on the family may move the family beyond a rigid or stalemated position into a more flexible mode of family functioning characteristic of earlier stages of their family life. The early and ready occurrence of this phenomenon is indicative of flexibility in the family system and a favorable therapeutic outcome.

Additional Guidelines

Additional guidelines for family assessment (Weber et al. 1985) include the following:

- Establish structure in the interview to counter the common tendency of dysfunctional families toward chaos, a high level of blame, and *silencing* of their members. *Reframing*—the restatement of a problem in a positive rather than a negative way—and *diffusion of attacks* by demonstration of a dyadic or triadic view of the problems are effective techniques to establish an empathic atmosphere.
- Maintain objectivity, avoid side taking or premature closure of topics, and elicit the views of all family members.
- Address the transactional patterns that are clearly burdensome to many family members and therefore more amenable to change (Gordon and Davidson 1981).
- Understand role of different family members within the family unit. The roles of *scapegoat*, *tyrant*, *martyr*, and *baby* are common in families with symptomatic children and adolescents.
- Uncover the explicit and implicit rules that govern family interaction.
- Determine the family's problem-solving behavior.
- Understand the nature of boundaries, splits, alliances, and coalition formations in the family.
- Assess the level of concordance between the developmental and chronological stages of the family.
- Assess the concordance between the value system of the family and the surrounding community.
- Help the families transcend the repetitive, immediate, and trivial problems and recognize the underlying patterns and main issues.

Goals of the Diagnostic Interview

A significant goal of the family diagnostic interview is to help the family recognize and acknowledge its strengths as a family and the assets of family members, particularly the *index patient*. The commonly observed emphasis of the family on negative attributes of the index patient is only a manifestation of the family's negative view of itself as a family that is projected onto the index patient. The recognition of the assets of the index patient, which is usually resisted by the family as a whole, is generally followed by recognition of many assets and resources of the family, and enhancement of the family problem-solving capacity due to a heightened optimism and confidence.

The Role of Closure

The closing of the diagnostic family interview is an important component of the assessment. When the diagnostic family interview is part of an overall comprehensive evaluation, it is best to delay the therapeutic recommendation until the closing conference. Under other circumstances, the family diagnostic interview should be closed by highlighting the points of convergence among the problems of the index patient, the information gathered from different family members, the transactional patterns in the family system, and the referral information. The clinician should attempt to integrate and summarize data while highlighting the family's assets, positive attributes, and affectionate feelings for each other, which would enhance their optimism and confidence for undertaking a therapeutic endeavor. An experienced family therapist attempts to highlight the family's assets, knowing well that the family is aware of its conflictual interactions and relationships but barely cognizant of those assets that are the key to therapeutic success. An inexperienced family therapist tends to focus on family problems to reveal his or her observational acumen; this may inadvertently make the family feel severely disturbed and discouraged.

Family History and Its Role in the Diagnostic Process

Significant experiences in the past may influence family orientation and mythology and directly or indirectly relate to the family problems. Such information includes the early death or suicide of a grandparent when a parent was very young, significant financial losses, or other events that were traumatic for the family. For example, an overly solicitous father of a young man revealed that the year before his son's bar mitzvah, the son was involved in a serious accident requiring prolonged hospitalization and cancellation of the plans for his bar mitzvah. The paternal oversolicitousness toward the son was related to the impact of the accident, which was unknown to the new stepmother, who was irritated by her husband's inappropriate oversolicitousness.

The gradual unfolding of historical information in the family session is an important aspect of the family interview and generally reveals the affectively charged and dynamically significant past experiences of the family. This phenomenon of *living family history* (Ackerman 1958) exceeds the validity of the historical data obtained in a formal chronological, developmental history. The living family history may reveal past deprivations, successes, failures, hidden strengths, and weaknesses of the family that may be related to the current crisis (Sholevar 1985).

Most family therapists gather historical material as it arises in the family interview and occasionally probe specific issues in the past that appear likely to be related to current problems. The information can be gathered along chronological or analogical lines. Multigenerational family therapists gather such information within a multigenerational context. The revelation of family data may disclose that some of the current dysfunctions are a prolonged attempt at solving past problems, at times spanning many generations.

Family Life Cycle/Developmental Issues in Families

Collecting diagnostic information about disruptive childhood disorders within a developmental framework is essential for a child/adolescent psychiatrist. In cases of oppositional defiant disorder and conduct disorder, history of criminality or mental illness in the parents, prenatal maternal smoking and substance abuse, the level of parental-infant bonding, attention to and reinforcement of prosocial behavior, presence of "coercive" family processes, and the adequacy of parental monitoring practices are important areas of inquiry (see Chapter 18, "Family Therapy With Children: A Model for Engaging the Whole Family"). Assessment of the level of cooperation and alliance between the family and other social systems, such as school and peers, has received increasing attention (Henggeler et al. 1999; Sholevar 2001; see also Chapter 18, this volume). Inquiry into the exposure of family members to domestic violence or to violence in the community can help the psychiatrist to assess the level of stress or potential for violence in the family (McAdams and Foster 2002).

In cases of attention-deficit/hyperactivity disorder (ADHD), parental level of positive attentiveness, enhancement of attentiveness and focusing capacity in the child, reinforcement of prosocial and adaptive behavior, and protection of the child's self-esteem are some of the important areas for evaluation. The predominance of a negative interaction between parents and child should alert the child/adolescent psychiatrist to the disruption of a positive parent-child relationship as a result of inadequate management of the disorder (see Chapter 18, this volume). Poor management of parents' own childhood ADHD may make them especially vulnerable to transmit some unadaptive and counterproductive parental practices from their past experiences to the present.

The concept of the family life cycle proposes that family issues are different at various stages in a way analogous to the life cycle of individuals. This model describes a series of stages and their corresponding family tasks (Sholevar 1995). The most commonly accepted models by Carter and McGoldrick (1980a) and Zilbach (1989b) describe the stages of coupling, becoming three with the arrival of the first child, and then a family with young children. These stages are followed by a partial or more complete separation of the adolescent family members from the family, succeeded by the death of one spouse or partner, and ending with the death of the other partner. During different stages of the life cycle, the family structure is rearranged to facilitate the adaptation and mastery of family members. The concept of the family life spiral and its intergenerational dimension proposes overlapping issues in different generations. The family assumes a centripetal shape around birth and the early life of the children and a centrifugal shape as the children move into adolescence (Combrinck-Graham 1985). The family life-cycle models are used differentially by different family theorists, and they describe the emotional problems characteristic of periods of the life cycle that manifest themselves when the family becomes stagnant. The family crisis when older adolescents leave home is a common clinical problem (Duvall 1962; Haley 1973; Terkelson 1980; Zilbach 1988).

Establishment of a Therapeutic System and Joining Operations

Minuchin (1974a) has termed the therapist's methods of creating a therapeutic system and positioning himself or herself as its leader as *joining* operations. The joining maneuvers are a prerequisite for subsequent family change and are necessary because the clinician encounters an organized family system. Such maneuvers include making contact with each family member in such a way that each feels heard, understood, and respected. Attention to the needs of younger, less articulate, or disruptive family members is an important aspect of joining. The accommodation by the therapist to the family system is necessary to *join* them. *Mimesis* is the accommodation of the therapist to the family's style, affective range, and tempo of communication. The therapist should accept the family's organization and experience the strength of its transactional pattern, the pain and pleasure of different family members, and the family's resistance to the interventions. The therapeutic challenge to the family should not endanger its return for the next session. Therefore, the initial joining maneuvers may be away from the therapeutic goal and in the service of the temporary alliance with the family members and rules.

The therapist's accommodation to the children and to their style of communication is an important but neglected area for many family therapists, who tend to be more responsive to the adult family members. Attention to children's communication, play, and art products can enhance their alliance with the clinician. Working with different family subgroups can be an important restructuring tool (Scharff and Scharff 1987; Zilbach 1986).

Definitions

The following definitions are commonly used by clinicians:

Joining is more related to the initial phase of the treatment and establishment of a family diagnosis in contrast to the restructuring methods that belong to the therapeutic phase proper.

Maintenance is a joining operation that refers to the accommodation techniques that provide planned support to the family structure. For example, the therapist may exhibit respect for a strong relationship between a mother and her children by making his or her contact with the children through the mother, or by praising the complementarity between husband and wife when the husband defers to the wife's leadership. The maintenance operation may involve the active confirmation and support of the subsystems, such as the executive parental position.

Tracking is an accommodation technique by which the therapist follows the contents of the family's communication and encourages the members to continue with their expressions, asks clarifying questions, makes approving comments, and requests amplification of certain points. Tracking can apply to the actions or verbal communication of the family.

Psychodynamic Family Data

In addition to attention to observable and conscious communications, the psychodynamically oriented family therapist is equally attentive to the manifestations of the unconscious life of the family. The unconscious system is considered the repository of repressed object relations derived from past and present family experiences and rooted in the basic need for attachment to others. The psychodynamic family therapist pays special attention to the creation of a *holding environment* in the treatment—a mode of functioning that contains the emerging family anxiety, thereby minimizing the need for projection and suppression. Two other important aspects of psychodynamic family therapy are attention to transference phenomena among family members and the clinician's own countertransference feelings. The emergence of a strong transference reaction toward the therapist in the diagnostic sessions is generally indicative of more severe psychopathology and possibly requires early transference interpretation. The therapeutic use of countertransference feeling as a tool requires constant scrutiny and self-examination by the therapist to understand the nature of the family's communication (Scharff and Scharff 1987).

Psychodynamic family therapists are particularly allied with psychodynamically oriented psychiatrists because of their mutual emphasis on the concordance between the developmental level of behavior in the troubled person and transactions in the family. Two special levels of arrest in relational development are excessive infantile dependency among family members and excessive oppositional and defiant behavior and power play. The goal of the treatment is to enhance cooperation, reciprocity, and tenderness characteristic of a more "mature genital phase" level of interaction and development among family members.

Family Interactional Diagnosis

The family diagnosis is a working hypothesis that encapsulates the clinician's observations of the family interactions, structure, and presenting problems. The dysfunctions in the above areas may be correlated with diagnosable disorders in a child or *primary relationship disorders* in the family, with no symptomatology in individual family members. The clinician's assessment places particular emphasis on the family as a whole and the course of the family in the future; this view contrasts with other approaches that are oriented toward the past and problems, particularly in an individual.

Assessment

Minuchin (1974a) emphasizes the following six major areas in family assessment:

1. The family structure, its preferred transactional pattern, and the available alternatives
2. The role of the symptoms in the maintenance of the family's preferred transactional pattern

3. The family system's flexibility and capacity for autonomous restructuring by reshuffling the system's alliances and coalitions to deal with stress
4. The family system's resonance and sensitivity to individual members' actions and feelings and their threshold for the activation of corrective or repressive measures
5. The family life context, including sources of support and stress in the family network
6. The family's developmental stage and its concordance with the family members' chronological stage

The interactional diagnosis is achieved by the process of gathering different classes of verbal and nonverbal information. The diagnosis has to be made after the therapist has entered and joined the family because the diagnosis cannot be made from outside. The therapeutic joining with the family would introduce alternative transactional patterns that are an important indicator of prognosis and therapeutic outcome.

Therapeutic Contract

The contracting phase is an important step prior to initiating formal family therapy. It refers to agreed-on issues and goals for treatment between the therapist and the family. In addition to accepting the family's wish for help with their presenting problem, the therapist recommends the broader goal of alteration in the family interactions underlying the problem, such as disciplining methods used with the children. Later on, the goals can be expanded to include the disagreement between the parents, such as in their views on child rearing or on other issues.

Many treatment failures are due to inadequate contracting between the family and the therapist. The problems of contracting include covert disagreement between the therapist and the family, within the family, or between the family and referral sources (e.g., the Department of Human Services or the court system).

Family Evaluation Scales

Family evaluation scales may be used to augment the clinical interview by providing standardized, self-report data that can highlight the areas of family dysfunction. A comparison of family evaluation scales is available elsewhere in this book (see Chapter 13: "Family Assessment"). There are several commonly used scales.

The Beavers-Timberlawn Family Evaluation Scale (Lewis et al. 1976) is an observer-rated scale that addresses the structural dimensions of power hierarchy, parental coalition, family mythology, goal-directed negotiations, permeability, conflict, self-disclosure, and invasiveness. The controls and sanctions that are measured are overt power and responsibility. The Family Adaptability Cohesion Evaluation Scale (FACES III; Olson et al. 1978) is a self-report instrument that addresses the structural dimensions of systems feedback, negotiation, the family roles, boundaries, coalitions, space, decision making, and time. The controls and sanctions include assertiveness, control, discipline, rules, and independence. The Family Assessment Device (Epstein and Bishop 1981) is based on McMaster's problem-centered model of family therapy. This self-report instrument assesses the structural dimensions of problem solving, communication, roles, and general functioning. The Family Environment Scale (Moos and Moos 1981) measures social climates of all types of families, with subscales in such areas as family cohesion, expressiveness, conflict, independence, and achievement. It has been used widely in many research projects. The Card Sorting Procedure (Reiss 1981) is an observer-rated instrument that addresses the structural dimensions of configuration, coordination, and closure.

Case Example

The following initial family interview not only describes the basic family evaluation process but also demonstrates two additional factors: 1) the impact of ethnic characteristics of the family and 2) the interface between family evaluation and hospitalization.

> Present in the sessions were Ricardo, a 15-year-old; his 9-year-old sister, Lisa; the mother, Ms. F; and the mother's boyfriend, Mr. J. Ricardo had been hospitalized for the third time in the past 3 years at the same hospital for conduct problems and dangerous behavior. His father moved back to the Dominican Republic when Ricardo was a few months old and subsequently died when Ricardo was 7 years old. Ricardo visited his father for several months, at 1- to 2-year intervals, before the age of 7. The consulting family therapist, Dr. S, was told that Mr. J had moved out of the house and probably was no longer involved with the family. Therefore, Dr. S was not sure whether Mr. J would attend the session.
>
> ### Opening Phase of the Interview
>
> The mother was a slender, attractive woman; Ricardo was a large, overweight boy; Lisa was a well-dressed, attractive girl who carried herself regally; and Mr. J was a tall, muscular, handsome, and exceptionally articulate African American who was casually dressed but carried a briefcase.
> Dr. S was introduced to all the family members by Ricardo's psychiatrist and social worker and shook hands with everyone as they entered the room. Mr. J inquired immediately about where Dr. S was going to sit and was encouraged to choose his own seat. The family seated themselves, with Mr. J

on the outside, the mother next to him, and Ricardo next to the mother. Lisa immediately moved away from the family to write on the blackboard; she continued to draw circles, write the names of her friends in the circles, erase them, and rewrite them. She only interrupted this activity to answer direct questions in a pleasant, cooperative, and eager fashion. Mr. J started the session by asking about the location of the offices of Ricardo's psychiatrist and the social worker and sent his regards to another hospital staff member. He then directly asked Dr. S, "What are we going to talk about?" He wanted to know if we were going to talk about such matters as "the child's issues, adult-child issues, adult issues, or the circumstances around hospitalization." Dr. S responded by smiling and saying, "All of the above."

As soon as a comment was made about Lisa, Dr. S used the occasion to ask Lisa how she was doing, what grade she was in, what her activities were, and if she had any friends. Lisa clearly was pleased and proud that she was doing well in school, had many friends, and was free of any problems. Mr. J then proceeded, in a very long, articulate speech, to state that Ricardo was doing well and learning well in the hospital classroom, He said he believed hospitalization was a way of getting Ricardo out of the neighborhood to prevent his hanging around with the wrong crowd. He was not interrupted by Ms. F or anyone in the family, although after 10 minutes Ricardo started to show signs of restlessness. At that point, Dr. S inquired if the reason for hospitalization was to get Ricardo out of a bad neighborhood or if there were some behavioral problems requiring hospitalization. Mr. J became somewhat quiet at that point, which allowed Dr. S to inquire about Ms. F's point of view. Ms. F. spoke in broken English, despite having been raised in the United States, and appeared very passive. Mr. J attempted to interrupt Ms. F on several occasions, but Dr. S encouraged her to go on and asked Mr. J gently to allow Ms. F to finish her statements. In response to direct inquiries, Ms. F eventually revealed that Ricardo was hospitalized because of dangerous behavior such as throwing large bags of garbage down from a roof where young children were walking by and recklessly using a BB gun around his young cousins, which frightened the family.

Commentary

It was quite clear that the mother is a very passive and ghostlike figure in the family and that Mr. J is a very central and dominant force. Dr. S was puzzled by the contradiction between the preliminary information, which indicated that Mr. J had moved outside of the family and was uninvolved with them, and the observations about his central position in the family.

Second Phase of the Interview

Dr. S inquired if Mr. J lived with the family. Mr. J became momentarily anxious but explained that he had moved away from the family because he was disappointed that Ms. F had not become more of a person, obtained a job, furthered her education, and *blossomed*. Mr. J and Ms. F continued dating while living apart, but, according to Mr. J, Ms. F still had not yet *blossomed*. Mr. J's underlying assumption was that Ricardo's nonaccomplishments, poor school performance, noncompliance, and maladjustment were related to the mother's unproductivity, lack of goals, and insufficient self-definition.

Commentary

The second phase revealed a major point of stress in the family. Mr. J, who had been the central and dominant figure in the family for 3 years, moved out around the time of Ricardo's hospitalization. Furthermore, it revealed an underlying conflict between the adults that had caused Mr. J's departure. At the same time, Mr. J's behavior in the session and his continued involvement with the family and Ricardo exhibited his strong commitment to both the children and Ms. F.

The plan for the next stage was to include Ricardo in the process and solicit his point of view, further explore the differences between Mr. J and Ms. F, and assess the two adults' ability to negotiate their differences.

Third Phase of the Interview

Dr. S noticed Ricardo's mild restlessness but praised him for his patience and invited him to join the group and share his ideas. Before Dr. S addressed the teenager's problematic behavior, Ricardo proudly described his adjustment to the hospital classroom and his positive response to medication (Mellaril). The problematic behavior was then discussed, and Ricardo subtly acknowledged that before his hospital admission his behavior had been dangerous. Next, in the *living family history*, the family described the circumstances leading to Ricardo's hospitalization and Mr. J's departure from the family's house; they revealed that both events occurred approximately at the same time.

The family then became confused and could not accurately identify the dates of Ricardo's hospitalization and Mr. J's departure. Mr. J then stated strongly, "Ricardo was hospitalized before I left the house," revealing his strong guilt feelings about the possibility that his moving out could have precipitated Ricardo's decompensation and hospitalization. Once the sequence of events was clarified, Dr. S explored the feelings of different family members about Mr. J's departure. Ricardo said that he was "feeling depressed" about Mr. J's moving out. He explained that his depression was extremely deep but volunteered that he was not suicidal. Having established the connection between Ricardo's strong depressive reaction and Mr. J's departure, Dr. S asked Lisa about her reaction. Lisa became openly attentive at this point and stated that she was very depressed and said she had had a disturbing dream. Dr. S quickly inquired about the dream, which occurred within 6 months of Mr. J's departure. In the dream, Lisa returns home from school and to her great delight finds that Mr. J is back home, although she expects him to be absent. Lisa described and enacted in the session her ritualized greeting for Mr. J. She shook her head, swung her braided hair from side to side, and tapped her feet. In her dream, Lisa acts the same way when she returns home and finds Mr. J is back; she reenacted this scene. The family united in a joyful moment of laughter, which was understood to be reminiscent of better days when they were all happily united at home.

Ricardo clearly connected the regression in his behavior—the maladaptive and dangerous behavior—to his deep feeling of depression in anticipation of Mr. J's departure. Lisa shared Ricardo's feeling of depression about Mr. J's leaving. Dr. S inquired about Ms. F's reaction to Mr. J's departure. She gave a faint, affectless smile saying that she did not have any feeling about it, implying that the event did not have much effect on her. Mr. J was listening quietly and attentively. Ms. F's comments came through as a clear *putdown* and lack of appreciation for Mr. J's enormous contributions to the family and the child rearing.

Commentary

The mother appeared to be in denial of her feelings of loss and grief, which enhanced Ricardo's acting out and Lisa's excessive psychological departure from the family into her peer group and school. Dr. S suspected that Mr. J felt that his contributions were not valued by Ms. F and possibly the family.

Fourth Phase of the Interview

Mr. J revealed his deep devotion to the children and his wish to help them along, describing himself as an exceptionally caring man. He said he acted as a father figure to many children in his large family and neighborhood. His interest in children dated to the departure of his father when Mr. J was very young. His mother became solely responsible for the total care of the children while being the breadwinner and wage earner for the family, and Mr. J assisted his mother with the children.

Dr. S emphasized Mr. J's importance to the children and to the family as a whole, as well as his competence and interest in caring for and connecting with the children, and touched on Mr. J's frustration about Ms. F's lack of progress in becoming a more competent person, woman, and mother, as well as partner for him. However, Dr. S wondered why all of Mr. J's expectations for the family could not be achieved, considering his enormous attachment, dedication, and skillful contributions to the family. Following up on Mr. J's deep interest in being a father figure to Ricardo and the other children, Dr. S praised Mr. J's commitment to self-improvement and success, excellent physical health, and muscular build before Mr. J revealed that he was carrying his gym shoes in his briefcase. Dr. S then asked Mr. J. if he took Ricardo to the gym so that they could work out together.

At the conclusion of the session, Lisa psychologically rejoined the family, Ricardo's behavior was placed in the context of the tensions and conflicts in the family, and Ms. F became somewhat animated, recognizing the value in meeting Mr. J's expectations. Accomplishing Mr. J's goals would have helped her become a competent leader in the family. Mr. J was very proud and pleased that his enormous contributions to the family were recognized, that he was not viewed as someone who had deserted the children, and that he had not been instrumental in bringing about Ricardo's decompensation. Mr. J asked for Dr. S's business card and inquired where he was teaching as the family prepared to leave the room.

Discussion

The family was using the defensive maneuver of isolating the context of the events leading to the presenting problem from the problem itself. They denied intrafamilial conflicts and externalized the origin of the problem into the bad neighborhood and negative peer pressure. Connecting the two events—Ricardo's hospitalization and Mr. J's leaving—made it clear that the tensions eventually leading to Mr. J's departure had been building for several months and therefore predated the deterioration in Ricardo's behavior. In this way, the presenting problems were placed into their true context, which was the inability of Ms. F and Mr. J. to negotiate their differences. Mr. J was further humiliated by his own family and by his peers for acting as a *sucker*, raising the children of someone who did not do her share in the family.

During the session, it was revealed that Ricardo's father moved back *to the islands* because he was depressed. His death, in the Dominican Republic, occurred while he was in his 30s and seemed to be related to multiple depressive episodes with the possibility of suicide.

The interconnection between genetic predisposition to depression—with possible seasonal features—and conduct disorders and depression in Ricardo was emphasized as an issue requiring exploration and resolution in family and individual treatment. The strong reaction of Ricardo to Mr. J's departure was possibly also related to his unresolved grief over the loss of his father, further complicated by Ms. F's inability to deal with loss.

An important contributing factor to Mr. J's conflict with Ms. F was the cultural context of the family. Being an African-American man, Mr. J was deeply committed to *upward mobility*, self-enhancement, and improvement in one's circumstances. Ms. F, in contrast, reflected the more relaxed cultural expectation of a woman in a Dominican family. Furthermore, her poor acculturation and limited accommodation to the American culture left her isolated, vulnerable, and lacking in skills. She was clearly inhibited and ambivalent about enhancing her skills and pursuing success rigorously, despite having been enrolled in school to become a beautician.

Mr. J's high expectations of Ms. F were partly rooted in his comparison of Ms. F with his mother, who was a hard-driving, competent woman functioning as a mother and father to the children. Compared with Mr. J's mother, Ms. F appeared as highly lacking, which made Mr. J feel anxious about being attracted to her.

The interface between psychiatric hospitalization and family functioning was apparent in multiple ways. Ricardo, as well as the family, considered the hospital as a second line of support when the family was no longer able to contain Ricardo's problems. The family clearly viewed the hospital as a Hispanic family would view the grandmother (*comadre*) for the care of the children when the family is no longer able to deal with the problems. Ricardo felt very comfortable returning to the hospital when the home situation proved depressive and a void was created by the departure of Mr. J. The task of inpatient family therapy was to enhance the familial resources to reabsorb Ricardo rather than *adopting* him or declaring the family hopeless.

Conclusion

The initial family interview is a highly valuable tool for determining the interpersonal and interactional characteristics of the family and its contributions to psychopathology in a child or an adult family member. Furthermore, the family interview allows the child psychiatrist to demonstrate the hidden resources of the family, enhancing the family's positive expectancies and countering the feelings of despair and antagonism.

Chapters on Related Topics

The following chapters describe concepts related to initial and diagnostic family interviews:

- Chapter 13, "Family Assessment"
- Chapter 14, "The Family Life Cycle: A Framework for Understanding Family Development"
- Chapter 15, "Functional and Dysfunctional Families"
- Chapter 16, "Diagnosis of Family Relational Disorders"
- Chapter 18, "Family Therapy With Children: A Model for Engaging the Whole Family"

13

Family Assessment

Bruce D. Forman, Ph.D.
Jodi Aronson, Ph.D.
Mark P. Combs, Ph.D.

Introduction

The starting point in treating the family is with a thorough assessment and diagnosis. Assessments in psychiatry are less clear than in physical medicine, due in large measure to the divergence of theory regarding etiology and treatment of psychological or behavioral disorders that characterize the mental health field. Consequently, there has been little agreement over what constitutes necessary and sufficient parameters for inclusion within a competent and acceptable assessment of families in clinical practice.

As the need for reliance and accountability has increased in the psychiatric profession, family research has demonstrated the need for measures that assist in assessing and treating. Hence, there has been growth in such measures, as evidenced by Lindholm and Touliatos' (1993) identification of 946 instruments in more than 50 journals spanning a 60-year period from

---

Portions of this chapter are reprinted from Forman B, Hagan B: "Measure for Evaluating Total Family Functioning." *Family Therapy* Volume XI, November 1984. Used with permission.

The authors wish to thank Linda Schwoeri, Ph.D., for her fine editorial assistance with this chapter.

1929 through 1988. A corresponding survey of marriage and family therapy practitioners by Boughner et al. (1994) revealed that despite the emphasis on standardized use of assessments, their utilization by practitioners did not reflect an emphasis on standardization.

Much of the assessment of families used by family therapists is conducted on an informal basis. That is, assessments are made via diagnostic interviews and by observation of family interactional patterns, as well as the clinician's preference for one particular theory over another. As accountability and reliance on third-party payments increasingly have become realities of professional survival, clinicians are turning more to formal professional procedures. It is therefore necessary for practitioners to understand more about the formal assessment process to ensure that procedures are used in a manner consistent with professional standards.

Test Construction

The preparation of tests has long fallen within the purview of the discipline of psychology, with a concomitant massive body of literature. Use of any test presupposes acceptance of the theory on which the instrument was based. This remains a fundamental axiom of psychological tests. Psychological testing for psychodiagnosis in psychiatric practice has been an accepted protocol for decades. Yet, within the specialization of family treatment, the use of tests has not been as readily integrated into practice. However, interest in formal family assessment has grown as family interventions have joined the mainstream of mental health practice.

There are two essential characteristics customarily associated with test construction: reliability and validity. **Reliability** refers to the consistency of the instrument, or how often the results are the same. Reliability includes three areas. First, *stability* is how well the results hold up over time in test-retest reliability coefficients. Second, *homogeneity* is how similar the items are within a test. If a test is measuring a human attribute, it follows that all the items should be relatively similar. Homogeneity is sometimes referred to as the internal consistency of a test. A number of mathematical procedures have been used to compute a test's internal consistency. Third, *generalizability* is the extent to which a test can be administered to different categories of people with much the same result. A reliable test should be usable with equal confidence with males and females.

Validity may be defined as a test's ability to measure that which it is purported to measure. We are only concerned about validity once we are satisfied that a test possesses adequate reliability. There are three basic types of validity. The first, *content-related* validity, is done by sampling items to ensure that they are representative of the domain in question. For instance, a test for depression should include items concerned with behavior that is characteristic of a mood disorder.

The second type of validity is *criterion-related*. Here, test performance is checked against a criterion that is a direct measurement. Thus, a test for depression may be validated against independent psychiatric ratings or another test already shown to be valid for assessing depression. When the criterion against which a test is validated is obtained at about the same time the test is administered, it is referred to as *concurrent validation*. When there is a difference in times the measures are taken, we refer to this as *predictive validity*.

The third type of validity, *construct-related validity*, is the degree to which a test measures a theoretical concept or trait. A theoretical construct such as family cohesion is translated into behavioral referents, which are then operationalized via test items and subscales.

Background

Assessment of family functioning has been approached via numerous methods and instruments. Most methods may be subsumed within three categories: unstandardized measures of total family functioning, subsystem assessment, and standardized total family assessment. *Unstandardized measures of total family functioning* include interview schedules, rating scales, and schemas that lack psychometric developments such as indices of stability, internal consistency, and validity. These unstandardized measures of "total family functioning" refer to equivocal combinations of unintegrated elements and processes that the authors believe most important for understanding how the family operates. There are several observation or interview formats for use in family diagnosis and treatment planning (see, e.g., Brown and Rutter 1966; Geismar and Ayers 1959; MacVicar and Archibold 1976; Meyerstein 1979; Morgan and Macey 1978; Watzlawick 1966).

Standardized total family assessment procedures include measures that are designed to assess the entire family system, or at least those dimensions the authors believe explain a significant portion of the activity of the family as a unit. This category represents efforts that have integrated domains of family behavior with multiple aspects (i.e., control, support, and communication) while adhering to accepted rules of behavioral measurement. Our purpose in this chapter is to provide critical evaluations of the instruments and their psychometric properties subsumed under the classification of standardized total family assessment.

Family Assessment Instruments

Beavers-Timberlawn Family Evaluation Scale

The Beavers-Timberlawn Family Evaluation Scale (BTFES) was developed by Beavers, Lewis, Gossett, Phillips, and their colleagues (see, e.g., Beavers et al. 1972) to assist in identifying interactional patterns characteristic of healthy family functioning. The measure consists of 13 single-item scales subsumed under five theoretical domains: Family Structure (Overt Power, Parental Coalitions, Closeness), Autonomy (Self-Disclosure, Responsibility, Invasiveness, Permeability), Affect (Expressiveness, Mood and Tone, Conflict, Empathy), Perception of Reality (Family Mythology), and Task Efficiency (Goal-Directed Negotiations). Ratings are assigned during 10-minute observations of videotaped family interactions pertaining to the five central domains.

Each of the 13 scales consists of a statement regarding the definition assigned to a particular family dimension, such as Overt Power. Ratings are made on a 9-point continuum (1, 1.5, 2, etc.) ranging from a general absence of the dimension being measured in the relationship to a completeness or fullness of the dimension. Although the authors admit to numerous areas of scale overlap, each scale is believed to express an essential construct used in assessing family system functioning. Several studies have reviewed and extended the BTFES (Brock 1986; Coombe 1987; Green and Herget 1989b) both supporting and questioning its overall utility in work with families. The BTFES is not frequently cited and has not received much attention in the literature, which suggests that researchers and practitioners are using other measures more extensively.

Family Adaptability and Cohesion Evaluation Scales

The Family Adaptability and Cohesion Evaluation Scales (FACES; Olson et al. 1978) is a self-report measure designed to operationalize the Circumplex Model of Marital and Family Systems (Olson et al. 1979). The Circumplex Model was derived from the Simulated Family Activity Measure (SIMFAM; Straus and Tallman 1971), a laboratory research method for studying family interactions. SIMFAM was designed to assess five aspects of family functioning: Power, Support, Communication, Problem-Solving Ability, and Creativity. The method employs a standard condition, which is ascertained by family members engaging in the task of discovering rules for a shuffleboard-like game.

The Circumplex Model is a circular matrix employed in locating a family's style of functioning along two major dimensions, family cohesion and family adaptability. Each dimension is conceptualized by a 4-point continuum ranging from disengaged (low) to enmeshed (high) cohesion, and from rigid (low) to chaotic (high) adaptability. The circular matrix, therefore, provides 16 possible positions for describing types of marital or family systems (i.e., from rigidly disengaged to chaotically enmeshed). Family cohesion is defined as an emotional, intellectual, and physical oneness that family members feel toward one another. Family adaptability refers to the family's ability to shift its power structure, roles, and rules of relationships in response to unfamiliar or stressful conditions. A moderate balancing of both dimensions is viewed as necessary for optimal family functioning.

The original FACES was a 111-item instrument with 16 subscales (six items each), 9 of which assessed cohesion (i.e., emotional bonding, independence, family boundaries, coalitions, time, space, friends, decision making, and recreation), and 7 of which measured adaptability (including assertiveness, control, discipline, negotiations, role rules, and system feedback). In addition, a 15-item modified version of Edmonds' (1967) Social Desirability Scale was included. Each participant received a score for each subscale, total scores for both the adaptability and cohesion dimensions, and a response validity score, or 19 scores in all. A Family Composite score was obtained by summing individuals, while a Discrepancy score was derived by comparing responses of different family members.

The FACES items were selected from an original pool of 204 short statements formulated to describe high, balanced, and low levels of family cohesion and adaptability. Clinical validity was assessed by 35 marriage and family counselors, who rated each item on a 9-point scale representing low to high cohesion and adaptability. The responses of 410 college students, who rated the items in terms of applicability to their families of origin, were then factor analyzed by using a varimax orthogonal rotation. The cohesion items produced 11 factors: factors 1 through 4 accounted for 63.5% of the variance. The adaptability items produced 6 factors: factors 1 and 2 accounted for 78.6% of the variance.

Reliability estimates were provided by 201 families, each consisting of a mother, a father, and an adolescent, making a total of 603 family members. Social desirability was not correlated with the total cohesion score (see Table 13–1), indicating a greater tendency to give "idealistic" responses to the cohesion items. The internal consistency (alpha) of the total scores for cohesion and adaptability were $r=0.83$ and 0.75, respectively. Because the split-half reliability for each subscale was very low, the authors recommended use of total scores for decisions regarding cohesion and adaptability rather than individual subscales.

Several changes have been made to the FACES, and FACES IV is the newest version. FACES III, the version cited and currently utilized most frequently, consists of a 20-item instrument designed to measure both co-

Table 13–1. Summary of assessment instruments for total family functioning

Instrument	Beavers-Timberlawn Family Evaluation Scale (BTFES)	Family Adaptability and Cohesion Evaluation Scales (FACES)	Family Assessment Device (FAD)
Standardization sample	N=23 families	N=603 individuals from 201 families	N=503
Number of items	13	111	53
Number of scales	13	16 plus a social desirability scale	7
Internal consistency	Interrater reliability: 0.65–0.90 Xr=0.77	Cohesion: x=0.83 Adaptability: x=0.75	0.72–0.92 x=0.78
Stability			
Scale intercorrelations			0.37–0.67 (0.01–0.23 with General Functioning held constant)
Validity	a. Discriminated families with a healthy adolescent member from families with a psychiatrically impaired member b. Used to categorize healthy, neurotic, behavior disordered, and psychotic member families	a. Factor analytic b. Low correlation with social desirability for adaptability scales (r=0.03), moderate correlation for cohesion scales (r=0.45) c. Face validity of items rated by family counselors (n=35)	Correctly identified 67% of 21 nonclinical families and 64% of 78 clinical families

Family Assessment 283

Table 13–1. Summary of assessment instruments for total family functioning *(continued)*

Instrument	Family Assessment Measure (FAM)	Family Concept Assessment Method (FCAM)	Family Evaluation Form (FEF)
Standardization sample	$N=433$	Several hundred families in various studies	$N=132$ individuals from 200 families
Number of items	115	80	136
Number of scales	7 plus 2 response bias scales	9 plus 3 scales derived from combining all family members	18
Internal consistency	0.80–0.93 $X=0.86$		$C=0.69$ (combined husband/wife)
Stability		Five studies (clinical and nonclinical samples) over 2 weeks to 4 months FCQS: $Xr=0.67$ (real); 0.71 (ideal) FCI: $Xr=0.80$ (real); 0.87 (ideal)	0.40–0.94 for 15 families over 2–6 weeks
Scale intercorrelations	0.55–0.79	Congruence Score (representing arithmetic average of family members) for Mother × Father: $Xr=0.66$ (real); $Xr=0.67$ (ideal)	Husband × Wife 0.30–0.76 Median=0.50
Validity	Correlated with the Locke-Wallace ($r=0.53$ and Philadelphia Geriatric Morale Scale ($X=0.44$) for measuring retirement adjustment	Validity studies include measures of adjustment, social desirability, discriminative ability with clinical and other samples, and factor analytic studies	

Table 13–1. Summary of assessment instruments for total family functioning *(continued)*

Instrument	Family Environment Scale (FES)	Family Functioning Index (FFI)	Structural Family Interaction Scale (SFIS)
Standardization sample	$N=285$ families	$N=399$	$N=196$
Number of items	90	15	85
Number of scales	10 plus Incongruence Score	6 plus Total Score	13 (Primary) 10 (Secondary)
Internal consistency	Items scale: $Xr=0.52$ $Xkr20=0.73$ Item-Item: $Xr=0.20$	0.07–0.96 (Husbands) 0.21–0.95 (Wives)	0.25–0.74 (Primary) −0.08–0.56 (Secondary)
Stability	0.68–0.86 for 9 families with 47 individuals over 8 weeks 0.52–0.89 for 241 families over 1 year	0.83 for Total Score for 29 families over 5 years	
Scale intercorrelations	$Xr=0.20$	Husband × Wife=0.72	−0.002–0.604 (Primary) −0.014–0.424 (Secondary)
Validity	a. Differentiated clinical from normal families b. Assessed changes attributed to psychotherapy	a. 0.39 correlation for total score × professional rating of family b. Significantly differentiated clinical and normal families	a. Scale intercorrelation reflects many theoretical assumptions b. Successfully discriminated between families with and without a learning-disabled child

Table 13–1. Summary of assessment instruments for total family functioning *(continued)*

Instrument	Simulated Family Activity Measure (SIMFAM)
Standardization sample	
Number of items	5
Number of scales	5
Internal consistency	0.43–0.96
Stability	
Scale intercorrelations	
Validity	a. Construct validity has been demonstrated via support for theoretically derived hypotheses b. Correlated with self-report measures of family cohesion (0.41) and adaptability (0.50)

Note. FCI=Family Concept Inventory; FCQS=Family Concept Q Sort.

hesion and adaptability. Like the original measure, FACES III was normed on 2,453 adults and 412 adolescents and has fair internal consistency and good face validity (Fischer and Corcoran 1994). In a review of the literature of standardized assessments (Piotrowski 1999), the FACES ranked as the third most popular listing in 109 citations from 1974 through 1997. Discussions of FACES III that address convergent and discriminant validity were reviewed by Perosa and Perosa (1982) with respect to cohesion and adaptability, aspects that in their opinion needed additional research. Other reviewers point out the linearity versus proposed curvilinearity of the tool as posited by the originators (Crowley 1998).

Family Assessment Device

The initial McMaster Family Assessment Device (FAD) was a 53-item self-report measure developed by Epstein et al. (1981, 1983). The FAD is based on the McMaster Model of Family Functioning (MMFF), a clinically oriented conceptualization of families that views family functioning as related more to transactional and systemic properties of the family unit than to intrapsychic attributes of individual family members. Designed as a screening instrument, the FAD collects information on various structural and organizational dimensions of the family system. This information is then integrated into a more extensive data collection process. Currently, the FAD is a 60-item questionnaire.

The FAD measures six dimensions of family functioning identified by the MMFF:

1. Problem Solving (PS): the family's ability to resolve problems at a level that maintains effective family operations
2. Communication (C): the content and quality of information exchanged among family members
3. Roles (R): established patterns of behavior that provide for resources, nurturance, support, personal development, and family system maintenance
4. Affective Responsiveness (AR): the ability of family members to experience appropriate affect over a range of stimuli
5. Affective Involvement (AI): the interest and value family members place on each other's activities and concerns
6. Behavior Control (BC): the manner in which a family exercises and maintains behavior standards

The FAD consists of seven scales in all, one for each of the six MMFF dimensions described above and an additional General Functioning scale that assesses the overall health or pathology of the family. All family members over age 12 may complete the FAD questionnaire, and the responses are made on a 4-point scale of agreement ranging from "strongly agree" to "strongly disagree." The scales contain between 5 and 12 items each. Originally, the FAD was developed from test responses of 503 individuals to the questionnaire (see Fischer and Corcoran 1994 for discussion).

The FAD has been translated into seven languages and is considered one of the most extensively researched psychometric tools (Ridenour et al. 1999). The Italian adaptation was considered to need improvements (Roncone et al. 1998).

Family Assessment Measure

The Family Assessment Measure (FAM; Skinner et al. 2000) is designed to measure strengths and weaknesses in family functioning with reference to a process model, utilizing a 4-point scale of agreement. FAM-III includes a 50-item general scale concerning the family as a whole, a 42-item dyadic scale concerning dyadic relationships with specific family members, and a 42-item self-rating scale regarding one's own functioning within the family. Each of these scales may be used independently, but their combined use provides a comprehensive view of family functioning.

Each scale assesses the seven constructs contained in the FAM authors' Process Model of Family Functioning (Skinner 1984; Skinner et al. 2000):

1. Task Accomplishment: the achievement of important biological, psychological, and social goals
2. Communication: the content and clarity of information exchanges
3. Role Performance: the performance of defined activities aimed at completing essential family tasks
4. Affective Expression: the exchange of feelings among family members
5. Affective Involvement: the degree and quality of concern for and interest in one another
6. Control: the process of interpersonal influence
7. Values and Norms: rules by which values are put into practice and the standards against which behavior is evaluated

Standardization on 815 adults and 475 children showed internal consistency (alpha) coefficients of 0.86 or greater. A number of studies attest to the FAM's discriminant validity (see, e.g., Forman 1988). The FAM is short and can be completed in 20–30 minutes. The scales can be used separately, which gives it an advantage for rapid screening, since administration of separate scales takes considerably less time than the complete test. Until recently, the FAM was not commercially available, limiting access by most clinicians. While the instrument is easy to administer and score, effective use requires familiarity with the Process Model of Family Functioning. Studies have shown that it is a useful tool but did not rate in the top 10 measures as Piotrowski (1999) found when reviewing the most-used standardized tools.

Family Concept Assessment Method

The Family Concept Assessment Method (FCAM; van der Veen 1960, 1969) provides a standardized assessment of a person's perception of his or her family and its cognitive, social, and emotional structures. The instrument can be used to characterize the family as it presently exists (the real family concept), as it might be ideally (the ideal family concepts), or even as the concept of one's family of origin. The test consists of 80 items that were constructed to apply to the entire family unit and not just to an individual family position or relationship. The entity to be rated, "my family/we," remains the same.

There are two principal versions of the Family Concept Assessment Method: the Family Concept Q Sort (FCQS) and a multiple-choice format known as the Family Concept Inventory (FCI). The FCQS presents the rater with 80 items on separate cards in random order by which to describe the family. Each item is rated on a nine-point continuum from "least like my family" to "most like my family." Since only a specified number of cards can be placed in each pile, the rater must abide by a forced response distribution format. The 80 items were selected from an original pool of 150 items on the basis of their relevance to as many different psychological and interpersonal aspects of family living as possible. Eleven mental health professionals rated the degree of relevance and appropriateness for each item. The FCQS was then administered to the parents of five families and was readministered 4 weeks later. The results encouraged further investigations employing the instrument.

The FCI, however, consists of 80 items listed in a test booklet, with each item rated from 0 (least like the family) to 8 (most like the family). The respondent may choose whichever rating is deemed an appropriate response for any given item by circling the corresponding numeral, thus eliminating the forced response distribution format. In addition to this format revision, 21 of the original 80 FCQS items were modified in the FCI to clarify, simplify, or otherwise improve their meanings. A Spanish-language edition is also available.

Global scores derived from the FCAM include measures of Family Congruence, Family Satisfaction, and Family Effectiveness. The Family Congruence scores indicate the degree of agreement between the real and/

or ideal family concepts of the various family members, either in pairs or as an entire unit. The Family Satisfaction score refers to the correlation between a person's real and ideal item scores. Family Effectiveness is a summary score of family adjustment based on 48 of the 80 items. These items were selected by 27 clinicians as exemplifying behaviors important for healthy family life.

Scores derived from FCAM show good discriminatory powers with a number of contrasting populations (Bagarozzi 1986, 1987). Higher family concept scores have consistently indicated better adjustment for parents of nondisturbed versus disturbed children, as well as psychiatrically healthy adolescents compared with their disturbed siblings (van der Veen and Novak 1974). The FCAM was also used to report family perceptions of the parents of adolescent runaways and nonrunaways (van der Veen and Waszak 1975). The correlation between the combined parents' real and ideal family concepts was markedly higher for the parents of nonrunaways ($r=0.73$) than for the parents of runaway adolescents ($r=0.30$).

Since its initial construction in 1960, the FCAM has enjoyed considerable usage. However, over two-thirds of the 50 studies employing the FCAM consist of unpublished manuscripts such as theses and dissertations. Difficulty in obtaining these works greatly diminishes their utility for most researchers and practitioners. Nonetheless, the instrument has been used in a number of accessible, published investigations (e.g., Hurley and Palonen 1967; Reiter and Kilmann 1975; Wattie 1973, 1974). In addition, an annotated bibliography of the completed studies has been compiled for inclusion in the FCAM manual (van der Veen and Olson 1983).

Family Evaluation Form

The Family Evaluation Form (FEF), a self-report measure of family life whose development incorporates both relational and empirical procedures, was constructed by Emery et al. (1980). The item-content domain of theoretical constructs regarding family functioning adopts concepts gleaned from clinical and research literature, prior instrument development, and reports by adults of daily life events. The FEF consists of 136 items, yielding 18 relational or content-relevant subscales termed Conflict/Tension, Open Communications, Emotional Closeness, Extra-Familial Support, Community Involvement, Children's Relations, Children's Adjustments, Inconsistent Discipline, Mother/Father Dominance, Marital Satisfaction, Financial Problems, Nurturance, Independence Training, Behavioral Control, Explanation of Rules, Strict Discipline, Homemaker Role, and Worker Role. The final seven scales are designed to be scored twice—once for the ratings of one's self and again for the rating of one's spouse. The items are rated predominantly on a seven-point continuum (0 = not at all; 7 = extremely), determined by how congruent the item is with the rater's perception of family, spouse, or children.

The FEF authors selected by consensus 213 items thought to serve as potential measures of each construct; the items were then administered in pilot form to a nonrandom sample of 26 parents. Scales were created by grouping the pilot item mean scores (theoretically designated as belonging to a given scale) and calculating item-to-subscale correlations. Only items having the highest correlation with their rationally assigned scales were retained.

Normative data were gathered by mail from a random sample of 200 white families (stratified by income) residing in a suburban New York county. Eighty-eight families, or 44% of the originally designated population, completed and returned the forms. Forty-four families submitted forms by both parents, 34 families submitted forms by one parent only, and 10 forms were submitted by single-parent families, for a total of 132 completed FEF forms. The mean number of children was 2.2, with a range of one to six children per family.

Test-retest reliability coefficients of individual scores in the 26 subscales were calculated for 15 families from the same community who completed the FEF twice within a 2- to 6-week interval. Stability coefficients ranged from a low of 0.40 for Communication to a high of 0.94 on Emotional Closeness, with the coefficient for 19 subscales exceeding 0.75. The FEF authors caution limited interpretation of these statistics because of the small sample employed.

The domains of family functioning assessed by the FEF are generally broad in scope and include areas such as family interpersonal relationships, sibling relations, and children's adjustments, as well as more traditional measures such as marital satisfaction and child-rearing practices. The FEF is equally applicable to the mother or father, to double- and single-parent families, and to a broad range of family sizes. Unfortunately, results of FEF administrations do not provide input on perceived family functioning by the children.

Family Environment Scale

The Family Environment Scale (FES) is a 90-item, true-false questionnaire constructed by Rudolf Moos (1974) and is considered to be the most widely cited assessment tool, with more than 465 references between 1974 and 1997 (Piotrowski 1999). The FES was designed to measure the interpersonal relationships among family members, the directions of personal growth emphasized by the family, and the basic structural organization of the family. The FES comprises 10 relational subscales that assess three dimensions of family functioning. These three dimensions are Relationship Dimension (Cohesion, Expressiveness, and Conflict); Personal Growth Dimension (Independence, Achievement Orientation, Moral-Religious Emphasis, Intellectual-Cultural Orientation, and Active-Recreational Orientation); and System Maintenance (Organization and Control). The FES is intended to provide a conceptual framework for organizing disparate observations within a family and represents an extension of Moos' work on other social environments (Moos 1974).

Similar to the FCAM, the FES has been adapted into several major forms. The most frequently employed, the Real Family Form (Form R), is used to characterize the family environment as it exists presently. The Ideal Family Form (Form I) is designed to measure the family as the members would ideally like it to be. The Expectation Form (Form E) permits an assessment of how individuals expect the typical family to function. Finally, the Short Form (Form S) for the FES was designed to permit reasonably rapid measurements of either large families or groups of families. Form S is composed of the first 40 items of the regular 90-item form (Form R). The FES also yields Family Incongruence scores, both for any given pair of family members and for the entire family.

The present style of the FES evolved from an original pool of 200 items (Form A), many of which were adapted from other social climate scales developed by Moos and his associates (Moos 1974; Moos et al. 1974). Each item was chosen for its suitability to identify an environment that would exert pressure on a family to move toward one of the three main dimensions of family functioning (i.e., Relationships, Growth Orientation, or System Maintenance). Form A was administered to a relatively broad sample of 285 families, including clinical, nonclinical, and ethnic minority families. Family size was somewhat evenly divided among families and ranged from three to seven members. Psychometric criteria used in construction of the final 90-item form (Form R) included low to moderate subscale intercorrelations, maximum discrimination among families, and an overall item split that avoided items characteristic only of extreme families. Although the authors report that each of the psychometric criteria was met in all three samples of families, the specific results are not directly provided (Moos et al. 1974).

Reliability estimates for the FES were established for the revised 90-item, 10-subscale Real Family Form (Form R). Average item-to-subscale correlations and subscale internal consistencies were calculated from data provided by 240 families ($N=814$) of the original 285 families participating in the FES construction sample. The item-to-subscale correlations ranged from 0.45 (Independence) to 0.58 (Cohesion), with a mean of 0.52. Internal consistency for the 10 subscales was computed with the Kuder-Richardson Formula 20. The mean coefficient was 0.73; the coefficient varied from a low of 0.64 to a high of 0.78, with seven of the subscales obtaining coefficients over 0.70. Test-retest reliabilities of individual scores on the 10 subscales ranged from 0.68 to 0.86 (see Table 13–1). In addition, average subscales intercorrelations were about 0.20, indicating that the subscales measure distinct but related aspects of family functioning and social environments.

The FES has been used to explore differences between the perceived family environments of normally functioning families and families undergoing psychological distress. A consistent finding among families with one or more dysfunctional members is a tendency toward less cohesion and expressiveness, poorer organization, and the experience of greater conflict (Scoresby and Christensen 1976; White 1978). Janes and Hesselbrock (1976) reported that the children of a schizophrenic parent perceived their families as significantly lower on Intellectual-Cultural Orientation and Active-Recreational Orientation. Also, the greater seclusion implied by low scores on these scales differentiated the childhood families of both black and white heroin users (Penk et al. 1979) from the normative score comparisons (Moos et al. 1974).

In a study of adolescent runaways, Steinbock (1978) compared the perceptions of three groups (those who became runaways, those who were in crisis but did not run away, and a control group) and their parents. Although the parents in the three groups did not differ in perceptions of their families, the runaway adolescents perceived much less cohesion and independence but more conflict and control in their families than did either their parents or the control group of adolescents. The FES has also enjoyed some success in demonstrating a relationship between family environment and the outcome of treatment for alcoholism. Both Finney et al. (1980) and Moos et al. (1979a) reported that the more supportive the family, as indexed by high Cohesion and Active-Recreational Orientation and low Conflict, the more positive the prognosis for the alcoholic family member. Other research has used the FES and points to its concurrent use with other tools and with many ethnic populations and ages; such research includes international studies (e.g., Lau and Kwok 2000; Westernick and Giarratano 1999).

Despite the encouraging direction of this research, it must be noted that evidence supporting the specific behavioral relevance of the dimensions tapped by the FES is still tentative. Increasingly, the FES is also being used in university settings and is frequently cited in dissertations. Another area of use has been in response to family stressors, as in the field of medical issues (e.g., Thompson et al. 1999). Concurrent validation with more estab-

Family Functioning Index

The Family Functioning Index (FFI), developed by Pless and Satterwhite (1973), was designed to provide a rapid indication of families in need of assistance with coping with stressful events. This instrument was adapted from a semi-structured interview schedule administered to a random sample of parents with school-aged children ($N=399$) in a suburban New York county. An almost equal number of these children were considered either healthy or suffering from some form of chronic physical disorder. The FFI was constructed on the basis of 15 theoretically and empirically derived questions, which the authors believe reflect the multidimensional nature of family functioning, and which were asked of the mothers during the final portion of the interview. Factor analysis of the mothers' responses resulted in six factors: Marital Satisfaction, Frequency of Disagreement, Happiness, Communication, Weekends Together, and Problem Solving. Correlations between these components and the total index score were computed independently for both mothers and fathers. Correlation coefficients ranged from a low of 0.07 for problem solving to a high of 0.96 for marital satisfaction for the fathers, while correlations for the mothers ranged from 0.21 to 0.95 on the same components, respectively.

Test-retest reliability, with a 5-year interval, was established by drawing a randomized and proportionately stratified sample of cases (Satterwhite et al. 1976) from the original subject population (see Table 13-1). The FFI was readministered to those subjects who had neither experienced a change in marital status nor had enrolled in subsequent family therapy. For the 29 families meeting these criteria, the Pearson product-moment correlation coefficient between the original and retest FFI total scores was 0.83 ($P=0.001$). The authors report that no special significance is attached to the 5-year interval period, beyond that ordinarily assigned to a shorter retest interval. In addition, although a 0.72 correlation between independently obtained FFI scores for husbands and wives reportedly contributes both to the reliability and the validity of the measure, no information is provided on the sample size or its description.

An additional feature of the FFI is the availability of *parallel forms* for each spouse, with appropriate wording. The format of the 15 items varies, with some questions answered on a continuum (e.g., 1=very disappointed; 5=very pleased), and others in an ordinal format (e.g., more, same, less). The information pertaining to total family functioning is obtained solely from the parents. As with other tools, the references and use have not been robust, and few studies in the literature have reported on the FFI's usefulness since the 1980s and 1990s, when it was reviewed in professional journals.

Structural Family Interaction Scale

The Structural Family Interaction Scale (SFIS) was constructed by Linda Perosa (1980) as part of a doctoral dissertation. The title of this instrument may be somewhat misleading, since the SFIS was intended not merely to assess interactions but to operationalize Salvador Minuchin's (1974a, 1974d) model of family system functioning. Minuchin conceives of family functioning in terms of two central dimensions. The first, Boundaries, ranges along a continuum from diffuse (Disengaged) to overly rigid (Enmeshed). The second dimension of Minuchin's structural model of the family involves the manner in which families adapt to stress and conflict. The family's capacity to adapt depends on its ability to maintain firm but flexible system boundaries, permitting realignment to changing circumstances.

The SFIS utilizes an 85-item questionnaire to specify a family's position within these two central dimensions. Sixty-five of these items are considered primary, yielding 13 subscales containing 5 items each. The subscales are termed Enmeshment, Disengagement, Overprotection, Neglect, Rigidity, Flexibility, Conflict Avoidance, Conflict Expression Without Resolution, Conflict Resolution, Parent Management, Triangulation, Parent-Child Coalition, and Detouring. The SFIS also includes 20 secondary items that retain the same stem as the 65 primary item statements but have been modified from general words like "parent" to more specific terms such as "mother" or "father." These subscales attempt to refine the information provided by the primary items on the family as a unit by measuring family subsystem functioning. The 20 secondary items form 10 subscales of 2 items each: Mother Overprotection, Father Overprotection, Mother Neglect, Father Neglect, Parent Conflict Avoidance, Parent-Child Conflict Avoidance, Parent Conflict Expression Without Resolution, Parent Conflict Resolution, and Parent-Child Conflict Resolution. Responses to all 85 items are made on a 4-point scale of agreement ranging from "very true" to "very false."

Initially, a list of 200 items derived from an outline of Minuchin's concepts was presented to six family therapists, along with a categorized description of those concepts. The therapists chose the category each item best fit and rated the degree of congruence. Interjudge reliability for each item ranged from 0.817 to 1.00, with a mean of 0.95 for the final 95 items chosen for the pilot instrument. The data, which were obtained from 50 volunteer families from a western New York metropolitan area, were used to select the 65 primary statements included in the revised 85-item SFIS.

The SFIS was administered to 50 new families (Perosa et al. 1981), in which both the parents and two children completed the instrument ($N= 196$). Twenty-five of the families included a learning-disabled child, while 25 children were *without* special disabilities. The average age of the children in the first group was 12 years, and 12.8 years for the second group. The sample consisted of Caucasian and almost exclusively two-parent families.

Using Cronbach's (1960) alpha, internal consistency for the 13 primary subscales ranged from a low of 0.25 for Neglect to 0.74 for Parent-Child Coalition. Nine of these subscales achieved a coefficient of 0.50 or greater. Internal consistency ranged from –0.08 for Parent Conflict Avoidance to 0.56 for Father Neglect; coefficients for 8 of the 10 subscales fell below 0.50. Average item-subscale correlations were more stable for both the primary and secondary subscales. Primary subscale scores ranged from 0.50 for Neglect to 0.70 for Parent-Child Coalition, while secondary subscale scores ranged from 0.70 for Parent Conflict Avoidance to 0.83 for both Parent Conflict Resolution and Father Neglect. No test-retest reliability figures are available. The scale has been revised since its initial development.

According to the authors, evidence of validity is provided through interrater agreement that item content is consistent with construct definitions and that scale intercorrelations are in predicted directions. Although there can be little dispute that interrater agreement is high, it is difficult to accept this limited form of construct validity as empirical evidence of the instrument's effectiveness in measurement. A general tendency for scale intercorrelations to reflect theoretical assumptions is borne out in the data provided by the authors. To date, there have been several studies that support the usefulness of this scale.

Simulated Family Activity Measure

The Simulated Family Activity Measure (SIMFAM), devised by Straus and Tallman (1971), was originally designed to assess five aspects of family functioning: Power (an index of family leadership); Support (an index of the social solidarity of the family); Communication; Problem-Solving Ability; and Creativity (an index of ideational fluency and flexibility). The SIMFAM uses direct observations and videotapes of family interaction under a set of standardized conditions, engaging family members in the task of discovering the rules for a shuffleboard-type game.

The SIMFAM requires a 9×12-foot court marked out on the floor with masking tape, pucks or balls, pushers, two blackboards, a light board, colored armbands, and a scoreboard. The light board displays a red and green light for each player. The game or task is divided into eight "innings," separated by rest periods during which the family may discuss strategy. The number of players is normally set at three, typically the father, mother, and one child. The family's task is to discover the rules of the game by observing the patterns of red and green lights they receive as feedback to the different scoring strategies they employ. A green light indicates a participant has followed a rule correctly; a red light indicates a rule has been violated.

Basically, the SIMFAM uses just two sets of rules. During the first four trials, the green light is flashed whenever a player hits a ball of the same color as that player's pusher and armband against one of the backboards. This constitutes a normal problem-solving situation insofar as the rules and feedback apply directly to the actions of the family members. The last four trials represent a crisis or stress condition. During these trials, red lights are displayed for every scoring attempt with the exception of two green lights given randomly to keep motivation high. Motivation is further enhanced through the use of artificial scores recorded on the scoreboard. It is virtually impossible for the subjects to know whether or not the posted scores and lights agree, since the game is played rapidly and the ambiguous rules make almost any score plausible. Although the game normally ends with the family in crisis, several variations exist. For instance, Russell (1979) altered the SIMFAM format to allow for a recovery period in which the family's ability to reorganize and adapt to new rules was assessed.

The SIMFAM appears highly flexible since the basic procedures may be systematically varied, and a wide variety of ratings and scores can be obtained from the repertoire of observed family behavior. The SIMFAM has been employed primarily as a method of assessment for the Circumplex Model of Marital and Family Systems (Olson et al. 1979) (see, e.g., Circumplex Model or Family Functioning discussed earlier in the subsection "Family Adaptability and Cohesion Evaluation Scales"). Two of the variables that the SIMFAM was originally designed to measure, support and creativity, have been assessed as facilitative concepts to Cohesion and Adaptability. The aspects of power and problem solving have been absorbed within the two central constructs of the Circumplex Model; however, Olson et al. (1980) modified the model to include Communication as a major dimension.

Family Assessment Dimensions

Family assessment instruments can be compared by assigning the scales contained within each measure to the categories of a schema developed by Fisher (1976). Fisher reviewed the literature dealing with clinical assessment of families and organized the criteria employed by 29 authors or groups (i.e., Family Service Association; Group for the Advancement of Psychiatry) into a list of significant areas of functioning. From this list he developed a composite of five dimensions considered necessary for assessment of entire families: Structural Descriptors (e.g., roles, alliances, communication patterns); Controls and Sanctions (e.g., power and leadership, dependency, differentiation); Emotions and Needs (e.g., rules of affective expression, need satisfaction, affective themes); Cultural Aspects (e.g., social position, cultural heritage, cultural views); and Development Aspects (e.g., appropriateness to developmental stage or life cycle of the family). Fisher organized these dimensions into a *two-level hierarchy.* The first level includes cultural and developmental aspects that, Fisher argues, provide a context for understanding the remaining three behaviors identified in the second level. Limitations of this schema include the lack of attention to the psychometric qualities of assessment methods employed and the equal weight given to all research, including studies relying on clinical interviews and single-concept measures. Despite these flaws, Fisher provides a cogent framework for arranging data on the functioning of whole families.

Table 13–2 provides information on 10 assessment measurements based on Fisher's schema of family dimensions.

Individual subscales of the instruments discussed are categorized according to the dimensions identified in Fisher's schema in Table 13–2. The table shows that the subscales emphasize these dimensions to varying degrees. The dimension receiving greatest attention is Structural Descriptors, which could suggest that it accounts for a substantial proportion of variance in family functioning. Alternatively, this dimension may simply be the easiest to identify. Developmental Aspects were not represented among the subscales but are readily obtained and need not be included in the formal assessment process since they are purely informational. Of greater value would be a qualitative evaluation of how well the family manages issues relevant to its current phase.

Several commonalities appear among the instruments, although markedly different labels are given to similar constructs. The structural descriptor "cohesion" is represented either by name or by function in nearly every assessment method. The concept of cohesion actually spans several dimensions and refers to a broad, abstract characteristic. Therefore, the strictness with which the various scale constructs or nomenclatures are interpreted will determine the degree to which cohesion is seen as underlying a particular instrument's scale structure. Moreover, two of the instruments ascribe major importance to cohesion in their theoretical base. One of these instruments is Minuchin's model of family functioning, where it is referred to

Table 13–2. Instruments categorized by Fisher's schema on family dimensions

	Structural descriptors	Controls and sanctions	Emotions and needs	Cultural aspects
BTFES	Parental coalitions Mythology Goal-directed negotiation Permeability Conflict Self-disclosure Invasiveness	Overt power Responsibility	Closeness Expressiveness Mood and tone Empathy	
FACES	System feedback Negotiation Roles Family boundaries Coalitions Space Decision making Time	Assertiveness Control Discipline Rules Independence	Emotional bonding	Interests and recreation Friends
FAD	Problem solving Communication Roles General functioning	Behavior control	Affective responsiveness Affective involvement	
FAM	Task accomplishment Communication Role performance	Control	Affective expression Affective involvement	Values and norms

Table 13-2. Instruments categorized by Fisher's schema on family dimensions *(continued)*

	Structural descriptors	Controls and sanctions	Emotions and needs	Cultural aspects
FCAM	Consideration vs. conflict Open communication Togetherness vs. separateness	Internal vs. external locus of control	Family actualization vs. inadequacy Family loyalty Closeness vs. estrangement	Community sociability Family ambition
FEF	Conflict/tension Extrafamilial support Children's relations Homemaker role* Open communication Worker role*	Inconsistent discipline Mother/father dominance Behavioral control* Explanation of rules* Strict discipline* Independence training*	Children's adjustment Marital satisfaction Nurturance* Emotional closeness	Community involvement Financial problems
FES	Cohesion Organization	Conflict Control Independence	Expressiveness	Moral-religious orientation Intellectual-cultural orientation Active-recreational orientation Achievement orientation
FFI	Frequency of disagreement Communication Problem solving Weekends together		Marital satisfaction Happiness	

Table 13–2. Instruments categorized by Fisher's schema on family dimensions *(continued)*

	Structural descriptors	Controls and sanctions	Emotions and needs	Cultural aspects
SFIS	Enmeshment Disengagement Flexibility Rigidity Conflict avoidance Conflict expression without resolution Conflict resolution	Parent management Triangulation Parent-child coalitions Detouring	Overprotection Neglect	
SIMFAM	Problem solving Communication Creativity	Power	Support	

Note. BTFES=Beavers-Timberlawn Family Evaluation Scale; FACES=Family Adaptability and Cohesion Evaluation Scales; FAD=Family Assessment Device; FAM=Family Assessment Measure; FCAM=Family Concept Assessment Method; FEF=Family Evaluation Form; FES=Family Environment Scale; FFI=Family Functioning Index; SFIS=Structural Family Interaction Scale; SIMFAM=Simulated Family Activity Measure.
*Scored twice: once for self and once for spouse.

as "Boundaries." The other instrument, the Circumplex Model, derives conceptual support from the inclusion of, and emphasis on, cohesion in the assessment methods. Unfortunately, empirical verification has not been very successful. Russell et al. (1984) found virtually no correlation between the cohesion scale of the FES and the SIMFAM, and instead suggested that the FES scale actually measures the concept of support. Although the methodology employed in the study could have contributed to the disappointing results, efforts to cross-validate these instruments with one another and against additional criteria should eventually lead to refinement and improvement of total family assessment capabilities.

Discussion

Two major criticisms leveled at the field of family assessment a decade ago are still true (Halvorsen 1991). First, there is disagreement about what constitutes the key concepts that should be considered when assessing families, as well as accepted definitions. Second, there is inconsistency in the design of and attention to details in psychometric evaluations of instruments. While there are many differences between the assessment methods presented in this chapter, significant similarities also exist. The majority of family assessment methods were compared and contrasted according to dimensions suggested by Fisher (1976), and were reported by Forman and Hagan (1984). The 1980s witnessed the proffering of few new instruments to assess overall family functioning. Instead, efforts have been devoted to further refinement and validation of those already in use. While there have even been cross-validational studies in which several instruments were studied for areas of commonality (e.g., Bloom and Kindle 1985; Bloomguist and Harris 1984; Perosa and Perosa 1982), there is only a modest estimate of convergent or discriminant validity (Doherty and Hovander 1990). As a result of the studies of the 1980s, clinicians can be more certain of what is being measured and can make judgments and predictions with greater confidence than was true less than a decade ago. However, there is not a good fit between the definition of family constructs and the instruments, making it essential that clinicians understand what the instruments can and cannot do and exercise caution in usage.

It should be apparent from the discussions in this chapter that each assessment method is based on a set of presuppositions as to which dimensions of family behavior are important. When a clinician selects a particular assessment method, he or she tacitly endorses those areas of family functioning prescribed and proscribed by the test author(s). Hence, the clinician should select only those assessment methods that are consistent with his or her orientation and beliefs about which theoretical constructs are most effective for working with families.

Chapters on Related Topics

The following chapters describe concepts related to family assessment:

- Chapter 12, "Initial and Diagnostic Family Interviews"
- Chapter 16, "Diagnosis of Family Relational Disorders"

14

The Family Life Cycle

A Framework for Understanding Family Development

Joan Zilbach, M.D.

> **W**hat is meant by a family.... The very omnipresence of the family renders it almost invisible. Because we are immersed in a family we rarely have to define it or describe it to one another. (Degler 1980, p. 3)
>
> Although the arena of human passion is ordinary family life, only recently has this context come under actual observation and been taken seriously. It is becoming more evident that families undergo a developmental process over time, and human distress...symptoms appear when this process is disrupted. (Haley 1973, p. 42)

Introduction

We are born into and live immersed within our families, experiencing their *omnipresence*, as Degler notes in the above passage. Because we live within our families, and are therefore so close to them, we must work to attain enough objectivity to become aware of the family developmental process and to be able to describe and define the family life cycle. The concept of family development has been present from the beginning of therapeutic work with families in the mid-1950s (Zilbach 1968). However, family therapy has not always been acknowledged or defined in detail.

In 1968, I wrote a paper on family development that was influenced by Erikson's individual model, my experience in child psychiatry, and my early work in family therapy. Family development, as such, had been more extensively explicated in the field of family sociology (Duvall 1977; Hill and Rodgers 1964). In addition, some family investigators had used family development as an integral part of their conceptual framework for their family research (Goodrich 1991; Rapoport et al. 1977; Rausch et al. 1963). Haley (1973) and Minuchin (1965) also included family development as part of their theoretical framework. The volume on the family life cycle by Carter and McGoldrick (1980a) was a major influence.

Carter and McGoldrick and the other authors mentioned above all use some variant of a linear stage model. Another author, Lee Combrinck-Graham takes a different approach, using a spiral rather than the linear-stage model (Combrinck-Graham 1985). The model I have developed is also presented in a linear fashion for purposes of clarity. However, various nonlinear modifications may occur, with certain "later" phases preceding earlier ones.

The Family

> We often think that when we have completed our study of one [individual] we know all about two, because "two is one and one." (Eddington)

The family is not a sum of "ones," composed simply of the total of individual family members. The family is a natural group of nonstrangers, a "unity of interacting persons" (E.W. Burgess 1926). A family, consisting of a unity of interacting personalities, is a living, changing, growing organism:

> The actual unity of family life has its existence not in any legal conception, nor in any formal contract (like marriage) but in the *interaction* [emphasis added] of its members. For the family does not depend for its survival on the harmonious relations of its members, nor does it necessarily disintegrate as a result of conflicts between its members. The family lives as long as interaction is taking place and only dies when it ceases. (E.W. Burgess 1926)

The family is a primary biopsychosocial entity that functions as a single psychic entity (Zinner and Shapiro 1974). The family is a whole unit, with family characteristics of its own, *beyond* and different from the characteristics of individual family members. The psychic boundaries of individual family members must be blurred, if not erased, in order to comprehend the family as a unit. The family as a whole is not an unchanging static unit, but rather is always *on the move*, developing and undergoing change. I emphasize this concept of continuous family development because it is the foundation of my developmental model of the family life cycle.

Development is defined as an orderly sequence of changes or phases that occur over time in which the progression, the unfolding of one expectable change of organization or function originating from a previous change, determines the next stage (Zilbach 1986). Developmental progression occurs in cells, groups, children, families, institutions, and larger societal processes with a beginning, a middle, and an end phase; all of these units experience a series of expectable phases in which life cycle stage markers identify their concomitant tasks. In this chapter I discuss the family unit, within a family developmental life cycle, and the series of family stages and stage markers that correspond to the life cycle.

The *family life cycle* remains the dominant theoretical model at the turn of the twenty-first century. This model has been increasingly used to help understand the complexities of normal development as well as the impact of a range of clinical phenomena on the course of a family life cycle.

The family unit is a special type of small, natural group that undergoes a sequence of developmental stages. Unit development is concurrent with but distinct from the psychosexual, psychosocial, and other types of development of individuals within the family. Every family member is simultaneously undergoing individual development while the family as a group is pursuing its own developmental path. We often try to understand a family, which ranges from two or more members in size, in terms of the sum or interaction of individual developmental paths; such a portrait of a family becomes very complex and confusing.

Some aspects of families are complicated; others are simpler than they may seem at first glance. An impartial observer can blur the boundaries of the individuals within the family and consider it as an objective and comprehensible entity. One can hear from one's own family or from other families statements to the effect of "My family can do that now; we're in that stage," or "We can do things like that now, we're that kind of family and in that time of family life!" These are statements of the family as a unit that show implicit recognition of family life cycles and developmental stages with particular tasks to be accomplished. Like other developing institutions, the family life cycle progresses through early, middle, and late stages. Although each specific family unit comes to an end, the larger or extended family attains continuity in its family history, traditions, and practices. This continuity in turn strengthens new generations and family units.

At each stage of family development there is a marker or signal and a core family task that must be accomplished in some fashion by all members. Through task accomplishment, family development proceeds and carries into each subsequent stage the characteristics of the previous periods. Predictably, the family unit will experience progression or regression in the course of its life cycle. Impediments to family development are described later in this chapter (see the section below entitled "Clinical Examples").

Stages of the Family Life Cycle

In the following sections, I discuss the stages of the family life cycle, including the marker and task that accompany each stage. I would like to note at this point that the concept of life cycles is applicable to many kinds of families and does not presuppose Western, two-parent, two-sex nuclear families. The stages of family development apply to "alternative" families and also to some other cultures. It would be presumptuous to say that the stages described below apply to all cultures; such a claim awaits investigation. However, there is enough evidence to suggest the applicability of these stages to the kinds of families that therapists encounter in daily life and in clinical practice.

Courtship

Courtship is a kind of preparatory period that precedes the actual start of the family life cycle. This stage can be called a courtship, an engagement, or another variety of prefamily social practice.

The implications of courtship (and of the family life cycle in general) for women are not discussed in this publication. The model has been developed (I hope) without prejudice to the possibility of changing outcomes for women. The reader should at least keep in mind Carolyn Heilbrun's description of the implications of courtship to women in *Writing a Woman's Life*:

> For a short time, during courtship, the illusion is maintained that women, by withholding themselves, are central. Women are allowed this brief period in the limelight—and it is the part of their lives most constantly and vividly enacted in a myriad of representations—to encourage the acceptance of a lifetime of marginality. And courtship itself is, as often as not, an illusion: that is, the woman must entrap the man to ensure herself a center for her life. The rest is aging and regret. (Heilbrun 1988, p. 21)

Early Stages—Forming and Nesting (Creation) (Stages I and II)

Stage I: Coupling

The beginning of a family unit is the establishment of a common household by two people who may or may not be married. The central or core family task of Stage I is to facilitate movement from individual independence to the couple's interdependence. The interdependence and *joining* of the couple establish a household. *Basic family functions* must be initiated in this stage. Basic and other family functions that are essential aspects of family life will be discussed later in this chapter.

One person may establish a household without coupling, and a single person may accomplish the initiation of basic family functions.

Stage II: Becoming Three

The second stage of the early years of family life begins with the arrival and subsequent inclusion of the first dependent member of the family. The dependent member may be a child or another adult family member. The core family task at this stage of family development is to progress from coupled, dyadic interdependence to the incorporation of dependence within triadic interdependence.

With increasing frequency, the first dependent member may be a parent, sibling, or another adult from outside the family. In other models of the family life cycle that are child-focused, the birth of the first child and his or her subsequent incorporation into the family unit is regarded as a universal event for families. A more accurate and inclusive model of Stage II centers on the incorporation into the family unit of the first dependent member, whatever his or her age.

In some alternative families, becoming *three* is actually becoming a *twosome*. The single-parent family consists of a single mother or father who has chosen to have a child by adoption or other methods, such as donor insemination. The single-parent family completes Stage I and accomplished family tasks individually. Stage II dependents are incorporated within the dyadic unit rather than triadic interdependence.

Middle Stages—Family Expansion/Separation Processes (Stages III, IV, and V)

Stage III: Entrances

Although there are many paths that families follow in the middle stages of development, *entrance* can be identified as a universal task or stage marker.

This third stage begins with the partial exit of a dependent member from the immediate world of the expanding family by entrance into the larger extrafamilial world. Like Stage II, our Stage III model assumes a child as the primary dependent member; therefore, the first extrafamilial environment is usually a school. However, if the first dependent member is not a child, the exit may be to a hospital, nursing home, or other extrafamilial institution. The family's task in Stage III is to help members begin expanding and separating from the family.

Stage IV: Further Expansion

The family task in Stage IV is to foster the continuing *expansion* of partial separations. Stage IV is marked by the entrance of the last remaining dependent member of the family into the larger community.

Stage V: Exits

The end of the middle stage of family development is marked by the first complete *exit* of a dependent family member from the family unit. In this stage, the establishment of an independent household completes the previous partial expansion, separation, and independence processes of a family member. The newly established independent household may include marriage or alternative forms of cohabitation. Whatever the form of the familial unit, it necessitates the establishment of basic intrafamilial family functions by the exiting family member. The central family task of Stage V is to facilitate the establishment and functioning of a household unit; that is, to *launch* a family member and his or her family unit into their own path through the family life cycle. In clinical practice, many referrals of family units that we encounter are in the middle stages of family development.

Late Stages—Finishing (Stages VI and VII)

Stage VI: Becoming Smaller and Extended

Ultimately, the moment comes for the exit of the last dependent member or child from the family to the extrafamilial world to establish an independent household. The family task of Stage VI is fostering the continuing expansion of independence. This stage of family life may include grandparenthood. Most of the emphasis and much of the task work for all family members in this stage concern the expansion of certain family processes rather than diminishment, shrinking, or emptying. The terms *shrunken family* or *empty nest*, which have been used as descriptors for this stage, have a negative connotation that is not accurate for a normative or nonpathological model. Feelings of emptiness may predominate in some families that have difficulties negotiating the tasks and other work of this stage of family development. However, expansion and creative growth are often part of the experience for many families in this later stage of family life.

Stage VII: Endings

> The family lives as long as interaction is taking place and only dies when it ceases. (E.W. Burgess 1926)

The last stage of family development includes the death of a spouse or life partner, if this has not occurred earlier, and continues up to the death of the other partner. The *sibling* family structure exists until the death of the last sibling. At that point, a family has come to an end; family history, myths, and traditions continue on in the new family units that have been spawned and created in the course of family life.

The beginnings of family units are simpler to define and study than endings. Even the complicated middle phases of the family life cycle, with their extensive family patterns and intricate pathways, are easier to recognize than family endings.

Stage VII inevitably includes grieving for lost family members. The grief of the family unit is also a powerful context for individual mourning, and when any part of the grieving process is incomplete, all family members suffer in some long-lasting, poignant, and sad manner. The important family task of Stage VII is to progress from support and expansion of independence to working through final separations. During these last years of the family's life together there are many changes, decreases, and diminishments. Often enough, however, there are remarkable, albeit mostly unnoticed, enhancements and progressions. Some families experience a downward plunge to nothingness with extremes of complication and pain; fortunately this is not the only pattern for later family life.

During these later years, the parental unit undergoes many changes. The couple's function as parents sometimes diminishes to almost nothing. As a family member described the present stage of his family to me, "When we—the children—all left, my mother and father stopped speaking to any of us and to each other. That was the end of the family, and it was most unfortunate." For more successful traversals of this stage, new concepts and methods must be discovered and explored for parenting in the later years of life.

Some families experience resolution of issues and achieve familial integration only at this stage. A family role reversal of achieved independence to dependence may occur after the death of one parent, but this reversal is not limited to parents. However, household integration of a parent or inclusion of another family member does not automatically signify dependence. The rearrangement may include a higher level of integration. As difficult as it is to accept and conceptualize what happens after the death of the second parent, the family members of new units must mourn, for this particular family unit is at an end.

Many joinings and separations occur in the course of the family life cycle: the move from individual independence to couple interdependence; incorporation of dependence within triadic interdependence and partial separations; exits corresponding to the development of new independence; and expansion and the creation of family units. In this last stage, the final separations occur with closure and completeness. Death may have been a part of family life at earlier times, but the death of a surviving spouse or partner, and finally the death of the last sibling, mark the closing of the family cycle. By this time, the new families of the children will be in various stages of their own family life cycles and development; each in its own way will resolve the death of the original family.

Basic Family Functions

The *basic functions* of every family must be facilitated from the moment of its creation, similar to an infant organism. Families have fundamental needs that must be met for survival and continued existence. These needs of the interacting family entity, including the need for space (psychosocial shelter and housing), provisions and supplies (food), finances (employment and money), and healthare, are met in ways that become characteristic of each family unit—the *basic family functions*. The care of children and other dependent members, including all aspects of individual emotional development, is a basic function of all family members in the course of the entire family life cycle. Because these functions are *everyday activities*, they are easily and often dismissed or do not receive continuing attention. However, the establishment, continuance, and maintenance of the family unit depend on the operational substrate of basic family functions.

It is important to recognize that basic family functions are performed by *all* family members as a group, including children of any age. Thus, the work of the family unit is greater than the work of an individual family member. Some family functions have their origin early in family life; others emerge later. As these functions change over time, they can be adequately, partially, or inadequately performed or diminished in their development and fulfillment.

There are two major divisions of basic family functions: the *primary intrafamilial processes* that potentially create and enhance closeness and intimacy between family members, and the *extrafamilial processes* that create and enhance bonds outside the family and foster familial expansion into the community and the larger society.

The primary intrafamilial processes are 1) psychosocial space (shelter and housing); 2) household supplies, particularly food; 3) finances (money and employment); and 4) health. These are primary family functions because without their establishment and continuance in some fashion, a family unit cannot exist.

The extrafamilial processes involve various aspects of socialization and enculturation. This group of family functions includes the provision of education, transmission of values, provision for leisure activities, and other activities that connect members to the community.

The primary intrafamilial processes begin in Stage I of the family life cycle and continue with necessary changes at each subsequent life cycle stage. Extrafamilial functions gain importance in the middle phases of the family life cycle (for further details of basic family functions, see Zilbach 1978).

The family life cycle model was expanded in the late 1990s by its application to a variety of social and clinical situations. Simultaneously, it was criticized for its view of families as a uniform entity, its insensitivity to cultural diversity (Logan 1996; Shapiro 1966), and its failure to account for the sexual orientation of the couple (Morgan 1997; Rice and Greenberg 1994).

Recent studies have examined the life cycle course with African-American single-parent families (Logan 1996), Chinese-American families (Hamilton 1996), and Latino families (Shapiro 1966). For example, Latino families emphasize responsibility to others and the formation of affectionate ties with alternative caregivers, and Chinese-American families emphasize *filial piety* and respect for parents; these family interactions have clear implications for the family life cycle course.

Studies have been conducted on the impact of a number of diseases on the family life cycle. The disruptive influence of Crohn's disease (Wright 1999), cancer in adults or children (Veach and Nicholas 1998), infertility and adoption (Salzer 1999), and disabilities (Marshak et al. 1999) are examples. Rolland (1994) has proposed a comprehensive model to sensitize clinicians to the impact of disease. The differential course of *launching* in families with mentally retarded (Kraus and Seltzer 1998) or schizophrenic members (Stromwall and Robinson 1998) is an example of such a variation.

Multiple attempts were made between 1995 and 2000 to revise and rethink the family life cycle model. These attempts include examining hidden theoretical assumptions in the model (Dilworth-Anderson and Burton

1996); introducing feminist rather than traditional views of the family (Rice and Greenberg 1984); and simplifying the model to the three stages of coupling, expanding, and contracting (Gerson 1995). The most intriguing proposal is to include the narrative metaphor and narrative accounts in the examination of the family life cycle (Erickson 1998). This proposal parallels the recent evolution of narrative therapy.

In the next section, I provide case examples to illustrate aspects of the family life cycle and basic family functions in clinical practice.

Clinical Examples

Examples of clinical application of the family life cycle in this chapter will focus on the early stages. Other examples throughout the life cycle can be found in other publications, particularly those by Zilbach, including *Young Children in Family Therapy* (Zilbach 1986); "The Family Life Cycle," in *Children and Families* (Zilbach 1988); and *Children in Family Therapy: Treatment and Training* (Zilbach 1989a).

Divorce and remarriage are such frequent occurrences that it seems useful to address the significance of families formed by stepparents and stepchildren in the family life cycle. Stage I development of such a couple involves the interaction and simultaneous existence of Stage I, combined with whatever stage(s) the other, earlier family units may be in. As the *new* (remarried or blended) primary couple in a *remarried, reconstituted*, or *blended* family, the couple must inevitably traverse Stage I. This includes the necessary establishment of *new* basic family functions while being influenced by the other family members, including the stepchildren. An example that includes stepchildren highlights some common experiences in Stage I development when young children are involved. The basic family function of providing shelter and housing, which establishes psychophysical external boundaries and interior living space, is demonstrably affected by the formation of a new family unit of stepparents and stepchildren.

> After a period of *going together* (gestational stage), Arthur and Barbara decided to *join* their households, and they bought a house (Stage I—Coupling). Arthur and Barbara both had joint custody of their respective school-age children. There were many discussions about allocation of space, particularly play space and bedrooms, that became quite repetitive. The new couple was puzzled about the *stuck* quality of these decisions. The couple had agreeably resolved various other issues (e.g., money, space, and the house itself), and they had expected that this relatively nonconflictual process would continue after the actual purchase was completed. But in the area of space allocation, the couple encountered the stepchildren.
>
> Arthur and Barbara were able to recognize that their desire as a new

couple for their *nest* in the choice of space for the master bedroom in the new home had to be combined with the play space and other needs of the various stepchildren units. The impasse occurred when one of the two sets of needs—the Stage I need of a new nest and the Stage IV need for a stepfamily home—threatened to dominate. Resolution and decision making occurred when rather than making an *either-or* decision, the family could recognize both sets of family stage needs.

Both Arthur and Barbara had been in individual treatment prior to and during the course of their earlier divorces. Their confusion as they joined their families did not seem to them to be a serious problem, and they decided to seek joint consultation. Because both families were involved, they chose a family therapist, who asked them to bring in all of the children. During the evaluation about the present state of the basic family functions, information about the couples' difficulties in organizing the space in their new house was elicited. The children described their needs, which were dominated by Stage IV. The parents eloquently described their new couple needs: they wanted a master bedroom in the area the children wanted as a big playroom! The therapist observed that the whole family unit was in developmental transition and proceeded to identify the needs generated by this state. The therapist used arguments about the allocation of physical space to demonstrate family needs. The parents and children had an animated discussion about various aspects of their developmental transition and difficulties. Consultation was terminated after a few sessions and resolution took place amicably and without further serious difficulty.

Family housing—the space within the family home—is the psychosocial functional interior of the family unit. The need for explicit change in the interior space of the family and the intensity of the process is analogous to the inevitable change that occurs in the expanding personal interior space of the pregnant mother. Thus, the need for change in interior housing space is not necessarily propelled only by concrete *reality*, but rather by the family developmental force of Stage III—Becoming Three, expressed in this area of basic family functions. Within the framework of family development, these physical manifestations of psychosocial change become both observable and understandable. The family feels an urgency that propels change.

"We must have a place for the baby," Mrs. B said a bit desperately and with considerable intensity. Within their house there was an existing room that seemed to have good space possibilities for the needed nursery. This room was small but adequate and sunny; it was in disarray at that time, containing an overflow of books, clothes, and other adult sundries. The practicalities of extensive remodeling in order to provide nursery space for the new baby were reviewed and seemingly dismissed. However, the need to make space for the baby persisted and became a big project that required dismantling large areas of the house and took considerable attention just before the birth and physical displacement and discomfort in the immediate postdelivery period.

However, the enthusiasm of both Mr. and Mrs. B remained high and fairly constant with the expressed theme of "making things new and different, spanking clean and shiny, for this special time in our family life!"

All of the other basic family functions—household supplies and food, finances and employment, and family health—also undergo change when new family units are being formed. These changes may not be as obvious as the need for housing space described in the preceding example. In addition, each family function has a complex relationship to the others. In the following example, it appears that as one family function changed, others seemed to follow. But this may also be an artifact of narrative description, which is sometimes inadequate to describe the intermixed, intertwined, and simultaneous events of family development.

A young artist and his graduate student wife had lived together for several years. The basic family functions of shelter and housing, finances and employment, household supplies and food, and family health were well established in Stage I. In this stage, as the couple established a joint household, changes occurred as they worked out the development of their couple interdependent functions. The wife moved into the husband's art studio apartment. Their external family boundaries of shelter and housing were essentially satisfactory in his art studio, though they moved some internal walls. These internal changes, rather than a total physical move, seemed to satisfy the need for new couple space. She had steady employment, which provided sufficient basic family finances. Additional income from his artwork was sporadic but allowed them some monetary and economic flexibility. She also pursued her chosen graduate studies on a part-time basis, which worked well with their respective schedules because of the extensive time demands for his creative and artistic pursuits. Both members of the couple provided household supplies and food, cooking, and other tasks, depending on which member was not occupied with work or school.

Before the birth of their first baby, the couple discussed and came to a mutual agreement as to how their new family would function. They planned that the wife would return to work shortly after the birth of the baby, since she provided the most stable income, and the husband would do the major portion of primary child care. The delivery was uneventful, and the baby was healthy. But in the first months of life the baby developed a number of protracted, troublesome, and somewhat serious infections, and there was some additional concern about the baby's mental development. There seemed to be some evidence of developmental lag or possible retardation.

What was the status of the basic family functions at this phase of family development, Stage II, particularly regarding the baby? The inclusion of a baby, a dependent family member, had of course increased the needs in all the primary family functions. The basic income supplied by the mother's employment had remained stable, though the supplementary income from the father's artwork had decreased, since time previously given to artistic production was now partly taken up with primary child care. There was also increased financial need because of the additional family member, and particularly because the baby had numerous lengthy infections requiring frequent and expensive medication. Because of these and other increased expenses, there was pressure on the father to sell more of his artwork. This had not been an issue in Stage I. He was not immediately willing to do this because it required marketing time, and he preferred to create rather than market during the time he was not spending in child care. His sparse free time was designated solely for artistic work.

At first it appeared that the basic family functions of shelter and housing and household supplies and food were adequate. However, further discussion revealed that the father often lost track of time when involved in his artistic work. In addition, the baby's space, the nursery, had been constructed and placed at some distance from the work area of the father to protect the baby from the toxic art materials.

When the father was fully absorbed in his creative endeavors, the cries of the baby went unheard, and provision of adequate food, medication, and other stimulation was neglected. The father and mother, though willing and agreeable, had not made the necessary adjustments to the needs of the new and totally dependent family member, the baby.

All of these family functions had been discussed before the birth of the baby and solutions mutually agreed on. The baby was planned: both father and mother had agreed that children were important for both of them. This family's difficulty in developing satisfactory patterns for adjusting to and meeting the needs of the early phase of Stage II was not revealed effortlessly but rather through specific family developmental inquiries.

When different arrangements for childcare were made to supplement the father's primary care, recurrences of the baby's infections diminished in number and length. The development of the baby accelerated and reached an age-appropriate stage when other caregivers and the father provided adequate nutrition and stimulation. The father was also able to devote some time to selling his artwork, and the couple's finances improved. Besides these interlocking changes, the mother decreased her responsibilities that were unrelated to childcare. An incipient case of *failure to thrive* was prevented, and the issue of developmental lag or retardation was resolved.

Finances and employment, household supplies and food, and family health were addressed up to this point. But there were to be changes in shelter and housing as well. An auxiliary space was made in order for the baby to be closer to the father on *safe days*, when he was using nontoxic materials. Changes and readjustments thus occurred in all of the basic family functions, and the family developmental difficulties of Stage II were thereby resolved.

Family referrals are not common at Stage II. The above case involving a child was seen in a family consultation at a health agency. Stage I referrals are more frequent for marital or couples therapy. In later stages, the initial request may be for couples therapy and children are often not mentioned in the initial referral but appear later if the whole family is considered essential to the evaluation process. When a developmental model of the family life cycle is used to understand families and their treatment, the whole family must be included in the evaluation and treatment process (Zilbach 1989a).

The family life cycle encompasses family development from the beginning of the life of a family unit to its conclusion. The work of the family as a unit is complicated and may seem overwhelmingly complex. However, a developmental model of the family life cycle helps us to understand families and create family therapeutic interventions.

At the turn of the twenty-first century, the family life cycle has maintained its prominent position with all theoreticians in family therapy. It has been expanded to incorporate cultural diversity (Hamilton 1996; Logan 1996; Shapiro 1966) and the impact of multiple clinical disorders (Dwyer 1996; Krauss and Seltzer 1998; Rolland 1994; Veach and Nicholas 1998; Wright 1999). The proposed revisions have been made to enhance the sensitivity of the model to cultural diversity, gender roles, and the impact of clinical conditions.

Chapters on Related Topics

The following chapters describe concepts related to the family life cycle:

- Chapter 4, "Psychodynamic Family Therapy"
- Chapter 17, "Family Therapy With Children and Adolescents: An Overview"

15

Functional and Dysfunctional Families

W. Robert Beavers, M.D.

Introduction

The distinction between functional and dysfunctional families is one that can stir up strong, if not mixed, feelings in many people today. As we enter the new millennium, how do we define *functional*? or *dysfunctional*? or for that matter, *family*?

Any labeling of families can produce mistrust in some group in our culture. Many feminists, for example, believe that functional families are really dysfunctional; that is, they operate on assumptions that are destructive to the dignity and potential of females. And families who have a severely mentally ill member must find it a double blow to first struggle daily to care for that person and then have their family labeled *dysfunctional* according to some definitions of the term.

Even the concept of *family* is controversial. How is *family* defined in the United States today? Certainly many people now believe that yesterday's stereotype of a mother and father living in a neat house with 2.3 children who visit grandma and grandpa on the farm each summer is naïve and unbelievable. Can't a family consist of two same-sex lovers? Does a single parent with five children and a friend who lives with her constitute a family? Is a family dysfunctional when poverty and deprivation force it to use unorthodox efforts to survive? Further, how should mental health professionals approach these issues? Is functioning in families correlated with functioning in individuals? If it is, how is it related?

The subsequent material may not offer a definitive answer to any of these significant questions. But the discussion is forged with an awareness of these ambiguities, changes, and controversies. It is one researcher/clinician's attempt to organize some of what the research group he works with believes. As will be noted later in the description of well-functioning families, an awareness of the incomplete and subjective quality of human truth is necessary for successful negotiation and adaptation. It is certainly necessary for any ongoing productive dialogue.

For many years our research group has defined *family* by asking family members whom they consider family. We base our operating definition on their answers. This allows for flexibility in research and in clinical work.

Functional is defined as that which is *adaptive* for the family's members. This is verified by subjective reports, as well as by evidence of success or failure with goals the family either is expected to have (e.g., protecting and nurturing children) or have stated their wish for (e.g., achieving economic success).

Dysfunctional, as it applies to the family, is related to emotional pain and frustrated goals as well as to the inclusion of a symptomatic member. A systems approach to illness and health requires the awareness that we live on many levels, including the biological, personal, dyadic, family, institutional, and cultural. Each of these levels influences the other. The family that is coping well, even though it has a member with severe schizophrenia, can be as functional as a family with no serious individual problems that demand special adaptation.

A Family Model

In earlier work, Lewis et al. (1976) established that family functioning was indeed correlated with individual functioning. This was determined by studying families with adolescent members whose illnesses had been diagnosed as neurotic or behaviorally disordered. Further, there was a correlation between the performance of small tasks, such as planning a family activity, and the more important performance of the larger task of raising children and providing support and nurture for them as well as other family members.

The following is an overview of the research that co-workers and I have done over a 25-year period on functional and dysfunctional families, along with a description of these family groups and their characteristics. This discussion is concluded with a summary of attitudes and behaviors that distinguish well-functioning from dysfunctional families.

The family field has reached a reasonable consensus on the most important variables necessary for family health. Any one of several models would be sufficient for the general reader to obtain satisfactory, family-systems grounding. I have chosen to provide the reader with results from our own research and the clinical approach to the issue of family functioning, and then generalize beyond these data to include some findings of other experts in the field. The Beavers' systems model is integrative but emphasizes variables that can easily be summarized and evaluated for both research and clinical purposes (Beavers 1988).

Several underlying principles, including the following, contributed to the characteristics of this model:

- Family functioning is best described on a *continuum*, rather than by discrete *types*. Most of the dangers inherent in psychiatric labeling are a result of trying to pigeonhole our varied and complex universe—trying to make it fit our simplistic, if rational, explanations. A concept such as family types, for example, encourages noncontextual, nonsystems thinking. Visualizing qualities, patterns, and functioning abilities as existing on various continuums promotes the conception of health and disease *in relation* to other people and other processes (Beavers 1982).
- The model provides for measurement of competence or functioning ability in whole families engaged in performing current tasks. When family members are asked a question such as "What would you like to see changed in your family," the resulting behavior is valuable in determining the current negotiating capacity of that family.
- The model should be compatible with major clinical concepts of family functioning that have been derived from family therapy. For example, Minuchin's structural concepts (Minuchin 1974a, 1974d) and Bowen's emphasis on differentiation of self (Bowen 1978) fit this model easily. They are consistent with an assessment approach generated out of clinical material and guided by systems concepts.
- Families also have various *styles* of functioning that may be unrelated to adaptation or competence. Useful family models must take these stylistic differences into account (Kelsey-Smith and Beavers 1981).

Competence and style are quite different; capable families vary greatly in their ways of doing things. This variation is, paradoxically, only possible because of a singular similarity in the processes found in these competent or functional families everywhere we look. The central core of functional families is the ability to negotiate differences and resolve conflict between members. Therefore, it is not surprising to learn that the negotiating process between unique and differing people will result in many ways of handling necessary family tasks.

Functioning depends on adaptation throughout the family life cycle. Early in the course of a family, an optimal style is one that my co-workers and I termed *centripetal* (Beavers 1977), following Stierlin's use of this term (Stierlin 1974). Centripetal family members look for satisfaction within the family, seek harmony, and discourage conflict. These behaviors promote nurturing in infants and small children.

Later in the family life cycle, such a style would be maladaptive, leading to difficulties with children leaving home. Helping young people become independent and find satisfaction outside the home is a vital task for family members and the overall family system to accomplish. With a house full of teenagers, the optimal style is more *centrifugal* (Beavers 1982). Centrifugal family members seek satisfaction outside the family unit. Conflicts are more open and acknowledged. Such a style promotes a natural evolution of a family to one in which parents find joy in activities other than parenting. The children can grow up and find satisfaction in others, who eventually become more important to them than their own parents.

One difficulty in pursuing this family life cycle as ideal is seen clinically after a divorce and the remarriage of the male to a somewhat younger female, with whom he begins a new family. When a child from the previous marriage comes to live in the new family, stylistic requirements for the two sets of offspring may conflict. Teenagers benefit by a centrifugal orientation, whereas infants demand a centripetal style. Unless there is recognition of the complexity of needs in these families, where teenagers share parents with infants, adaptation can be thwarted and often a teenager is singled out as *out-of-step* or labeled *bad*.

In addition to such family life cycle demands, there are a variety of social and contextual variables requiring successful family functioning to be associated with negotiated adaptation to these outside circumstances. Capable families, therefore, create whole groups of varied family types to achieve this goal.

In our research, we see many unorthodox but functional family structures. We find functional single-parent families made up of individuals related by love rather than kinship and families comprising multiple generations or missing a generation (e.g., where the grandmother has assumed the role of the mother). These families are more frequent within the context of poverty, joblessness, and severe material and emotional need (Beavers et al. 1986). *Form follows function* in good families as well as in good architecture. Figure 15–1 is presented as an aid to conceptualizing functional and dysfunctional families.

On the horizontal axis are characteristics of family groups functioning from low to high levels; on the vertical axis, the groupings are related to style. The associated individual diagnoses have been supported by data

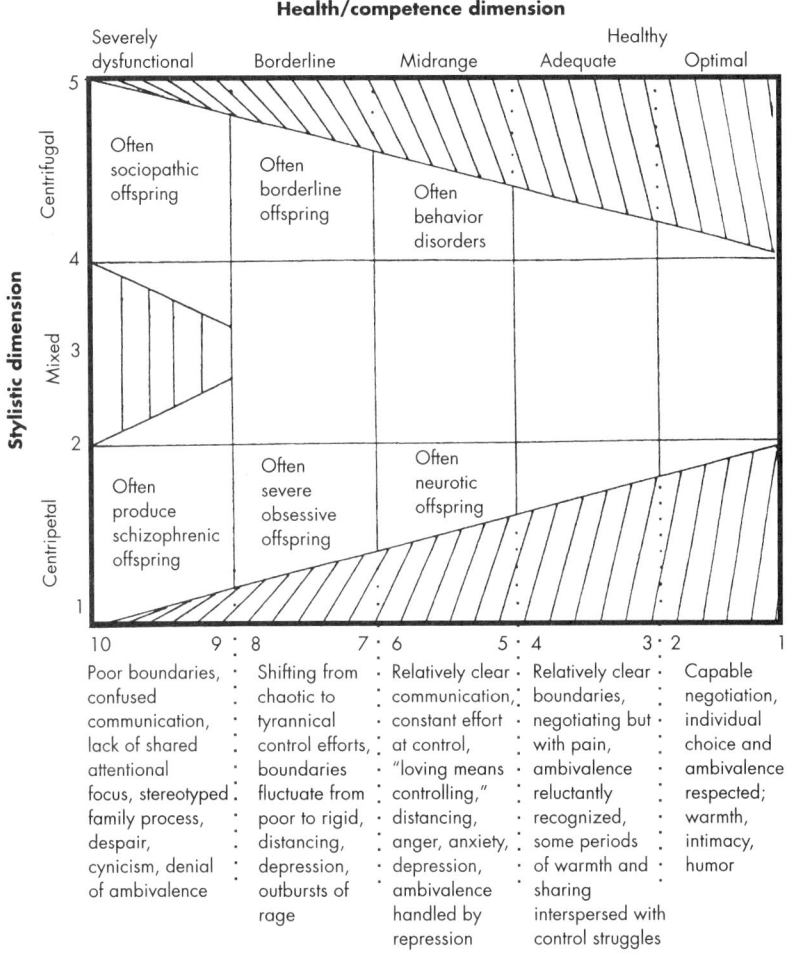

Figure 15–1. Conceptualizing functional and dysfunctional families.

from self-reported family data (Hampson et al. 1989) correlated with psychiatric diagnoses made in a large urban hospital emergency room.

Nine Clinically Useful Groupings of Families

The following are general descriptions of nine family groups assessed by using two sets of reliable interactional scales; one for competence and one for style (Beavers and Hampson 1990). We used 10 minutes of observed interaction after asking the family to "discuss among yourselves what you would like to see changed in your family." We also developed the self-report family inventory for individuals to use in describing their family (Hampson and Beavers 1988). This *inside* approach can also be scored to place the family on the diagram.

Group 1: Optimal Families

Optimal families are well-functioning families that are seldom seen by clinicians, yet serve as our model for effective and adaptive functioning. In these families, as described earlier, intimacy is sought and usually found, a high level of respect for individuality and the individual perspective is the norm, and capable negotiation and clear communication are the results. There is a strong sense of individuation with clear boundaries; hence, conflict and ambivalence (at the individual level) are handled directly and overtly and (usually) are negotiated efficiently. The hierarchical structure of the family is well defined and acknowledged by family members. Yet flexibility and a high level of adaptation to individual development and external stresses are also evident.

Group 2: Adequate Families

Adequate families show some characteristics of the optimal families in terms of the importance of family life, caring for members, and relatively low incidence of individuals' psychiatric disturbance. However, they show diminished negotiation skills, they are more control oriented, and parents often resolve conflict by intimidation or direct force. The parental coalition is usually effective, though less emotionally rewarding. Sex-role stereotyping and some dominance patterns are more characteristic throughout the family (including the marital couple itself). Males are typically prescribed to be powerful, unemotive, and conventional, while females are relatively less powerful, highly emotive (sometimes depressed), and more traditional in providing or seeking nurturance. Hence, compared with those in optimal families, interactions produce less intimacy and trust, less respect for personal individuality, and less spontaneity in minute-to-minute exchanges. While there is some pain, some loneliness, and some feeling of being misunderstood, these families can function quite well, although with less flexibility and adaptation than in optimal families. Previous studies showed these families able to produce children with competence equal to that of optimal families. These parents care about parenting, and work hard at it.

Groups 3, 4, and 5: Midrange Families

While optimal and adequate families are rarely seen in clinical practice, midrange families usually rear sane but limited offspring. Both parents and children are susceptible to emotional or behavioral disorders. These control-oriented and rigid systems revolve around power, status, and the belief that people are basically evil and untrustworthy and need to be controlled. Although there are few flagrant boundary violations or invasions, there are frequent projections. Ambivalence is frequently handled by denying one strong emotion and using repression or projection for the other, as in statements such as "You never have a good time when we go out, but I always do." There is room in these families for some rebuttal and clarification. The parental relationship is generally conflicted and not supportive. It is not uncommon for each parent to have a *favorite* child, often following Oedipal (father-daughter, mother-son) patterns (Beavers 1977).

Group 3: midrange centripetal families. Midrange centripetal families manifest great concern for rules and authority. They expect overt, authoritarian control to be successful in restraining the base impulses of family members. Since the expressions of hostility and overt anger are disapproved of and expressions of love and caring are approved of, intense and clear expression of frustration and anger are infrequent. Therefore, conflict resolution, clarity of expression, and competent negotiations are compromised. One sees only modest spontaneity shining through the web of concern for rules, order, and authority. Sex stereotyping is very strong in these families: dependent, emotional women and "strong," silent, authoritarian men are predominant. Hence, the marital relationship takes on the appearance of a male-led unit, with mildly depressed females carrying out most household and child-rearing duties.

These families promote internalizing and repression as means of dealing with distress and upset. Anxiety, depression, and somatizing disorders are usually seen. The patients' concern for propriety and authority make them *good* psychiatric patients who pay their bills, work hard, and keep their problems well-hidden until next week's session.

Group 4: midrange centrifugal families. Like midrange centripetal families, midrange centrifugal families attempt to control by authority and intimidation; however, the parents are much less successful in controlling themselves or their children. Family members deal with this lack of control through frontal assaults and blame—pervasive in the family from time to time—and manipulation. Anger and derogatory blame are more frequent than professions of warmth and tenderness. The parental dyad is openly conflictual. The parents spend little time in the home; the coalition is tenuous; and unresolved power and control struggles are commonplace. Children learn to survive through maneuvering and blaming others. They move out of the family earlier than the norm and have difficulty with authority figures. Typically, emotional problems are made manifest through *acting-out* behavior disorders, such as sexual precocity, moderate substance abuse, and vandalism.

Group 5: midrange mixed families. Midrange mixed families have a mixture of centripetal and centrifugal behavior. The attempts at control are consistent, but the effects vary at different times or with different children. Couples in this group experience role tension and struggles; they can present well socially but they frequently blame and attack each other. Often one child will manifest internalizing symptoms, while another may be openly defiant and hostile.

Groups 6 and 7: Borderline Families

Borderline families are characterized by chaotic power struggles, with persistent (though ineffective) efforts to build and maintain stable patterns of dominance and submission. It appears to outside observers that the members have lost sight of any satisfaction to be had in family life, and search instead for control. Family members have little ability to attend to and accept emotional needs in themselves or others. There is little spontaneity or warmth catalyzing these families' interactions. Pain, amorphous personal boundaries, and futile attempts to establish rigid control are more characteristic of these groups.

Group 6: borderline centripetal families. In borderline centripetal families, the chaos and discomfort are more verbal than behavioral, and control battles are usually covert, internalized, or somatized by members. The parental coalition is dramatically skewed, often with one parent verbally controlling and the other passive. Generational boundaries become diffuse, with increasing tendency for covert parent-child coalitions or triangular patterns of dominance with one (scapegoat) child. Open rebellion and overt rage are discouraged, so family members must retreat and protect themselves through patterned rituals or attention seeking. Severely obsessional and anorectic individuals are frequently found in these families.

Group 7: borderline centrifugal families. Borderline centrifugal families are much more open than borderline centripetal families in the expression of anger, with direct assaults and frequent leave-taking. The parental coalition is loosely connected, and stormy battles occur with high regularity. There is a sense of *no-man's land* in this group. Children are left with little or no nurturance or support. Each individual is on his or her own to try to derive whatever advantages can be gained by manipulation or reckless attention seeking. Unresolved ambivalence is quite evident and usually expressed behaviorally. Assault and defiance mask depression and despair. Children learn to manipulate within the unstable but oscillating system;

many receive a psychiatric label of *borderline personality disorder* as they carry these tendencies into the outside world.

Groups 8 and 9: Severely Dysfunctional Families

Severely dysfunctional families are the most limited in negotiating conflicts, adapting to developmental and current crises, resolving ambivalence, and choosing goals. The greatest need is for communicational coherence. There is a lack of shared focus of attention and contribution to discussion, accompanied by a peculiar distancing that prevents satisfying or clarifying encounters. Hence, boundaries are diffuse and relational clarity is minimal. There is also no clear leadership, so family functioning appears chaotic, disjointed, and even random. However, since control is attempted through a variety of covert and indirect methods, there are drearily repetitive themes in these families. What appears chaotic to the outsider may be *more of the same* attempts at maintaining rigid balance, as viewed by insiders. There is virtually no spontaneity or satisfying personal exchange.

Group 8: severely dysfunctional centripetal families. Severely dysfunctional centripetal families have a tough, nearly impermeable outer boundary, allowing little independent or autonomous growth; time is an unwanted stranger. Hence, children are handicapped in their progression through normal sequences of emotional and personal development. The parental coalition as a functional unit is nonexistent; its appearance is maintained awkwardly through polite role-playing, although the spouses' inability to support each other is obvious. The parental coalition is often supplanted by a significant parent-child coalition, a mother-son or father-daughter pair. This family group is often associated with a history of many losses poorly mourned, occasional dramatic rule-breaking during an outburst of rage on the part of one member, dissociation, emotional blunting, and alcoholism. If a member has a psychiatric diagnosis, it is probably a psychosis.

Group 9: severely dysfunctional centrifugal families. Severely dysfunctional centrifugal families, as locked into their stylistic pattern as the centripetal families are, show a loose and tenuous outer boundary. There is frequent absence, desertion, or running away, and even a lack of clarity about who the family is. Members express hostility and deride each other for their faults: since the principal medium of exchange is action rather than words, there is frequent abuse, neglect, and assault. Like the centripetal family, however, relational and communicational clarity is never achieved. Since expressions of tenderness, vulnerability, and dependency are met with contempt and derision, no one addresses these needs or has them satisfied. People frequently hurt each other (emotionally, sometimes physically) and are usually insensitive to others' pain. Since the necessary nurturing provisions are minimal in these families, character development is severely limited and is often antisocial in nature. Guilt is pervasive but has no effectiveness in regulating behavior. Members feel bad but do not know how to behave in order to feel good.

Qualities That Identify Functional and Dysfunctional Families

This section of the chapter presents summaries of qualities that distinguish functional from dysfunctional families. The information is derived from many studies of nonlabeled, healthy, "normal," or functional families (Beavers and Voeller 1983; Beavers et al. 1986; Hampson et al. 1990; Lewis et al. 1976) and clinically referred families (Hampson et al. 1989; Mishler and Waxler 1968). The families represent a variety of ethnic and socioeconomic circumstances. The characteristics of functional families can be separated into 1) expressed or implied beliefs and 2) observable patterns.

Expressed or Implied Beliefs

Relative—Not Absolute—Truth and Subjective Reality

One of the most helpful beliefs of well-functioning family members is that people's minds are limited and finite. For this reason, human beings never possess the absolute truth. All human mental apparatus, though marvelous, is subject to error. Our perceptions, memories, deductions, and conclusions are fallible; therefore, honest differences usually are an opportunity for synthesis, rather than necessary indications of struggle (see Beavers 1985).

In contrast, many dysfunctional family members seem to believe that their opinions or beliefs are omnipotent ("my eye is God's eye"). People who have this point of view seem to believe that if their perceptions, memory, or conclusions are challenged, then their very being is challenged, and they must conquer or be vanquished. This most unfortunate belief leads to the fear of encounter and, hence, to avoidance of conflict or, alternatively, to the continuance of frustrating battles. Usually, these certainties are derived from one's family of origin. Either a revered or a despised parent can be the source of absolute truth. The revered parent passes it on directly; the despised parent offers such a negative absolute that a child believes anything to the contrary. In many areas—for example, politics, religion, child rearing, or family governance—families can pass on opinions that deny uncertainty and human limitation.

Well-functioning families, however, recognize that everything in life is uncertain. They seldom get into the dreary habit of directly contradicting others, struggles that punctuate dysfunctional family interaction.

This valuable belief in the uncertainty existing in the human enterprise can be learned. Central to such learning is an environment that is relatively nonthreatening. The therapist must model this awareness of human uncertainty. Direct challenges aimed at fervently held viewpoints are not necessary and are usually counterproductive. One possibility is to say something like the following: "You know, it's a wonder anybody can keep a family going these days. There are so many challenges to being a spouse, a parent, or even a kid. I have come to believe that nobody knows how to be a spouse, just as much as nobody knows how to raise kids." Subsequent discussion helps family members learn from each other and begin a more adaptive negotiating process.

Uncertainty about what one knows and appreciation for the useful subjective quality of people's perceptions go hand in hand. Sometimes I tell the tale of the 8-year-old boy who came running into the house shouting, "I just saw a fierce dog that was as big as a house." His father took his belt off and beat the boy, saying, "I won't have any lying in my house." As I ask family members their opinion of the father's actions, they come to see that his literal approach misses the opportunity to understand the reality of the boy's fear and to consider that he is expressing a deeper truth (Beavers 1985).

Decency of Most People

There is a close relationship between good family functioning and the shared belief that people close to you have decent motives, that their intentions are basically neutral or benign. Individuals need not hold a global, philosophical belief in the goodness of man; in fact, family members may believe that large portions of the world's population intend evil. They do need to believe, however, in the potential trustworthiness of their own spouse, parents, and children (W.R. Beavers 1977). This belief allows people to err and disagree without the threat of abandonment or harm. Human frailty is not translated into evil. When husbands forget birthdays or when wives want to work (or husbands want them to work), imperfections or differences can be perceived as easily as human perversity. When children set fires, utter obscenities, destroy a plant, or torment a pet, it is easy to explain these aberrations by a belief in the basic badness of people. Though this can make for a satisfyingly simple certainty, it also dooms efforts at problem solving.

Several satellite beliefs are necessary to support the concept of people's basic decency. One must assume that sexuality, anger, vindictiveness, willfulness, and deep ambivalence are a part of the human condition—not good sometimes, but hardly evidence of intrinsic malevolence.

Ambivalence is worthy of special mention here, because I have never seen a respect for ambivalence in dysfunctional family members! "You don't love me" is a frequent response to pain produced by a spouse. It is important to know that people are, indeed, ambivalent about anything that is finite and yet needed—such as loved ones, jobs, and friends. Ambivalence can be resolved, but it can never be eliminated. Healthy, functional family members know this and tolerate outbursts of bad feelings from a spouse and children without using such negative experiences to *prove* evil intent.

The opposite belief, that of people's basic malevolence, produces distancing and causes what I have termed the *war in the nursery*, with parents defining their love by how much they control and discipline. Parents who believe their job is to beat basic badness out of a child can engage in flagrant child abuse, justified as being a responsible parent.

Human Encounters Rewarding

Discovering that human encounters are rewarding means combining a healthy respect for uncertainty with the belief that family members are not malevolent, which leads to the development of a climate of trust and cooperation in families. If people can trust each other and cooperate reasonably well, their experiences may lead them to believe that human encounters are usually rewarding. In other words, people will become optimistic. This is a mindset that supports the idea that hard work can be effective and that there is reason to hope even when situations are bad, such as those times when a spouse errs or a child is alienated and hostile. Hope is essential to any successful endeavor, and functional family members have it (Beavers and Kaslow 1981).

A Systems Point of View

Well-functioning family members intuitively recognize and operate from what can be called a systems point of view. This view includes at least three basic assumptions: 1) any individual needs a group—a human system for individual definition, coherence, and satisfaction; 2) causes and effects are interchangeable; and 3) any human behavior is a result of many variables, rather than one single cause (Beavers 1977).

Healthy family members know that people do not prosper in a vacuum; human needs are satisfied in an interpersonal matrix. As children develop and mature, they leave their families, not for isolated independence but for other human systems. Whether they enter college or the military or marriage, or become "swinging singles," these people will continue to need community. For this reason, they must develop interpersonal skills to adapt to the next system. Some theoretical concepts found in mental health literature (Beattie 1987) give short shrift to this reality (just as disturbed families do) by defining maturity as a hypothetical independence that is close to being alone. Well-functioning families do not make this error; they define maturity as the evolution of new relationships that provide reciprocal, satisfying intimacy. Adults develop skills in meeting the needs of others as well as their own. Humans are accepted as social animals that grow up, leave home, and necessarily establish new close relationships.

This awareness promotes an open system, one with rules compatible with (though not necessarily the same as) those found in the larger society. People in dysfunctional families, with peculiar rules obtained from their family of origin, find it hard to leave home and establish a new family.

The second quality of a systems view of the world recognizes that causes and effects are interchangeable and are equally significant. Dysfunctional family members are awash in confusion, looking vainly for clear, identifiable causes for their frustration and pain. As a result, they often retreat to vague or mystical answers, hinging on fate or destiny, to explain personal and family problems. Other dysfunctional families seek oversimplified causes for human problems. For example, they may decide someone within the household is a bad seed (scapegoating) or born evil. Evidence of human perversity drives people to flounder forever in their efforts to control whatever evils they believe exist.

Well-functioning family members know, for example, that hostility in one person promotes deception in the other, just as deception, in turn, is bound to promote hostility. Efforts at tyrannical control increase the possibility of angry defiance, as much as uncooperative defiance invites tyrannical control. Stimuli are responses, and responses are stimuli. This is a process with shape and form but with no clearly defined individual villains or victims.

The third assumption—that human behavior results from many variables—is clear to healthy family members. Dysfunctional families usually consider only one explanation of a human problem. A child of 3, for example, spills milk at the table. There are a number of possible explanations. Perhaps the event was accidental—then no motive should be attached to the behavior. Perhaps it has interpersonal meaning—the child had a personal score to settle with a parent. Maybe the child's anger is unrelated to parents. Or a tired or anxious child just made a mistake. Or the problem could be a mechanical one: the glass is too large, and little hands are unable to hold it. Each of these approaches is used almost exclusively by one or another type of dysfunctional family. Well-functioning families, in contrast, use all of these notions and more. They are not locked into stereotyped responses from theories of simple causation. Their responses to an event vary with the context in a highly pragmatic fashion. Functioning families have problems galore; they also have tools to deal with the problems.

Meaning to the Human Enterprise

A great deal of energy and sense of purpose is tied up in neurotic interaction. Freud once remarked that neurosis was a *private religion*; Berne (1964), who simplified psychoanalysis to excessive proportions, spoke of the *games people play* with the same implications. Fighting back because of the insult of the night before can be a reason for getting up in the morning. Taking care of a depressed spouse can provide some meaning to existence.

But what do well-functioning family members do to provide a reason for working, for making and keeping commitments, for continuing the various processes of being a successful human with a social network? One usual answer if singularly emphasized—caring about loved ones and supporting their needs—generally leads to dysfunctional family interaction rather than to health. Parents are threatened by children's growth and development, and children fear leaving home because their meaning and purpose are intertwined with that of other family members. Even the mutual support that healthy couples provide one another is not enough to sustain purpose.

Individuals in optimally functioning families have meaning that transcends their own skin and the boundaries of their family members. It may be provided by conventional religion or by a passionate cause, such as protecting the environment, preserving capitalism and the American way of life, or fighting nuclear proliferation. The content of the belief can vary tremendously, but it is the belief that provides and directs energy; it also enhances a sense of community with others outside the family. The absence of such a belief system supported by some significant segment of the larger community leads to anomie (Beavers 1977).

It has been my happy experience to work with many families and couples and to observe, as many of the old neurotic struggles and games are seen through and put aside, a new energy and power emerging that requires direction. When this happens, an interest in a once significant religious structure is rekindled, or a cause that has been given lip service is now supported by action, or entirely new sources of transcendent meaning are found and acted on. Often several family members are active. Sometimes one is more active, and the others operate as supportive stabilizers.

Observable Patterns of Behavior

Observable behavior patterns are, of course, related to shared attitudes. Attitudes are internal representatives of interpersonal patterns—usually from the family of origin—and function to develop interpersonal behavior. Conversely, one can often deduce attitudes from observing behavior. However, observation is more trustworthy than reports of beliefs, and the congruence between the two is most important in determining family competence. The behavior patterns to be described include those that 1) reflect a modest, overt, power difference, 2) illustrate the capacity for clear boundaries, 3) operate mainly in the present, 4) respect individual choice, 5) share positive feelings, and 6) negotiate skillfully.

Reflecting Modest Overt Power Differences

Including the word *overt* in labeling power differences has developed from our observations of couples and families, both healthy and dysfunctional, over many years (Beavers 1988). Indeed, one can argue that any family member has as much power as another, since helplessness, passivity, and dependency are all powerful in their own way. Raters of families, when forced to decide which members of a family are more powerful or more in control, often do not agree, but they *can* agree on the degree of overt power difference. These differences are observable.

It is worth noting that the more prevalent an overt power difference, the more effective are covert methods of control through weakness, irresponsibility, or dysfunction in individuals. Demanding control over another leads to being controlled if the other reciprocates with helplessness.

Ideally, two people who choose to live together as partners could have precisely equal covert power. That is, neither would use power maneuvers, such as giving imperious hand signals, drowning out the other's voice, or making the other feel guilty as a means of controlling him or her. In real life, perfect partnerships seldom, if ever, happen, but healthy couples are on the low end of a scale of overt power differences. Most of the time these partners respect each other's perceptions and negotiate their problems, and if they seriously disagree with each other, they do so without practicing one-upmanship.

Only in situations of equal overt power can there be *intimacy*—the experiences of being open or vulnerable and of being able to share one's innermost feelings and thoughts. At any age, with anyone, overt power and intimacy are highly correlated. Parents know this intuitively, and when they wish to share a close moment with a 5-year-old, they will move to eye level with the child.

In relationships of unequal overt power, the dominant individual ("top dog") is fearful of exposing weakness. Conversely, the subordinate individual ("bottom dog") is fearful that anger, assertiveness, or wishes for equality or domination will surface. Therefore, each person is necessarily isolated to a significant degree.

The sexual encounter is probably the best and most dramatic example of the relationship between power and intimacy. With equality, risk taking and dialogue are possible. The twin threats to sexual satisfaction—*spectatoring* and *performance anxiety* (Kaplan 1974)—are minimized. The embrace, to be healing, must include equality between the partners; otherwise, there is inevitably a loss of dignity and some reduction of humanity in the sexual act itself.

The sexual encounter also gives us a valuable example of how equal overt power can be developed and maintained through *complementarity*, which can offer cooperation, joy, and effectiveness without subjugation or an overt power difference.

Such a finding is relevant to the broader social issues concerning the rights of women and the possible threats to men as women have attempted to become more powerful. Equal covert social power is beneficial, not damaging, if there are complementary rather than symmetrical role relationships. In both long and short time frames (months and years as well as minutes and hours), optimal couples demonstrate complementary roles—such as teacher and taught, speaker and listener, aggressive role definer and supportive partner, breadwinner and homemaker, volatile reactor and one who "cools" down the conflict rather than adding to the fire. This complementarity allows for equality without hostile competition or rivalry. Complementary roles need not be stereotyped; they need not slavishly follow cultural expectations. But they must exist whenever overt power is equal, so that relating can be shared enjoyment rather than a struggle.

Some current cultural definitions of equality insist on a symmetrical role. For example, working partners should share housework and house care equally. Couples in optimally functioning families do not have such symmetry, but symmetrical relationships of this sort are found regularly in dysfunctional families, along with continued unresolved conflict. Complementarity and role differentiation appear necessary to allow pleasant interaction with shared dignity. A metaphor for this situation is a sport such as basketball. On unskilled teams, everybody tries to get the ball and shoot baskets; on skilled teams, players cooperate—playing complementary roles—and morale improves as the team becomes a winner.

It is through a variety of complementary roles that well-functioning family members evolve relationships with equal dignity, respect, and, on balance, equal overt power. This was one of the strengths of the *traditional* family—role definitions assigned a variety of family responsibilities to male and female parents and children.

At the present time, well-functioning families have few guidelines that define *power* areas of responsibility. (Few, in my experience, wish to have the same kind of family as they did growing up!) Therefore, it is necessary to demonstrate much greater negotiating skills than those that were required in previous generations of well-functioning families. Equally powered, symmetrical relationships lead to unresolvable conflict and severe emotional pain. This was demonstrated in our studies of both heterosexual and homosexual couples. The most functional couples have negotiated areas of primary competence and subsequent responsibility, with each partner being the leader in some, the helper in others.

Setting Clear Boundaries

Well-functioning family members are capable of telling the difference between one person's feelings and wishes, and the other's. This ability is extremely important in working together, in making decisions that are supported by both, and in being with the other and feeling good. The living cell is a fine metaphor for family functioning. The cell boundary has integrity, yet it is most permeable to the outside world, allowing effective interchange.

It is important to note that the discarding of acknowledged boundaries is not what defines family pathology, nor is the stubborn insistence on maintaining boundaries any paragon of health. In the midst of passion, whether sexual or angry or ecstatic, boundaries are lost. Sometimes it is delightful, sometimes it is horrendous. Functional family members experience this just as dysfunctional ones do, but the fortunate and effective can regroup, clear up the boundaries, and have effective dialogue with shared dignity and autonomy.

Family members quarrel. Some do it openly. Some do it covertly. Some are loud. Some are quiet. But none quarrel and maintain clear boundaries! When feelings ride high, there is a juicy jumble of claimed and projected present and past, childhood memories and old hurts, frustrated wishes and dreams. During these times, one must not expect a great deal of *sense* through reasonable dialogue and clear boundaries. When the passion has cooled, however, well-functioning family members can redefine where each ends and the other begins, and a productive resolution is possible. In dysfunctional families there is an ongoing inability to develop or maintain clear boundaries.

A drearily frequent maneuver of the dysfunctional family is to make what I termed *the unholy bargain*, which consists of the following: "I have strong mixed feelings, like all people. You have strong mixed feelings, too. It is very painful and requires lots of growing up to acknowledge these feelings and resolve them. Why don't we make an unholy bargain? You give me half of your mixed feelings, and I'll give you the other half of mine. That way, neither of us has to grow up. We can blame each other rather than ourselves for any difficulties. Of course, the only problem is that for the next 40 years we will fight like hell." Examples abound: "I like to go out; you like to stay home." "I like people; you withdraw." "I like sex; you never want it." In such a fashion, couples can live together for years, have sex, have children, have tragedies and triumphs, and never have the experience of feeling adult, responsible, and free (Beavers 1985).

Operating in the Present

Most of the problems that plague members of dysfunctional families can be traced to experiencing the world as it was in childhood and assuming that the world's rules and people are clones of that particular childhood. This thought process forces people to interpret the present situation as repetitions of the past, rather than *in the light of* the past.

The parents in families have families, and these families made a powerful impact. They are responsible for creating specific attitudes, expectations, and ways of operating that make up individual personality.

Much family humor consists of some awareness of this history. Sometimes with delight, sometimes wryly, we see ourselves, our spouses, and our children repeating patterns we knew as youngsters. We can track threads of behavior for three, four, even five generations, and wonder at the continuing mysteries of how nature and nurture come together.

The trick in dealing well with present life situations is to know as much about the past as one can, remember it as well as one can, and use it as a guide, not a directive. Well-functioning family members can usually do this because they possess the ability to watch themselves interact, to critique, and to experiment with new ways of achieving goals. Using the past as a guide, rather than as a prophecy, goes hand in hand with adaptation.

Spouses in dysfunctional families are also influenced by their families of origin, of course. They often have unhappy memories of growing up. They are much more apt to continue relating to their own parents as a child is, or they will make a radical, self-conscious break with their parents. Either position makes it much more difficult to work through early relationships and clearly see them as different and separate from the relationship one has with a spouse.

The parents of well-functioning families relate to their own parents with comparative ease, incorporating them in some fashion into their present lives, and deriving satisfaction from their parents in a way that seems to add to, rather than diminish, the pleasure in the spouse's company. A similar happy experience can be observed with most couples in the latter phases of treatment. Usually, as treatment progresses, these spouses reach out to their own parents, if they are alive, to establish something solid and understandable. If a parent is dead, there will be a hunger to talk, with a spouse and therapist, of that parent and to resolve some painful mixed feelings.

An acceptance of continuity from generation to generation seems to be an intrinsic part of well-functioning families. Some family things do not change through time, and some things need to be changed. A present marriage can be better than the one that preceded it. Hope for making a better now is based both on memories of the past and on current experiences.

The greatest threat to operating mainly in the present is the presence of unmourned grief in family members. Well-functioning families are more apt to talk of grief and lost family members when presented with a stimulus that suggests the possibility of death (Lewis et al. 1976). Here is a clear-cut circularity—if families function well, they are apt to mourn well and go forward. If a family is caught up in unmourned loss, relationships suffer, living in the present may be impossible, and mourning is difficult (Paul and Paul 1968).

It is a most important aspect of family work to determine whether addressing an unmourned loss will release the previously unavailable competence of family members and make a significant difference in adaptive negotiating abilities. This seems to be especially true in families with substance-abusing members (M.D. Stanton 1977).

Respecting Individual Choice—Autonomy

Our society places a premium on behavioral manifestations of a personal sense of autonomy. The autonomous person knows what he or she feels and thinks, takes responsibility for personal behavior, and interacts with others with a reasonably clear notion of choices.

From a developmental standpoint, the well-functioning family is involved in a continuing effort to assist children in developing a sense of separateness and autonomy, while assisting adults in maintaining such separateness at the same time.

An effective way to observe the degree of autonomy present in a family is to see how much respect there is for individual opinions and choices. Fortunate families have evolved a system with rules that allow and even encourage the identification and expression of personal perceptions and wishes. This is, of course, a necessary ingredient in successful negotiating.

The qualities mentioned thus far are most important in encouraging choice. If an effective human system requires the least possible overt power difference, the capacity for clear boundaries and belief in the basic decency of the self and partner and in the inevitable subjectivity of any human truth, people will make decisions more easily, resolving ambivalence rather than dithering or projecting. It is, of course, necessary for individuals to resolve ambivalence in order to have autonomy.

Dysfunctional family members often attack personal choice as willful, selfish, and wrong. Many strive to work on their marriage by attempting to be more selfless. It is possible to help these poor souls function more capably by defining human warmth as "human need, honestly expressed, with the recognition of the other's limits" (Beavers 1977). When warmth is described in this fashion, it places responsibility where it belongs. To enjoy an enterprise, one must derive benefit and pleasure from it. Conversely, when a person is experienced as enjoyable, and is given evidence of this, satisfaction is given and received.

Put another way, resolving one's mixed feelings and making choices is a necessary contribution to a loving relationship. Well-functioning family members know this and generally operate this way. They usually state to each other their significant personal desires while remaining aware of the limits of the situation and the people involved.

One well-functioning family, for example, was in transition from the conventional father-breadwinner, mother-homemaker system to a system in which both adults were working, and the children grown. The wife had been content with the family-earning capacity, tailoring her wishes to the husband's income. As her work level decreased in the home, however, she became aware of a greater desire to work outside for more money and for other benefits it could bring. The husband was able to take this transition in stride by defining what was most important to him; namely, the emotional support he got from his wife. Their negotiations made it possible to keep what was most important to each of them.

These transitions often flounder, because people have difficulty in resolving their own mixed feelings, and fall back on intimidation. In a similar situation, spouses in dysfunctional families rarely define wishes and needs clearly. They often try to fit themselves and their spouses into some kind of stereotype, such as the long-suffering or outraged husband or the liberated or subservient wife. They both wind up feeling cheated, regardless of the role they feel pressured to occupy. Such *cartooning*, or becoming a caricature of the real, complex human reality, is an intrinsic part of dysfunctional families.

Sharing Positive Feelings

A striking, observable quality of well-functioning families is the shared fun, the enjoyment of day-to-day encounters and projects. When the business of living is kept current, with little in the way of unresolved conflict, encounters are effective, optimistic, and fun. Most people enjoy what they do well, and relating to family members is no exception. The mixture of personal skills and good humor while dealing with the serious challenges of a family's life cycle is most impressive in well-functioning families.

Negotiating Skillfully

All of the attributes of well-functioning families are brought to bear on the continuing process of negotiating conflicts and differences. In this way, families develop creative and viable solutions to problems and opportunities.

Families have conflicts. Individuals have ambivalence. Both are ubiquitous and not related to illness or health or to functioning or not functioning.

It is the ability to resolve conflict and move toward agreed-on goals that makes families functional—just as it is the ability of an individual to resolve ambivalence and become effective in attaining chosen goals that makes that person functional.

These qualities of family and persons are related. All of us have psyches that are developed by the family system we came from. Our abilities to resolve personal conflict, as well as interpersonal conflict, are powerfully influenced by the negotiating abilities of our family of origin.

Conversely, the ability of one family member to resolve personal ambivalence and become effectively goal directed is a powerful influence on increasing his or her present family functioning abilities. We live on many levels, and each level influences the other.

Future Directions for Study in Family Competence

Many of the basic patterns of adaptive behavior for families have been confirmed and reconfirmed by research and clinical experience. The current dissent and controversies about family health issues center on challenges to conventional concepts regarding *roles* of men, women, and even children in optimal or desirable families.

It is this author's view that many of these controversies represent presystemic thinking, with an attendant disregard for the discoveries of the past 25 years regarding overt power differences, intimacy, and negotiation.

They are, therefore, supported with more polemics and political firepower than with research and the clinical data.

Yet, we are all products of our culture and inevitably share some of the shortsightedness and blind spots present in any culture. We have seen more studies of family health in economically blessed and socially secure families than in inner-city and minority families.

We continue to see strong reactions to those who challenge the idea that the *status quo* (whatever is) is by definition *normal*. An example of this is the furor over Hillary Clinton, the wife of our 42nd president (and currently a U.S. senator). She is an accomplished attorney, an effective and knowledgeable political observer, and a fervent advocate for children. She has been described as everything from an example of lost family values to a vivid example of the new woman. There seems little doubt that Ms. Clinton is an embodiment of a changing view of women and of women's role in family and society. This changing view is seen across economic classes, across racial and ethnic differences, and across the world. When leading a group of family therapists into China in 1988, the author found the same yearnings in women and an uneasiness in men similar to that which we see in our country.

Future research in family competence will focus on these changing definitions of male and female roles, letting successful families teach clinicians and researchers how adaptation takes place in the year 2000 and beyond.

Child nurturance and guidance are constant needs, as are the needs for emotional support and intimacy for adults. The competent family's structure and appearance will change with cultural changes. Good research is humble, eager to learn from that which is studied. No one knows how to be an optimal parent or how to be an optimal spouse. We have millions of people doing their best to find out in an atmosphere of ever-increasing social change.

Chapters on Related Topics

The following chapters describe concepts related to functional and dysfunctional families:

- Chapter 10, "Gender-Sensitive Family Therapy"
- Chapter 13, "Family Assessment"
- Chapter 14, "The Family Life Cycle: A Framework for Understanding Family Development"
- Chapter 16, "Diagnosis of Family Relational Disorders"
- Chapter 23, "The Divorcing Family: Characteristics and Interventions"

Functional and Dysfunctional Families

- Chapter 24, "The Remarried Family: Characteristics and Interventions"
- Chapter 25, "Marital Enrichment in Clinical Practice"
- Chapter 26, "Sex Therapy at the Turn of the Century: New Awareness and Response"
- Chapter 27, "Family Variables and Interventions in Schizophrenia"
- Chapter 28, "Depression and the Family: Interpersonal Context and Family Functioning"
- Chapter 33, "Family Therapy With Personality Disorders"

16

Diagnosis of Family Relational Disorders

David J. Miklowitz, Ph.D.
John F. Clarkin, Ph.D.

Introduction

Do families have relational "disorders" or "diseases" that can be identified and reliably classified, or do mental disorders reside only in a single individual? Can clinicians identify familywide relational dysfunctions from signs and symptoms typically presented in a family evaluation and apply a diagnostic label that captures these disturbances, in the same way that we might for an individual? Why would we want to make these familywide diagnoses?

We review in this chapter historical attempts to classify family or marital relational disorders in existing psychiatric classification systems, such as the *Diagnostic and Statistical Manual of Mental Disorders*, 4th Edition (American Psychiatric Association 1994), and its text revision (DSM-IV-TR; American Psychiatric Association 2000a). We conclude that the systems of diagnostic classification used in the field, rather than relying exclusively on the diagnosis of single individuals, would be enhanced by the development of criteria for classifying family "relational disorders" that capture the dysfunctions present in two or more individuals.

We also discuss two relatively modern relational diagnostic systems, one developed by the authors of this chapter in the context of a DSM-IV literature review (Clarkin and Miklowitz 1997) and the other by the Group for the Advancement of Psychiatry (GAP; 1991, 1995) Committee on the Family. Finally, we recommend 1) conducting empirical field trials of the reliability and validity of these systems, 2) linking family-based diagnoses to individual diagnoses wherever possible, and 3) using family diagnoses as sources of information for treatment planning.

What Is a Mental Disorder?

What is a mental disorder? There has been and remains confusion and controversy over the definitions of "mental diseases" (a frankly medical-model term) and "disorders" (the term used in DSM-IV-TR; see also Blashfield 1984). The introduction to DSM-IV-TR includes the following definition of mental disorder:

> In DSM-IV, each of the mental disorders is conceptualized as a clinically significant behavioral or psychological syndrome or pattern that occurs in an individual and that is associated with present distress (e.g., a painful symptom) or disability (i.e., impairment in one or more important areas of functioning) or with a significantly increased risk of suffering death, pain, disability, or an important loss of freedom....Whatever its original cause, it must currently be considered a manifestation of a behavioral, psychological, or biological dysfunction in the individual. Neither deviant behavior (e.g., political, religious, or sexual) nor conflicts that are primarily between the individual and society are mental disorders unless the deviance or conflict is a symptom of dysfunction in the individual. (American Psychiatric Association 2000a, p. xxxi)

This definition of mental disorder was influential in guiding the definition and inclusion of syndromes in DSM-III-R (American Psychiatric Association 1987; Williams 1988), and later in DSM-IV, and thus is most relevant in considering the status of family relational disorders and their inclusion in the DSM system. Note that in this definition, a mental disorder always resides in a single individual. However, one could also conceive of a *family mental disorder* characterized by group dysfunction of clinical significance. This disorder could be related to underlying behavioral, psychological, or biological dysfunction. Such a disorder would reside not in the individual but in the family as a unit, even if it reflected in part the collective influences of dysfunction in one or more members of this unit.

Why Diagnose Families?

Why should modern classification systems move from individually based diagnoses to diagnoses based on *groups* of people? Before addressing this question, we must first ask an even broader question: Why diagnose at all?

Classification Versus Diagnosis

The terms *classification* and *diagnosis* have both specific uses and a hierarchical relationship. *Classification* is the arrangement of organisms, objects, or ideas into relatively homogenous groupings. Classification is at the heart of any scientific enterprise and provides 1) a nomenclature for communication among those in the field, 2) a basis for information retrieval, 3) a nexus for descriptive information, 4) a basis for making predictions, and 5) the basic concepts for theory formation (Blashfield 1984).

In contrast, *diagnosis* is "the art or act of identifying a disease from its signs and symptoms" (*Webster's Tenth New Collegiate Dictionary* 1998, p. 319). Thus, diagnosis is a lower-order term that is subsumed by and is only one type of classification—that of diseased or disordered states. Diagnosis in medicine has typically served three primary functions: 1) to allow health professionals to communicate with each other using a common language; 2) to enable the attending health professional to develop hypotheses about the etiology and prognosis of a condition; and 3) to suggest treatments that are tailored to this specific syndrome. In contrast to the many historical attempts at *classifying* family dysfunctions (see below), *diagnosing* family-based relational disorders is a comparatively new enterprise.

Advantages of Diagnosing Families

Diagnosing families as opposed to individuals has the advantage of encompassing a variety of pathological foci. If diagnostic criteria for family disorders were developed that could be reliably applied and were based on empirically validating "field trials," then family-oriented clinicians would be able to communicate among themselves using a common language. Clinicians would also have a sense of the origins of certain family (or couple) dysfunctions and what might happen to a given family in the future, and could select treatments that specifically address the relational problems encompassed by the diagnostic label. For example, research criteria in use since the mid-1970s suggest that a marriage is "distressed" when 1) communication difficulties exist that may have characterized the couple from the premarital period, 2) marital dissatisfaction and/or divorce are likely if the marriage problems are not treated, and 3) there are probable benefits of behavioral or cognitive-behavioral marital treatments that emphasize communication and problem-solving skills (Dobson et al. 1988; Jacobson and Margolin 1979; Markman 1981; Spanier 1976). Can more specific relational problems be articulated and operationalized that would offer a similar wealth of information?

Family clinicians already have informal systems of classifications that are used somewhat haphazardly. Families are often referred to as "dysfunctional," "codependent," "enmeshed," or "schizophrenogenic." However, few clinicians mean the same thing when using these terms, and the current use of a common vocabulary may mask real differences in theoretical assumptions, orientation, and treatment methods. An agreed-upon diagnostic system with an associated empirical database would force clinicians to operationalize their terms and base their treatment decisions on common understandings of what is helpful in what situations. In time, the more recent accomplishments for individual psychiatric disorders may spread to the field of family therapy—that is, the operationalization and manualization of specific treatments for specific relationship conditions.

There is a further advantage in developing systems for classifying family problems. Many individual psychiatric diagnoses imply blame of the individual, without considering the relational context that might promote the patient's behavior or pathology. Thus, a child may be labeled with "oppositional defiant disorder" without recognition that the parents are beating or otherwise maltreating the child. Likewise, a woman may be labeled "dependent personality disorder" without recognition that her husband has been avoidant and chronically unfaithful to her. A family relational diagnosis allows us to add important information to the diagnostic formulation of a given individual. More generally, it helps us to move from one-person understandings of disorders to the recognition that disorders can have their foci in the behavior of multiple individuals.

Assumptions of Family-Based Typologies

Family-based typologies rely in part on certain assumptions for success. First, in order to believe that treatment of a family would be best served by applying a diagnostic label, we must believe that the family or marital disorder is superordinate to disorders in any of the individual members. There is no point in applying a label to a group if all of the group dynamics can be explained by one or more individual pathologies. For example, an individual who shows communication dysfunction in the family setting may or may not show a similar level of dysfunction when interacting with persons outside of the family. If he or she does show such cross-situational consistency, we must consider the alternative hypothesis of an individually based disorder that would be present with or without the family's influences.

Thus, family diagnosis is based in systems-oriented recursive thinking. In other words, transactions among family members are bidirectional and mutually initiated and create tensions, distress, and psychopathology in the system as a whole and in its individual members that cannot be fully explained by an individual's behavior. In fact, a family may show relational pathology even if there are no diagnosable psychiatric disorders in any of its individual members. Likewise, we need not assume that the family diagnosis singularly caused the individual disorders of each member of the family; individual disorders may have biological or genetic origins. Rather, family and individual diagnoses are viewed as independent but mutually influential.

Second, we must believe that a family relational disorder is serious enough to warrant treatment, either in conjunction with or as a substitute for individual treatment of the disordered member or members. We must believe that without treatment, the consequences for individual family members and the family unit as a whole may be quite negative, perhaps leading to the onset of or exacerbations of individual psychopathologies, social and/or occupational dysfunction, increased family tension, and possibly family dissolution.

Third, even if a family or marital relational disorder can be presumed to have directly resulted from pathology in an individual member (e.g., a marriage that was previously happy but becomes dysfunctional following the onset of Alzheimer's disease in the husband), we must still believe that treatment of the family or marriage is an important and useful contribution to the treatment plan of this disordered individual. That is, we must believe that *not all* families in this situation would develop these relational problems, and that the reactions of family members to pathology in the individual, while understandable, are not as adaptive as they could be.

Disadvantages of Diagnosing Families

There are disadvantages to the diagnosis of mental disturbance in both families and individuals; this is well articulated in the psychiatric literature. But there are more specific disadvantages to diagnosing families. First, thinking in terms of "group problems" may lead to some unusual outcomes: Should we have diagnostic criteria for a "Boy Scout troop communication disorder," "sibling competition disorder," or "university faculty problem-solving dysfunction"? Worse still, will diagnosing groups of people further "us versus them" thinking? There is always the danger that we will justify our dislike for another group of people by applying a diagnostic label, as some say (e.g., Szasz 1960) we have always done for individuals we do not like.

Second, there is not yet convincing evidence that family dysfunction both precedes and is directly related etiologically to individual psychiatric disorders. Whereas some longitudinal studies show that family communication dysfunction is present prior to the onset of major psychopathologies such as schizophrenia (e.g., Goldstein 1987), there is still controversy about whether these styles of communication are etiologically significant. Should we say that an individual has the comorbid condition of depression and a family communication disorder, even if we have no evidence that family communication styles are a primary cause of depression?

Certainly, DSM-IV and other diagnostic systems have acknowledged the lack of evidence to connect individual diagnoses that co-vary with each other. For example, consider a patient with the dual diagnosis of substance dependence (on DSM-IV Axis I) and borderline personality disorder (on Axis II). Can we assume that the Axis II disorder preceded or was etiologically related to the Axis I disorder? Knowledge of the exact cause-effect relation of these two disorders is not necessary in order to prescribe a treatment plan that may include pharmacological, behavioral, and psychotherapeutic components.

Third, the problem of diagnostic "thresholds" must be addressed for a family-based diagnosis to be valid. How much distress or dysfunction must a family or marital couple show before we consider it to be within the clinical range? For example, how many examples of problem-solving failures must we observe before we conclude that a family has a dysfunction in its ability to solve problems? Once again, this problem parallels an issue in the diagnosis of individuals: How depressed/anxious/psychotic must an individual be before a label is applicable? This is an issue that must be addressed in empirical studies. The risk, of course, is of overdiagnosis in the absence of clearly operationalized diagnostic criteria.

A fourth, more insidious problem is the possibility of discriminating against certain cultures and basing diagnoses on middle-class, urban, white views of family functioning. For example, direct, self-disclosing, and/or assertive communication originating from a son to his father, while viewed as healthy in an Anglo American family, might be viewed as disrespectful in certain Asian cultures (see McGoldrick et al. 1991 for an extensive discussions of these issues). If we devise diagnostic criteria that define certain patterns of interaction or dominance hierarchies as dysfunctional, do we then diagnose families from specific cultures as more frequently dysfunctional than others? Of course, the error can go in the other direction as well. We can devise criteria that strongly take into account cultural variations in family life and label certain family patterns as dysfunctional only if they occur in a culture in which they are uncommon. This decision could result in an underdiagnosis of relational disorders in certain societies and make reimbursable treatment less available to members of this culture.

Finally, the availability of criteria for family diagnoses may encourage family-oriented clinicians to apply a relational diagnosis in every case in which a family brings in one or more disturbed children or adolescents, simply to justify family therapy. The saying, "When all you have is a hammer, the whole world becomes a nail" applies here. Clearly, a disorder in an individual does not in tautological fashion suggest that a family disorder is present; nor does the presentation of a family or couple for treatment automatically justify a relationship-based diagnosis. Rather, the clinician must be ready to assess the family's communication styles as independently of the individual pathologies as possible, and be ready to acknowledge that any given family may show dysfunction in each of its individual members but that the dysfunction may still fall short of the diagnostic criteria for a family disorder.

These limitations notwithstanding, several attempts have been made to classify (as opposed to diagnose) family relational problems. These are reviewed below, and a critique of these methods presented at the end of the section. In later sections, we review modern attempts to develop family diagnostic systems.

Historical Methods of Family Classification

Early Studies of Schizophrenia

Early studies of schizophrenia by Lidz et al. (1957) resulted in one of the first typologies for family dysfunction. This typology described the intrafamilial circumstances that accompanied and were believed etiologically related to the onset of schizophrenia in a child. Lidz and his colleagues noted two predominant patterns: 1) *marital schism*, where the parents openly and directly fought each other and forced one or more children to take sides; and 2) *marital skew*, where one parent was overly dominant and the transactions of the family were oriented toward satisfying this parent's emotional and physical needs. In both cases, preschizophrenic children were thought to develop enmeshed, symbiotic attachments to one parent, interfering with the development of good self-esteem and appropriate sex-role identification.

Nameche et al. (1964) described families with schizophrenic members differently by focusing on the absence of appropriate expressions of emotionality. *Emotionally divorced* families were those in which the parental pair were disengaged and emotionally disconnected. *Pseudomutual* families were those in which the parents made strong efforts to maintain the appearance of normality, to the point that family transactions became rigid, stereotypical, and highly predictable. Underneath this facade was presumed to be a great deal of emotional distress and unacknowledged conflict. Again, one or both parents were thought to turn to the preschizophrenic child as a source of the emotional nurturance lacking in the marriage.

These typologies, as well as others that emerged around the same time (e.g., Jackson 1960), were never really designed as diagnostic systems, but instead were meant as clues to the psychosocial etiology of schizophrenia. However, it has never been clear that these family processes distinguish families with schizophrenic members from those without schizophrenic members, and no longitudinal studies have examined whether these patterns are present before the onset of schizophrenia in the index child. Thus, these subtypings of families fall short of providing a usable taxonomy for families with schizophrenic members. Nevertheless, they were important in generating hypotheses for later attempts to understand schizophrenia (see Goldstein and Strachan 1987).

Modern Studies of Families of Schizophrenic Patients

Modern studies of families of schizophrenic patients very often employ two constructs occurring both in the clinical and in research literature: *expressed emotion* (EE) (Vaughn and Leff 1976) and *communication deviance* (CD) (Wynne et al. 1977). (For a review of EE and CD, see Chapter 27, "Family Variables and Interventions in Schizophrenia," in this volume; see also Miklowitz and Stackman 1992.) These constructs describe families of patients with severe psychiatric disorders (often schizophrenic patients) on dimensions like degree of criticism, hostility, or emotional overinvolvement (EE) or degree of unclear, fragmented, or amorphous communication (CD). These constructs also were never intended as classification criteria but rather as predictive indices. However, EE and CD may provide the clinician with information about families with respect to 1) how certain patterns of communication come about, 2) the short-term prognosis of the psychiatric disorder, and 3) psychosocial treatments that are likely to be of help to the patient and/or family. For example, schizophrenic patients from high-EE families are more likely than those from low-EE families to relapse within a 1-year period of follow-up (for reviews, see Butzlaff and Hooley 1998; Miklowitz et al. 1984). Nonschizophrenic but vulnerable adolescents from high-CD families are more likely to develop disorders within the schizophrenia spectrum in adulthood than adolescents from low-CD families (Goldstein 1987). High-EE families also appear to benefit from psychoeducational family interventions, particularly in the reduction in relapse rates for the patient and improved communication within the family (for review, see Chapter 27, "Family Variables and Interventions in Schizophrenia," in this volume; see also Goldstein and Miklowitz 1995).

Thus, the constructs of EE and CD may eventually form the basis of usable classification schemes for families containing a mentally ill person. Initial attempts to employ these constructs as aids in classification are discussed in a subsequent section of this chapter (see "The DSM-IV Methods: Future Directions").

Anorexia Nervosa

Anorexia nervosa was the subject of early attempts to classify familywide disorders. Minuchin et al. (1978) were among the first to describe what were essentially classification criteria for familywide disorders as they applied to members of families with anorexia nervosa (which they referred to as "psychosomatic families"). Minuchin and his colleagues described four criteria that they believed distinguished anorexic families from those with other psychosomatic illnesses and from families with other types of emotional disturbance or normal control subjects: 1) enmeshment (overinvolved relationships); 2) overprotectiveness; 3) rigidity (an overcommitment to the family status quo); and 4) lack of conflict resolution (i.e., avoiding acknowledging or trying to solve problems). However, these criteria were rather vague and not fully operationalized. In Minuchin's research, classifying families on the basis of these attributes was typically based on individual self-report rather than observation of the family.

Family Dimension of Medical Disorders (Medical Family Therapy)

Reiss (1981) studied medical disorders as an aspect of family relational disorders. He described a series of dimensions on which to evaluate the family and its relation to its external environment, and applied these dimensions quite fruitfully to studies of families with a member with end-stage renal disease. According to Reiss (1981; see also Reiss and Klein 1987; Reiss et al. 1986), there are three orthogonal dimensions of family problem-solving behavior:

1. *Configuration,* or the degree to which the family can see patterns or coherence in what appears to be a confusing situation, and the family's resulting confidence in their ability to master the situation
2. *Coordination,* or the family's belief that it must face a problem situation as a unified, cohesive, well-integrated whole

3. *Delayed closure*, or the degree to which a family is able to change its definitions of and solutions to problems in response to new information (the inverse of Minuchin's notion of rigidity)

Reiss developed scores on each of these dimensions on the basis of the family's reactions to a pattern recognition task.

In hemodialysis patients with end-stage renal disease, high delayed closure scores for families predicted fewer medical complications at a 15- to 24-month follow-up, but high levels of coordination predicted early death (Reiss et al. 1986). Reiss and his colleagues cautioned that these three family attributes, while appearing to be healthy dimensions of family functioning, may in certain cases indicate pathology. High coordination, for example, may suggest low levels of individual autonomy, poor boundaries, or enmeshment.

Reiss has essentially described *dimensions* of family functioning rather than *classification* of family relationships. His approach, however, takes advantage of longitudinal and empirical methods and suggests certain criteria that could be used to classify families who may or may not cope well with problems generated by medical illness in one or more members.

Classification of Distressed Marriages

Other writers have concentrated on characterizing marriages as distressed or nondistressed, and those that may or may not require conjoint treatment. These classification schemes differ from the schemes described above in that there is no presumption (with the exception of Dobson et al. 1988 discussed below) that one member of the couple has an individual psychiatric disorder.

Early Descriptive Typologies

Early descriptive typologies were employed in the work of Lederer and Jackson (1968b; summarized in Berman and Lief 1975), who described four different levels of functioning in marriages, within which were different styles of coping with marital or family situations. These levels of functioning ranged from "stable-satisfactory" marriages (highest level), to "stable-unsatisfactory" and "unstable-unsatisfactory" marriages (middle levels), to the lowest level of functioning, consisting of "gruesome twosomes" and "paranoid predators." These levels of functioning were not so much diagnoses of couples as much as descriptions of their interactional patterns. For example, "psychosomatic avoiders" (unstable-unsatisfactory category) were described as couples that could not express anger openly, and in which one member develops a psychosomatic or substance abuse problem as a way of guarding against unconscious hostility in the relationship. In contrast, "paranoid predators" huddle together as a way of protecting themselves from a hostile world, which may make members of the couple superficially happy but severely disrupts the development of the children, much like the "pseudomutual" style described in families with schizophrenic members (Nameche et al. 1964).

Whereas Lederer and Jackson (1968) described levels of functioning in marriages, Cuber and Harroff (1966) described marital types based on core emotional features of the relationship:

- *"Conflict-habituated,"* in which there is conflict combined with strong controls over emotional expression and fears of aloneness
- *"Devitalized,"* in which the emotional environment is numb and apathetic but relatively free of conflict
- *"Passive-congenial,"* in which partners live together and occasionally support each other, but within a basic stance of disengagement
- *"Vital marriage" or relationship*, which is what we all strive for: exciting, enthusiastic, and rewarding, as well as stable and interdependent
- *"Total" marriage*, the pinnacle of all marriages, in which each partner must have the engagement of the other to enjoy all activities (Berman and Lief 1975)

Other marital typologies have been devised, such as pairings based on interlocking personality styles (e.g., the obsessive husband with the histrionic wife; Ard and Ard 1969), and schemes based on couples' behaviors on cooperative and/or competitive tasks (Hoffman 1981; Ravich 1974). Few of these schemes are based on empirical research, and little is offered in terms of recommendations for specific types of interventions. Furthermore, none are designed as classification systems per se and, as a result, do not employ specific diagnostic criteria or specify the types of individual pathologies that might accompany each marital type. Rather, these schemes describe marital dynamics that can be addressed in treatment if the marriage is dysfunctional, as defined by either the couple or the clinician (who of course may not be in agreement).

Classifying Marriages Containing a Depressed Member

More recently, Dobson et al. (1988) elaborated a classification system for marriages in which one member is depressed. This system tries to help the clinician select between individual cognitive-behavioral therapy (CBT) for the depressed person versus behavioral marital therapy (BMT) for the couple, two treatments whose efficacy for depression has been well documented (e.g., Blackburn et al. 1981; Jacobson et al. 1984b). Four types of couples were described (Dobson et al. 1988):

1. "Classic" couples have at least one member with depression and the marriage is distressed, in which case both CBT and BMT are recommended.
2. "Denial" couples have a member who is depressed but neither member reports significant marital problems, although by all outside accounts, including standardized assessments, the marriage is distressed. In this case, CBT may be the initial treatment for the depressed partner, while BMT may be "phased in" without directly confronting the denial of the couple.
3. "Systemic" couples acknowledge marital distress, but on assessment at least one member is found to be depressed, usually as a direct result of the distressed marriage. In this case, BMT is usually recommended alone, as individual CBT for the depressed person may be difficult to rationalize to the couple.
4. "Social support" couples acknowledge depression in one member, but the report of the couple, as well as all assessments, indicates no severe marital problems. In this case, individual CBT is recommended, and occasional sessions of BMT may enhance the nondepressed partner's ability to support the depressed partner.

The matching of couple subtype to recommended treatment is a highly laudable goal. In fact, this direction is being taken by clinicians for many individual disorders in DSM-IV. For example, there are now practice guidelines to match different forms of depression to different types of pharmacological or psychosocial treatment (American Psychiatric Association 2000b). The system of Dobson and his colleagues deserves to be further elaborated with empirical study, to ensure the following: 1) the reliability of making these kinds of distinctions can be established; 2) the patterns of interaction that distinguish these couples can be identified; and 3) it can be established that each type of couple—and the depressed member within each type of couple—benefits from a different combination of pharmacological and psychosocial treatment, and perhaps other treatments.

Historical Attempts at Classification: What's Missing?

The foregoing review is not an exhaustive coverage of all of the clinical or empirical attempts to classify family and marital problems, but the classifications reviewed are illustrative of the advantages, as well as disadvantages, of attempting to do this kind of work. There is a certain intuitive appeal to having a descriptive label—one that has been articulated in the clinical or research literature—to apply to a particular couple or family. But the typologies described earlier have not been shown in most cases to meet the validity criteria that a diagnosis should have, in terms of identifying likely etiological mechanisms, giving prognostic information, or predicting responses to certain treatments. Of course, few disorders in DSM–IV can be said to meet all of these criteria. However, classifications of marriages and families suffer from a lack of empirical study, to the extent that we cannot yet justify their regular use in practice. For example, do all families of anorexic patients share the features of enmeshment and/or lack of conflict resolution, or only some? How do families of schizophrenic patients with and without high communication deviance differ in treatment responsiveness?

Few empirically based criteria exist for defining marital or family disorders. How much denial about marital problems must be present and for how long before we call a couple with a depressed member a "denial couple"? Can we apply these classifications reliably? Can we fully distinguish one marital subtype from another?

In the next sections, two diagnostic classification schemes are described that begin to address some of these problems. These systems attempt to emulate the development of DSM-IV (Widiger et al. 1991) by basing diagnostic categories, and changes in diagnostic categories, on empirical studies and field trials.

A Classification Scheme Associated With DSM-IV

In the planning of DSM-IV, there was a recognition that relational disorders might be usefully incorporated into the existing individually based DSM system, perhaps as V codes or as a sixth diagnostic axis. There already existed ill-defined categories in DSM-III-R such as "parent-child problem," "marital problem," or "other specified family circumstances." However, it was clear that introducing criteria for relational disorders, even if well rationalized, added a level of complexity not present for individual disorders. Thus, several extensive literature reviews were undertaken to determine what family attributes existed that had sufficient empirical justification to be classified as "disorders," and that could be operationalized such that precise and reliable "presence versus absence" judgments could be made.

A Search for Reliable and Valid Constructs

Our method (Clarkin and Miklowitz 1997) began with a thorough review of the research literature on family and marital assessment studies, with particular emphasis on studies involving direct measurement of family interactions. The search was for *constructs* that met the following conditions:

- Were clear definitions of different types of marital and family *communication* disturbances that could be described with well-operationalized criteria.
- Were identifiable simply from interviewing or watching the interactions of the couple or family, particularly with the support of assessment instruments.
- Were useful in distinguishing distressed from nondistressed marriages (defined by standardized criteria) or families containing a psychiatric patient from those without one.
- Were longitudinally predictive of the functioning of one or more members of the family or the family unit itself.

In conducting our literature search, we looked in particular for identifying constructs that could be assessed with reliable and validated instruments. The reliability of individual diagnoses in DSM-III and DSM-III-R was greatly enhanced by the availability of structured diagnostic interviews (e.g., Structured Clinical Interview for DSM-III-R; Spitzer et al. 1988), and it is likely that this will prove true of DSM-IV diagnoses as well. The close relationship between explicit criteria and the generation of instruments to assess these criteria reliably has corollaries in the family field. A number of family researchers have generated instruments to reliably assess salient dimensions of family function versus dysfunction, as reviewed elsewhere (Clarkin and Glick 1989; Jacob and Tennenbaum 1988).

Because our focus was on communication, we did not include other types of family dysfunction, such as incest or family violence. However, these topics were undertaken by teams commissioned by DSM-IV (e.g., O'Leary and Jacobson 1997) and by the GAP Committee on the Family (see discussion later in this section).

Nature of the Criteria

We developed two sets of criteria: spousal communication disorders and family communication disorders (Tables 16–1 and 16–2). The criteria sets overlap to some extent but are not isomorphic. For example, on the basis of the EE literature, we concluded that emotional overinvolvement was an empirically supportable criterion for disturbed family relations but not for marital relations.

In line with what has been done for many of the disorders in DSM-IV, each type of communication disorder is accompanied by several modifying attributes:

Table 16–1. Criteria for spousal communication disorders

For at least 3 months, there has been evidence of *functional impairment* in one or more members of the couple (i.e., interference with job functioning, poor parenting, psychiatric symptoms in one or both spouses) and *at least two* of the following:
1. Couple does not clarify mutual requests, provide information, or accurately describe problems.
2. Spouse(s) verbalizes underlying attributions, assumptions, and expectations that are negative (e.g., the other spouse is globally negatively intentioned) or exaggerated (e.g., "couples should never fight").
3. Communication is characterized by negative affect (i.e., anger, hostility, jealousy), critical remarks, disagreement with spouse, and nonacceptance of what the mate has communicated.
4. Low frequency of self-disclosure of thoughts, feelings, and wishes.
5. Couple demonstrates inadequate problem solving, characterized by poor problem definition, lack of task focus, mutual criticism and complaint, and negative escalation.
6. Couple displays sequences of negative communication characterized by criticism, disagreement, negative listening, and refusal to agree.
7. Couple avoids conflict by withdrawal, lack of discussion, and subsequent non-resolution.

Associated Features
Low reported marital satisfaction, depression in one or more spouses, threatened and contemplated separation and divorce, concentration and job-performance difficulties.

Source. Adapted from Clarkin and Miklowitz 1997.

- *Functional impairment.* This impairment takes the form of at least one of the following: 1) serious personal dissatisfaction; 2) disruptive behavior, including family violence or abuse, separation or divorce, or lack of effective parenting; or 3) Axis I or Axis II individual disorders in at least one member of the family or couple.
- *Duration.* The signs of the family's or couple's disorder must be present for at least 3 months and not represent a transitory reaction to a life event.
- *Associated features.* These features, which include reports of marital dissatisfaction, divorce, and disruptive behavior in children, are not requirements of the diagnosis but may signal its presence.

We also felt it important that disturbance be seen in more than one domain of communication. A single sign of dysfunction (e.g., avoidance of and withdrawal from conflict in a couple) is not sufficient in this system to diagnose a relational disorder; at least two signs must be present, and it is ex-

Table 16–2. Criteria for family communication disorders

For at least 3 months, there has been evidence of *functional impairment* in one or more family members, as exemplified by psychiatric symptoms or low social and/or academic competence in one or more children, low job functioning in one or both parents, or psychiatric symptoms in parents; and *at least two* of the following:
1. Family is unable to communicate clearly, cannot communicate closure, or cannot share a focus of attention (communication deviance).
2. Family communication is characterized by unidirectional hostility or frequent criticism from one member to another, or by bidirectional, negatively escalating cycles of pejorative or critical comments (high expressed emotion with criticism and/or hostility).
3. Parent-offspring relations are characterized by overprotectiveness, "emotional overinvolvement," overconcern, unnecessarily self-sacrificing behaviors, intrusiveness, or overdependence (high expressed emotion with overinvolvement).
4. Parent-offspring interchanges are marked by negatively reinforcing "coercive cycles" that tend to perpetuate antisocial or aggressive behavior in one or more family members.
5. A broad array of family problems cannot be solved because of the family's inability to agree to try to define, generate, or evaluate and implement solutions to existing problems.

Associated Features
Adolescent acting-out and disruptive behavior ("externalizing disorders") or withdrawing, self-punitive behavior ("internalizing disorders"); major psychiatric disorders in one or more family members (i.e., schizophrenia, major affective disorders); poor parental morale; marital distress; parenting dissatisfaction.

Source. Adapted from Clarkin and Miklowitz 1997.

pected that frequently, many more will be evident. This requirement is analogous to the DSM-IV requirement that depressed mood be accompanied by at least four associated symptoms before the diagnosis of major depressive disorder is warranted. Thus, a couple with a communication disorder might direct many negative remarks toward each other *and* be unwilling or unable to solve other problems that we have raised in our discussions. A family with a communication disorder might be one with unclear, fragmented communication in which the observer cannot draw conclusions about the topics of interest, *as well as* a family in which dyadic relations between parent and offspring are marked by overconcern or overprotectiveness.

It is important to emphasize that each criterion was selected on the basis of a substantial literature demonstrating its reliability and discriminant and/or predictive validity (Clarkin and Miklowitz 1997). For example, a large number of studies suggest that distressed couples are characterized by negative reciprocity (i.e., mutual fault finding, cross-complaining) as well as the verbalization of global, negative attributions about partners' behaviors (Billings 1979; Gottman et al. 1976a, 1976b; Margolin and Wampold 1981; Rausch et al. 1974; Revenstorf et al. 1984). Based on these and many other experimental studies, negative escalation and negative, verbalized attributional styles were both selected as criteria for a spousal communication disorder. A similar method was used for specifying criteria for a family communication disorder.

We developed our criteria while DSM-IV was in the process of being published. There must be substantial field testing of these criteria before their inclusion in any diagnostic manual, including future versions of DSM, could be justified. However, specification of these criteria is a first step in providing a direction for future field trials.

Relation of Individual Diagnoses to Family Diagnoses

The utility of any relational diagnostic system is enhanced by the gradual linking of specific types of family communication patterns to the occurrence of specific individual psychiatric disorders. That is, the "associated features" of individuals in each type of disordered family need to be more clearly specified and articulated. Unfortunately, evidence for the co-variation of individual disorders with specific family pathologies is weak at best.

We have begun to delineate family dysfunctions that co-vary with certain individual disorders. Table 16–3 lists some of the criteria in our system and the individual disorder(s) for which each criterion has been most consistently studied. There is no presumption here that these family dysfunctions are 1) etiologically related to the specific psychiatric conditions listed, 2) ubiquitous characteristics of the family environments accompanying these disorders, or 3) specific to these conditions and not also present in other disorders. However, an important gauge for validating these diagnostic systems is demonstrating that the occurrence of some of the criteria for spousal or family relational disorders is associated with, even if not limited to, definable types of individual disturbance.

The Group for the Advancement of Psychiatry Method

When DSM-IV was in the process of development, the GAP (1985, 1991, 1995) Committee on the Family also prepared a set of diagnostic criteria: The Classification System of Relational Disorders (CORD). The GAP Committee argued that relational disorders should be placed on Axis I,

Table 16–3. Examples of associations between disordered family/marital communication processes and specific psychiatric disorders

Relational construct	Individual disorder	Representative study
Family-based dysfunctions		
Communication deviance	Schizophrenia, bipolar disorder, at-risk adolescents	Goldstein 1987; Miklowitz et al. 1991; Wynne et al. 1977
Parental overprotectiveness	Schizophrenia, borderline personality disorder, depression	Parker 1983; Zweig-Frank and Paris 1991
Coercive parent-child processes	Aggressive children	Patterson 1982
Couple-based dysfunctions		
Negative affective expression	Depression, alcoholism, bipolar disorder	Gotlib and Whiffen 1989; Jacob 1987; Simoneau et al. 1998
Poor problem solving	Depression, alcoholism	Biglan et al. 1988; Jacob 1987
Low self-disclosure	Depression	Billings et al. 1983
Negative, global, internal attributions about partner	Depression, negative-symptom schizophrenia	Camper et al. 1988; Hooley et al. 1987

while a separate axis—the Global Assessment of Relational Functioning (GARF) scale—should be used to describe levels of relational functioning along a continuum of severity (see subsection below on the GARF scale).

The GAP method differs from our method presented above in that the CORD criteria are focused on specific family problem areas, such as sexual or physical abuse, divorce, sexual dysfunction, failures for infants to thrive, and separation disorders. The GAP committee provided reasonably detailed criteria and associated features for these disorders. For example, the CORD criteria for "conflictual disorder with and without physical aggression" not only describe the central diagnostic features of couples or families with intense conflict but also list predisposing factors (e.g., alcohol and drug use), associated features (e.g., depression), prevalence, cultural- and gender-related factors, and course of the disorder.

Global Assessment of Relational Functioning (GARF) Scale

The most salient outcome of the GAP Committee on the Family's work to date is the development of a dimensional rating scale, the GARF, for evaluating the overall functioning of and level of pathology in any given family (GAP 1995). The GARF scale (Table 16–4), which the originators view as a potential replacement for Axis IV (psychosocial stressors) in future versions of DSM, is currently listed in Appendix B of DSM-IV-TR, "Criteria Sets and Axes Provided for Further Study." It is designed to alert clinicians to evaluate the residential context of patients with a psychiatric disorder (GAP 1995). The GARF is analogous to the DSM-IV Axis V rating of global functioning of the individual—namely, the Global Assessment of Functioning Scale (GAF) rating (Endicott et al. 1976).

The correlation between the GARF and the individualized GAF ratings is established in several ways. First, like the GAF rating, the GARF rating is made on a 100-point scale with descriptors for every 20-point interval (see Table 16–4). Second, the GARF is designed to be applied by clinicians with relatively little experience (in this case, little formal training with families). Third, the family can be rated for any of several time frames: the family's current functioning, best and worst functioning in the past year, or functioning after a period of treatment. Finally, the GARF is designed to be rated from observation of the family in intake or treatment sessions; it is not dependent on specific evaluation procedures or paper-and-pencil methods.

When rating family functioning, the clinician is directed to consider three areas of family group functioning: problem solving, family organization, and emotional climate. Thus, a family in the 61–80 range of the GARF scale is seen as having 1) unresolved problems that do not disrupt relationships, 2) good family organization but with some deprecation of members

Table 16–4. Summary of Global Assessment of Relational Functioning (GARF)

Rating of 81–100

Occasional conflicts resolved through shared problem solving.
Shared understandings of roles and responsibilities.
Emotional atmosphere of optimism, warmth, and caring.

Rating of 61–80

Some issues unresolved by problem solving.
Decision making is competent, but members' efforts at control of one another are sometimes greater than necessary and/or are ineffective.
Some irritability, pain, and frustration evident in emotional climate.

Rating of 41–60

Communication and problem solving quite frequently disrupted or inhibited.
Excessive rigidity or significant lack of structure at times.
Pain, anger, or emotional deadness interferes with emotional climate.

Rating of 21–40

Frustrating failures at problem solving; tyrannical or ineffective decision making.
Uniqueness of individuals ignored by rigid or confusingly fluid coalitions.
Frequent distancing or open hostility.

Rating of 1–20

Communication is repeatedly disrupted; relational routines negligible.
Boundaries between relational units cannot be identified or agreed on.
Despair and cynicism pervasive; no sense of attachment or mutual concern.

Source.   American Psychiatric Association 2000a; Group for the Advancement of Psychiatry 1995.

and "scapegoating," and 3) a range of appropriate emotions but with some tension. A family in the 21–40 range of the scale is seen as having 1) ineffective problem-solving skills in relation to life cycle transitions (e.g., loss), 2) excessively rigid or confusingly fluid coalitions, and 3) obvious distancing or open hostility.

The definition of the family unit to be rated on the GARF—unlike Axis V of DSM-IV, on which the object of the rating (the individual) is clear—is rather broad. The authors of the scale mention individuals related by legal and/or biological connections (i.e., marital pair, nuclear or extended family); individuals who cohabit; persons in the same social network who are involved in couple/family problem-solving, organizational, or affective issues; and even members of health care treatment networks. Thus, the definition of the relational unit to be rated can become vague and possibly far-fetched. Nevertheless, the GAP committee may have done the field a great service by developing a scale that can be applied to the myriad of relational units that individuals in society actually inhabit.

The GAP Committee on the Family (GAP 1995) is presently conducting field trials with the GARF. These field trials, conducted in the United States and Europe, involve both cross-site videotape ratings and observer ratings of families newly arrived at certain clinics. Interrater reliabilities for videotape ratings have been quite good, with intraclass correlations in the 0.81–0.94 range (Dausch et al. 1996). There are now concurrent validity data on the GARF as well. As judged from their interactional behavior during problem-solving discussions, high-EE families containing a member with bipolar disorder have lower GARF scores (poorer relational functioning) than low-EE families (Dausch et al. 1996).

The inclusion of the GARF in DSM-IV (and DSM-IV-TR) Appendix B reflects the increasing recognition that individual disorders must be understood within a relational context. Of course, adding new axes to the DSM system may increase the probability that clinicians will ignore them, the way they have often ignored Axis V. Furthermore, although the cross-site reliability findings of the GAP Committee on the Family are encouraging, there remains the question of whether researchers or clinicians can reliably apply the GARF in practice.

The DSM-IV Methods: Future Directions

There are many compatibilities between our relational diagnostic scheme and the GAP Committee on the Family's methods (the CORD system and the GARF rating). For example, the GARF rating scale is based on three aspects of family functioning (problem solving, organization, and emotional climate) that are also identified as significant dimensions of family functioning in our review (Clarkin and Miklowitz 1997). However, our literature review suggests that there are other constructs that may be related to but go beyond the three GAP committee dimensions (see Tables 16–1 and 16–2). For this reason, the combination of a relational disorder diagnosis and a GARF rating may be the most optimal way of classifying a given family.

Both our method and the GAP Committee on the Family's methods need substantial field-testing before they can be made available for general use. First, as is currently being done with the GARF, a series of videotape reliability studies must be conducted to establish that relational disorder criteria can be applied with high levels of agreement. Second, a series of epidemiological and validity studies must be conducted to determine the following conditions:

1. How many couples and families meet criteria for these relational disorders
2. Whether couples and families that do meet diagnostic criteria differ from those that do not on dimensions such as levels of psychiatric disturbance in individual members, job functioning, or parenting skills
3. The etiological precursors of relational disorders (e.g., genetic predisposition, violence, abuse, or other traumatic events)
4. The predictive validity of the categories (or dimensional ratings) for the short- and long-term psychological health of individual family members
5. Whether treatments that address the dysfunctions that led to the original diagnosis (or GARF score) result in improvements in the functioning of individuals within this unit

Why Diagnose Families? A Question Revisited

If we do succeed in establishing the reliability and validity of these systems of relational diagnosis, we still have a key question to address. Does diagnosing a family or a marriage help the persons who have come to us for treatment? This is not a question with a clear answer. If we do not have a system of interventions that target specific types of marital or family dysfunction, it is doubtful that we are helping anyone by applying a label. However, if we can articulate targeted interventions for specific disorders, a diagnosis may be quite useful in developing a treatment plan.

For example, if a couple meets criteria for a spousal communication disorder, such as negative attributions and low levels of self-disclosure, a marital therapy with cognitive and communication-oriented components, such as those designed by Baucom and Epstein (1990) or Jacobson and Christensen (1996), may be most effective. If we know that the family of a son with schizophrenia or major affective disorder has bidirectional, negatively escalating cycles and maternal overprotectiveness, empirically supported psychoeducational approaches to family treatment, such as those designed by Falloon and Liberman (1984), Hogarty et al. (1986), Leff et al. (1989), or Miklowitz and Goldstein (1997; Miklowitz et al. 2000), may be recommended. Finally, a couple or family that meets the criteria for a relational disorder but defines its problems as stemming directly from the psychiatric disorder of one family member may benefit initially from individual therapy for this member; this could be followed by easing into a nonthreatening, relatively structured family approach that makes no causal assumptions about the origins of the individual disorder. This matching of diagnosis to treatment, which is just beginning to be accomplished for the individual DSM-IV disorders (e.g., American Psychiatric Association 2000a, 2000b), must be further articulated and specified for the family disorders.

Conclusion

The family field has long groped for reliable and valid constructs, categories, and dimensions that describe family functioning. This process has not historically gelled into a predominant method of classifying or diagnosing families either for experimental or for clinical work. The work presented in this chapter is a step in this direction.

Much field-testing of new criteria for family relational disorders must be accomplished before their inclusion in future versions of DSM is justified. But if this basic supporting empirical work were to be accomplished, the field of marital and family therapy would obtain a legitimacy that it does not now enjoy. More importantly, families that seek professional help would benefit from the availability of agreed-on methods of diagnosis and treatment, rather than being limited to the method championed by the particular practitioner they consult.

Chapters on Related Topics

The following chapters describe concepts related to the diagnosis of family relational disorders:

- Chapter 15, "Functional and Dysfunctional Families"
- Chapter 27, "Family Variables and Interventions in Schizophrenia"
- Chapter 28, "Depression and the Family: Interpersonal Context and Family Functioning"
- Chapter 31, "Alcoholic and Substance-Abusing Families"
- Chapter 32, "Family Intervention With Incest"
- Chapter 33, "Family Therapy With Personality Disorders"

IV

Family Therapy With Children and Adolescents

17

Family Therapy With Children and Adolescents

An Overview

G. Pirooz Sholevar, M.D.

Introduction

Family therapy with children and adolescents is synonymous with family therapy because the family consists of multiple generations and the children embody the aspirations, dreams, vitality, and future of the family. Both the gratifying and traumatic experiences with one's parents and families of origin are reenacted with *one's own* children. Although family therapy as a field has paid much lip service to the importance of children in the families, many family therapists in practice lack the necessary skills, knowledge, or attitude to work with families with young children or adolescents. Many family therapists are in effect marital therapists who have attempted to broaden their reach by including the children or the members of the families of origin. Early in the family therapy movement, one would hear that the difficulties with the children were reflective of the marital problem and that their correction required only remediation of faulty parental marriage. These formulations ignored a truly dynamic family model whereby the interactional patterns were established by exchanges and events that occurred among all family members. The formulations also ignored how developmental progress became impeded within the family system. There was even less knowledge of biological factors in disorders such as attention-deficit/hyperactivity disorder (ADHD) or depression.

The presence of a number of prominent family therapists who were highly gifted in working with children ushered in the specialized practice of working with families with young children. Prominent among this group were Nathan Ackerman, Carl Whitaker, and Salvador Minuchin. Some of the knowledge and skills gained from the practice of such pioneers are reflected in the chapters in this book. Chasin and White provide a creative framework for including children in family therapy sessions, particularly in the initial interview (see Chapter 18, "Family Therapy With Children: A Model for Engaging the Whole Family").

History

Ackerman, Whitaker, Minuchin, and Bell are four pioneers who were especially gifted in working with families of young children and adolescents. Bell (1975) is the first family therapist who included children in family sessions. Ackerman (1950, 1954, 1958) was particularly gifted in demonstrating and describing the methods of reaching a silent, sullen, scapegoated adolescent who is directing destructive behavior toward himself and others. He was equally expert in recognizing the interconnections between a parental emotional divorce and a symbiotic relationship between a mother and child, a relationship that leads to a high level of dysfunction and psychopathology in the offspring. Ackerman was also expert in demonstrating the shared defensiveness of the family against the expressions of passion, aggression, and dependency in the family—inhibitions that take away the lifeblood necessary for developmental progression in all family members, particularly the children. Carl Whitaker (1975, 1976a, 1976b) had an exceptional ability to get down to the level of children, including infants. It is a deeply touching moment to watch Whitaker on videotape crawling on the floor on his hands and knees attempting to relate to a toddler who is making a "BM" in his diaper. Whitaker formulated the existence of unexpressed, defensive feelings and trauma in the life of the family that deprive the group of supportive and warm interactions. Whitaker's de-emphasis on theory and "rules" in the session helped the status of the children within the family who did not have the sophistication to use the rules to their benefit.

The work of Minuchin et al. (Minuchin 1967; Minuchin et al. 1974a) in the correction of enmeshment in families proved to be particularly helpful to the families with young children who exhibited behavioral or psychosomatic disorders in a crisis situation. Minuchin's description of psychosomatic families (Minuchin et al. 1978) had a profound impact on the field of family therapy and was readily adopted by pediatricians, psychiatrists, and other mental health professionals working with psychosomatic disorders.

More recent contributions to family therapy with children have come from the work of Patterson et al. (1982, 1992), Forehand and McMahon (1981a, 1981b), Alexander and Parsons (1973), Joan Zilbach, and David and Jill Scharff. The first two groups of contributors added immeasurably to our knowledge of conduct disorders and delinquent behavior. Zilbach (1986) provided a systematic way of including young children in families. David and Jill Scharff's (1987) formulations are particularly applicable to families with adolescents.

Theoretical Concepts

All schools of family therapy provide theoretical concepts specifically applicable to family therapy with children and adolescents. The failure of separation and individuation in enmeshed family organization as described by *structural family therapists* reveals that a highly interactive family process is usually reflective of parental shortcomings that do not provide enough distance and objectivity to allow for differentiation of the children. This lack of differentiation in the children as a result of a high level of enmeshment interferes with their utilization of the school and social systems to gain further maturity (see Chapter 2, "Structural Family Therapy").

The overinvolvement between a child and parent in the context of a highly distant parental marriage is emphasized in *strategic family therapy*. The conceptual formulation and intervention strategies allow the reduction of involvement between the overinvolved dyad, particularly if the uninvolved parent is available for reengagement with the child and the family unit. The triadic-based family therapy is particularly effective in families in which a child is used as a "principal" in a fight with one of the parents and in which the feud is fueled by the second parent in a collusive fashion (see Chapter 3, "Constructing Therapy: From Strategic, to Systemic, to Narrative Models").

The concept of *projective identification* describes the projection of unresolved parental conflicts onto a child who assumes an identity based on a historically assigned role. This assumed identity interferes with appropriate identity formation based on maturational forces and situational requirements (see Chapter 4, "Psychodynamic Family Therapy," for further discussion). The transference reaction from the parents onto the children is the motivator for many dysfunctional interactions in current family situations. Traumatic events in the early history of the family or of the parents, such as child neglect, physical abuse, or sexual abuse, can result in the repetition of such traumatic situations. Conversely, the defensive restriction of the child's normative activities can be based on early traumatic events. For example, a mother whose sister had drowned as a child did not allow any of her four children to learn how to swim or go in the ocean because of the fear of drowning.

Parentification assigns a parental role to the children and deprives them of age appropriate experiences. The prominence of sadomasochistic interactions in the early history of the parents can result in parental masochistic personality development. The parents then seek to reestablish a sadomasochistic relationship with their child in order to recreate earlier traumatic experiences, as an attachment to painful affects (Kissen 1995). A frequent giveaway of the nature of this type of relationship is when the parents refer to the child as their "punisher" or "monster." The inappropriateness of such labels can reveal the origins of the behavior that are generally hidden in the parental motivation (see Chapter 4, "Psychodynamic Family Therapy").

Behavioral family therapy uses social learning theory to explain the impact of either faulty reinforcement practices or no reinforcement practices in the families. Either can result in a variety of interactional patterns that are detrimental to the development of the children. In such cases there are frequently both the lack of a cooperative and reciprocal relationship between the parents and a high preponderance of psychopathology and aggressive behavior at the parental level. These interactional patterns can result in the *coercive family processes* described by Patterson (1982) that result in aggressive and unmanageable behavior in the children.

Projective family mechanisms and *triangulation*, described by Bowen (see Chapter 5, "Multigenerational Family Systems Theory of Bowen and Its Application"), are major sources of the lack of differentiation and immaturity that are transferred across the generations. Triangulation results in the exploitation of the child in parental conflicts as the parents look for ways to reduce the anxiety and tension in their relationship. The parents very often use the child as the recipient and target for this tension, which leaves the child in an undifferentiated state.

Contextual therapy (see Chapter 6, "Contextual Therapy") describes the invisible loyalties to the families of origin that deprive the family of procreation of the healthy entitlement to nurturance necessary for its developmental progression.

Acute or chronic family disintegration may result in the use of hospitalization to bring about temporary or prolonged realignment or reintegration of the family. Unfortunately, there has been a tendency in residential and hospital settings in the past to "adopt" the children rather than enhancing the capability of some of the families to reabsorb their children. The current emphasis on the combined use of family intervention in a hospital and residential setting can enhance the likelihood of the child's returning to the parents or foster parents and can interrupt the "extrusion" of the child as a way of coping with family dysfunction (see Chapter 29, "Family Intervention and Psychiatric Hospitalization").

An important task for family therapists is to enable family members to separate from their adolescent offspring. Few family therapists truly recognize the intricate network of developmental failures in the family and the adolescent that undermines the separation-individuation process. One of the finest examples of application of the separation-individuation process can be found in the investigations of Helm Stierlin (1974), who has described the modes of binding, delegating, and expulsion as three ways that families bring about a pathological separation in order to overcome their fear of prolonged fusion. In the binding mode, the excessive binding of the family can force the growing adolescent into a psychotic or suicidal behavior to free himself or herself from the family unit. In the expulsion mode, the adolescent is rejected and extruded by the family to achieve their goal of separation. The mode of delegation is an intricate one by which the family allows the adolescent to depart from the family unit "on a long leash" and to return periodically to share the tales of his or her exploits in order to compensate for the restricted life of the parents.

Application

Family intervention that includes children and adolescents has become an essential treatment modality in outpatient, inpatient, residential, and day treatment centers and in schools. In any of these services, the clinical space for seeing a family should be welcoming to the young children and adolescents and should combine many of the positive features of a living room, with additional possibilities for play activities. The interventions with families should address both the immediate and the long-standing family dysfunctional patterns. In addition to the resolution of conflict between family members, important goals include the enhancement of parent management skills and the resolution of parental individual psychopathology. Family therapy can prove an effective therapeutic intervention with acute disorders, particularly in a crisis situation for families with young children. However, the treatment of more serious and long-standing disorders, such as ADHD, conduct disorder, parental depression (and its impact on the children), and substance abuse in adolescents, may require a combination of family intervention with pharmacotherapy, marital therapy, individual therapy, or multimodal-multisystemic interventions. The theoretical concepts and strategies for dealing with depression, divorce, substance abuse, incest, and hospitalization are described in other chapters.

Frequently, family therapy with children goes through two phases. In the first phase, which may take approximately 10–20 sessions, the symptomatic behavior of the child becomes the focus of treatment and the child may oppose the treatment situation on behalf of the parents. This phase results in an improvement in the child's behavior through enhanced school performance, peer group relationships, sports activity, and interest in peers of the opposite sex. Encouraged by the therapeutic results with the child, the parents frequently develop a higher aspiration for the additional goals of improvement in marital dysfunction or resolution of parental psychopathology. This ushers in the second phase of treatment. At times, a third phase of the treatment can become necessary when one of the parents decides to pursue a more ambitious therapeutic goal in order to reach a higher level of productivity, maturation, and creativity.

A common phenomenon resulting in therapeutic mismanagement is when the parents succeed in diverting the therapeutic focus away from the initial goals for the children and into a premature exploration of marital complaints. This phenomenon can be a resistance against the child-centered phase of the treatment and can frequently result in diffusion of the therapeutic goals and in ineffective treatment outcome both with the child and with the parents' marital problems. Montalvo and Haley (1973) recommended that the therapist recognize the resistance in such maneuvers and refrain from entering into marital therapy until either the problem with the children is satisfactorily resolved or there is a clear recontracting for marital, rather than child-centered, family therapy. Frequently, family therapy with children can reveal the well-recognized phenomenon of child neglect by parents. When family support is potentially available, family intervention can result in mobilization and rehabilitation of resources to provide the child with the attention necessary to resume his or her developmental progression. When such resources are not present, it may be necessary to search for an alternative living situation with the help of the Department of Human Services, including departments of youth and families and foster and adoption services. Such therapeutic options may be particularly appropriate for children who are being considered for admission to a residential treatment center.

Family Therapy With Different Childhood Disorders

Conduct Disorders and Their Family Context

The high prevalence of conduct disorders in the general population and their occurrence in families with a history of antisocial personality, depression, or criminal behavior have been the focus of family-based investigations and interventions. The role of the parents in the genesis of antisocial behavior in the offspring was initially described by Johnson and Szurek (1952). The work of Minuchin et al. (1967) described the structural and functional deficiencies in families with aggressive children from a deprived socioeconomic background. Minuchin described conduct problems in both enmeshed and disengaged families, although the substantial part of the investigation of structural family therapists centered on working with enmeshed families.

A significant but underappreciated attempt at family therapy with adolescents with conduct disorder was undertaken by the Multiple Impact Therapy (MIT) group in Galveston, Texas (MacGregor 1962, 1967). The novel intervention by this group included two days of family therapy by a large group of professionals who alternated among different family members during the brief but intensive therapeutic encounter. Their classification system of dividing the children into groups of defiant, conduct disorder, prepsychotic, and "intimidated" youth predated the more recent classification systems and made a significant bridge between individual and family psychology. Their description of family dynamics in each of the four groups of adolescents is highly consistent with subsequent investigative findings about children who have conduct disorder or oppositional defiant disorder.

Coercive Family Processes and Parent Management Training

Patterson et al. (1982) used social learning theory to describe *coercive family processes* by which parents with poor management skills initiate overly punitive and aggressive reactions toward their children but withdraw in the face of strong opposition from the child. The coercive processes result in a high level of aggressive and uncontrollable behavior in the child. Patterson's more recent research (Patterson 1990a; Patterson and Chamberlain 1994) reported the relationship between aggressive behavior in the children and depression in the parents, particularly single mothers. The *parent management training* (PMT) programs developed by Forgatch and Patterson (1989) and Forehand and McMahon (1981a) provide the theoretical rationale and intervention methodology with this population (see Chapter 19, "Parent Management Training").

These families are generally burdened with an extensive history of antisocial and criminal behavior, alcoholism, substance abuse, depression, separation and divorce, disruption of education, unemployment, and related economic hardships. There is a high rate of family aggression that results in impulsive punitive parental reactions in excess of what can be justified by the child's behavior. The child's equally explosive and aggressive response to the parental intervention results in a retreat of the parents from the disciplinary course. The repetition of this process, entitled *coercive trap*, teaches the child that in the long run aggressive behavior can result in the withdrawal of punishment, which in turn reinforces the disruptive behavior in the child. Depression in the parents of children with conduct disorder commonly occurs as a result of failures in the parenting and further interrupts the parental management practices.

The intervention takes place primarily within the home situation, but its results can be generalized to school and other situations. *Parent management training programs* and *functional family therapy* have demonstrated effectiveness in the reduction of conduct disorders in adolescents and the prevention of conduct disorders in their siblings, as well as the reduction in parental depression and psychopathology (Sholevar 1995, 2001).

Functional Family Therapy

Functional family therapy (FFT) is a method of treatment for conduct disorder. This method, developed by Alexander and Barton (1976), integrates systems, behavioral, and cognitive intervention strategies. Its effectiveness has been demonstrated in a controlled research study of adolescent delinquents with status and index offenses. It has proven effective both in reducing recidivism rates (Alexander and Parsons 1973) and in reducing adolescent delinquent behavior (Friedman 1990). Functional family therapy views problems from the perspective of the *function* they serve in the family system. The research underlying FFT has shown that families with delinquents have higher rates of *defensive interactions* in the parent-child and parent-parent communications and exhibit a lower rate of mutual supportive interaction. The goal of treatment is to improve family communication by enhancement of supportive and reciprocal interactions among family members. The focus is on increasing the adolescent's social competence, problem-solving skills, self-regulations, and autonomy through positive family relationships. It addresses the total context, which includes the monitoring of behavior in the family, the peer group and its influence on the family interactions, and the adolescent's individual developmental needs.

Family Coordination

The investigations of Reiss (1971, 1982) have focused on the role of cooperation and cohesiveness in the family's *coordination*, which is related to the genesis of conduct disorders in the children. Their laboratory-based investigations have demonstrated the weaknesses of *coordination*—the ability of the family to see themselves as a group with unity—and *cooperation* in conduct-disordered families.

Multisystemic Therapy

Since 1990, greater attention has been paid to the complexity of conduct disorders, with significant emphasis placed on the interlocking systems, including individual, familial, peer-group, school, and neighborhood and community variables.

Multiple treatment interventions have addressed the multiplicity of factors that operate in a variety of disorders, including conduct disorder and substance abuse (Henggeler 1997; Henggeler and Schoenwald 1998; Henggeler et al. 1998a, 1998b; Liddle et al. 1995). The multisystemic therapy (MST) of Henggeler has been extensively studied in the past decade, although his approach has not yet been replicated by other independent investigators.

MST is an intensive family- and community-based treatment that addresses the multiple determinants of serious antisocial behavior in juvenile offenders. MST emphasizes that the adolescent is nested within a complex network of interconnected systems that encompass individual, family, and extrafamilial systems such as peers, schools, and neighborhoods. The interventions are intended to bring about change in the uses of natural environment by using the strength of each system. The major goal of each intervention is to empower parents with the skills and resources needed to independently address the difficulties that arise in raising teenagers, and to empower youth to cope with the family, peers, school, and neighborhood problems. The usual duration of treatment course is approximately 60 hours of contact over 4 months. The therapists carry a low caseload and are available to the family on a 24-hours-a-day, 7-days-a-week basis.

The treatment is based on a family preservation model of service delivery. The treatment outcome includes a significant reduction in long-term rates of rearrest; significant reduction in out-of-home placement; extensive improvement in family functioning; and decreased mental health problems for serious juvenile offenders. Even when placement out of the home has become necessary for the youth, the length of the stay has been below that of the comparison group.

Similar results have been reported with substance-abusing youth. The results, although encouraging, have not yet been replicated by other independent investigators.

Psychodynamic Approaches

Psychodynamic approaches in family therapy address the broad range of dysfunctions in family relations that can produce conduct disorders. A variety of events in the course of family development can result in *narcissistic* and distorted self-object relationships in the family. The narcissistic disturbances can include feeling insignificant, unloved, unworthy, and incompetent. A defensive grandiosity can be adopted to reduce the painful affects of being neglected, unloved, or abused. The interplay of such forces in the parents, between the parents, and between the children and parents can result in a maze of projective identifications, lack of empathy, and disregard for everyone's needs, including the children's developmental needs.

The interventions focus on defensive grandiosity (that has led to a child-environment mismatch) (Bleiberg 1995), distorted self-image, and the disturbed object representations that underlie the defensive interpersonal interactions. The feelings of being a victim of neglect, violence, and sexual abuse, and the attempts to victimize others as a way of identifying with the aggressor (A. Freud 1936/1966), are commonly observed in multiple family members and should be addressed repeatedly and sensitively. The goals of treatment are enhanced awareness and sensitivity of family members to each other's contemporary needs and protection of their relationship from distorted self-object representations that were based on past experiences and that made them overly self-protective and insensitive to the impact of their actions.

Attention-Deficit/Hyperactivity Disorder

In multiple studies of ADHD, Ritalin and other stimulant medications have produced a dramatic change in the on-task behavior of the child. Once the child has been medicated, the behavior of the mother exhibits the same dramatic change in terms of reduction in negative behaviors such as being critical and controlling. However, no increase in positive parental behavior, such as an increase in the level of praise and affection, has been reported with the use of Ritalin. Such parental behavior seems most responsive to family interventions rather than dependent on pharmacological agents. The family intervention can help teach parents to respond positively to their children by using praise, affection, and reinforcement (Goldstein et al. 1997; Wagner and Reiss 1995).

Nonshared Environment in Adolescent Development

In the comprehensive and well-designed study of *nonshared environment in adolescent development* (Reiss et al. 1994, 2000), researchers attempted to directly measure the environment to locate differences between siblings' exposure and experience and the impact of these differences on their development. They attempted to determine along which parameter siblings differ in their exposure to an experience of the environment and which shared or nonshared differences were associated with differential developmental outcomes in individuals.

This study included several hundred families that were divided into the following six groups: 1) those with monozygotic twins (siblings were 100% genetically similar); 2) those with dizygotic twins; 3) ordinary siblings in nondivorced families; 4) full sibs in stepfamilies (all 50% related); 5) half sibs in stepfamilies (25% genetically related); and 6) unrelated sibs in stepfamilies (0% related). Nonshared valuables could be any social, biological, or physical factors that affected psychological development. The environment measured here refers to the shared and nonshared environmental components that account for the portion of variance that remains after subtracting the variance accounted for by genetic factors and error (Reiss et al. 1994, 2000).

The emerging data suggested that at least certain nonshared variables had systematic influence on developmental outcomes (Dunn et al. 1990). For example, some data pointed to the importance of differential parenting between siblings. Children who received more affection and less control from their mothers were less likely to show signs of internalizing behaviors as rated by mothers. Children who received more paternal affection became more ambitious educationally and occupationally (Baker 1990; Reiss et al., in press).

Adolescent Substance Abuse

Significant developments in the treatment of substance abuse have been made and are described fully in Chapter 31, "Alcoholic and Substance-Abusing Families."

Acute and Chronic Medical Illness and Somatoform Disorders

Acute medical disorders are described in Chapter 2, "Structural Family Therapy," and Chapter 35, "Medical Family Therapy." Chronic medical illnesses in children and somatoform disorders are also described in Chapter 35.

Affective Disorders and Children of Depressed Parents

Both affective disorders and children of depressed parents are described in Chapter 28, "Depression and the Family: Interpersonal Context and Family Functioning."

Reaction of Children to Parental Divorce

The reaction of children to parental divorce is described in Chapter 23, "The Divorcing Family: Characteristics and Interventions."

Research

There have been an increasing number of controlled investigations using families of children and adolescents who have a variety of disorders. These investigations include family therapy for children with "psychosomatic disorders" (Minuchin et al. 1978); parent management training for children with conduct disorders (Forehand et al. 1981; Patterson 1982, 1992); and functional family therapy for families with delinquent children (Alexander and Parsons 1973). There have also been investigations of treatment effectiveness with substance-abusing adolescents (Chapter 31, "Alcoholic and Substance-Abusing Families"). The dramatic response of anorexic children to structural family therapy was reported by Minuchin et al. (1978). The replication of these findings by independent investigators has been quite limited, but the structural family approach has been adopted enthusiastically by a large number of family therapists who find this approach to be quite effective with young anorexic adolescents who still live at home. The application of this methodology to the older and more chronically disturbed populations with eating disorders has been unsubstantiated.

Parental management training (Patterson et al. 1982, 1992; Forehand and McMahon 1981a) and functional family therapy (Alexander 1973) have exhibited significant beneficial effects in adolescents with conduct disorder. Beneficial impact on the prevention of conduct problems in the siblings, and reduction of parental depression has also been noted. The PMT approaches of Patterson and Forehand have been successfully replicated by independent investigators in multiple settings.

Conclusion

Although family therapy started in the 1950s and was primarily rooted in the treatment of families of adult schizophrenic patients, a number of pioneering family therapists were keenly interested in the meaningful inclusion of the children in family treatment. Ackerman, Whitaker, and Minuchin influenced the practice of family therapy significantly by challenging practitioners to include young children and adolescents in family therapy sessions and so establish a true intergenerational dialogue. All schools of family therapy have made significant theoretical and technical contributions to the treatment of families with young children and adolescents. Frequently, the families present the children as the symptom bearers for family referral due to either the involvement of the schools or the relatively lower stigma of having a symptomatic child rather than an emotionally disturbed parent. However, in the process of effective family therapy, the children can quickly become asymptomatic and the marital dysfunction or parental psychopathology can become the center of a more prolonged treatment.

There has been a recent move to look beyond family therapy, to a combination of family intervention with individual treatment, psychopharmacotherapy, special education, peer group activities, and group therapy to enhance the remedial reach of the interventions. Multimodal and multisystemic approaches to treatment may be necessary for chronic and severe disorders.

Future directions in family therapy should differentiate between true family relational disorders involving children, and the impact of parental psychopathology on the younger generation. The latter phenomenon has been particularly well investigated with the phenomena of conduct disorders, depression, incest, and child neglect. Such an approach will facilitate preventive intervention with populations at high risk; such intervention programs have proven successful with children of parents with affective disorders (Beardslee et al. 1997).

Chapters on Related Topics

The following chapters describe concepts related to family therapy with children and adolescents:

- Chapter 14, "The Family Life Cycle: A Framework for Understanding Family Development"
- Chapter 18, "Family Therapy With Children: A Model for Engaging the Whole Family"
- Chapter 19, "Parent Management Training"
- Chapter 23, "The Divorcing Family: Characteristics and Interventions"
- Chapter 24, "The Remarried Family: Characteristics and Interventions"
- Chapter 28, "Depression and the Family: Interpersonal Context and Family Functioning"

- Chapter 31, "Alcoholic and Substance-Abusing Families"
- Chapter 32, "Family Intervention With Incest"

18

Family Therapy With Children

A Model for Engaging the Whole Family

Richard Chasin, M.D.
Tanya B. White, Ph.D.

Introduction

The diagnostic and therapeutic value of including children in family therapy is abundantly documented (Ackerman 1966; Augenbaum and Tasem 1966; Bloch 1976; Dowling and Jones 1978; Johnson et al. 1999; Keith 1986; Villeneuve and LaRoche 1993; Zilbach 1986). However, family therapists frequently avoid holding such meetings because they can be technically difficult (Johnson and Thomas 1999). This chapter focuses on concepts and methods to help the therapist meet that challenge. It also provides a model for a first

---

This chapter relies heavily on previously published work (Chasin 1981, Chasin and Roth 1990; Chasin and White 1988; 1989; Chasin et al. 1989; K.D. Fishman 1991). The authors are very grateful for the excellent editorial assistance of Linda Schwoeri.

family session. The concepts, methods, and model interview are intended neither as definitive theory nor as prescription for action, but as ideas that might inform any family therapy session that includes children.

Theoretical Concepts

Emphasis on Strengths and Goals

In the traditional medical model, the therapist begins the client contact by inquiring about the chief complaint and the presenting problem. However, in recent years an increasing number of family therapists have departed from this tradition and deliberately avoid an early focus on the family's problems. They strive from the opening moments to create a positive frame about the family and its therapy by reinforcing family strengths and discovering the family's goals for the future (de Shazer 1985; Johnson et al. 1999; Lipchik and de Shazer 1986; Penn 1985). The emphasis on future goals rather than past failures tends to establish a hopeful set and prevents the family from becoming mired in guilt, failure, and demoralization (Chasin and Roth 1990; Chasin et al. 1989).

This approach discourages *pathologizing*, *blaming*, and *scapegoating*. Family members who are usually named as the source of problems are thereby spared additional shame, alienation, and anger. This is particularly important for children, who often expect a family consultation to be a time when their deficiencies will be pointed out and they will be punished for them. In this new approach, when problems finally do emerge, they may be externalized (Epston 1989; White 1984, 1989, 1995). During family sessions, a boy who soils may not be called *encopretic* (the source of the problem), but rather he and his family are regarded as victims of encopresis. This framing prepares the family to attack a problem, not its members.

Therapeutic Alliance

It is frequently difficult for the therapist to establish and maintain an adequate therapeutic alliance with all family members, especially when they are at widely varying levels of development. With families, it is ordinarily safer to establish an alliance with the adults in a preliminary parent interview and to alert them that the family sessions may feel child centered. In the full family meetings, the therapist may then feel safe to emphasize the alliance-building effort with the children.

During the whole family sessions the therapist can endanger therapeutic alliances by being either too brilliantly successful or too miserably ineffective with the children. If unruly or reticent children are easily managed by the therapist, their parents may feel shamed and incompetent. However, if resourceful children are alienated, the therapist may find it hard to regain a positive alliance with any family member.

Developmental Esperanto

Esperanto was designed as a language that could be easily learned and used by people with different native tongues. It has never been broadly adopted. People at widely different developmental levels may share one language but not understand each other because they speak it differently. However, there are ways to bridge the communication barrier. In fact, virtually every important fact or idea for a clinical session can be shared simultaneously by children and adults through careful attention to language and the creative use of play. To include young children, one may need to use simple words and phrases, delivered in a somewhat higher pitch and volume. Brevity, repetition, and phrasing questions that require only simple answers (Snow 1972) are all useful strategies. The therapist can also take cues from the parents, many of whom understand quite well what type of language will provoke a response from their children (Benson et al. 1991; Garnica 1977; Stith et al. 1996; Taffel 1991; White 1982). When preschool children are present, we try to speak in a manner that a 3-year-old with average language abilities can understand. In some instances, play or pictures can augment verbal explanations.

> Two-year-old Jesse's mother had read to him *C Is for Curious: An ABC of Feelings* (Hubbard 1990). Afterward he exclaimed, "Tigger jealous!" when the family dog jumped on his mother while she was cuddling Jesse. His parents could effectively use the words *curious* and *jealous* when role-playing his feelings (and theirs) after he bit another child in his family day care program.

Therapeutic Contract: Explicit Rules, Expectations, and Agreements

It can be terrifying for anyone to play a game without knowing the rules, particularly if the stakes are high. We believe that the therapist should establish a contract about behavior during the family meeting. There are only a few sources available to the therapist who is interested in limit setting as a safeguard. In his writing about the psychoanalytic treatment of children, Moustakas (1959) encourages definitive limit setting to provide a sense of security to the child, stating that "limits provide the structure within which growth can occur." He suggests time limits as well as rules about safety, physical abuse, and leaving and returning to the room. Satir (1964), in discussing her conjoint work with parents and children, mentions a number of rules that should be followed during treatment to protect office equipment, as well as to provide structure during the sessions. Zilbach et al. (1972) comment that the therapist has the "obligation to set and enforce standards of behavior" (Lee 1986). Because lack of structure can generate anxiety and lead to normal but problematic insecurity in the adults and disruptive limit testing by children, we try in our contract to establish that

- There will be no coercion. All participants are free to not answer any question or follow any suggestion, except when the safety of people or property is at risk.
- Physical safety is the joint responsibility of everyone. Anyone can act to prevent physical harm in the session.
- The room and equipment belong to the therapist. The therapist decides what is used and how.
- Parents set all other limits for their children. Parents are asked to allow only what is permitted at home.

Further agreements may be made about confidentiality, videotaping, and other matters relevant to the session. Even after a contract has been made, it is important for the therapist to continue to be clear about structure, so that at any point in the meeting the family will know what the therapist wishes or expects them to be doing.

Therapeutic Environment

The therapist's office is not often addressed in the literature. This is unfortunate, because surroundings in the therapeutic situation may influence comfortable and open communication between adults and children. Offices that are specifically set up either for adults or for children are usually not good spaces in which to conduct whole family interviews. Rooms designed for adults may not be sufficiently childproofed, and the child may feel alienated by the formal furnishings and lack of toys. The parents and therapist will be nervous about delicate equipment that may be within the reach of naturally curious children. If the walls are thin, the therapist may inhibit useful but raucous exchanges during the family session so that people in the adjoining room are not distracted by the intruding noise.

Settings that are designed for individual child therapy often feel uncomfortable to adults, who may feel cramped in small chairs and uneasy about the presence of paints and clay that could soil the clothing they wore to work before the session. For most children, the abundance of exciting toys typically on display in such an environment is likely to be more fascinating than the interview process. The room is often too small for individuals and subsystems to establish comfortable distances from one another; crowding can be persistently stressful for disengaged families and can impede boundary formation with enmeshed families.

Layout

The best workspace is relatively bare and contains only moveable chairs and a few cushions (Bloch 1976; Chasin 1981; Zilbach 1986). An ideal office would probably include

- An *observation area* that is big enough to accommodate professionals and family members simultaneously, as well as keep recording equipment out of the reach of children.
- A *waiting room* with an adjacent bathroom that can serve as a time-out space. It should be cut off both visually and acoustically from all other areas so that family members can temporarily withdraw from the interviewing activity.
- A *discussion area* that is designed for discussion and quiet play. This space should be furnished with simple objects, such as moveable chairs and large pillows. It could comfortably accommodate children drawing or using hand puppets.
- A bare *play area* that is a safe place for large-scale play such as directed enactments and spontaneous wrestling.

Most of the toys and equipment should be kept out of sight. The therapist decides which ones to bring into the room, and when. Too often a therapist will assume an attitude of denial and passivity about an unsuitable workspace and will neither comment on it to the family nor attempt to do anything about it. Even when little can be done, it will foster the alliance with the family if the therapist points out the problems of the space and works with the family to minimize its hindrances.

Toys

In order to promote communication, toys should meet the following criteria:

- They should be *safe*. They should not be dangerous or make loud, frightening noises.

- They should lend themselves to play that children and grown-ups can all interpret.
- Generally, it is easier to make sense of what a child does with mother and father dolls or hand puppets than it is to find meaning in what he or she does with a device that generates colorful sparks.
- They should lend themselves to active and creative play rather than obsessive, repetitive routines. Although any toy can be used spontaneously or obsessively, some toys, such as checkers or even doll houses, may draw children away into evasive rituals. By contrast, a *bataka* (a fat, soft, harmless bat) rarely engenders that risk.
- They should promote interaction between children and adults. Baby dolls will usually serve that purpose better than will an intrinsically fascinating Nintendo game designed for children to use individually when alone. Building blocks can encourage cooperative construction of both fanciful and real environments, including floor plans of homes into which the family will move or the future apartment of a parent who is preparing to separate from the family.

Categories of Play

Therapists who work with young children rely on the revealing and therapeutic nature of the child's most natural activity: play. Yet, all play is not equally revealing or therapeutic. In this section we describe the types of play that we have found to be most illuminating and engaging in family sessions, emphasizing those forms of play that tend to be underused.

For the purposes of this discussion we classify play by three continua: *distanced-involved*, *nondirected-directed*, and *imaginative-factual*. Child therapists are typically trained to employ play techniques on the left side of these three continua: distanced, nondirected, and imaginative. Although these techniques have great value and are not to be abandoned in family work, we believe that techniques representing the right side are insufficiently used.

Distanced Versus Involved Play

Child therapy in the psychoanalytic tradition (Axline 1969; Winnicott 1971) tends to use drawing materials, clay, doll houses, and small rubber dolls in *distanced play*—play in which objects are often held at arm's length, literally, and sometimes experientially. Their manipulation by the child is interpreted by the therapist as revealing projection of intrapsychic or interpersonal issues. This interpretation then serves as the basis of intervention on the part of the therapist and the parents (Larner 1996). In the less-used *involved play*, which we advocate, the child *is* the toy and the action usually requires little interpretation. The child may play a role in an enactment using no toys, or perhaps (in a slightly distanced form) using only hand puppets (Gil 1994). Such play is particularly well suited for work with families, as it can be used by both children and adults, and it ordinarily communicates emotionally engaging information in an intelligible way.

Nondirected Versus Directed Play

There is a significant difference between directed play, the type of family therapy with children that we advocate, and nondirected play, traditional play therapy. By definition, *direct play* therapy requires us usually to be more directive. We will often decide when to play, what to play, how to play, who joins in, and who watches. Even with these decisions in the therapist's hands, there will be plenty of room for spontaneity. If the therapist is too nondirective, an impulsive family may become chaotic and a repressed one may be unable to act in the face of so much freedom. Individual child therapy with a psychodynamic orientation typically relies heavily on *nondirected play* techniques. Using this method, a therapist may provide a stockpile of materials and tell the child to do whatever he or she pleases with them. While potentially rich, the resulting play may require great patience and skillful interpretation. We encourage the use of *directed play* that is actively guided by the therapist. For instance a child might be asked to play a particular role in a specified scene: "You're Dad at the dinner table and your brother is Mom, who has just arrived home late from work. Make up a skit that shows us what would happen if your parents got along exactly the way your mother wants them to." This form of play is very efficient, pertinent, and informative in an individual or a family setting.

Imaginative Versus Factual Play

Imaginative techniques generally involve the playing out of fantasies. Children may become kings and queens, monsters or animals; they may travel to nonexistent planets or brave wild, terrifying jungles. In contrast, factual play documents the actions and feelings of real people as they are now or could realistically be in the future, as in the following example: "Dad, be your daughter, and Mom, be the dentist. Show us what will happen at her checkup next week." Factual play can be an easily comprehensible alternative to using words to explore real events.

The more traditional, distanced, nondirected, and imaginative types of play are certainly valuable in many therapy contexts, including that of family therapy. Free drawing, as outlined by Zilbach (1986), is an example. The children work on their drawings while the adults are engaged in conversation to which the nonparticipating children may be closely attuned. Through the drawings, children may express their concerns about family relationships and "communicate family issues that might otherwise remain underground, or at least take much longer to be raised by adults" (Zilbach 1986, p. 98). The drawings are interpreted both diagnostically and as clues to progress in family work.

However, there are many virtues to recommend the directed, involved, and factual type of play in the context of family therapy (Onnis et al. 1994). To the extent that play is directed, it is efficient and to the point. To the extent that it is involved, families become actively engaged and display high levels of energy. To the extent that it is factual, it is directly informative about everyday life.

Role-Playing

Role-playing usually exemplifies the three types of play that we have found most beneficial in family work: it is always involved, it is usually directed, and it lends itself to factual situations.

Many therapists who work with families have employed role-playing in some form or another (Bernal et al. 1972; Coppersmith 1985; Forehand 1977; Haley 1976; Madanes 1984a, 1984b; Minuchin 1974a; Neill and Kniskern 1982; Onnis et al. 1994; Papp 1981; and Satir 1964). In fact, this therapy has been used by representatives of most approaches to family work.

Particularly notable among its virtues are the enthusiasm with which family members impersonate each other and the honesty with which they represent everyday life as it affects them. Of course, in these impersonations, each family member may develop empathy for the person he or she plays and may gain fresh perspectives by observing his or her own behavior as it is played by those affected by it. The following vignette is an example of involved, directed, factual role-playing:

> In the initial contact with the parents, the therapist was told that the identified patient, Pat, age 9, was suicidal and intensely jealous of, and competitive with, her younger sister, Sue, age 6. Pat told her recently separated parents that she would remain silent in any individual or family session. After an initial interview with the parents that established an urgent need for accurate assessment, the therapist chose to see the girls together, assuming that Pat could not resist talking in the presence of Sue. After joining with both girls, the therapist introduced the idea that puppets could play the roles of family members. The girls became involved with the puppets

immediately. At first the tone of the play was humorous, with much joking about the puppets' messy hair. "I'm not looking my best today," Pat said on behalf of one puppet, giggling. Eventually each girl had a chance to play Mommy's response to Pat's unhappiness. Then the therapist, playing Pat, asked:

> **Therapist** [*as Pat*]: You know what I'm especially not happy about? Daddy's going away. Why did he go away?
> **Sue** [*as Mommy*]: I don't know. You'll have to ask him.

Pat later played herself and spontaneously stated that Daddy went away because he fought with Mommy too much. The therapist suggested that the girls do a "Mommy and Daddy fight."

> **Pat** [*as Daddy, with a deep, pompous voice*]: Did you see anything in the paper today about acid rain?
> **Sue** [*as Mommy, in an annoyed tone*]: Don't ask me that. I never look at the paper. You should know that by now!
> **Pat** [*as Daddy*]: Well, you'd better start looking.
> **Sue** [*as Mommy, angrily*]: Don't tell me what to look at.
> **Pat** [*as Daddy*]: You're my wife.
> **Sue** [*as Mommy*]: You shouldn't tell me what to do even though I am your wife. We're not related except by marriage. *[The parent puppets hit each other throughout the scene.]*
> **Therapist:** That was very good. Want to do another one?

At this point Pat decided to be Mommy. Sue stated that Mommy should start the fight this time.

> **Pat** [*as Mommy*]: What were you doing last night?
> **Sue** [*as Daddy, in a deep, long-suffering voice*]: Working at the office.
> **Pat** [*as Mommy, in a sarcastic tone*]: With Carla?
> **Sue** [*as Daddy*]: No, I was working with Bill.
> **Pat** [*as Mommy*]: He doesn't work there any more.
> **Sue** [*as Daddy, obviously evasive*]: I mean I was working with what's-his-name.
> **Pat** [*as Mommy*]: I'm going to get my hair done tomorrow. I expect you to stay with the girls.
> **Sue** [*as Daddy, importantly*]: No. I've got an appointment.
> **Pat** [*as Mommy*]: I'm going right now. Good-bye.
> **Sue** [*as Daddy*]: Pat, I want you to take care of Sue. I have to go to a conference.
> **Pat** [*as herself, with original little girl puppet, speaking in a high-pitched, panicky voice*]: No, you have to stay here.
> **Sue** [*as Daddy*]: Well, get Sue. We'll all go to the conference.
> **Pat** [*as herself*]: No.
> **Sue** [*as Daddy*]: Well, I'll have to put you in bed. *[The father puppet angrily stuffs the girl puppets in a box.]* Get in your bed. *[Starts to leave.]*

Pat *[as Mommy, just coming home, accusingly]:* What are you doing?
Sue *[as Daddy, defensively]:* Ah, just going to check on something outside. Now that you're here, mind if I go to the conference?
Pat *[as Mommy]:* I do mind! I just came back for my purse.

Discussion

The girls were highly attuned to the parental battle. Their mutual awareness that they had been abandoned by their angry, self-involved parents was now obvious. Pat's distress about having to care for her younger sister when she was not getting sufficient nurturing herself was also apparent. It was evident that Pat was not suicidal but that her self-destructive claims and behavior at home were a cry for help. The role-plays were highly informative to the therapist and to the parents, who saw a videotape of them. It also served to unite the sisters, because through helping, each became aware that the other knew what was going on in the family; neither was alone in her distress. The bonds between them were strengthened by this method of revealing their shared misery.

A Model Format for a First Family Session That Includes Young Children

The following model is presented as one way to prepare for and carry out a first interview with the whole family when a child is the identified patient. It is also intended to illustrate the theoretical concepts described above and to provide an example of positive attitudes, intelligible language, informative play techniques, clear structuring, and careful sequencing. All of these might be applicable to any family session that one might carry out at any stage of assessment or treatment, regardless of the initial presenting problem. The model covers nine phases: 1) preliminary contact with the parents, 2) orientation, 3) rule setting, 4) joining, 5) stating goals, 6) goal enactment, 7) optional enactment of undesired outcome, 8) problem exploration, and 9) reflections by the therapist and recommendations to the family.

Before the Family Session: Preliminary Contact With Parents

If at all possible, the initial phone call should involve both parents. Together, they can best provide information on which to base decisions about the first session. Most importantly, no matter who is the *index patient*, the therapist will need to decide during that phone call whether to begin by seeing the parents alone, the whole family, or some other individual or subgroup.

Usually, we begin with the parents (or other responsible adults). If symptoms are mild and acute, a single session with parents may be sufficient to empower them, through support and advice, to experiment successfully with fresh approaches to the problem. If so, the child may not be seen and thus will be spared the burden of clinical contact. If symptoms are severe or long-standing, a preliminary meeting with parents can be used to take a careful and extended history of the family and its past attempts to solve the problem. This information is most efficiently gathered without young children present. A preliminary meeting with parents also provides an opportunity for the therapist to assess the parents, particularly with respect to their commitment to the work that may lie ahead, and gives the parents an opportunity to ask questions and express concerns about the expected course of assessment and treatment.

There are many important exceptions to the parents-first rule. We usually see the family first if the initial phone contact or referral has indicated that 1) it is the family's wish to be seen first as a family; 2) adequate background information has been, or can be, transmitted over the phone, obviating the need for an initial parent interview; or 3) the parents feel secure enough to present the family directly to us. We may see a child first if the child so requests. Finally, we see a child or children without parents first in an emergency situation in which the parents are unavailable.

However, the therapist who interviews the parents first has already gathered considerable information and begun to establish an alliance with them. That therapist can afford to concentrate more on the children in the whole family sessions, because the parents, having already been seen, are less likely to feel neglected. The therapist will also be prepared by the parent session for some of the special problems and opportunities that will present themselves when the whole family is interviewed.

Orientation

During orientation, the therapist explains the reason for the family meeting. We have seen experienced therapists begin interviews by asking the children, "What did your parents tell you this meeting was about?" or "Why do you think we are here?" Sometimes parents had not prepared children at all for the meeting and occasionally had even lied to them about it. In those cases, the session got off to an awkward start, with the parents feeling exposed in their incompetence or dishonesty.

We prefer that the therapist begin the session by introducing himself or herself and asking the family members how they would like to be addressed. Once introductions are over, the therapist takes responsibility for the session by immediately telling the family members why he or she has assembled everyone and what it is that they can expect. This requires the therapist to disclose the substance of prior contacts with the parents and other informants and to indicate the purpose of the whole family session.

> **Therapist** *[to each parent and then to each child]*: What name would you like me to call you? *[Family members reply. Mother is Ellen and Father is Dan. Children are Eric, age 7, and Polly, age 5.]*
>
> **Therapist** *[to everyone]*: My name is Dr. Alexander. You may call me Alex if you would like to. My work is to help families find ways to make things better for themselves when everything is not all right. Ellen and Dan called me on the phone the other day and told me that you have a good family but that everyone in the family was unhappy in some way. They said Polly has been sad and has scary dreams. They told me that her teacher says she is unhappy in school, too. When I heard all that, I asked Dan and Ellen to visit me here in this room.
>
> **Therapist** *[continuing]*: We met a few days ago and talked about Polly. They said they were also a little worried about Eric, who seems angry a lot. They even said they themselves disagreed a lot with each other and fought sometimes. After we talked, I told them that I would like to meet with everyone in the family. What we are going to do here today is to talk and play so that you can find new ways for the family to be happier.

In this opening step, the content that is shared and the simple phrasing that is used by the therapist are designed to model respectful candor and reflect the therapist's wish that all members of the family understand and participate in the meeting. A conscious effort should be made throughout the sessions to ensure that each member of the group is treated with equal respect. If the parents or older children talk over the heads of the younger ones, the therapist can indicate that full engagement of the children is important by translating the remarks made by older family members into language the children can understand.

> **Father:** My wife and I have difficulty coordinating our schedules to accommodate the children's need to be chauffeured to their various activities. We have had many discussions with them about taking responsibility for being ready on time but we still receive little cooperation.
>
> **Therapist** *[to the children]*: Dad says he and Mom work hard to be able to take you to your lessons. They want you to be all set to go when one of them is ready to drive you somewhere.

Contracting

Whether or not some contract was made in a prior parent session (and we would hope it was), the therapist and the family now need to agree on rules for the session. The therapist should explicitly set out the rules we have outlined in the section titled "Theoretical Concepts" for the whole family. At the minimum, it is wise to make agreements about noncoercion, safety, limit setting, and the use of the space and equipment (Lee 1986).

> **Therapist** *[to everyone]:* Before we begin I want to suggest some rules.
> First, you should not answer a question or do anything I ask unless you feel ready to do it. If you do not feel ready to answer a question or do something I ask, just don't do it. It will be all right. If you wish, you can tell me that you are not ready by saying *pass* or *not now* or something like that.
> The second rule is that we all try to make sure that everyone is safe. If somebody is doing something that might cause a cut or a bruise, anyone here can help to stop it from happening.
> The third rule is that I decide which of my toys we can use and when we can use them.
> The last rule is that Dan and Ellen are responsible for deciding how Eric and Polly behave. If Eric or Polly does something that is not allowed at home, then Ellen and Dan should do here just what they would do at home.

After suggesting each rule the therapist asks, "Is that clear and OK?" and then waits for agreement before proposing the next rule. In some cases, the therapist may also need to make agreements about other matters, such as confidentiality and videotaping. It is indeed a challenge to establish boundaries and define expectations briefly enough not to exhaust the patience of the family but clearly enough so that the rules are understood by everyone who can possibly comprehend them.

Without rules the family may experience iatrogenic anxiety and their behavior can be distressing and misleading. For example, we have seen children so badgered by an ordinarily permissive parent to "answer the doctor's question" that the doctor regrets ever having asked it. With the *noncoercion* or *pass* rule in place, the therapist can say, "Your son has just passed. Thank you for trying to help me, but it is my problem, not yours. I need to think of questions he is ready to answer."

Joining

After the rules are established, the therapist can begin to interact more extensively with the family. The word *joining* rather than the phrase *alliance building* has been used by family therapists for this early period of exchange because the therapist does not simply ally, but *temporarily* becomes part of the family, or, more precisely, becomes a member of a new system, the therapist-family system (Minuchin 1974a, 1974d). While many therapists tailor their joining methods to each individual family, we almost always join by asking family members to tell us their strengths. By always using the same approach, we learn a great deal from families right away because we can apply a yardstick of extensive comparable experience. Furthermore, this method is almost always agreeable to families, and it starts the session off on a distinctly positive note.

> **Therapist** *[to everyone]:* If I am going to help you find a way to figure out how to make things better, I first need to know what *power, strength, and ability* you all have. I'll ask each of you to tell us about something that you are good at doing, something that you know how to do and are proud about. I'd like to start with Eric.
> **Eric:** I have good friends.
> **Therapist:** What is it about you that makes it possible for you to have good friends?
> **Eric:** Kids like me. I don't tell them lies and junk.

The father might mention that he works hard and supports his family no matter what. Mother might indicate that she too is a hard worker and that she protects her children. The daughter might say she is nice, that she is no trouble to anyone.

The therapist continues until each of the family members has described two or three positive characteristics. Young children often interpret this inquiry as referring to things they like, rather than to abilities. However, for anything a child likes, the therapist can suggest a skill that such a preference reflects. For example, if the child says he likes to run, the therapist might ask whether he or she is fast.

When this mode of joining is used, *the family is relieved that the therapist is not dragging out the worst problems immediately.* Indeed, the family's morale is enhanced by discussing its strengths. In multiproblem families with poor self-esteem, especially if the family is poor and a member of a minority, the members may expect disrespectful treatment from therapists. They are sometimes deeply moved when a therapist is interested in celebrating their strengths.

Stating Goals

Once rules have been agreed on and rapport has been established through joining, the interview may go in one of a number of directions. Some interviewers prefer to work in an organic, seamless way, without predesigned, well-demarcated, explicit steps. They may use something that happened in the rule-setting or joining phase as a springboard to the next topic. We prefer to maintain clear expectations and to state precisely what we are attempting to do in each phase of the interview. Although it probably does not matter just how obviously the interviewer changes direction, the choice of the next step is vital for the success of the evaluation.

At this point, most clinicians ask the family to say what the problem is. Some therapists think that unless one starts with and maintains a focus on *the problem*, the family will lose its motivation. However, we believe that even after effective joining, many family members still feel quite unsafe. By focusing on the problem now, the therapist may foster a negative set in which people will feel guilty, demoralized, and inept. Such a negative set, especially at this delicate juncture, endangers hopefulness and may undermine the family's exercise of its strength. Other therapists might assign the family a general, exploratory, standardized task (e.g., Burns and Kaufman 1972) designed to reveal some aspect of family functioning or self-perception. There are many such exercises available to therapists. The difficulty with using one at this time is that family members may not grasp the object of performing a task that may seem totally unrelated to their distress.

A less risky step than moving to problem exploration, and one that is more obviously pertinent than most standardized tasks, is to ask the family members to *specify their goals*. Experienced clinicians know that such a task is often extremely difficult to accomplish. Families are much more likely to be obsessed with their distress than they are to have specific objectives in mind. Furthermore, many members are eager to complain to the therapist and are in the habit of attacking one another. In short, they may not be in a mood to be goal directed. Undoubtedly, this is true for some families. Nonetheless, seeking out family goals early in the evaluation has so much to recommend it that we think it is the best next step in most situations. For example, a 10-year-old, wishing for more closeness in a family that spends very little time together, may have as a goal that the family will eat dinner together more often. Her wish may open the door to the expression of longings by other family members and may stimulate in the therapist's mind hypotheses about general family needs and ideas about potential interventions. Since eliciting goals is more easily said than done, we offer a few guidelines:

1. *The instructions should be clear and the task simple to fulfill.* For example, the therapist may say, "I am going to give each person a chance to tell me one or two ways the family can be better than it is now. Remember what I said about the rules. You don't have to say anything if you don't

want to. But each of you will have a chance if you want it. Who would like to start by saying one way the family could be better?"

2. *Statements of goals are most helpful when they are concrete enough to be imagined and general enough to have some breadth of meaning.* The therapist may need to reframe the young child's overspecificity ("So you want a stuffed animal, something warm and cuddly like a stuffed animal"). The therapist may also lead adults from the general toward the specific ("Could you try to tell us what might happen if, as you say, there was no more fighting?").
3. *The therapist should encourage each family member to turn any complaining or blaming into a goal.* For example, a complaining sibling may be told, "You don't want your brother to hit you. OK. What do you want him to do instead?"
4. *The therapist should remove all pressure for comprehensiveness,* as in this example: "You don't have to say all the ways things could be better now. You'll have plenty of chances to tell me about other things later."
5. *The therapist should not pressure the family for completion of the task if any of the following conditions apply:*

- They seem incapable of putting anything in a positive frame, even after gentle encouragement.
- The task seems to undermine their motivation—for example, if a peripheral father says, "How can we talk about dreamland stuff when these savages are destroying the family?"
- The family is going through overwhelming stress (e.g., the recent death of one of its members) and it seems insensitive or disrespectful to deal in "desires." In such situations the therapist might move ahead to *problem exploration*, saying, for example, "I don't think it was such a good idea for me to ask you first about what you want. What I think we should do instead is find out what it is that you are not happy about in your family. Afterward, we can talk about what will make you happier."

Goal Enactment

Once goals have been stated, the therapist can direct enactments of those goals—set the scene of a desired future. Ideally, separate enactments will be directed for each member's goals. The enactment of goals has distinct advantages. First, it promotes specificity and concreteness of objectives. When it is demonstrated what the family might look like and sound like when the goals are met, everyone can have exactly the same image of what each person wants. That image will be "worth a thousand words." Second, it gives the family members a chance to rehearse how they want to be without necessarily feeling pressured to change in that way. For example, the therapist may say, "Remember how your son showed us the way he wanted you to help him make things. Of course, this may not have anything to do with the problem you came about, and it may not be anything that we are going to work on in therapy, but let us complete the exercise anyway."

Suppose Johnny's goal is for the family to get him a stuffed animal. The therapist can encourage enactment by saying, "Johnny, you don't have to be fancy. You think the family would be better if you had a stuffed animal. That's a fine goal. Here is a pillow. Make believe it is a stuffed animal. Can you show me who would give it to you, what you would do with it, and how the family would be better if you had it? Let's start with who would give it to you." If he points to his mother, the therapist may say, "Make believe you are your mother and that your mother is you. Give her the animal just the way you would want her to give it to you."

In some situations the therapist may decide against separate enactments and instead design and direct the family in a single role-played minidrama that incorporates the goals stated by each family member. Even though inventing and directing such a dramatized integration of family goals is often difficult, it may deeply engage the family and sometimes appears to foster rapid change. The following vignette provides an example of such an enactment (Chasin and White 1988; Fishman 1991):

> George, 11, the index case patient, seemed depressed to his parents and teachers. In the second phase of the interview, each family member stated goals. Father said he wanted George to show more enthusiasm as an indication that he wasn't depressed. Mother wanted the boys to help at mealtimes and wanted dinner to be calmer, with intellectual exchanges and no fighting. She wanted Alice to sleep through the night instead of having nightmares and coming to her bed. George wanted his brother, Bill, to do more with him.
>
> The therapist constructed and directed a scene in which the family's goals have been achieved. He did this by explaining privately to each family member what role he wanted him or her to play. For example, Bill was instructed to show interest in George's ideas if the family included George in their discussion. No family member knew what the whole scenario would look like until it was played out. The enactment proceeded as follows:
>
> The whole family is at home. George has arrived and is expressing to his father and Bill wild enthusiasm about his recent visit to a computer fair. Bill says he is eager to go there with George the next day. The mother, on that cue, announces dinner and thanks the boys for preparing it. During dinner the father mentions a newspaper article about someone who attempted murder and was released on $500 bail. Everyone has something to say about the event.
>
> The therapist dims the lights for bedtime. Alice lies down on a couch with a blanket, as if safe in her bed. The therapist assures her that she is very

comfortable. She now overhears the rest of the family talking softly about how nice it is that she has been sleeping through the night recently. Her father jokes that the electric bills are lower; her mother and both brothers comment on how good it is that they can all get a good night's sleep now and that Alice is so grown up.

When the therapist turns up the lights and announces that it is morning, Alice bounds excitedly from bed and rushes to her mother to tell her about a wonderful dream she had that night about swimming without her water wings.

When the enactment was over, the family members seemed lighthearted and pleased with themselves. Following some further exploration of family problems, the therapist told them that there was no need for further meetings at this point. At follow-up 4 months later, George's and Alice's symptoms had disappeared. However, the father seemed depressed and unenthusiastic about his work—he had been putting off a career decision for a year.

As in the following case, a goal enactment scene can lead quite naturally into an effective therapeutic intervention (Fishman 1991).

Andrew and Ted—the two older brothers of out-of-control, 4-year-old Bobby, who was affected by encopresis, wished that he would grow up so that they could play with him.

> **Dr. Chasin** *[to the older boys]:* You want him to go to the bathroom like a big boy, and you want to talk to him like a big boy, and you want to play with him like a big boy. So you want him to be part of your club, huh? You have a big boys' club in your house.
> *[Dr. C asks Bobby to stand on a chair and show them how tall he would like to be. The brothers seem pleased when Bobby climbs up.]*
> **Dr. C:** Now let's make believe you're very big, OK? And see what happens. *[Dr. C, Andrew, and Ted all kneel down.]* Now let's turn it upside down; let's make believe that Andrew is the baby. *[Andrew and Ted regressively begin to roll around on the floor and hit each other with pillows.]*
> **Dr. C** *[to Bobby]:* OK, now look at those babies, look how they're carrying on. You can tell them to stop because you're bigger.
> **Bobby:** Stop! Stop! *[The older boys stop immediately.]*
> **Dr. C** *[to Andrew]:* Now pretend to poop in your pants.
> **Dr. C** *[to Bobby]:* You tell him what to do.
> **Bobby:** Do it inside the toilet! *[Andrew pretends to obey.]* Now pee-pee in the toilet. *[Andrew and Ted pretend to pee, giggling.]*
> **Bobby** *[continues commandingly]:* Hold it! Hold it! *[They stop.]*
> **Dr. C** *[standing next to Bobby while coaching him]:* You're a terrific grown-up.
> *[Andrew and Ted resume hitting each other with pillows.]*
> **Bobby:** No more hitting. *[The boys freeze.]*
> **Dr. C:** They're getting good at holding it.

Soon afterward the therapist suggests an enactment that he thought might lead to an understanding of Bobby's dilemma and greater bonding among the somewhat disengaged sibling subsystem. The therapist suggests they play "a very strange game called *Poops*; everyone is a *poop* in this game." He suggests that they all jump into a make-believe toilet.

> **Dr. C:** We're all poops. What happens after we go down the toilet?
> **Andrew:** We drown. Aaah. *[All three boys have jumped off a bench onto the floor, where they roll around, laughing, bobbing up and down.]*
> **Dr. C:** We're swimming in the sewer somewhere. *[The boys collide, squealing.]*
> **Ted:** Watch out what you're doing! Look out.
> **Dr. C:** We're going into the ocean. Did you ever swim in the ocean?
> **Andrew:** Yes.
> **Dr. C:** I bet you didn't know poops had this much fun after they left the toilet. *[The boys continue to bump into each other.]*
> **Andrew:** Get off me, you poop.
> **Dr. C:** I want to interview each of these poops. Now did you go into a toilet?
> **Andrew:** Yep, I almost drowned.
> **Dr. C:** You almost drowned, but what happened? You seem to be quite alive right now. Did you go into the ocean?
> **Andrew:** No, I think I've been resting in the sewer drain for about 50 years. I'm almost faded, you see.
> **Dr. C:** I see, you don't have quite a good color. Now what about you?
> **Ted:** I am an old hand. I've been in the sewer for about 30 years. Sixty years!
> **Dr. C:** All right, and are you a poop over here? Did you go into that toilet, poop?
> **Bobby:** Yes, I just went down a big tube, yesterday.
> **Dr. C:** And what's at the bottom of the tube?
> **Bobby**: Poops. *[The three boys laugh and jump on one another.]*
> **Dr. C:** All his brother poops. A whole family of poops.

The encopresis stopped soon after the session.

Optional Alternative to Goal Enactment

Some families will not enact goals but are willing to create a scene that shows how things will be in the dreaded future if nothing changes. This alternative can be painful, but is almost always worth the strain. In role-playing the *dreaded future*, the same principles and practices of enactment apply as in the enactment of an improved future. The principal virtue of enacting the dreaded future is that it provides detailed information about the family's current problems without blaming anyone for past or current misdeeds. It is usually a nightmare fantasy, not a damning, well-documented indictment.

A secondary benefit is that explicit visions of a dreaded future defeat denial and stimulate motivation for change.

If the therapist feels that one of these enactments turned out to be the maligning of a particular family member, the therapist may invite that person to set the record straight, that is, indicate how the *maligning* version may seem unfair and misleading. Ordinarily, however, it is best to allow these *enacted fears* to stand unchallenged and to remind the family that these worries are simply concerns about the future and not portrayals of actual current or past events. If the therapist does permit protests about *unfair representations*, corrections should be briefly stated and not pursued.

In the following vignette, fears about the future were of paramount concern. Only a few symptoms of anxiety existed at the time the family sought therapy.

> The mother requested a consultation for herself and her anxious 3-year-old daughter, Beth, who in the next few weeks would be facing several events, which the mother felt Beth could handle separately. In combination, however, these events threatened to overwhelm the little girl. Beth was to witness her single mother giving birth to a sibling; lose a grandparent to illness; visit her divorced father, who had just moved to another city; and face a few other new and potentially frightening experiences.
>
> At first the mother played Beth going from one event to the other, getting increasingly frightened and flustered. Beth laughed, but showed interest and curiosity. Beth said she would like to try playing out these occurrences. The therapist suggested that she use toys and puppets to enact her role in each event, in the order in which the events were likely to occur. The therapist used different parts of the room to symbolize each event and walked Beth through them in sequence. Beth then reenacted each one by herself, with a sense of relaxation and mastery over her anticipated itinerary. It was like learning a nursery rhyme. Enacting and reenacting the dreaded future functioned as a desensitizing, therapeutic intervention.

Problem Exploration

By the time the phase of exploration occurs, the therapist already has a great deal of information. Family members have discussed their strengths, expressed their wishes, and experienced their goals psychodramatically. Thus, the phase of problem exploration can begin with a sense that the therapist is informed and the family feels understood. Furthermore, the therapist is in a good position to determine what kind of problem exploration will be most likely to succeed with the family. One object of this phase is for the therapist to fill in whatever gaps of information remain after the prior phases. By the end of the problem exploration phase, the therapist should have answers, or at least good hunches, about the following (White 1989, 1995):

A Model for Engaging the Whole Family

- Whether there exists a problem requiring urgent attention
- What principal cycles or redundant sequences of behavior are associated with family distress or developmental impasse
- When and in which contexts these problems emerge, and where and when they do not emerge
- What attempts have been made to solve problems and with what results
- What beliefs seem to prevent the family from discovering a solution
- The degree to which the family has been able to frame the problem as an external force that oppresses all its members

In most instances, this phase should begin either with a relatively non-threatening but revealing family task or with a series of inquiries in which each family member is asked to describe the problem, when it arose, where and when it is most and least evident, who plays a role in it, how it affects the family, what each family member thinks about it, and what has been done to resolve it. This exploration would include the therapist's attempt to create with the family a description of the problem not as a problem originating from one member but as an agent that burdens the whole family.

Reflections and Recommendations

At the end of the whole family interview process, which may take one to three separate sessions, the family members need to learn what the therapist thinks of them and what to do next. Such a statement should not be put together hastily. It is often useful to take time-out before composing it. Some family therapists work with a co-therapist or even a team that brainstorms together. The therapist, and sometimes the whole team, will impart their reflections and suggest possible ways to proceed.

A closing statement will ordinarily include the following:

- Respectful acknowledgment of the family's strengths
- A brief summary of the family's wishes and fears
- At least two or three hypotheses that benignly connect the family's current problems with well-intended (but currently ineffective) family patterns of thought and behavior
- An externalizing description of the problem that can mobilize all family members to act in opposition to it
- One or two suggested courses for future action, with a brief rationale for each

In the case of Pat and Sue, a closing statement to the family might have included the following:

This is a family in which everyone seems very bright and thoughtful. However, everyone may be upset now that Father has gone to live apart from other family members, and everyone wants to feel less frightened, angry, and insecure. When you [Father and Mother] separated, much happened that caused you to fight more with each other and ignore your children. Good friends became so worried about each of you that they told you each to "look after yourself," sometimes causing you to be less considerate of others in your family. But this attention to yourselves got out of hand at times and became like an octopus with a tentacle grip on every family member, squeezing thoughtful and generous feelings out of them. It even affects Pat and Sue, who are now less helpful to each other. There are a number of ways you may be able to struggle against this octopus and be kind to yourselves and to others at the same time. As you do this, you may feel less lonely and sad. I think that Mom and Dad need a therapist to help them loosen the grip of the octopus while they learn how to live apart. I think the girls understand the family situation very well and can work together with a therapist to find their own ways to fight off the octopus and the fear and sadness that comes with it.

Conclusion

In this chapter we have offered theoretical concepts and demonstrated specific methods to guide the family therapist when including young children in therapy sessions. Although young children can be challenging, the rewards to be gained from their involvement are considerable. These benefits depend on having an office with an adaptive layout that has been properly prepared with appropriate toys, and a skilled and sensitive therapist who can provide structure, emphasize strengths, build an alliance with all members of the family through clear, simple language, and encourage everyone to be involved in setting goals and discovering ways to undo obstacles to achieving them. We recommend using play techniques that are involved, directed, and factual in the family sessions so that everyone understands everyone else, no matter how diverse the developmental levels. Role-playing, while sometimes hard to perform, is almost always easy to understand, allowing each family member's fears, hopes, and perceptions to become known to everyone else in the room without interpretation by the therapist. We have described a model for a first family session with young children that maintains a positive set, emphasizing family strengths and externalizing problems. It contains the steps of *contracting, joining, stating goals, enacting goals* (or an alternative, *exploring problems*), and *making a summary reflection and recommendation*. We hope that the concepts, methods, and the model presented here will help clinicians who have had reservations about conducting a family session with young children feel more confident to do so now.

19

Parent Management Training

Ellen Harris Sholevar, M.D.

Introduction

Children and adolescents have always broken laws and committed crimes. Throughout history, their punishments parallelled those meted out to adults and the law made few distinctions between adult and child offenders. Similarly, there was little concern about the motivation for offenses.

Development of Psychoanalytic Theories of Behavior

At the turn of the century, Sigmund Freud and a number of other pioneers proposed new ways of conceptualizing and understanding human behavior, models that became the influential psychoanalytic theory of our times. They focused on subjective, intrapsychic conscious and unconscious processes while de-emphasizing family and societal influences. Freud concerned himself primarily with the treatment of adults, but his followers, including his daughter Anna Freud, began to develop treatment strategies for children and adolescents that were based on modifications and refinements of the same psychoanalytic principles. As a result of this movement, there was increased interest in the etiology of antisocial acts of children.

Increase in Studies of Antisocial Behavior in Youth

In 1935, August Aichorn wrote a pioneering book entitled *Wayward Youth* (Aichorn 1935), which for the first time began to look at causes and offer a formulation of the aggressive and antisocial offenses of children and adolescents. This was followed by *Searchlights on Delinquency: New Psychoanalytic Studies*, edited by Kurt Eissler (1949). In 1951 Fritz Redl and David Wineman wrote *Children Who Hate: The Disorganization and Breakdown of Behavior Controls* (Redl and Wineman 1951). Redl and Wineman described the failure of ego controls in these conduct-disordered youth and documented success in treating adolescents in a residential treatment setting. The following year, Johnson and Szurek (1952) described the "superego lacunae" that were transmitted through the families of antisocial youth. Despite the exciting developments in the young field of child and adolescent psychiatry and psychology, the enthusiasm of these new ways of understanding child and adolescent behavior gave way to disillusionment about the effectiveness of psychoanalytically oriented approaches in treating this difficult group of youngsters. The juvenile justice system continued to apply the harsh solutions of a penal model to punish or reform the majority of youthful offenders.

Development of Social Learning Theories

Working with a different theoretical orientation, Homans (1961) in social psychology, Sullivan (Zaphiropoulos 1985) in psychiatry, and Skinner (Bachrach 1985) in experimental psychology all made seminal contributions in their modeling and aggression studies. Bandura (1973) then consolidated their findings into social learning theory. Social learning theory, however, was primarily concerned with the behavior of mentally healthy individuals. In an effort to provide more effective treatment, later researchers refined and modified this theoretical model to the study of antisocial youth.

In the first chapter of *Coercive Family Processes*, Gerald Patterson (1982) described his early training in a variety of techniques that were relatively ineffectual and the impact that reinforcement theories, social learning theories, and operant psychology had on his thinking about the aggressive children he studied. He later adapted Bandura's social learning approach and developed coercive family process theory to explain the aggression seen in the children studied by the group at the Oregon Social Learning Center (OSLC).

Development of Parent Training Strategies

Other investigators (Forehand and McMahon 1981a) independently developed similar therapeutic strategies based on training parents. Kazdin (1996) termed the parent management training (PMT) approach "highly promising" in the treatment of conduct disorder and noted that "no other technique for conduct disorder has been studied as often or as well in controlled trials as has PMT" (p. 85).

Family Dysfunction in Conduct-Disordered Youth

Studies reveal family dysfunction in conduct-disordered (CD) youth. Children and adolescents with conduct disorders have families who differ from those of non-CD children in a variety of ways. Children of parents with major affective disorders showed an increased rate of behavior problems (Beardslee et al. 1983). Mothers and fathers of children with conduct disorders showed increased rates of antisocial personality disorder, and fathers were more likely to abuse substances (Lahey et al. 1988). Mothers showed higher scores on Minnesota Multiphasic Personality Inventory (MMPI) scales assessing antisocial behavior, histrionic behavior, and disturbed adjustment (Lahey et al. 1989). These families lacked family management skills (Loeber and Dishion 1983; Rutter and Giller 1983). How does this family dysfunction mediate oppositional-defiant and CD behavior in youth in the family? The section below offers an answer to this question.

Coercive Family Process Theory

Gerald Patterson (1982) used a social learning model to elucidate what he termed *coercion theory* and shifted from thinking about learning to thinking about performance—that is, describing present conditions that led to aggression. In addition, sophisticated multivariate techniques were needed for organizing concepts and specifying which ones were related. Structural equation modeling was cited by Patterson as a statistical tool. Patterson and other investigators (Forehand et al. 1981; Patterson 1982) documented that antisocial children were more aggressive in *bursts* or *chains*, and that this aggressive behavior was intended to have an impact on another person and was not random but contingent. Parents of CD children exhibited a higher rate of aversive behavior toward their children and gave poorly formulated and poorly delivered commands often delivered in a threatening or angry way. A lower rate of positive attention to the child's prosocial behaviors was seen in these parents. Patterson postulated that the function of the behavior of the coercive child is to terminate aversive intrusions by other family members, a negative reinforcement model that led to the "coercion trap" and began to change the family structure and lead to serious long-term problems.

Patterson gave central importance to aversive events that were frequent and often of low amplitude. He postulated that within the family, these were the building blocks that, over time, lead to more serious aggressive behaviors. Similarly, he emphasized the attributions and state of arousal that predispose to aggressive behaviors. The term *nattering* was used to describe threatening or scolding by parents that did not lead to punishment. Nattering and beatings were used frequently by parents of antisocial children. In contrast, more effective parents either ignored or took effective steps to stop coercive child behavior.

According to Patterson, the irritable behavior in families with antisocial children is a bilateral trait; in other words, the interaction between the parent and the child is both a "style of interacting with people" and "a means of coping with problems." It was not clear whether this pattern occurred in settings outside the home. Studies in the home over a 1-year period suggested a high degree of consistency in the following types of adverse behaviors: counterattack, punishment acceleration, and continuance. *Crossover* referred to the increased probability that the family members of antisocial children would respond to a neutral or prosocial behavior with an attack. The problem child was most likely to start a conflict with the mother, by a ratio of 2 to 1 over other family members. There was also a high probability that once a family member attacked, another family member would counterattack. This was observed most often between the parents and the problem child in the family and was much less significant in child-sibling interactions. In *punishment acceleration*, a negative exchange was followed by a behavior that increased the probability that another deviant behavior would follow. *Persistence* was the tendency for *chains* or *bursts* of aversive events to continue regardless of the reaction of other family members. Once this process began, the basic structure of the interactions between family members was altered.

Robinson and Jacobson (1987) pointed out, "Coercion theory is concerned with the temporal sequence of events that constitute the topography of family interaction, and not with the internal structuring of information." Modeling is not invoked as a cause. Patterson de-emphasized cognitions, agreeing with Freud that most people cannot give a good reason for their behavior. Patterson quoted Bem (1967) as demonstrating that changes in behavior are more likely to determine changes in attitude than the reverse.

Patterson was also influenced by Bronfenbrenner's (1977) concept that family interactions occur in an "ecological matrix." Patterson cited factors such as grandparental discipline practices, stress, transition, marital adjustment, parental social disadvantage, troubled neighborhoods, and parental psychopathology that provided "setting events." "Setting events" (Kantor 1959) lead to "coercive processes" and a breakdown of the "consistent and contingent" parental approach essential for fostering prosocial behaviors.

Coercion and Neglect Model

Wahler and Dumas (1987), who viewed the family antecedents of conduct disorder in a somewhat different way, defined a coercion and neglect model. They viewed categories of child problem behavior as either conduct or dependency problems with overt and covert subtypes. The irritable parent living in an irritable community context with an irritable infant was likely to engage with the child in a coercive and inconsistent way. This produced a child with overt conduct problems. An unresponsive infant with an irritable parent became a child with overt dependency problems. When there was an unresponsive parent living in an unresponsive community with an irritable infant, a neglectful pattern of interaction and covert conduct disorder developed. They postulated that the same situation with an unresponsive infant produced a covert dependency problem. Wahler and Dumas (1987, p. 620) postulated new principles of stimulus-response:

> In our opinion, two functions are likely to be documented: (a) An "uncertainty" principle may account for some aspects of the child's coercive interpersonal style. According to our view of the principle, children react to indiscriminate parental attention as aversive stimuli. When faced with this sort of social context, a child will resort to those behaviors that generate predictability. Of course, coercive responses such as nagging and yelling are highly effective means of capturing predictable forms of parental attention, typically of the unkind nature. (b) If we remove time as a dimension of triadic operations, it may prove useful to conceptualize setting-event functions as instances in which maternal response is governed by the relational properties of two simultaneously present stimuli.

Definition

The definition of PMT is an empirically based and fruitful therapeutic intervention used with parents of children with conduct disorders. The therapist works from a social learning model in a structured paradigm with parents to remediate parenting skill deficiencies. Parents are trained to encourage prosocial rather than antisocial behavior in their children.

Antecedents of Parent Management Training

Early therapeutic interventions by Patterson (1982) and his group at the OSLC focused on helping parents to positively reinforce prosocial behaviors without any use of discipline or punishment. This was relatively ineffective until the component of mild punishment was added, further refining the treatment strategy.

Effective discipline was characterized by three sets of skills: The first was tracking and classifying problem behaviors, the second was ignoring trivial coercive events, and the third was using an effective backup consequence when punishment was necessary. Parents of antisocial children were likely to classify as deviant the behaviors rated as typical by clinicians and most parents. They were also more likely to engage in aversive behaviors such as *nattering*, which actually increased child aversive behaviors. Effective punishment decreased aversive child behaviors. If parents of well-behaved children failed to use consequences to back up their commands and requests, children became progressively less compliant. Parents of antisocial children were unable to obtain even routine compliance and often resorted to physical abuse in an effort to gain compliance. Parents of antisocial children tended to be both inconsistent and explosive in their punishment. The parent-training model seemed to be useful in changing the behavior of younger children referred for extreme antisocial behavior and for both boys and girls. Ineffective discipline was followed by antisocial behavior in measurements made 2 years later and after.

Methodology and Technique

Oregon Social Learning Center Approach

The OSLC developed methodologies and techniques for the PMT method, which sought to train parents to use mild punishment in a contingent manner to encourage prosocial behaviors and discourage antisocial behaviors. Treatment was conducted primarily with the parents. Parents were trained to interact differently with their child and to identify, define, and observe problem behavior in new ways. Treatment sessions covered social learning principles and the procedures that follow from them. Techniques included positive reinforcement, mild punishment (e.g., time-out, loss of privileges), negotiation, contingency contracting, and other procedures. Basic elements included

- Pinpointing and accurate labeling of child behavior
- Refocusing from exclusive preoccupation with antisocial behavior to emphasis on prosocial goals

- Daily tracking of specific child behavior
- Administering tangible social reinforcement
- Using alternatives to physical punishment (i.e., differential attention, response cost, time-out)
- Communicating effectively (e.g., clear commands, undiluted praise)
- Learning to anticipate and solve new problems

Other elements included the following:

- Treatment sessions provided opportunities for parents to see how the techniques were implemented, to practice using the techniques, and to review the behavior change programs in the home.
- The therapist used instructions, modeling, role-playing, and rehearsal to convey how the techniques were implemented.
- The immediate goal of the program was to help parents develop specific skills. Parents began by applying their new skills to relatively simple behaviors that could be easily observed and were not enmeshed with more provoking interactions.
- As the treatment progressed, the focus shifted to the children's more severely problematic behaviors.
- The program was carefully designed to reinforce or punish consequences and to permit evaluation to determine if the program was working.
- It was essential that for the most favorable outcome, PMT had to be effective and therapists had to employ skills for dealing with parent resistance, marital conflict, and familial crises.
- Well-trained, experienced therapists were most effective in promoting a positive outcome.

Case Examples

Patterson and his colleagues (Patterson et al. 1975) described Maude, a troubled 10-year-old girl referred by her school:

> Maude stole, lied, and was disliked by her peers because of her bullying behavior, which included shouting orders at others and kicking and striking them. At home she was difficult to manage and fought regularly with her two sisters. Her parents no longer expected her to do any chores and had even considered institutionalizing her.
>
> Maude's parents agreed to participate in PMT. After her parents mastered the introductory material of the training course, they entered into a contract with Maude that identified, in order of importance, behaviors of hers that concerned them most. Time-out and a point system were agreed on as punishment and reward, respectively, for specific behaviors. Rewards were also set up for earning a specific number of points. Initially the time-

out procedure was ineffective, so the therapist worked with the parents to modify the plan. By the third week of the contract, the incidence of noncompliance by Maude was greatly decreased and the parents were relieved and pleased with the results. They then began to work with Maude to change her other less adverse behaviors and even began to consider working on their own chronic marital problems.

The present author, an experienced child/adolescent psychiatrist, evaluated a 14-year-old boy, Nate, who had been referred by his parents for behavior problems:

Nate refused to do homework, was almost failing in school despite above-average intelligence, and was often asked to leave class because of disruptive behavior. Nate had begun to associate with friends having similar problems and was caught shoplifting with a friend. With his parents he was noncompliant, had many angry outbursts, and sometimes lied about his activities. He was also inattentive and was taking stimulant medication that decreased his impulsiveness but had not altered his disruptive behavior problems significantly. Nate had been in weekly individual outpatient therapy for 10 months but had not improved. When evaluated individually, he admitted to the psychiatrist that he was doing poorly in school but appeared to have little interest in participating in therapy and denied most of his problems. However, he was willing to continue taking stimulant medication and agreed with his parents' desire to work with the therapist in order to help him.

The middle-class parents were concerned and willing to participate in PMT. At the first session, they spoke with the therapist for 2 hours, providing an extensive history. They were then given introductory material (*Parents and Adolescents Living Together*, Part 1 [Forgatch and Patterson 1989]) to read before the next session.

In the second 2-hour session, the principles of social learning theory and the importance of pinpointing, defining, and observing behavior were discussed. The therapist and the parents considered an important, but limited, specific problem and agreed on a plan to increase Nate's compliance with parental expectations. They also developed a system for the daily tracking of his behavior with consequences for noncompliance. Praise and rewards were planned for Nate, whenever the parents observed desired behavior.

The parents planned a meeting with Nate to present the contract to him. Although they were pleased with the plan, they said that in the past they had not tried to set firm limits but had given in and tried to placate the youth. They were concerned about the effects of setting limits. What if their requests led to more impulsive and defiant behavior from their son? Possible negative outcomes of the plan and their concerns were explored. Despite having misgivings, they agreed to try.

In the third session the parents expressed surprise and pleasure that the plan had worked well. Nate had cooperated with the plan. The parents had checked his behavior daily and followed through with praise—they had not found it necessary to punish him. Focusing on prosocial goals, communicating effectively, using differential attention, and learning to anticipate and solve new problems were discussed at this session. They also examined two specific issues: The father felt that the therapist was blaming the parents by working with them rather than the son; the mother felt that keeping charts was too demanding for her. The parents also brought up their concerns about communicating with the school and getting frequent reports on academics and behavior. A plan was formulated to be implemented by the parents that focused on clear communication with the school and included consequences for the youth for both improvement and regressions. The therapist also identified additional resources for parents, from which they could obtain further information and support.

In the next two sessions of 1½ hours each, the parents continued to work on setting clear limits, giving mildly aversive punishments for lack of compliance, and noting and commenting on prosocial behaviors. A special family vacation for the parents, Nate, and his younger brother was planned (and later took place). The parents continued to express concern about Nate's ongoing disruptive behaviors and were coached on the school intervention program.

Between the sessions, the parents continued to track and monitor specific behaviors and to identify consequences. The therapist also telephoned them several times to check on progress and identify problems.

The parents did not wish to continue regular sessions; they believed they understood the basic concepts and were making progress. They kept in touch with the therapist by telephone and came for another session again 2 months later. The parents reported significant improvement in Nate's behavior at home and reviewed new modified school plans with the therapist.

Two months later, at another session, the parents expressed surprise at the significant improvements in their son's home and school behavior. The teen was doing homework on a regular basis with close monitoring by the parents, academics and behavior at school were significantly improved, and he was more compliant at home. The mood of the home and the attitude of the parents had improved. The father decided to get into therapy to address some of his own concerns. Nate's stimulant medication was discontinued because of the side effects.

Two months later parents and son came for a family meeting. Nate was doing well in academics, had found a new group of *nice* friends, and was described by his parents as "confident and calm." The boy was surprised to discover that he was able to do his homework regularly and be successful in school. He wasn't sure why that happened but was very pleased. Three months later the parents reported continued improvement.

Forehand-McMahon Parent Training Program

The Forehand-McMahon Parent Training Program (Forehand and McMahon 1981a), like the OSLC approach, was based on social learning principles and designed for the parents of young children ages 3 to 8 years.

In the first of two phases of treatment, the parents were trained to eliminate commands, questions, and criticisms that are correlated with increased deviant child behavior and to increase the frequency of social rewards. Training was also provided in this phase for praise statements and contingent attention for desirable behaviors. The parenting skills of *attends*, *rewards*, and *ignoring* were taught and a daily 10- to 15-minute homework assignment known as the *Child's Game* was used in which the parent practiced the new skills with the child in a free play situation.

In the second phase the parent was trained to use time-out procedures for lack of compliance within a defined time (5 seconds) of a command's being given. Commands were to be specific and direct, given one at a time, and followed by a pause of 5 seconds. If the child was not compliant, a time-out procedure was used for a minimum of 3 minutes. Homework in the second phase consisted of the parent's practicing commands.

After the parent had mastered phase two and was successful in using the time-out procedure, a final session was held to review the progress and summarize the gains made. The number of sessions varied with the length of time it took for the parent to master the material being presented and usually ranged from 5 to 12 sessions.

Measurement Indices

The need for measurement indices was supported by evidence (Eyberg and Johnson 1974; Forehand et al. 1980) that there were significant discrepancies between reports of child behavior from parents or teachers and reports from systematic in situ observations using a standardized instrument (Family Interaction Coding System [FCIS]; Burgess and Conger 1978; Forehand et al. 1975; Patterson et al. 1969; Reid and Hendricks 1973; Wahler and Dumas 1986). Observing behaviors rather than relying on parent or child self-report influenced Patterson to develop ideas and techniques about how to describe and conceptualize what was observed. As described by Patterson and his colleagues (Patterson et al. 1982), the following indices were developed and used by the group at the OSLC:

- The FICS (Reid 1978) had the highest reliability of any complex home observation coding system. This 29-category observation system was designed to sequentially sample ongoing family interactions.
- The Total Aversive Behavior (TAB) indice consisted of 14 noxious-behavior categories. This score served as the main criterion score for evaluating treatment outcome for socially aggressive children. The 90th percentile for the TAB score data for each age level defined the normal range.
- The Parent Daily Report (PDR) was a 34-problem behavior checklist designed to assess the frequency of occurrence or nonoccurrence of symptoms during the prior 24-hour period.

Outcome

The outcome of PMT therapy has been best demonstrated by applying home measurement indices. In the past 20 years, Patterson and colleagues have seen more than 200 families for outpatient treatment of aggressive children between the ages of 3 and 12 years. The effectiveness of treatment was evaluated by the OSLC group as well as by other investigators. The OSLC group presented data to suggest that parent and teacher impressions of changes in child behavior as a result of treatment may be significantly biased. Thus, they prefer to rely on the home observation instruments described above such as the FICS and the TAB combined with the PDR.

Patterson and colleagues (Patterson et al. 1982) reported on a group of problem children treated with 17 hours of PMT and compared them with a waiting-list group who were referred to community practitioners (at the master's and doctoral level) using a variety of treatment modalities, including an eclectic approach, behavior modification, family therapy, and other approaches. The OSLC-treated group showed a 63% reduction in child deviant behavior compared with 17% for the community controls. In addition, 70% of the OSLC subjects had TAB scores within the normal range at termination, while only 33% of the community treated controls had scores at that level.

Other investigators have replicated these results. Webster-Stratton and Dahl (1995) and Wells and Egan (1988) found parent training therapy to be more effective than waiting-list controls and systems family therapy.

Questions about PMT remain. Kazdin (1997) points out that most studies are short term, focus on preadolescent children, do not attend to cultural or ethnic issues, and use relatively short follow-up periods. He notes that PMT has been used with a variety of diagnostic problems, including autism, mental retardation, and learning disabilities, in addition to the disruptive behavior disorders. Most studies have been done with youth having disruptive behavior disorders. Ho and colleagues (Ho et al. 1999) used PMT with Chinese nurses treating disruptive Chinese youth in Hong Kong. These investigators found efficacy for children with conduct problems. The writer of this chapter is unaware of studies using PMT with other ethnic or racial groups outside the United States. Eyberg and colleagues (1998) pointed out that research documenting long-term gains with the use of PMT was limited. He studied the role of booster sessions and other techniques to bolster the durability effect of treatment gains.

Conclusion

At the time of this writing, violence in the United States is epidemic, and the violent death of our young men and the "vile weed" of Patterson is bringing untold suffering to many of our young people, their families, and our society. The PMT approaches described in this chapter are not a panacea but hold promise for helping children and adolescents with disruptive behavior disorders and other problems. This chapter does not purport to be exhaustive but merely hopes to provide an introduction and pique the curiosity of the interested reader.

Chapters on Related Topics

The following chapters describe concepts related to parent management training:

- Chapter 8, "Psychoeducational Family Intervention"
- Chapter 17, "Family Therapy With Children and Adolescents: An Overview"
- Chapter 18, "Family Therapy With Children: A Model for Engaging the Whole Family"

V

Couples Therapy

20

Couples Therapy

An Overview

G. Pirooz Sholevar, M.D.

Introduction

The turn of the century finds couples therapy in a strong position. The empirical foundation for the field established in the past 20 years enabled it to improve some of its methods, learn from its mistakes, and modify some of its exaggerated claims. Multiple clinical approaches have moved toward an intelligent integration, combining their strongest elements to produce innovative, multifaceted, pluralistic, clinical systems.

More people seek therapy for marital-related problems than for any other reasons (Veroff et al. 1981). It is estimated that 50% of those who enter psychotherapy do so primarily because of marital disorders; another 25% have marital difficulties in addition to other problems. Although marital affairs are usually pointed to as the reason for divorce, it is clear that for both men and women, the major factor for marital dissolution is a disparate sense of growing apart, followed by fighting and finally affairs (Gigy and Kelly 1992). Given this plethora of marital issues, the scope of couples therapy has also broadened to address these factors.

Whereas three decades ago, the function of a marital therapist was to preserve marriages at all cost, today, couples therapy has become a highly effective instrument to help spouses achieve a higher level of personal development and maturity, whether the outcome is staying married or obtaining a divorce. A recent development has been the preventive application of marital therapy knowledge in marital enrichment programs, with the goal of increasing marital satisfaction and personality growth in spouses.

If the alarming rise in the divorce rate can be taken as a sign of both the fragility of marriages and the large number of unhappy ones, the field of marital therapy will continue to grow. In spite of the high prevalence of marriage-related emotional problems, surprisingly few training programs in psychiatry, psychology, or social work offer adequate didactic and supervised clinical practice in marital therapy. Reasons for this relative neglect of marital therapy training are unclear but may include the discipline's lack of a unified theoretical base, the domination of Western psychiatry by individual psychology, and the absence of a well-accepted diagnostic code. The uncertainty regarding the availability of reimbursement for couples therapy through medical insurance, the historically low professional status of marriage counseling, and the diverse professional backgrounds and disciplines of marital therapists may also be contributing factors. The effectiveness of couples therapy in a wide variety of disorders, however, has brought it to a more central position in the range of psychiatric interventions.

History

Marital counseling and couples therapy are truly children of the twentieth century. Attempts to strengthen marital relationships and to resolve marital conflicts, however, are as ancient as the institution of marriage. The function of helping young married couples resolve their marital conflicts traditionally belonged to the older, extended family members, whose perspective on marital stress was based on their own experiences. With the declining influence of the extended family around the turn of the twentieth century, clergy and physicians were called on to assist troubled couples. Both were natural groups to address marital problems because they had contact with family members at significant stressful times in the life cycle of families and had the advantage of ongoing rapport with the family before problems surfaced.

Professional marital counseling emerged in the 1920s and 1930s. The Marriage Consultation Center was established in New York City in 1929, the Marriage Council of Philadelphia was founded in 1932, and the American Institute of Family Relations was established in California in 1939 to offer counseling specifically for marital problems.

The theoretical foundation for marital therapy was established by a variety of theoreticians. C. P. Oberndorf (1938) published a classic paper entitled "Folie à Deux," reporting on the existence of similar paranoid delusions in a husband and wife and proposing that a neurosis in a married person is strongly anchored in the marital relationship. He considered a complementary neurotic reaction in the marriage partner as an important aspect of the married patient's neurosis. B. Mittleman (1948) employed concurrent treatment of married couples and offered a psychoanalytic classification of marital problems based on a *complementary needs satisfaction* model of marriage. The empirical foundation of marital therapy was established when behavioral techniques were applied to marital disorders in the mid-1960s. Initially, desensitization and assertiveness training were applied, followed by the use of contingency management based on operant conditioning. Subsequently, cognitive and therapy concepts were broadly applied by behavior therapists. The 1990s marked the years of the integration of multiple theoretical models when eclectic interventions were applied by different practitioners and evaluated empirically.

The advances in the broader field of family therapy emerged in the 1950s. The concepts of homeostasis, communication, and family conflicts were applied to marital relationships. The dynamics of small groups in marital situations were explored in the 1950s.

Definitions

Couples therapy—the treatment of the couples relationship—refers to a broad range of treatment modalities that attempt to modify the marital relationship with the goal of enhancing marital satisfaction or correcting marital dysfunction. The marital dysfunction may assume the form of an overtly conflictual, dysfunctional marriage, or it may be covert but result in symptomatology or dysfunction in one or both spouses or their children. In couples therapy, the relationship is considered to be the *patient* rather than the individual spouses. This focus implies that two reasonably healthy spouses may form a symptomatic or dysfunctional marriage. The interlocking of the underlying "neuroticism" and emotional disorders of each spouse, however, is a common contributor to the formation of a dysfunctional marriage.

Couples Therapy

There is a general tendency to blur the boundaries between couples therapy and counseling for couples on theoretical and technical bases, but the core of the practices in couples therapy and counseling can be differentiated. Couples therapists employ varied extensive assessment techniques and utilize their systematic knowledge of personality, behavioral, cognitive, or communicational-systems theory to promote the therapeutic process. A thorough knowledge of the field of orientation enables them to assess the totality of the pathological and adaptive behaviors of the spouses and assist them through the use of marital, individual, or other therapeutic modalities. The goal of couples therapy can include the enhancement of the marital relationship and the treatment of any underlying emotional disorders in one or both of the spouses. Although the ultimate goals in marital treatment may remain unrealized, the eventual outcome should be a progression by the couple to a relationship on a higher developmental level.

Marriage Counseling

Marriage counseling includes a very broad range of technical interventions for reduction of marital disharmony. There are clear overlapping areas between marital counseling and therapy. These interventions can include giving advice on concrete problem solving. The focus and goals of the treatment are generally the resolution of the immediate presenting problems and the provision of the spouses with emotional support and enhancement of their self-esteem and optimism. The treatment goal does not include the restructuring of relational and personality structures.

Indications and Contraindications

Couples therapy is indicated in a wide range of situations in which relational dysfunction, symptomatology, or disability in a "married" person is present. The clearest indication for couples therapy is the presence of overt marital conflicts that result in the recognizable, severe discomfort of both spouses. Frequently, such spouses seek couples treatment because they fear divorce or because they recognize the limits of their effective problem management. In many situations, however, the presence of a marital disorder may be covert and may exhibit itself in symptomatology or dysfunction in one of the spouses or the children.

Poor communication and extramarital relationships are the most frequent reasons for referral for marital treatment. Marital therapy should be considered when individual treatment has failed, or is unlikely to succeed, because of the lack of an appropriate capacity in the patient, such as poor motivation or limited ability to negotiate a treatment contract. Marital treatment is also indicated when the eruption of symptoms in a family member coincides with the outbreak of marital conflicts, or when gross distortions of reality are held jointly by the couple, increasing the risk of marital instability in cases of individual treatment.

In the 1990s, couples therapy was increasingly applied to a wide range of psychiatric disorders, including depression, alcoholism, and schizophrenia, in recognition of the significance of the relational dimension of the mental disorder and the ability of marital therapy to enhance treatment efficacy.

Contraindications to couples therapy are relative and few. The premature exposure of the spouses to marital secrets, such as illegal actions of a spouse, homosexuality, or an extramarital affair, can result in abrupt interruption of treatment or termination of marriage. Therefore, the revelation of secrets in marital therapy should be encouraged only when a couple have committed themselves to treatment. Once a couple are involved in treatment, such secrets can be handled in the therapeutic context to enhance marital relationship and closeness.

If the spouses use the sessions consistently to attack each other and seek the therapist's assistance with their destructive efforts, conjoint marital therapy may become unproductive. The lack of commitment to continuation of the marriage may be another contraindication to conjoint marital therapy. Conjoint sessions, however, are useful in undermining the rationalization of ambivalent couples who claim they are living together merely for financial reasons or for "the children's sake."

Types of Couples Therapy

The most common types of couples therapy are individual therapy, conjoint couples therapy, and combined couples therapy. Group therapy with couples is practiced by some practitioners. Currently, conjoint couples therapy is the most favored type of couples therapy, in contrast to earlier times when concurrent couples therapy prevailed. There is little comparative research on the effectiveness of different modes of couples therapy, and what exists contains contradictory findings.

Individual Therapy

In individual therapy of marital disorders, the therapeutic focus is on the marital relationship and the conflicts with the marital partner. At the time of marital crisis, the therapist may choose to see the other spouse to gain a more comprehensive perspective on the immediate marital crisis. Individual therapy for marital problems can be recommended when one of the spouses is very resistant to psychotherapy, one of the spouses may be considering a divorce, or when the patient seeking treatment is suffering from a variety of other symptoms, such as phobia, in addition to marital dissatisfaction. Such therapy for marital problems can be quite helpful to the healthier spouses who exhibit highly integrated personalities with minimal self-destructive and masochistic tendencies. Individual therapy is a poor choice, however, in the presence of marital disturbance and severe psychopathology, such as psychosis and physical abuse.

Concurrent Couples Therapy

In concurrent couples therapy, both spouses are seen individually in separate sessions by the same therapist. The establishment of a strong therapeutic alliance with each spouse can be readily achieved and maintained in concurrent therapy. Concurrent couples therapy reduces interpersonal defensiveness and apprehension and promotes self-revelation and introspection in an empathic and therapeutic environment.

Conjoint Couples Therapy

Conjoint couples therapy is the treatment of both spouses in the same session by a therapist or a team of co-therapists. It has been the most commonly used mode of marital therapy for the past two decades, having been used by more than 80% of therapists. The advantage of conjoint therapy is that it focuses the therapeutic efforts directly on the couple's interactions where the problems manifest. This focus enables the therapist to recognize the subtle transactional configurations and feedback mechanisms that support marital dysfunction and symptomatology. The therapist can observe the marital interactional patterns, contradictions between overt and covert messages, and subtle reinforcements of coercive behaviors. Conjoint family sessions tend to mobilize optimally the rehabilitative capacity of the couple for constructive marital changes; however, the latent forces toward separation can also be mobilized, prematurely encouraging the couple toward a breakup.

The limitations of the use of conjoint couples therapy include impending divorce, in which the issues confronting the spouses may be radically different, or situations in which the couples have different therapeutic goals. At times, conjoint therapy can be used destructively by the spouses for the purpose of mutual blaming and power struggles, and a temporary or permanent shift to concurrent therapy may be advisable. In deeply divided couples in whom mistrust and resentment run deep, it may be technically impossible for the therapist to maintain an effective neutral posture while developing a therapeutic alliance with both spouses.

Combined Couples Therapy

Combined couples therapy refers to the mixing of conjoint and concurrent marital therapies, although it can include other combinations, such as couples' group therapy. Conjoint couples sessions can be held at regular intervals, at the time of marital crisis, or when progress in concurrent treatment is impeded. The combined treatment has the advantage of allowing the use of fantasies in individual sessions while providing easy access to transactional and communicational patterns in joint sessions.

Couple Group Therapy

Couples can participate with a group of other couples in couple group therapy. The couples can learn from each other, render marital support, and serve as models for marital role modification. Some couples groups include didactic teaching about marriage in addition to traditional group therapy process (Coché 1995). Couple group therapy is contraindicated when a spouse lacks sufficient ego strength—that is, has a borderline personality—and is threatened by the group.

Concurrent marital therapy was the most widely practiced type of marital therapy throughout the 1950s and 1960s. Currently, the majority of marital therapists tend to favor conjoint therapy, as it provides observable information on the crucial marital interactional patterns.

Theories of Couples Therapy

Psychodynamic Theories

Psychoanalytic theories emphasize the concepts of complementarity of needs, self, object, early identifications, introjections, and projective identification. In projective identification, the person with a faulty sense of self as a victim, who has internalized pathogenic persecuting introjects, splits off the criticizing internalized introjects and projects them onto others. These split-off introjects create a polarization in which the spouse is seen as a victimizer and the self is seen as the victim (see Chapter 4, "Psychodynamic Family Therapy," and Chapter 21, "Psychodynamic Couples Therapy," for a more detailed description). In marriage, persons may choose to act according to one polarized half of their conflicted selves and project the other half onto their partners (projective identification). The introjected parts of the self are disavowed, split off, and projected onto the other person, who complies with the wishes of the partner. For the projective identification to take place and continue, the object should periodically exhibit the behavior projected on him or her by the subject. The selection of a mate is strongly weighed toward choosing one who can provide optimal gratification for unconscious neurotic needs. Therefore, the internalized intrapsychic conflicts of the spouses result in a tradeoff, leading to marital conflicts. It has been pointed out that the marital relationship is profoundly shaped by mutual transference reactions between the spouses. Consequently, the treatment of the marital relationship should address the projections and introjections of the spouses, in addition to their real differences. The preponderance of projection in intimate relationships explains the difference between marriage and other relationships.

From the field of eligible or potential mates, individuals choose a partner reflecting their unfulfilled personality needs. Normal couples tend to share more similarity of needs and traits than do conflicted couples. For neurotic couples, the complementarity of needs is more extreme, and the developmental immaturity of the needs may be greater than in normal couples. Therefore, the needs may be so intense that the couples can be labeled mutually *compensatory* and overfunctioning in the areas where each spouse is extremely weak and conflicted. Another way of differentiating couples with healthy functioning from dysfunctional couples is by observing the types of objects they choose. Well-functioning couples tend to choose an object of the dependent anaclitic type. The object choice of neurotic couples is based on that quality that enhances one's self-esteem (narcissistic). The idealization may be extreme, and the object can become a substitute for some of the subject's unobtained goals.

Neurotic couples are psychodynamically similar and are attracted by shared developmental failures. Spouses adopt opposite patterns of defensive organization to deal with similar conflicts and with equivalent levels of immaturity. Therefore, they appear as different personality types while they share similar dynamic conflicts. The example of The Odd Couple in film and television is a graphic depiction of this phenomenon. The different traits that initially attract the couple can later become the focus of conflicts.

Marital conflict can occur in the absence of significant individual psychopathology in either or both spouses. This phenomenon, described as *marital neurosis*, occurs when a neurosis develops in one or both spouses in connection with the marriage. Marital neurosis should be distinguished from the *marriage of interlocked neurotic spouses*, both of whom exhibit neurotic character traits that give rise to neurotic interactions in the marriage.

The paramount goal in psychoanalytic marital therapy is restructuring and reconstruction of both spouses' internally based perceptions and expectations of, and reactions to, each other, which are patterned after their early experiences and interfere with their present communications and relationship. Marital partners need to develop a sense of self that is more differentiated and internally integrated and to experience the other spouse as a safe and real person. In terms of practice, psychodynamic therapists tend to be quite pragmatic and eclectic in the selection of actual therapeutic interventions. Although active and directive at times, the therapist's basic posture remains one of acceptance, to allow the emergence and integration of the unacceptable aspects of the inner perceptions of both spouses into their personalities. The therapist's interpretations should be more integrative than regressive, considering the relatively brief character of marital therapy. It has been proposed that both neurotic and normal couples are extremely prone to think and experience relationships in dyadic terms, and the triadic relationship in the conjoint marital sessions does not disturb the spouses' dyadic perception of the therapist. Therefore, the therapist can interpret effectively the marital transference between the spouses as well as the therapeutic transference manifestations in the sessions (Sonne 1986).

The major deficiency in psychoanalytic marital therapy is its insufficient attention to the current issues in marital interactions that serve as grounds for projections and that maintain the distortions engendered by the marital transference.

Marital Contract Theory

Marital contract theory, developed by Sager (1976), is one of the few theoretical systems specific to marital therapy. The word contract is used to describe a set of assumptions and expectations of self and partner with which each person approaches the marital relationship. Each contract is conceptualized by the person in reciprocal terms, and each person behaves as if the partner had explicitly agreed to this exchange. Because much of the contract is not shared and some parts of it are unconscious, there are considerable possibilities for confusion. Three levels of contracts are described: 1) *verbalized*—the part of the contract verbally stated to the other person; 2) *secret*—the part of the contract not shared with the partner because of the fear of consequences of the revelation; and 3) *beyond awareness*—preconscious or unconscious needs that are unknown to the person. Marital conflicts in this model evolve from incongruent or nonfulfillable contracts. Contracts may be unacceptable to the partners, or there may be internal conflict between the conscious and unconscious part of the contract. The contract may be nonfulfillable by anyone, including the particular partner. The complexity of marital dynamics and marital conflict is primarily due to the level of contract that involves each person's individual needs and is beyond awareness.

Intergenerational Systems Theory—Bowen Theory

The central theoretical construct of Bowen's theory is differentiation of self or its opposite fusion. Undifferentiated people remain attached to their families of origin and tend to fuse with other people in order to reduce anxiety. They seek spouses who operate on the same developmental level and repeat with their spouses the same style of relating that they had with their families of origin. The goal of marital therapy is for the spouses to differentiate from their families of origin by detriangulating themselves from their parental families. Other critical variables are the degree of emotional cutoff from the previous generation and the ability of the spouses to bridge the gap and resolve the emotional attachment.

Bowen uses three basic intervention strategies. The first is defining and clarifying the relationship between the spouses. He asks the spouses to talk directly to him in the most calm, low-keyed, and objective way. This intervention is usually sufficient to undermine the marital fight and fusion. The second strategy is the didactic teaching of the spouses about the functioning of emotional systems. Bowen distinguishes between feeling and intellectual properties. The third stage is taking an "I position" stand, in which the therapist is clearly defined in relationship to the marital pairs and asks the marital partners to assume the same position while making therapeutic voyages back to their families of origin.

Systems Theories

Systems theories—or more accurately, *communication* approaches to family therapy—encompass a diverse group of theories and practices. The group of systems theories described here is composed of strategic therapies, in which structural and triadic-based family therapists usually focus on two hierarchical generations. The systems theorists use systems concepts, such as *wholeness, circular causality, homeostasis, positive and negative feedback*, and *family interactional patterns. Interaction*, the central notion of the systems theory, is considered explanatory of marital conflicts. Conflicted couples communicate at report and command levels simultaneously. Contradictions between different levels of messages are the root of the symptomatic behavior.

Systems theorists differ from each other in their conceptualization of marital problems. For Haley, the central focus in marital conflict is the power struggle between the spouses, and the treatment process is a way of working out overt, shared agreements on previously undiscussed issues. For Watzlawick, the major problematic dimension is a cognitive one, in which the spouses fail to differentiate between a common difficulty and a serious problem or in which an inept solution to a minor problem becomes a severe problem itself.

Therapeutic strategies include redefining the couple's problem through the use of reframing and relabeling as well as paradoxical tasks that help change the spouses' outlooks and therefore their subjective experiences. The use of paradoxical tasks or therapeutic double-binds is based on the notion that rules or the realities are relative, and when the therapist permits or encourages the usual or symptomatic behavior, the patient tends to discontinue it. Strategic marital therapy has given rise to recent postmodern approaches such as solution-focused therapy and narrative solutions couples therapy (Eron and Lund 1996). The conceptual and technical aspects of these approaches are described in Chapter 4.

Postmodern or social constructionist family therapy has produced two collaborative couples therapy models—namely, solution-focused and narrative approaches. The solution-focused approach, based on the work of de Shazer et al. (de Shazer 1985; de Shazer et al. 1986), shifts the focus of the treatment to talking about solutions to the problems, *exceptions* to the present problems, and the future without the problems. It emphasizes the couple's strength and competencies. The narrative approach (Eron and Lund 1996) uses the reframing search immediately for both spouses to understand their *stuck* situation, separate themselves from their problems, and coauthor a new narrative for themselves through *collaborative conversation* with the therapist. The new narrative is based on how the spouses like to see themselves and be seen by others. The way they prefer to see themselves is usually very different from their problem-saturated way of viewing themselves when they arrive for treatment.

Behavioral Couples Therapy

Behavioral couples therapy (BCT) employs a range of learning theories and techniques based on operant and social learning principles in the evaluation and treatment of marital transaction and disorder. The scope of contemporary BCT was significantly enlarged in the 1990s. The foundations of BCT were established in operant conditioning, social learning, and social exchange models. Operant conditioning conceptualizes behavior in terms of its specific antecedents and consequences. The major emphasis of behavior analysis is on four basic types of behavior. Two types are reinforcements that increase or maintain the likelihood of the responses (behavior) they follow; the other two types are punishments that decrease the likelihood of their antecedent behaviors. The first type of behavior, *positive reinforcement*, is performed to reward a person with something that he or she wants. The second type of behavior, *negative reinforcement*, involves the reduction or elimination of an unpleasant stimulus. For example, the cessation of unpleasant behavior in one partner could increase the possibility of pleasing behavior in the other. The third type of behavior, *punishment*, is the presentation of an aversive condition in order to decrease or eliminate unwanted behavior. The fourth type of behavior, *time-out*, is a form of punishment that involves removing or withholding something the other partner wants. These four types of behavioral contingencies can form at least two major kinds of reinforcement patterns: reciprocity and coercion. *Reciprocity* involves the mutual exchange of reinforcement in a way the partners see as equitable over time. The second social reinforcement pattern is *coercion*, which involves the use of aversive control to force desirable responses from one's partner. Punishment and coercion may be effective in controlling one's partner temporarily, but sooner or later punishment begets punishment or avoidance.

Dysfunctional marriages can be differentiated reliably on the basis of the concurrent relative strengths of reciprocity and coercion, the absence of sufficient reinforcements, and the prevalence of punishment, time-out, and avoidant behaviors. Marital difficulties arise from faulty behavior change efforts such as the demand for immediate change in the behavior of the other person and the use of coercion for noncompliance from the partner.

Behavioral Techniques

Behavioral couples therapists vary widely in the techniques they employ. Each of the operant, respondent, and cognitive approaches includes a variety of procedures. Each approach focuses on changing concrete behaviors to maximize the interactions that both spouses find subjectively satisfying. Specific techniques are described in Chapter 22, "Behavioral Couples Therapy," and include building communication skills, taking assertiveness training, exchanging behaviors, and contracting of *quid pro quo* or *good faith* types for contingencies. The research suggests that quid pro quo and good faith contracts are equally effective. The current emphasis is on informal marital agreements.

Cognitive-Behavioral Therapy

This approach addresses the irrational, unrealistic, and unconscious beliefs of spouses about themselves and their partners who serve as the mediators of their unadaptive behavioral response to each other. The basic cognitive model postulates that the person responds to perceptions and appraisals of an event rather than to the objective characteristics of the situation. Self-instructional training can be used to interrupt destructive spouse interaction based on irrational assumptions. In the 1980s, behavioral marital therapies (BMTs) began to introduce an emphasis on cognition to enhance the effectiveness of treatment with a larger group of patients who did not respond to traditional BMTs (Christensen 1987; Weiss 1980). They explored the areas of attributions, selective attention, assumptions, expectancies, and standards (see Chapter 22, "Behavioral Couples Therapy," for more information on BMT and BCT).

The role of emotions was subsequently introduced in some of the new BCT approaches. Some exciting new models emerged in BCT in the late 1990s that incorporate some of the recent developments in the broader fields of couples therapy and family therapy. Emotionally focused couple therapy (Johnson 1999) is an empirically validated approach that focuses on distressed affects and constrained interactional patterns, expands a couple's interactional position, and fosters emotional engagement to unearth attachment-related affects and bonding needs. The goal of fostering a secure emotional bond is based on Bowlby's attachment theory.

Integrative couples therapy (Jacobson and Christensen 1996; Lawrence et al. 1999) has introduced strategies to help the couple to emotionally accept each other before trying to implement changes in communication and problem-solving patterns. Preliminary outcome data show increased relationship satisfaction after 1-year follow-up (Jacobson et al. 2000).

In his seminal work on marital dissolution, John Gottman (1999) based his approach on observation and painstaking assessments in his laboratory. Specifically, Gottman noted that, in his words, there are four horsemen of the apocalypse, referring to the demise of the marriage. These are 1) criticism, 2) defensiveness, 3) contempt, and 4) stonewalling. Gottman noted that once the cascade of interactions was indicated by these four indices, the marriage had difficulties, particularly with the inclusion of contempt and stonewalling. Gottman uses behavioral exercises that combine with cognitive approaches but relies on teaching couples how to broach issues and maintain dialogue and to recognize the escalations and cascade responses that impede and overwhelm couples.

Classification of "Marital" Disorders

There is no widely accepted classification system for marital disorders, partly due to the diversity of the theoretical concepts and techniques used by different marital therapists. Only two classification systems of marital disorders are described here.

Marriage Type

Cuber and Harroff (1992) proposed the following classification for marital disorders:

The Conflict-Habituated Marriage

The conflict-habituated marriage is characterized by constant strife, tension, and undermining of one spouse by the other. Significant dependence and loyalty often tie the spouses to their families of origin. The couple's fear of loneliness binds them together. Other terms for such marriages are unstable-unsatisfactory, schismatic, or pseudohostile.

The Devitalized Marriage

In the devitalized marriage, the family atmosphere is pleasant, but the actual source of emotional support is derived from outside interests and the social network.

The Vital Marriage

In the vital, or total, marriage, the couple is highly enthusiastic about joint activities and raising children. The mutual involvement is more multifaceted in the total marriage.

Personality Type

There are several classification systems based on personality styles and the psychodynamic factors underlying the personality traits. The marriage becomes symptomatic only when role flexibility, or capacity for adaptation and enjoyment, is moderately to severely compromised.

The Obsessive-Compulsive Husband and Hysterical Wife

This type is generally known as the pattern of *cold-sick* man and *love*sick woman. The marital union is based on the husband's wish to become energized through his wife and the wife's desire to become more organized through his companionship. The underlying fear of intimacy is identical for both partners; however, for the hysterical personality, narcissism is largely in the service of dependency, whereas for the obsessional person, dependency is in the service of narcissism.

The Passive-Dependent Husband and Dominant Wife

The husband's feeling of inadequacy leads him to an aggressive and seemingly competent woman, with the unconscious wish of gaining strength from her. Being controlled by her, however, he feels more inadequate and fights with her in a passive-aggressive fashion. The wife becomes hostile, due to her own unconscious, unmet dependency needs and her inability to dominate him.

The Paranoid Husband or Wife and Depression-Prone Wife or Husband

There is significant ego-restriction and limited coping capacity in both spouses. They both feel suspicious of each other but too inadequate to be assertive. So they become depressed.

The Mutually Dependent Marriage

The spouses are immature, dependent, passive, and competitive with each other for attention, and their overreactions to minor difficulties make their marriage stormy.

The Neurotic Wife and Competent Husband

This is the pattern of the *inadequate-overadequate* marriage described by Bowen. The woman is chronically symptomatic and unable to function adequately. The husband derives extreme feelings of adequacy and competence caring for his *ill* wife and countering his own unconscious feeling of inadequacy.

Denial of Conflict

There is an additional major category of marital disorders termed *stable-unsatisfactory marriage*, *skewed marriage*, and *pseudomutuality* by different theorists. Here, the spouses are extremely frightened by the possibility of marital breakup in case of disagreements. Therefore, they deny any conflicts to the point of distorting or reinterpreting reality. A delusional or unreal familial atmosphere prevails. The couple consults a psychiatrist only when severe emotional disorders surface in the children.

Spouse Abuse

Spouse abuse has been recognized as a major threat to the welfare of American families (see Chapter 10, "Gender-Sensitive Family Therapy").

Common Marital Problems

Communication Problems

Communication problems refer to a host of problems, which include lack of talking and affection, mutual blaming, mind reading, and lack of problem solving. Clear and positive communication between the spouses expressing care, requesting need satisfaction, and validating each other's identities is the cornerstone of a healthy marriage. For clear communication to occur, the couple should accept responsibility for sending and receiving clear messages, paying attention to multiple levels of communication, and commenting on the incongruities between the overt and covert levels of messages when they occur. Attention to the nonverbal aspects of the communication is essential for the full understanding of messages.

Disturbances of communication include the summarizing self syndrome (Gottman et al. 1977; Markman 1992), in which both spouses are invested in proving the superiority of their own viewpoint and repeatedly restate their position rather than listening to their partner. This type of interaction generally results in escalating quarrels.

Extramarital Affairs

In more than half the couples requesting marital therapy, one or both had been involved in extramarital affairs with another person. The nature, duration, significance, and outcome of the affairs vary widely. They might represent a temporary activity on the part of a spouse at the time of marital crisis or might indicate a deep lack of satisfaction in and commitment to the marriage. There has been an increasing tendency in the field to view extramarital affairs as situationally based, rather than as a sign of a neurotic disorder in the involved spouse. It is initially essential to hold at least a diagnostic individual session with each spouse to explore the existence of extramarital affairs and to maintain such information confidentially. The decision and the timing for revealing the affair(s) to the other spouse should be left to the spouses in the course of treatment. The treatment process should include the exploration of the reasons and the meaning of the extramarital affairs, the deficiencies and strengths of the marriage, and the function of the affair in relation to the marital relationship. The exploration and expression of feelings of ambivalence, guilt, anger, and narcissistic injuries are necessary for the satisfactory resolution of the affairs. The outcome in terms of the continuity of marriage is a function of the strengths and weaknesses of the marriage and the effectiveness of the therapeutic management rather than the quality of the affair.

Depression and Marital Dysfunction

The high level of coincidence between marital stress and depression in one or two spouses is increasingly recognized. The range of clinical manifestations of this complex phenomenon and their therapeutic management are discussed in Chapter 28 ("Depression and the Family: Interpersonal Context and Family Functioning").

Divorce and Divorce Therapy

Divorce and divorce therapy became important issues as the rate of divorce in the United States steadily increased in the twentieth century. There were 5.3 divorces per 1,000 population around 1980. After that decade, the rate began to decline. By 1997, the last year when national statistics were available, the rate was 4.3 divorces per 1,000 population. Divorce therapy has emerged as a clinical field or orientation in recognition of the need to help divorcing couples achieve a psychic or emotional divorce in addition to a legal one. The phenomenon of *psychic divorce* refers to the successful resolution of marital bonds so both spouses can emerge with their own separate identities and pursue an autonomous life in the future. Ahrons (1994) has used the term *good divorce* to describe divorce in those families that continue to be a family, maintain good relationships between parents and children, and raise the children in a multiparent binuclear family. The typology of postdivorce relationships between the spouses is described in Chapter 23, "The Divorcing Family: Characteristics and Interventions."

The goal of divorce therapy is to assist the divorcing couple to resolve their remaining conflicts—including grief reaction for marriage and spouse—so the divorce procedure becomes less acrimonious and future adjustment of the spouses and their children is enhanced. In the process of divorce therapy, the therapist attempts to develop a therapeutic alliance with each spouse, gain his or her trust and confidence, and help all parties with two sets of concerns: 1) the decision to divorce or not and 2) the negotiation of issues, such as child custody. The therapeutic strategies used by divorce therapists include understanding the perspective of each spouse on the issues, promoting a climate conducive to decision making by the clarification of issues, and assuming a direct and active role in prompting agreements on substantive matters.

The strategy and technical interventions of divorce therapy are different according to the stage of marital resolution. In the *predivorce, decision-making stage*, the therapist generally helps the couple to look at divorce as one of the alternatives to their problems and apprise them of the consequences of different options. The therapist attempts to promote progressive and constructive communication and enhance negotiation during this stage. In the *second stage of divorce restructuring*, the therapist helps the family with the multitude of emotional, financial, legal, childcare, and social arrangements necessary at the time of divorce. The involvement of the lawyers at this stage of the marriage may be necessary and in the best interest of the couple. However, the therapist should help the couple use the lawyer as a legal expert rather than as a weapon to fight each other or detour their anger into unrealistic expectations. In the stage of postdivorce recovery, the therapeutic task is to facilitate the growth of the divorced spouses as autonomous individuals with stable social relationships and satisfactory lifestyle independent of the former marriage. The achievement of psychic divorce is necessary for the accomplishment of this goal. *Psychic divorce* refers to the phenomenon of coming to terms with the ending of the marital relationship, which allows the spouses to pursue their independent courses. The lack of psychic divorce is usually manifested by preoccupation with the previous marriage and the ex-spouse, which results in feelings of anger and disappointment. The anger is in turn channeled through continuous fights over financial and custody arrangements.

Divorce Mediation

Divorce mediation refers to a particular type of intervention by a trained psychotherapist or lawyer with the goal of helping the couple resolve conflicts over custody, visitation, child support and financial settlement. It can be effective in addressing postdivorce disputes related to the above issues as well as ones emerging during the remarriage stage. There are similarities in the goals between divorce mediation and litigation, but the mediator acts as a neutral facilitator to help the couple resolve their problems. It is common that the solutions reached through mediation are written up by lawyers as a legal document. The mature spouses find mediation a constructive alternative to the adversarial legal process.

Marital and Sex Therapies

The behavioral treatment (marital and sex therapies) of sexual dysfunctions in married couples has yielded encouraging results. Sex therapy is optimally helpful within the context of marital therapy, because 75% of couples exhibit a combination of marital and sexual dysfunctions. The use of conjoint marital sessions and a heterosexual co-therapy team can be an invaluable part of the therapeutic intervention. Careful assessment of the marital communication patterns can shed light on complex sexual dysfunctions. Sex therapy outcome research has produced encouraging results, although it has not supported the exaggerated claims of many sex therapists (see Chapter 26, "Sex Therapy at the Turn of the Century: New Awareness and Response," for a full discussion of sex therapy).

Couples Therapy Research

There has been a quantum leap in the quality and quantity of couples therapy research in the past two decades. The first broad review of results of marital therapy in 1973 identified 15 studies in this area (Gurman 1973). The studies have proliferated since and are summarized in Chapter 37, "Couples Therapy Research: Status and Directions," in this volume.

The studies in the past two decades have been methodologically sound, and outcome criteria have become more rigorous. The nature of marital distress is increasingly being reconceptualized. In addition to an increasing number of BCT studies, a few on nonbehavioral interventions have been reported with favorable therapeutic outcomes.

In addition to outcome research on marital distress, marital therapy with spouses with several identified emotional disorders such as agoraphobia, alcoholism, depression, and sexual disorders has been the focus of rigorous investigation. The research data have been particularly informative on the nature and characteristics of marriage and response to marital therapy in those experiencing depression and alcoholism. When marital distress and depression are simultaneously present, marital therapy can be at least as effective as alternative treatment modalities.

Johnson (Johnson and Lebow 2000) has identified the lack of a theory for the nature of adult intimacy, marital distress, and therapeutic change as a major barrier to more satisfactory progress in marital therapy investigation. She proposes attachment theory as a potentially useful theoretical model that can provide a framework for understanding marital interactions as well as cognitive and emotional processes with an intimate adult relationship.

Gottman's (1999) longitudinal research makes considerable effort in approaching marital therapy from a scientifically based endeavor. His work has shed light on enduring myths endemic to couples therapy but clearly not supported by sound interactional and multifaceted research. His efforts point to the many factors that need further clarification for successful treatment.

Conclusion and Future Directions

Couples therapy has consolidated its role as an effective therapeutic tool for reduction of marital stress, enhancement of interpersonal relationships, and a preventive measure against future relational conflict and dysfunction in marriage. The past two decades (1980–2000) have been especially productive in the exploration of the contributions of marital dysfunction to the maintenance and possible causation of certain emotional disorders. The role of marital disorders in depression and alcoholism and the employment of marital therapy as part of a multimodal intervention to enhance therapeutic results of these disorders have been increasingly clear.

Schools of family and couples therapy have enriched each other's approach while continuing along their own differentiated path. The major beneficiary of this eclecticism has been BCT, which has enlarged its focus significantly by emphasizing the importance of cognition and emotions in understanding the nature of marital distress and providing productive change strategies. The recognition of the limitations of contingency contracting and problem solving as the basic model for BCT has helped to enlarge the treatment focus. The concept of skill deficiency in communication and problem solving as a major explanatory basis for marital distress has also been questioned through the observation of adequate skills in many distressed couples.

The psychodynamic approach to couples therapy has incorporated the methodology of BCT and cognitive therapy to a lesser degree, although some recent empirical studies have emphasized its efficacy with couples therapy. A major integrative development has been the approach of emotionally focused therapy (Johnson 1999; Johnson and Lebow 2000), which uses attachment theory and the concept of insecure attachment to get past defensive effects to reach for the underlying *soft* effects: attachment effects. Integrative couples therapy (Jacobson et al. 1996; Lawrence et al. 1999) has also recognized a major concept in psychodynamic couples therapy—namely, the importance of accepting the symptoms before attempting to change them.

There are many tasks to be addressed by couples therapy as we enter the new century:

- The search for a comprehensive theory that can incorporate the empirical findings of different couples therapy schools, such as BCT, and maintaining healthy or dysfunctional marital interactions.
- Operationalization of key concepts to allow empirical validation of their role in marital distress and therapeutic change. Such an approach is applicable to many concepts in all schools of family therapy. The psychoanalytic model can operationalize concepts such as *projective identification, the nature of marital transference,* and the *evolutionary course of intimate adult relationships.*
- Exploration of the relationship between individual (intrapsychic) personality patterns and marital interaction: to what degree do the intrapsy-

chic characteristics shape the marital interactions, and to what extent do marital interactions organize each person's behavioral patterns?
- A comprehensive perspective on the role of the wide range of emotions—positive and negative effects—as signals of affective communication system promoting.

Chapters on Related Topics

The following chapters describe concepts related to couples therapy:

- Chapter 10, "Gender-Sensitive Family Therapy" (with extensive discussion of spouse abuse)
- Chapter 14, "The Family Life Cycle: A Framework for Understanding Family Development"
- Chapter 21, "Psychodynamic Couples Therapy"
- Chapter 22, "Behavioral Couples Therapy"
- Chapter 23, "The Divorcing Family: Characteristics and Interventions"
- Chapter 24, "The Remarried Family: Characteristics and Interventions"
- Chapter 25, "Marital Enrichment in Clinical Practice"
- Chapter 26, "Sex Therapy at the Turn of the Century: New Awareness and Response"
- Chapter 28, "Depression and the Family: Interpersonal Context and Family Functioning"
- Chapter 33, "Family Therapy With Personality Disorders"
- Chapter 37, "Couples Therapy Research: Status and Directions"

21

Psychodynamic Couples Therapy

Derek C. Polonsky, M.D.
Carol C. Nadelson, M.D.

Introduction

Couples therapy has evolved over the past 40 years from an ill-defined, "experimental" form of treatment to one that has a well-articulated theoretical framework, specific indications, and a reasoned technical approach. In this chapter, we deal with couples therapy from a psychodynamic perspective, in which family and individual histories are used to understand current interactions. A psychodynamic approach focuses on understanding the unconscious reasons for behavior, as well as the process of reenactment of past experiences in current relationships, in contrast to approaches that focus primarily on modifying current behavior. By using information about individual developmental experiences, the therapist is in a position to clarify the meaning of repeated and often seemingly contradictory or ambiguous interactions. There is a balance between defining the problems as seen by the couple, looking at their past, elucidating individual conflicts with the families of origin, and integrating what is learned in order to help couples move beyond the unconscious factors that contribute to repeating patterns that deplete the relationship. The reasons that couples seek therapy are as diverse as the circumstances of their relationships. We have chosen to use more specific terms related to couples who are married, but we recognize the current diversity of couple configurations (e.g., unmarried, gay or lesbian couples).

Relational Circumstances

We list below the various circumstances under which couples may seek therapy:

1. *Premarital.* A couple may seek therapy prior to making stronger commitments to a relationship in which conflicts have arisen. The couple wishes to see if conflicts can be resolved.
2. *Married with problems in the relationship.* A married couple with a strong, long-standing relationship has recurrent conflicts, and the spouses are dedicated to resolving issues in therapy.
3. *Turbulent marriage.* A couple that has been together for a period of time seldom have good feelings about each other, and collaboration is difficult. Therapy is a way for a couple to see if the relationship can be saved or if separation and divorce are the best options. Therapy can also help a couple (and their children) with the process of separation.
4. *Remarried.* One or both partners have been married before and each may or may not have children from a previous marriage. Issues of parenting often cause conflicts, as do divided loyalties. These conflicts may be similar to marital difficulties with a prior marriage.
5. *Sexual difficulties.*

Theory

Psychodynamic Theory of Couples

In this section we describe the psychodynamic theory of couples and its application. In our work with individuals, we carefully scrutinize intrapsychic phenomena, look at conflicts and their resolution, try to understand the nature of peoples' object relations, and strive to clarify the transference. In work with couples, some of the same considerations are important. Intense transferences may develop between the partners that can be the source of misery and suffering for them. Often, therapists whose experience is primarily in treating individuals avoid considering couples therapy as an option because it seems to be an exercise in frustration, confused transferences, and uncertain alliances. Couples have long-term "ties that bind"—their shared history, family attachments, and children. Often these ties elicit reactions and responses that cause pain and hurt to each partner. Anger, hurt, and disappointment can overwhelm the positive aspects of the relationship and make it seem devoid of good feeling. The partners complain of feeling trapped and miserable.

There are no *normal* or *ideal* relationships. There is a range of individual styles that each couple attempts to mold into a relationship. For some couples intimacy with much sharing of feelings is valued. For others a parallel relationship with little emotional intersection is the preferred style. Independence and autonomy may be important, or reciprocal dependency may be the choice (Sager 1981). The task for the therapist is to help a couple understand what their needs are, to see where they are frustrated, and to help them think about possible solutions.

In the mid-1950s, Martin and Bird (1953) utilized what they called *stereoscopic* therapy. Each clinician saw one partner weekly, followed by the therapists meeting alone to compare notes and attempt to derive the actual nature of the relationship from each partner's narrative. The confounding observation, however, is that often one can have both partners in the same room, recounting the same event, and yet the listener is convinced that he or she is hearing two totally unrelated occurrences. With their stereoscopic technique, Martin and Bird failed to appreciate the importance of distortions applied by both narrator and listener while trying to elucidate an elusive truth. The truth is less important than the way partners experience each other. In therapy discrepancies of listening and telling need to be made clear and an attempt made to understand the unconscious process of distortion.

Dicks (1964) observed that many couples complained that their relationship was ungratifying and yet remained in it. He attempted to explain this and other aspects of marital dysfunction by emphasizing the character of each partner's object relations and the reenactment of the dynamics of the family of origin. In discussing the process of integrating good and bad objects to form a cohesive model of relationships, Dicks indicated that

> in the less fortunate outcome there will remain certain unresolved, not outgrown need-demands towards the parent figures, who were experienced as frustrating, hence as objects of hate. This hate is felt to be both inside the self towards the object, as well as outside the self, in the object towards the self. (Dicks 1964, p. 260)

Dicks proposed that the transferential ties to the parents distort a couple's experience of each other.

To understand the ties that bind, Dicks looked to the concept of *repetition compulsion*. Freud initially described the tendency of individuals to repeat patterns of behavior regardless of the pain or unhappiness the behavior caused. He theorized that by so doing, people kept their attachments to their families of origin more active and were thereby protected from experiencing the pain and disappointment that might result if they were to notice the more depriving aspects of their early relationships. The repetition compulsion defense, while it may be protective, is also severely limiting. Rather than bearing the pain of disappointment and moving on to more gratifying relationships in which needs can more meaningfully be met, the individual reenacts old patterns in current relationships and fails to find lasting satisfaction.

Phases of Marital Relationships

The early phase of a couple's marital relationship is usually characterized by idealization. Partners are blinded to characteristics of each other that resemble unpleasant aspects of members of the family of origin. These characteristics may later become sources of enormous irritation. In this phase, however, the relationship is experienced most positively.

As the relationship grows, people tend to recreate aspects of their relationships with the family of origin. This observation is certainly reasonable, because individuals form expectations about relationships from their first significant contacts with adults (i.e., their parents). Dicks expanded this view by conceptualizing the processes of *reciprocity* and *collusion*. *Reciprocity* refers to a complementary fit of couples, whereby unconscious needs support the re-creation of aspects of early experiences in both partners. Thus, a couple may complain about a lack of closeness, but unconsciously both partners may need the distance they experienced in their families of origin. When one partner becomes more engaging, the other may withdraw. *Collusion* refers to the partners' unconscious mutual agreement to go along with these reenactments. Thus, a woman who talked about how devoted she was to her husband explained as an example that for 14 years she had taken him a cup of tea to his study each night at 10 P.M. and that he had never once said "thank you." She colluded with him by continuing to do this and never once commenting on his lack of acknowledgment or expressing her disappointment and anger.

Dicks summed up reciprocity and collusion by stating that there is a need in each partner to wring out of the other the response that signifies to the unconscious that typical interaction model with the internal object or objects that have come to be vested in the marital relationship (Dicks 1964). In other words, regardless of one partner's expressed intention, his or her behavior or speech will be experienced by the other partner in a particular (distorted) way. A common example of this distortion occurs when one partner is convinced that his or her spouse is angry when in fact this is not the case. The perception of the spouse undergoes a transformation that has an effect on the couple's mutual interactions. Thus, if a partner feels that the spouse is angry, he or she may respond by withdrawing. This in turn affects the spouse, but neither partner is explicit about what is happening.

An important corollary of distorted perceptions is that there are *no victims;* both partners have some unconscious investment in entering into a relationship in which there are shared distortions about both partners' real behaviors and personalities.

Case Study

Mike and Denise were contemplating marriage but were concerned about their patterns of retreating from each other and their lack of closeness. Denise had grown up in a prominent family. Her parents divorced when she was 12, and their marriage had always been difficult. When she was 17, her mother developed a malignancy and died within a year. In the relationship with Mike she was terrified of being abandoned and constantly needed reassurance. He experienced this as controlling and intrusive.

Understanding Mike's history helped explain the complementary issues. His father died when he was 7, and he was expected to be the "man of the house" and was required to take responsibility for his mother and younger sister. When he was 21, he was engaged to a young woman who developed ovarian cancer and died within 6 months. This stirred up powerful feelings of vulnerability to loss and the belief that to be involved with someone held great danger. When he withdrew from Denise and she expressed her feelings of abandonment, he experienced her feelings as a demand to take care of her as he had done with his mother, his sister, and then his girlfriend.

In therapy both Mike and Denise focused on their experiences of loss, in response to which the clinician at times shifted the focus or format of treatment to "parallel" individual therapy. The purpose of parallel therapy was to help each partner grieve more openly and to learn more about the ways he or she adapted and clarify the meaning of their behaviors. Mike began to see Denise's vulnerability in terms of her earlier losses, and Denise realized that Mike experienced her feelings as burdens. As they developed more understanding, they were able to feel closer.

Framo (1982) observed that people choose partners with similar levels of emotional differentiation. Thus, despite other disparities in personality and style, they may be more similar than is initially apparent. Therapists may respond more to the style of each individual than to the underlying intrapsychic issues, and diagnostic labels may be applied that do not capture the nature of a couple's interaction or its developmental determinants. For example, husbands are often seen as obsessional and higher functioning than their wives, who are seen as hysterical, "flaky," or borderline. When the therapist gets to know the couple better, *the similarities of developmental issues and the shared conflicts are clearer.* The appearance may be more in style than in substance, and outward differences can belie basic similarities. More outspoken partners often express feelings that quieter partners do not identify as theirs.

Main (1966) observed that couple partners engage in forms of distortions that perpetuate partners' artificial experience of each other. He described the distorting processes of *collusion, mutual projection, and projective identification.* The collusive aspects of relationships are often difficult to understand in a therapeutic modality other than in couples therapy. A therapist who is treating an individual may have limited awareness of collusive processes, depending on what the individual is either able or willing to bring to the therapeutic sessions. What is important about collusions is that *both partners* are involved in the process. Main emphasized that partners' reciprocal engagement in collusion enabled them to deny individual conflicts.

If one spouse in individual therapy begins to understand these unconscious needs and begins to change, the relationship may become stressed. The treated partner is increasingly reluctant to continue with the collusive process. One of the authors (D.P.) recalls seeing a woman in individual treatment while her husband was seeing a colleague. His understanding of the husband was that he was a narcissistic, entitled man, and that his patient (the wife) was masochistic to continue living with him. In the course of therapy the wife continued to discuss her husband's behavior, but it appeared to have little effect on her. The therapist noticed that he was feeling and articulating her distress but that she appeared to be unaffected emotionally; he was inadvertently becoming the bearer and expressor of her emotions. Because she was so cut off from her feelings, she was destined to repeat the behavior without learning from her experiences. A joint meeting was arranged with husband, wife, and both therapists, and what could then be observed was the wife's repeated disqualification and ignoring any of the husband's caring responses. This was entirely missed in the individual meetings.

Main (1966, p. 433) wrote that "we are aware of the ubiquity of unconscious collusions between marital partners to defend against unconscious problems by building joint misperceptions[,] and we prefer to see both partners before making an extended diagnosis." With mutual projection, a partner may have feelings about his or her own personality that are very disturbing. Rather than owning feelings and personal characteristics, the partner will locate them in the spouse, in whom they will be criticized.

As noted above, the work of Martin and Bird (1953) was focused on trying to understand the *reality* of the interaction between two people. Who is telling the truth? By contrast, Main (1966) emphasized that *reality* is less important than trying to understand the need for distortion. The distortion, he felt, was secondary to understanding the defensive function it serves. Thus, a man who feels conflicted about his aggression and competence may be critical and undermining of his wife's successes. He may initially have been drawn to that quality in his wife because he felt uncomfortable about the quality's presence in himself. By criticizing her, his inner conflict is externalized and not consciously experienced. The effect on the relationship, however, is to deprive both partners of the pleasure of their competence and abilities.

As Main stated:

> the marital relationship may be so invaded by archaic object relationships and their destructiveness that reality testing against old fantasies may be swamped collusively so that the marriage may become only a repository of old conflicts. The end result of such projection is not divorce, but a painful dependence on the hated partner. In such a marriage, the partner ceases to exist in his or her own right. The couple now need each other for hateful fantasy reasons. They cannot part and yet cannot enjoy the marriage. (Main 1966, p. 445)

Unless attention is paid to the partners' unconscious and hateful need for each other, the therapist may miss the underlying reenactments and fail to help patients deal with difficulties related to early object relations.

Framo elaborated on Main's description of hateful dependence, stating that

> one's mate (or children) are perceived largely in terms of the individual's own needs, or as carrying for him his own denied, split off traits. Mates select each other on the basis of rediscovering lost aspects of their primary object relations which they had split off and which, in their involvement with the spouse, they reexperience by projective identification. (Framo 1982, p. 197)

A main source of marital disharmony is that spouses project disowned aspects of themselves onto the mate and then fight them in the mate.

Case Study

> Robin and Paul were both in their early 30s and had been married for 4 years when they came for therapy. Robin was distraught about Paul's repeated, intensely angry, and vituperative outbursts that often appeared "out of the blue." In the initial session, Paul said little, while Robin detailed many incidents.
>
> Robin was committed to the couples therapy, but Paul refused. She was seen individually for 3 weeks. Little pressure was placed on Paul to participate. Therapy focused on ways for her to disengage from the fights and maintain her self-esteem.
>
> When Paul suddenly called and requested an appointment, the therapist had wondered what had happened. The therapist speculated that Paul's reluctance resulted from a concern that he would be attacked and criticized,

although Paul readily acknowledged his behavior. Keeping this in mind, the therapist focused the early sessions on a discussion of Paul's family, learning more about his background, and minimized opportunities for criticism. Paul told of his parents' troubled relationship. His father (like Paul) had repeated, explosive, angry, outbursts directed at his mother. Paul was terribly upset by these and felt helpless to protect his mother. As he grew older, his father began to direct the attacks at him, with much derision and considerable unpredictability. Paul could not remember doing anything with his father that felt good. As he told this story, Paul began to experience more affect about his father and was soon in tears. The therapist was then able to tie together Paul's experience with his father and the behavior with Robin. Paul saw the connections and acknowledged that he was reenacting aspects of his relationship with his father with Robin.

In this context, Paul began to see therapy as an opportunity to express feelings he had buried. His relationship with Robin improved. Even his initial response to therapy—his anticipation of criticism and derision from the therapist—paralleled his experience with his father.

Without understanding Paul's past experiences and expectations, it would have been difficult to engage him in therapy. If a clinician had focused primarily on current behavior, the therapy might have inadvertently re-created the experiences that led to Paul's self-hating. Because the therapist initially helped Paul see the connection to the past in a supportive and nonchallenging mode and elicited the connected affect, Paul could appreciate the value of couples therapy. In subsequent joint sessions, Paul was encouraged to recount his understanding of the previous meetings and involve Robin. Robin knew his father and had heard accounts of the past behavior from Paul's mother, so she was relieved that he had made some connections between past and present. She had had little awareness, however, of Paul's sadness. This understanding was helpful in fostering a more empathic response to him.

Projective Identification

The concept of projective identification enables therapists to understand the bridge between unresolved individual intrapsychic concerns and the interaction, very often based on distorted perceptions, between partners. Projective identification attempts to incorporate the concepts of collusion and mutual projection to understand the ways in which perceptions one partner has of the other are modified, thus changing how partners relate to each other. Each partner begins to react to the distorted perception of the other, and the relationship becomes constricted. If one compares the relationship to the multifaceted mirrored balls that decorate discos, it is as if each partner is fixed in aligning one personality facet with the other partner and all others are obscured. When this happens, the partners experience each other in a less "real" way because so many qualities are not perceived. What starts as *intrapsychic* conflict is experienced as *interpersonal* difficulty. Couples therapy can refocus the locus of affect in order to clarify distorted perceptions.

The process is illustrated in the following apocryphal story. A man was driving on a country road and his car had a flat tire. Much to his chagrin, he discovered he did not have a jack. Since there was a house nearby, he decided to ask the occupants if he could borrow a jack. As he walked closer to the house he began to think that the owner of the house would probably not want to lend him the jack, and that he might be suspicious of a stranger. Reaching the house, he knocked on the door. When the owner opened it, the man yelled, "You can shove your jack," and stormed off. This example illustrates the way in which his perception of the owner of the house underwent a transformation in his mind, without the owner having any awareness of it. Characteristics were attributed to the householder without any basis in reality and colored the motorist's reaction.

This is a powerful and often-observed phenomenon in couples. Unowned affects or conflicts are projected onto a partner and are then reacted to as if they were the partner's real characteristics. The partner may have no awareness that this has occurred, but he or she notices a change in the relationship.

Main (1966) extended the idea of projective identification when he conceptualized an *emotional economy* in couples where one partner becomes the repository of split off, despised, hated aspects of the self, without which the other partner would have to own them himself or herself. This underscores the purposes of dysphoric relationships. Unless the therapist is aware of emotional economy, it is unlikely that he or she will clarify the underlying reasons for the couple's behavior.

Diagnostic Considerations

We have found it useful to conceptualize a diagnostic spectrum for couples, based on their functioning:

- *Highly functioning couples with focal problems.* Such couples are able to use insight in therapy, tolerate frustration, and integrate positive and negative attributes of each other in their relationship. These couples have usually functioned well and develop problems around a specific issue. Therapy is usually brief, and they are able to collaborate easily with each other and with the therapist.
- *Couples with repeated conflicts that impair their functioning.* These couples have greater conflicts and tend to act them out. The transference between them is intense and may be acted on, resulting in periods of considerable

stress. However, they maintain the capacity to handle conflict and they have the ability to be objective and reflective. Therapy may take longer and require more early reconstruction and working out of mutual projections and transferences. The couple retains a sense of commitment to each other, and the integrity of their relationship is not at issue.

- *Couples with severe, long-lasting discord.* These couples function with frequent, intense conflict that may lead to transient ruptures in their capacity to integrate positive and negative characteristics. The result may be that one partner is sometimes seen as all good or all bad, and balanced perception may be difficult. These couples may require structure, limits, and a good deal of support. However, if they are able to maintain an alliance with the therapist, despite their significant distortions, they may improve considerably.
- *Severely turbulent relationships.* The relationship and the treatment of these couples are stormy and difficult. There are periods of significant rupture in the sense of collaboration. Partners are experienced as predominantly bad objects, and there is little capacity to recall endearing and valued qualities that are present at other times. Often, therapy is slow and the alliance with the therapist is precarious. A therapy hour can become a replica of the disturbance at home, with diminished capacity to listen to each other or to the therapist. Collaboration is very difficult because distortions are profound or marked. There is little consensus about reporting events, and the therapist may find it difficult to understand an event that is perceived so differently by the two participants. Therapy is often difficult and unsuccessful. The couple may leave therapy with a sense of failure. Frequently, the therapist is identified as the bad object, and for a short while the couple may unite in this view. They may stop therapy, feeling sustained for a while in having joined forces against a common enemy. The therapeutic challenge is to help each individual recognize and express his or her feelings, rather than disowning them and projecting them onto the spouse.

Therapeutic Considerations

Couples therapy can be quite stressful because, unlike individual therapy, each partner is forced to be more "honest." It is not easy to conceal material in this setting as in individual therapy. In addition, while the therapist may attempt to understand unconscious determinants, a couple may have little ability to integrate this information and use it therapeutically. However, a therapist who they can perceive as a benevolent parent can help them. This helpful transference does not necessarily have to be interpreted. For couples who have had poor role models in their parents, the therapist can provide a model for interacting that is different and that leads to more satisfactory resolution. Initially, sessions may be difficult for a therapist, and he or she may experience heightened anxiety. In dealing with two people at the same time, the complexity of transferences and the blurring of intrapsychic and interpersonal issues are confusing. Countertransference aspects of couples therapy are important to acknowledge and consider.

Evaluation

The evaluation of a couple should include individual meetings where both partners can talk about their own experiences, perceptions, and wishes. Although many therapists who see couples insist on seeing the couple together at all times, our view is that this deprives the therapist of opportunities to gather useful information about the individual dynamics that are part of the couple's relationship. Individual sessions also provide an opportunity for partners to reveal or raise issues individually that they are not ready to discuss with the partner present. Individuals may require some special help to raise these issues within the couples meetings.

There may be times, however, when additional information learned in individual meetings can lead to difficulties. Secrets that the therapist and one partner share can be collusive and undermine the joint work. Our experience has been that the more information that is available, the more likely we are to be in a position to understand and ultimately to be more helpful. The therapist can usually work with individuals to understand the meaning and implications of revealed secrets and to explore whether and when to share the information with the other partner. This can be an important process, especially if the individual's perception of the partner's response is a projection.

Clinical and Technical Interventions

Activity

In the early phases of treatment, the therapist may need to be quite active to engage the couple and begin to form an alliance. Although couples are extremely anxious about the state of their relationship, they view the therapist as someone who will be able to help them contain an intolerable level of stress in a way that they have been unable to do. The therapist provides some structure and support. He or she can rephrase what each partner says in a way that facilitates clarification of distortions in communication. In fact, in the initial phase of the therapy, much time is devoted to clarifying the difference between what one partner intends and what the other perceives. Therapists who are more reflective and silent in their approach may elicit confusion about expectations, as well as uncertainty about how to understand what has caused the deterioration of the marriage and what do to about it. This can intensify anxiety to the point that the couple may end therapy or may allow the couple to focus their anger on the perceived inadequacies of the therapist so that they don't deal with their own concerns. We try to be actively involved with the couple in a collaborative discussion about the origins of their difficulties, and we share with them our speculations, inviting them to discuss their own views.

Directions (Active Interventions)

There are times when it is helpful to give a couple an assignment. Therapists need to keep in mind their understanding about both individual and interpersonal issues, and assignments can be used to provide some structure for the couple and help them gain understanding of the process of their interaction.

Case Study

In Kim and Don's relationship, Kim was angry a great deal of the time, but Don denied having similar feelings. He was instructed to keep notes about anything that was the least bit irritating about his wife. The following week he returned with a list on a 3-by-5 index card. This list was discussed in the joint meeting, resulting in some new understandings.

Case Study

Rick and Sadie, after a brief separation, decided to live together again. When they planned to clean out Rick's apartment in another city, they lamented about how difficult it was going to be for them to stay in the apartment that had so many negative associations to this difficult period. The therapist asked whether they had contemplated staying in a hotel. Since neither had, they discussed how they might structure the weekend differently. After the weekend it was possible to review the results and help them think about making this kind of choice more often.

Developing the Concepts of Repetition Compulsion, Mutual Projection, Collusion, and Projective Identification

The concepts of repetition compulsion, mutual projection, collusion, and projective identification should be explained to the couple. This helps partners understand the idea of reenactments in relationships and facilitates the therapeutic process. Initially, patterns from families of origin are discussed, and the ways in which these patterns are reenacted in the marriage are pointed out.

The idea of an *informational statement* versus a *reactive statement* is explained to help a couple move away from repetitive troublesome interactions that result in defensive withdrawal, anger, and isolation. For example, if one partner talks about something the other did in positive terms, we will ask the spouse if he or she is aware of it. Often we find that the relationship is experienced as critical and unsatisfying, and couples miss opportunities to notice what each partner does positively. Couples can be expert at pointing out the negatives in each other and need encouragement to notice what they like and value.

Whenever there is a "he/she makes me feel" statement, it is likely that projective identifications are playing a role, and each partner is not owning or acknowledging feelings. We interrupt and encourage partners to rephrase the statement starting with "I feel." We point out that only an individual has a feeling and another cannot make it happen. This paves the way for couples to notice perceptual distortions, and it provides a model for each to begin to own feelings.

Case Study

> Early in treatment, Mary and Bob colluded by trading projections. A representative interaction would be when Mary pointed out to Bob that he was not meeting his part of the housecleaning agreement. Since it happened to be Bob's birthday, he became furious and said that she had ruined his birthday. In this instance, Mary's usual pattern was to withdraw and become silent. When her tendency to internalize angry feelings and withdraw was clarified, Mary could point out that when an issue like Bob's not doing the housework occurred, it was not she who did anything to him (e.g., ruin his birthday). In fact, she was able to observe "this has nothing to do with me—you are always depressed on your birthday and it is because your mother never calls. If you want to confront anyone, confront her." Bob was forced to own his feelings, and Mary did not withdraw.

Shifting the Focus of Couples Treatment

At times the clinician might shift the focus of couples therapy to an individual, in the context of the conjoint meetings. Far from confusing the treatment, this is often a useful part of the process. By one partner's being provided an opportunity to clarify an issue, the spouse can observe the therapist talking with the partner about a difficult issue and model the therapist's behavior. This facilitates an appreciation of the inner experience of the partner.

Case Study

Dave and Harriet visited Dave's parents for Thanksgiving. Dave entered the session after the weekend and seemed to be quite downcast. The therapist asked about the time with his parents. Dave could not identify anything that helped to clarify his reaction. Harriet then commented that they had been at his parent's house for 30 minutes before anyone said hello, an experience that she felt was bizarre. It was so familiar to Dave that he did not even consciously notice it, although he reacted strongly to the rebuff.

When working with an individual issue in couples treatment, a partner may feel that the therapist is taking the position that he or she is the problem in the marriage. We encourage individuals to let us know if they feel they are getting undue focus and restate our belief that both partners bring emotional "baggage" from the past into their relationship. As each partner's psychodynamics becomes clearer, we have been impressed with the resonance of early developmental issues. It is logical that partners, as Framo (1982) suggests, would experience familiarity with someone who had similar early experiences.

Depression and Couples Therapy

The impact of depression in one partner on a relationship can be substantial. A depressed partner often experiences guilt, despair, and hopelessness and may not be aware that the depression has a significant effect on other family members. The spouse initially attempts to be supportive and understanding, then tries to "fix" the depression, and finally feels frustrated angry and guilty when the attempt to help fails. The relationship may undergo a transformation and be dominated by the depressed affect. Children are also much affected by a depressed or compromised parent. The history of parental depression is often remembered as a confusing time. The child may feel responsible for the change in the family. By helping to alleviate depression in the parent, the therapist has a positive, though indirect, effect on the children as well as on the nondepressed partner.

In the following case example, the wife had a long-standing depression. Although she understood the complex issues that were replayed in her relationships with men, she continued to experience feelings related more to past events. Her individual therapy was "successful" in that she developed insight and experienced affect. She modified her relationship with her parents, but when there were reenactments in the marriage, the original feelings were incapacitating.

Case Study

Joan and Art had been married for 4 years. It was the second marriage for both. They fought repeatedly, and each complained about the "pathology" of the other.

During their intense battles they each would lose the capacity to hold onto any good feelings about the other. They felt a profound sense of hopelessness and thought about divorce. For a while they were seen individually, because, when they were seen jointly, there was such distortion and intensity that little useful work was accomplished. In individual meetings, it was possible to focus on the details of their family histories and attempt to connect these histories with the current conflicts.

Joan experienced her parents as extremely critical and devaluing. There was nothing she could do that would elicit any positive response from them. Art's father was in the army for the first 5 years of Art's life. During this time, Art had a very close relationship with his mother, who admired him as "her little man." When Art's father returned, his parents had more children. The birth of his three brothers dramatically changed the position he held in the family.

In the marriage, Art criticized Joan relentlessly. He read widely in psychiatry and had elaborate formulations about her "primitive mental structures." He was convinced that she was "hopelessly borderline." Joan felt exhausted by his attacks. Based on her experience with critical parents, she was unable to counter the attacks. She became more depressed, sleepless, and had frequent bouts of crying. Although connections were made with the feelings in her family, not much changed in her reactions to Art. After a number of months, they talked about Joan's depression and she revealed that she had begun to medicate herself. Subsequently, the decision was made to begin treatment with fluoxetine (Prozac). Within weeks, Joan began to feel better and was able to use psychotherapy more successfully. Over time, she responded to Art more effectively and was not plagued by the intensity of her earlier feelings. When Art would attempt to engage her in familiar struggles, she was able to resist and to see what his role was in these altercations.

The shift in the marital dynamics was dramatic. When Joan withdrew from the old loop, Art was forced to deal more directly with his feelings. The changes in the marriage continued as each partner continued the process of owning feelings and talking more from the "I feel" perspective. They began to experience for the first time the beginnings of shared intimacy.

Integration of Sexual Therapy and Dynamic Couples Therapy

The development of sex therapy is detailed in Chapter 26, "Sex Therapy at the Turn of the Century: New Awareness and Response." Couples therapists should be familiar with these techniques and know how to integrate them into couples therapy. Couples often present with a problem defined as sexual and may need to be treated with a sexually oriented approach before making a transition to the other troublesome aspects of a relationship. Material that comes up in the course of sex therapy can enhance understanding of the couple's unconscious interactions.

Case Study

Paul and Rae Ann had been married for close to 20 years. They had two teenage children, and each partner had had several years of individual therapy as well as couples therapy. They requested therapy specifically to deal with Paul's premature ejaculation.

They had remarkably similar family histories. Paul's parents were described as quietly disapproving and critical. They offered little support and encouragement to Paul. They undermined his decisions and consistently behaved in a way that resulted in his feeling guilty. Rae Ann experienced her parents as more openly hostile and critical. They were often disapproving and devaluing. When she was 17 she became anorexic. She was hospitalized and received electroconvulsive therapy. In individual therapy, she was able to begin to appreciate the effect her parents continued to have on her life.

Paul and Rae Ann were committed to each other and were interested in focusing on Paul's sexual difficulty. Sensate focus exercises were begun and went very well. Both felt relaxed and relieved of pressure. They continued to progress and were instructed about the squeeze technique to help Paul gain ejaculatory control. This too went very well, and both were delighted with the changes.

When the therapist, using Masters and Johnson's terminology, talked about *vaginal containment*, Paul experienced profound anxiety. The next week, they reported having had a terrible time. Paul had become impotent, and said that it had all begun when I mentioned the "vaginal entrapment" (Paul's words).

During therapy they revealed that both had had dreams the night before they attempted to deal with psychodynamic issues. Paul's dream was that he came into the kitchen and placed his hand in his daughter's birdcage to feed the bird. The bird flapped all over the cage and then fell down dead, "all shrivelled up." Rae Ann's dream also took place in the kitchen. She was walking in and found one of the children playing with the food processor, which he had managed to get started without the safety lid, and was about to put his hand into the machine. Paul's "entrapment" slip and the dreams paved the way for the therapist to begin to deal with the issues of anger in the family. Both Paul and Rae Ann were terrified of feeling angry, yet each felt anger about their early experiences. The focus of the couples therapy shifted away from sex and concentrated more on psychodynamic issues. They were able to offer support to each other when they had encounters with the parents and begin to manage anger with each other directly. As this happened, the sexual issues began to shift. What started off as "only" sex therapy developed into long-term, psychodynamically oriented couples therapy.

Transference

In the process of therapy, transference also warrants attention as it is manifested between the partners as well as with the therapist. Distortions, collusions, and projections are pointed out and the effects are noted. It is helpful to clarify how a spouse reacts to characteristics that an accused partner may not actually possess but rather characteristics that are disowned and projected feelings of the spouse. When one partner experiences the other in distorted terms, the subject partner becomes "less real" (i.e., good qualities that he or she may have are not seen or felt).

Case Study

> As a small child, Nat had been given repeated enemas by his mother. This lasted from age 5 through 14. He was aware of little affect about these experiences, but in his marriage he experienced his wife as intrusive and controlling. He was unable to notice and be affected by her caring, valuing comments, and he interpreted almost all of her behavior as a reenactment of the coercion he experienced earlier with his mother. As the therapy continued, a similar transference developed toward the therapist. Nat resented the therapist's attempts at interpretation and clarification, and he felt that the therapist was forcing him to admit to feelings he did not have. Nat began to feel that the therapist, like his wife, was intrusive, coercive, and uncaring. The therapist was able to use this transference development to help him understand how his experience of peoples' intentions (and most importantly his wife's) was influenced by his past experiences.

When transference to the therapist interferes with therapy, it should be actively interpreted. This is useful both for the affected individual, who begins to integrate and understand his or her projections, and for the partner, who is an observer rather than direct participant. The observing partner sees an interactional pattern develop between the therapist and the affected partner that parallels his or her own experience; this allows the observing partner to see more clearly the altered perception of the other partner. This process is quite similar to the interpretation a therapist might offer in an individual therapy.

There may be times when one partner feels that he or she has become the focus of the therapy and complains that it feels unfair. At this time, the therapist needs to question whether the concerns are valid and deal with them. There may be times when therapists may need to explain their reasons for a more individual focus and to reassure the patient that the spouse will have his or her turn.

Countertransference

Countertransference can cause therapists pain and endanger the outcome of therapy. As we have noted, many therapists are overwhelmed by the complex alliances that occur when dealing with two people together and feel that couples therapy is a confusing process that they would rather avoid. Often they worry about the inevitability that they will feel more positively toward one partner and take sides, thus damaging the therapeutic alliance. Several issues need to be considered.

As with any form of therapy, therapists have to strive to be neutral or balanced in their approach to individual partners. By continually striving to understand the *meaning* of behavior, and by using past history as a key to unlock the paradoxes, therapists define their role as a facilitator of understanding rather than a judge of behavior. Therapists must remind themselves that there is no ideal form of relationship and that their work is to identify and clarify couples' issues, however entangled or disturbed. Often therapists feel that a couple's relationship is deficient and that their role is to make it over. In this endeavor, the therapist will inevitably be frustrated.

Therapists also need to notice when the couple's issues resonate with issues in the therapist's own relationships. Sagert (1967) cautioned against acting out in this form of therapy and encouraged therapists to use peer supervision groups to help identify countertransference problems. He described a colleague's difficulty in treating a couple where the husband had divorced his former wife and married a younger woman. In a peer supervision group, the therapist came to understand that he secretly enjoyed the older man's distress because he was jealous of his patient. The therapist, who had remained in an unsatisfying marriage, wished he had been able to do what his patient had done.

When working with some couples, the therapist may be affected by a profound sense of hopelessness about the relationship and by the obvious sadness that the partners cause in each other. This occurs particularly with more disturbed couples, whose capacity to hold onto positive objects may be very limited.

Conclusion

Couples therapy is most useful when therapists are flexible and imaginative in the use of different approaches. The psychodynamic model provides an understanding of the unconscious factors that influence a couple's behavior and partners' experience of each other. Unconscious behavior is an important tool for clarifying the paradoxes so often seen in marital interactions.

Close attention needs to be given to collusions and mutual projection in order to understand the need to be in a relationship about which there may be so many complaints. Over time, a couple can be helped to appreciate and integrate these ideas. Therapists may also integrate a variety of techniques that might be called "behavioral" or "systems-related." By suggesting a task (e.g., "Make a list of the things that irritate you about your spouse"), the therapist can help the couple to focus their attention on behavior that they do not notice and then help them develop a better understanding of its meaning.

Depending on the needs and wishes of the couple, treatment can be used in different ways. Symptom relief might be all a couple wants, in which case the therapy will be brief. The focus will be on modifying some behaviors that result in conflict. Partners may come to feel safer bringing up issues that seemed frightening to discuss on their own or that they were unable to discuss because they could not tolerate their partner's response. Partners experience some relief of their acute tension and feel that they have been helped.

If the couple has an interest in understanding more about the origins and meaning of their interactions, the therapy can become more intensive and insight-oriented. It can attend to issues in each partner's family and focus on unconscious reenactments in the relationship. As couples see connections with the past, they can become freer to explore the potential in the current relationship, without the repeated distortions. At times, one can discuss the idea of the *hopelessness* of childhood and the *hopefulness* of a couple's relationship. By this we mean that because children have little ability to understand their parents' problematic behaviors, they may experience feelings of hopelessness about effecting change. This sense of futility can be brought into a marriage. A partner can feel that he or she cannot affect the spouse, who is experienced as depriving in a way similar to the parents. By discussing hopefulness, the couple can be encouraged to think about potential collaboration to meet each other's needs and about the possibility of change.

Transference should primarily be studied between the partners rather than with the therapist (although this aspect should not be ignored). By using the understanding derived from a psychodynamic assessment of each partner, it is possible to interpret the meaning of distortions of perception that can interfere with a couple's ability to relate to each other. When a couple develops an understanding of distortion, the relationship changes in a fundamental way. Initially it might be difficult for the couple to retain this new understanding; however, the therapist becomes the keeper of newfound understanding and is able to remind the couple. In time, when the relationship is under stress, one partner may remember what was learned and remind the other, thereby circumventing old patterns.

Therapy is framed as a collaboration between the therapist and the couple. It is important to share with the couple the understanding that the therapist has gained of their difficulties, and to describe the process of reenactments from family of origin in a jargon-free language. Couples can collaborate in unraveling what each partner brings to their interaction from their family of origin. Often one partner can describe "unnoticed" behavior in the spouse's family. The family's behavior is so familiar to the spouse that certain conclusions may not be reached. It is not unusual to hear from one partner that his or her family was close, warm, and loving, only to have the spouse describe relationships that were intrusive, critical, devaluing, and demeaning. In fact, the couples therapy format often helps to understand previously undetected issues.

In Pat Conroy's book *Prince of Tides*, the husband described the complexity of interactions as follows:

> Again and again, I thought of Sallie and our children. I had married the first woman I had ever kissed. I thought I had married her because she was pretty, blessed with horse sense and sass, and unlike my mother in any way. But I had married a fine and comely girl, and with brilliance and craft and all the instincts of self-preservation jettisoned. I succeeded over the years, through neglect, coldness and betrayal, in turning her into the exact image of my mother. Because of some endemic flaw in my manhood, I could not just have wives or lovers. I required soft enemies humming lullabies of carnage in the playroom, snipers in floral print dresses, gunning for me from the bell towers. I was not comfortable with anyone who was not disapproving of me. No matter how ardently I strove to attain their impossibly high standards for me, I could never do anything entirely right and so I grew accustomed to that climate in inevitable failure. (p. 100)

Couples therapy, while initially more confusing than individual therapy, offers the possibility to see transferences unfold. It reduces the possibilities for therapists to inadvertently collude with an individual patient's denials and distortions, and it offers couples an opportunity to experience their relationship as sustaining, in contrast to the depleting sense of isolation that distorted perceptions and consequent reactive behavior produce. By integrating the understanding derived from a psychodynamic approach and paying attention to current realities, couples therapists are in a unique position to offer enormous help to their patients as they struggle to free their relationship of recurrent destructive patterns.

Chapters on Related Topics

The following chapters describe concepts related to psychodynamic couples therapy:

- Chapter 4, "Psychodynamic Family Therapy"
- Chapter 5, "Multigenerational Family Systems Theory of Bowen and Its Application"
- Chapter 6, "Contextual Therapy"
- Chapter 20, "Couples Therapy: An Overview"
- Chapter 33, "Family Therapy With Personality Disorders"

22

Behavioral Couples Therapy

Steven L. Sayers, Ph.D.
Richard E. Heyman

Introduction

It is tempting to write a chapter about behavioral couples therapy (BCT) solely from the standpoint of what BCT is *not*. BCT has been referred to by some of its most enthusiastic advocates as "technology" (Jacobson and Margolin 1979), which we believe is an unfortunate and somewhat misleading term. Many critics believe that BCT addresses only surface issues and ignores important intrapersonal and interpersonal dynamics. We hope that this chapter will show how a behavioral approach to marriage is anything *but* shallow and technological and instead is concerned with the most important determinants of relationship happiness.

We believe that BCT sounds dehumanizing and mechanistic to some as a result of early attempts to portray it in a scientifically rigorous manner. We feel very strongly that empirical studies should guide our clinical work but believe it is also important to describe our clinical methods in ways that fully illustrate how our science of relationships is relevant to real human relationships. Our goal is to illustrate how a behavioral approach can be useful from a scientific as well as a clinical perspective. It is also clear that over the last several decades BCT has been modified, challenged, and reinvented. We briefly present this debate and then outline the most integral and enduring characteristics of the behavioral approach.

Relationship Dysfunction From a Behavioral Perspective

Behavioral approaches to relationship discord can be distinguished from other approaches by 1) the theoretical models that explain marital dysfunction, and 2) the therapeutic goals and procedures specified within these models. The theoretical aspects of BCT employ several terms or concepts that need to be clarified. The way these concepts are described is often the cause of the mechanistic *feel* that has been attributed to the behavioral approach. We encourage readers to apply these concepts to their own case examples, even though the cases may have been conceptualized using a different theoretical model.

One note about the label *behavioral couples therapy*, or BCT. The early development of the behavioral approach to intervention in couples used the term *behavioral marital therapy* (BMT), and many articles were published using that label. Early in the 1990s researchers and clinicians began to recognize the general application of the approach to many different forms of intimate dyads and appropriately began to use the newer label BCT, even though the bulk of the literature involved married heterosexual couples. For the ease of reading and recognizing diversity in the couples we might treat with the approach, we have adopted the use of the more general term, BCT, throughout the chapter.

Basic Concepts

Although all are included under the umbrella of the BCT label, several distinct traditions have coalesced under the name BCT. Reviewing the BCT chapter by Epstein and Williams (1981), we were struck by how *behavioral* their descriptions are compared with those used by the *new-wave* BCT of the 1990s (Jacobson 1991a). One of our goals is to describe the changes in conceptualizing and practicing BCT in the past decade. In this section we review the theoretical viewpoints that defined early behavioral approaches to marital distress. Subsequent sections will detail the evolution of BCT, a process of assimilation of other theoretical approaches and techniques that has caused some to question how *behavioral* BCT is.

Operant Conditioning

Operant conditioning derives from the work of Skinner (e.g., Skinner 1953). (Although classical conditioning could be invoked in behavioral models of marital distress, it rarely is.) Most basically operant approaches posit that the probability of a behavior occurring increases or decreases depending on the consequences. External, observable behaviors are the primary events of interest. (Consult Weiss 1978 for a detailed operant behavioral analysis of marriage.) Current descriptions of BCT seem to take operant principles for granted as authors focus on expanding BCT's domain. However, the following traditional behavioral terms have a primary role in this conception of marriage.

Positive Reinforcement

Positive reinforcement is experienced when the consequences of an individual's behavior lead to an increase and maintenance of that behavior over time. That is, a consequence is reinforcing only if it increases the likelihood of the behavior's occurring in the future. An outside observer (i.e., a therapist!) may not be able to define a consequence as positive, and in many cases whether the consequence is truly reinforcing is known only after the fact.

Punishment

Another important behavior, *punishment*, transpires when an aversive consequence decreases the likelihood that a behavior will occur in the future. Much of the punishment that occurs between partners comes in the form of unpleasant or aversive communication. The effect, however, of a communication on the receiver should not be taken for granted. To understand the dynamics of the situation, a therapist needs to conduct a retrospective and prospective analysis of how one partner's complaints about his or her workday affects the other partner's behavior over repeated days, months, and years.

Negative Reinforcement

Negative reinforcement is a response that is often misunderstood or mistaken for punishment. Negative reinforcement occurs when the *cessation* of an aversive stimulus increases the likelihood of the response behavior. Imagine that a wife repeatedly reminds her husband to complete a task around the house. If she stops *nagging* him when he acquiesces, then his acquiescence has been negatively reinforced (assuming it makes him more likely to give in, in the future).

Aversive behaviors (such as nagging, complaining, and making physical or psychological threats) occur in many relationships because they tend to achieve the desired end, if one examines only the short-term outcome (i.e., acquiescence). However, although these aversive behaviors often lead to immediate compliance, they also lead to a great deal of unhappiness and resentment. In the long term, individuals find other ways to terminate or escape their partner's negative behavior, or they try to use aversive behavior to terminate the partner's aversive behavior. The phenomenon of using aversive behavior to terminate the partner's aversive behavior is known as *coercion* (Patterson 1982). A husband complains, his wife then criticizes him, he then finds fault with her, she then puts him down, and so forth. Each partner intends his or her aversive behavior to serve as a punisher (i.e., a way of decreasing the partner's preceding aversive behavior). In actuality, each person's aversive behavior increases in amplitude until one partner gives in—they are finally both negatively reinforced ("My hostile partner has finally shut up!").

Gottman and Levenson's (1986) formulation of the coercion model posits that the source of reinforcement is an individual's physiological responses. They presented evidence to show that negative interactional behaviors produce aversive physiological states; behaviors that reduce these states provide the negative reinforcement. Those coercive interactions that are not powerful enough to evoke strong aversive arousal would not be negatively reinforced. The researchers have labeled this process the "escape conditioning model." As one spouse finds a way of terminating, or withdrawing from, or otherwise escaping the aversive interaction, this response is negatively reinforced.

Christensen (1988) discusses a highly related pattern of interaction in which one partner demands intimacy, emotional interaction, or change from the partner, and the other partner withdraws from these demands in an ever intensifying and frustrating cycle. This demand/withdraw pattern is often expressed in gender stereotypes, with women in the demand role and men in the role of the partner who withdraws. Although there may be a general difference between the percentage of men and women who fit into each role, the key aspect of the pattern is that it is a mutually reinforcing trap for each partner (i.e., each is intermittently reinforced for his or her demand or withdrawal behavior), but the overall effect is to decrease relationship-enhancing behavior. Thus, over time, each partner becomes less satisfied in the relationship, and the couple is less likely to resolve the problems and conflicts that they face.

Negative Reciprocity

Negative reciprocity may be understood as an extension and perhaps a result of the frequent use of aversive behavior in coercive marital interactions. It is the tendency for negative (or aversive) behavior to be reciprocated (i.e., responded to *in kind*) by the partner. Negative reciprocity has been used to denote the concept of *contingent responding to negative antecedent communication with a negative response*. Contingency is evaluated statistically through sequential analysis of partners' communication. Negative reciprocity is one of the most consistently verified differences between happy and unhappy couples.

Shaping

Shaping involves the reinforcement of successive approximations of a target behavior. Many target behaviors, such as cooking dinner, are actually *chains* of more discrete behaviors. Spouses are asked to reward even small changes in their partners to encourage even greater development toward a desired end. Thus, a wife may be asked to show appreciation for her husband's minimal participation in dinner preparation. Although this strategy may be somewhat unsatisfactory compared with her overall desire for him to participate equally, a negative or neutral response would certainly discourage the desired change. The concept of shaping behavior (and accepting incremental changes) should be remembered by therapists as they attempt to modify a couple's interaction patterns.

Extinction

The behavior called *extinction* occurs when a previously reinforced stimulus is no longer reinforced. Extinction is a gradual process, because most behaviors are learned and maintained over multiple trials. If a husband stops demonstrating that he appreciates his wife's listening to him talk about his day, then extinction of the listening behavior would probably occur. Jacobson and Margolin (1979) posit that reinforcement erosion is a key source of extinction for important relationship behaviors. As the novelty and excitement of each spouse's behavior wears off, many relationship-enhancing behaviors may suffer extinction with the loss of effective reinforcement. As the relationship becomes more demanding and difficult in the face of life stresses and the arrival of children, the couple is less well equipped to face these challenges.

Functional Analysis

Functional analysis is a type of assessment conducted from a behavioral perspective. Target behaviors are selected, and the factors that control these behaviors are measured or assessed. Controlling variables can include situations, behaviors, cognitions, physiological states, affective states, or learning history. "Far from measuring just behaviors, behavioral assessment encompasses both what humans do and *why* they do it" (Hayes et al. 1986, p. 464). Although traditional psychological assessment interprets problem behaviors as *signs* of underlying factors, behaviorists interpret such data as *samples* of behavior.

Discriminative Stimuli

Discriminative stimuli serve as cues that a particular functional relation between behaviors is operative. For example, a husband's bid for affection might typically be well received. If his wife has just come from work and is making dinner while trying to keep the kids under control, his bid for affection is met with anger. Over time, he learns that the chaotic time preparing dinner (the discriminative stimulus) is not a time to look for affection.

Social Learning (Social Cognitive)

Bandura's (1969, 1977, 1986, 1997) *social learning* theory integrates operant conditioning, classical conditioning, and cognitive mediation into a unified theory. Bandura's (1986, 1997) latest expositions emphasized cognitive-mediational factors to such a degree that he relabeled it "a social cognitive theory." Bandura proposed that human behavior is equally and reciprocally influenced by cognitive, behavioral, and environmental factors. Several concepts central to Bandura's theory are important for understanding BCT methods.

Observational Learning (Modeling)

Observational learning occurs when "by observing others, one forms rules of behavior, and on future occasions this coded information serves as a guide for action" (Bandura 1986, p. 47). Not only can modeling from their families of origin shape spouses' behavior, but modeling of skills by the therapist can provide corrective learning.

Efficacy Expectancies

The concept *efficacy expectancies* refers to cognitions about whether a behavior can be performed. If a husband believes that he will not be able to resolve a difficult problem calmly using a suggested behavior, it may be difficult to get him to try the behavior (and if he does not try it, shaping the behavior will be impossible). In general, if the couple cannot see the feasibility of behaving in the way the therapist is suggesting, then *resistance* is typically the result.

Outcome Expectancies

Outcome expectancies, in comparison to efficacy expectancies, are cognitions about what the result would be if a behavior were performed. A wife may believe that even if she attended to her husband's needs more, he would still not show her appreciation (so she doesn't see the point in being more attentive). Similarly, in treatment situations, a couple may believe that even if they do discuss a problem constructively, it will not help their relationship (so they don't discuss problems).

Social Exchange

Social exchange models (e.g., Thibaut and Kelley 1959) use an economic metaphor for relationships—spouses want to maximize benefits and minimize costs. The simplest aspect of social exchange theory entails the potential benefits and costs of a particular exchange of behaviors. For example, if a wife walks the dog and the husband gives his wife a foot rub in appreciation, both have engaged in medium-cost, high-benefit behaviors toward the other. However, if the husband responds indifferently to his wife's walking the dog, she receives a medium-cost, no-benefit exchange, while he receives a no-cost, high-benefit exchange. This probably would not be a wise strategy, however, if he wants to maximize his long-term benefits. Over time, behavioral theorists suggest, successful marriages are characterized by high *mutual* benefits and low *mutual* costs; conversely, unsuccessful marriages deteriorate into partners searching for high *individual* benefits and low *individual* costs.

Negative Reciprocity

The concept of *negative reciprocity* can be viewed from the perspective of social exchange theory. *Negative reciprocity* refers simply to the negative response of one partner following the negative behavior of the other. Because negative reciprocity can be examined in a single interactional sample (unlike reinforcement concepts, which must be observed over time), it is the most widely studied concept in the marital observational literature (see below).

Early Treatment Applications

The earliest treatment studies in the behavioral tradition (e.g., Azrin et al. 1973; Stuart 1969; Weiss et al. 1973) heavily emphasized behavioral contracting. *Behavioral contracting* entails helping the spouses negotiate a mutual agreement in which both spouses agree to change their behavior in ways desired by the other spouse. In this way behavioral contracting was more explicitly *behavioral* than later forms of BCT; the couple was helped by controlling each other's environmental reinforcers (via the other partner). Although high levels of external structure are deemed acceptable or even desirable in certain institutions in our culture (e.g., schools and psychiatric hospitals), the institution of marriage is not one of them. Not only did many consumers find such approaches alienating (Weiss 1978), but later research found that behavioral contracting was not necessary to ensure treatment efficacy (Baucom and Hoffman 1986).

The Oregon Marital Studies Program model (Weiss 1978), developed by Robert Weiss, Jerry Patterson, and their colleagues, was one of the first, most fully elaborated, and most widely imitated *first-wave* [1] BCT programs (see Gottman 1979 and Weiss and Weider 1982 for histories of the program). The first wave of BCT was social-learning based; that is, it had more cognitive elements than strictly operant precursors to BCT (e.g., Azrin et al. 1973). This model entails a formal assessment phase that includes the discussion of presenting problems and relationship history. Furthermore, in order to obtain a sample of a couple's communication behavior, assessors observe the couple discussing problems, and the spouses also complete a battery of written assessment measures. The assessment findings and conceptualization are explicitly shared with the couple as part of developing a treatment contract. The first treatment module of the Oregon model focuses on teaching couples to track behavior and behavioral contingencies, identify controlling situations, and practice basic communication skills. The second module involves teaching them support and understanding skills that are necessary for empathic listening. In the third module the couples are taught problem-solving skills necessary for resolving conflict. The fourth and final module involves establishing behavioral contracts to provide contingencies for problem behaviors.

---

[1] Weiss and Weider (1982) divide *first-wave* BCT into three phases, with what we have labeled *pre-BCT* comprising the first two phases, and what we have labeled *first-wave* BCT as the third. See Weiss and Weider 1982 and Epstein and Williams 1981 for discussion of the various early BCT phases.

The first wave of BCT left several legacies, including commitment to empirical testing, integration of assessment techniques into the treatment process, and development of treatment protocols that could be tested and widely disseminated. On the negative side, there was consistent underemphasis on the therapeutic soft skills necessary for proper implementation of BCT and the arrogant belief that this "technology" could save nearly any couple (Weiss 1981). There was also the wholesale borrowing of tested techniques from other theoretical perspectives (e.g., communication training, empathic listening), which made BCT less discriminable from other approaches. In large part the theoretical and clinical developments made in *new-wave* BCT have attempted to address the first two problems. The theoretical *purity* of modern BCT, however, remains a hotly debated topic among researchers (Baucom and Epstein 1991; Gurman 1991; Johnson and Greenberg 1991; Markman 1991; Jacobson 1991b, 1991c, 1992).

Building an Empirical Base

We have just covered the theoretical underpinnings of BCT and described a typical treatment model from 1970s BCT. As mentioned earlier, BCT adherents have tried to test the assumptions of their models and the outcome of their treatments. In this section we review selected results on positive and negative reinforcement, since reinforcement is the central construct of behavioral models (Jacobson 1991c).

Operant Conditioning

A true test of operant principles would require sampling couples' behavior, examining the contingencies, observing their behavior again, and testing to see if the contingencies witnessed at one time increased the rate of the behavior hypothesized to have been reinforced. If the stimulus behavior did not increase, then by definition it was not reinforced by the contingent behavior. The data that lend some credence to behavioral principles in marriage come mostly from cross-sectional studies that compare distressed and nondistressed couples.

Regarding positive reinforcement, a vast literature using observational and quasi-observational methods has demonstrated that nondistressed couples, compared with distressed couples, engage in more positive and fewer negative behaviors (Heyman 2001; Weiss and Heyman 1990b). This *may* be a by-product of positive reinforcement, as positively reinforced behaviors are defined as those that increase and are maintained over time.

Testing reinforcement constructs requires the observation of *sequences*. Yet studies employing sequential analysis have primarily used problem discussions, not exactly an environment to promote positive behavior. A preponderance of studies have found that distressed couples reciprocate negative behaviors more readily than do nondistressed couples (Heyman 2001; Weiss and Heyman 1990b). Although these findings may indicate that negative behaviors are positively reinforced by a partner's negative behaviors (i.e., they may increase over time), negative reciprocity has been more adequately explained within a coercion model, which stresses punishment and negative reinforcement. With observations and marital adjustment measured concurrently, results also indicate that both distressed and nondistressed couples reciprocate positive behaviors, whereas only distressed couples reciprocate negative behaviors (Hooley and Hahlweg 1989; Margolin and Wampold 1981). Furthermore, Filsinger and Thoma (1988) found that although reciprocity of negatives predicted relationship dissolution 12 years later, *positive* reciprocity was predictive of relationship dissolution at 5-year, 12-year, and 22-year follow-ups.

Gottman (1979) has offered a behavioral explanation for this type of pattern: distressed couples are more stimulus bound (i.e., more responsive to both positive and negative contingencies). Although this is a sensible explanation, reinforcement concepts alone would not predict that inattention to immediate contingencies is functional. To the contrary, according to operant theory, the levels of positive behavior in high-contingency-focused couples should lead to increases in positive behavior and probably increased relationship satisfaction. It is also possible, however, that reciprocating positive behaviors is not a functional way to facilitate problem resolution.

Thus, these results do not argue against behavior theories of marriage; they suggest, however, that understanding marriage requires a more complex model than simple positive reinforcement and punishment. Successful couples may be those that are able to stay on task during arguments (i.e., demonstrate rule-governed behavior) rather than be keenly sensitive to the partners' message (i.e., demonstrate stimulus-bound behavior) (Weiss 1978).

Heavey and colleagues (Heavey et al. 1995) also found support for the negative effects of the demand/withdraw pattern over 2.5 years in a sample of 36 couples who completed all of the study's measures at the two time points. The study used videotaped and problem-solving discussions that were coded to examine the demand and withdrawal behavior that occurred during the discussions. The authors showed that withdrawal behavior on the part of the men and the existence of the demand/withdraw pattern during the discussions were associated with declines in the women's satisfaction at the second assessment point.

Correlates of Change in BCT

Despite this positive evidence suggesting that the focus of BCT change efforts (i.e., negative interactional behavior) is predictive of declines in relationship satisfaction over time, there is inconsistent support for the idea that changes in BCT are associated with improvements in satisfaction. Sayers and colleagues (Sayers et al. 1991) examined whether changes in interaction sequences accompanied improvement occurring in the context of BCT. Reductions in overall base rates of negative behavior (e.g., criticism), withdrawal behavior on the part of husbands, and negative reciprocity during problem discussions were all associated with increases in satisfaction. As suggested above, two other studies found little association between changes in communication and changes in satisfaction over the course of BCT (Halford et al. 1993; Iversen and Baucom 1990).

Social Learning

Although social learning concepts have been critical to BCT since its inception, the bedrock social learning concepts have received less attention by researchers. Although observational learning itself has vast substantiation (Bandura 1986, 1997), it has not been studied directly within a marital context. Modeling of skills, nevertheless, is an important part of skills attainment in BCT.

Pretzer and colleagues (Pretzer et al. 1992) have studied efficacy and outcome expectancies and important aspects of social learning theory, using a comprehensive cognitive questionnaire. They found that for men and women, positive efficacy and outcome expectancies were significantly related to better marital adjustment, better self-reported communication quality, and fewer distorted beliefs (e.g., that "disagreement is destructive" or that "one should know what the partner wants and needs without asking"). In addition, women's positive expectancies were associated with lower levels of depressive symptomatology and lower levels of specific negative communication behaviors.

Heyman (1992) attempted to reconstruct cognitions occurring during couples' problem-solving interactions. He coded several types of cognitions (e.g., attributions, expectancies, affective tracking) (Heyman and Weiss 1991). As hypothesized, abusive men were 1) more likely to predict that they could not perform an important behavior (i.e., negative efficacy expectancies about self) and 2) more likely to predict that the outcome of their behaviors would be negative (i.e., negative outcome expectancies about self). The groups differed even after the effects of marital adjustment were controlled for.

Levenson and Gottman (1985) made an intriguing use of the expectancy concept. They found that not only were spouses' physiological responses highly related to future changes in marital adjustment, but their physiological responses *while they were waiting for their discussion to begin* also were highly predictive of changes in marital adjustment over 3 years. They interpreted this finding to mean that spouses' expectancies (i.e., their predictions about how the conversation would go) produced physiological reactions that were similar to those recorded during actual discussions.

Social Exchange

Findings provide evidence for a social exchange explanation of marital dysfunction. Quasi-observational studies using the Spouse Observation Checklist (Wills et al. 1974) have found consistently that the ratio of positive to negative behaviors is substantially higher for nondistressed than distressed couples (Christensen 1987; Weiss and Perry 1983). Gottman (1999), using observational methods, determined that the ratio of positive to negative behaviors is 5 to 1. Furthermore, direct observation of couples indicates that negative reciprocity is a hallmark of distressed couples.

Social Support Transactions

Social support transactions describe some other interactional behaviors that could be important in evaluating and treating marital distress. The vast majority of early observational studies of marriage have relied on a laboratory-based, problem-solving discussion, although it is likely that solving a problem is only one type of discussion that a couple may have when interacting on a daily basis. Recently, the impact of social support transactions on marital dysfunction among spouses has received greater attention. Pasch and Bradbury (1998) examined the communication behavior of 55 newly married couples using two types of videotaped discussion tasks—a discussion of a marital conflict and a discussion of nonmarital difficulties. Couples in which the wives solicited less or provided less support during the support task were more likely to be classified as distressed 2 years later. There was also support for the idea that couples who were more negative during the problem-solving discussion were more likely to be distressed after 2 years. The findings underscored the importance of examining a broad range of interactions to assess the usefulness of social learning and social exchange models of marital distress, as well as the importance of promoting relationship-enhancing marital behavior (see also Pasch et al. 1997).

Treatment Outcome Studies of First-Wave BCT

There are many narrative reviews of BCT effectiveness (e.g., Baucom and Hoffman 1986; Beach and Bauserman 1990), but a meta-analysis of BCT outcome research (Hahlweg and Markman 1988) provides the best consolidation of the literature. This study used 17 BCT and 7 prevention-oriented studies, for a total of 613 couples from five countries. The researchers found, using the yardstick of statistical significance, that BCT was significantly more effective than either wait-list or nonspecific therapy controls. Specifically, 72% of BCT couples made significant improvement versus 28% of the control couples. This finding held for European as well as American couples. The BCT intervention maintained its effectiveness at follow-up periods of 1 year. Prevention programs were also successful; on average, couples who participated in a behaviorally oriented prevention program were better off at post-test than 79% of nontreatment or attention-placebo controls. The positive effects were generally maintained over time (over follow-up periods ranging from 6 months to 3 years).

However, the literature suggests much room for improvement in BCT when clinical significance tests are used (i.e., whether or not a couple has moved into the *nondistress*ed range of marital adjustment). Hahlweg and Markman (1988) concluded that a considerable number of couples were still distressed following BCT. The reanalysis by Jacobson and colleagues (Jacobson et al. 1984b) of four BCT studies found that only one-third of the couples treated with BCT crossed over from the distressed to the nondistressed range, with clinically significant success rates ranging from 21% to 58%. A more recent meta-analytic review also found that BCT was more effective in increasing marital satisfaction than no treatment (Dunn and Schwebel 1995), although BCT did not fair as well as insight oriented marital therapy (IOMT) (Snyder et al. 1991) in two studies involving direct comparisons.

Although the data from BCT outcome studies were originally viewed as supportive for the effectiveness of BCT, over the last few years BCT researchers have begun to view the glass as half empty rather than half full. The ineffectiveness of BCT with many couples has led researchers to modify considerably the original model, and we now turn our attention to the changes BCT has undergone.

Broadening of BCT's Focus—The 1980s

By 1980, the limitations of first-wave BCT were obvious to its originators. Most importantly, many theorists felt that research and clinical writings de-emphasized the role of cognitions in marital functioning. Weiss (1980) presented several reasons why BCT should address cognitions. Most important is that BCT does not help a substantial number of couples. Because spouses' behavior accounts for only 25%–30% of the variation in daily marital satisfaction ratings (see Christensen 1987 for a review), there is reason to look beyond overt behavior. Furthermore, in distressed couples there are important differences between spouses' intended communication and the actual impact on the partner. Much of this may be due to thoughts that mediate how behaviors are understood or received. Indeed, research suggests that distressed spouses rate the impact of a message less positively than do nondistressed spouses, even when the partners' rated intentions do not differ (Gottman et al. 1976b). Lastly, operant and social exchange models have difficulty explaining why happy spouses can be rewarding to each other for years and why unhappy couples can stay together in high-punishment, low-benefit relationships. It is likely that cognitions regarding how spouses view their problems and relationships help explain this phenomenon.

Jacobson (1984b) and Weiss (1984) offered the following reasons for believing that cognitions affected success rates: 1) cognitions could remain dysfunctional even after behavior change; 2) cognitions often interfere with attempts at modifying dysfunctional behavior patterns; and 3) dysfunctional relationship cognitions (such as standards and expectancies) are often independent of behavior exchange and thus would require direct attempts at modification.

Models of Cognition in Marriage

Baucom and colleagues (Baucom et al. 1989, p. 31) lamented that "the study of cognitions in intimate relationships has little coherent direction of movement, either from a research perspective or in terms of treatment of marital distress." They defined what they considered to be the most important cognitive variables in the study of marriage.

Selective Attention

Selective attention about negative behavior relative to positive behavior may be associated with marital distress in many relationships. Spouses cannot attend to and process all incoming information. What spouses choose to attend to is as important as how they process information that they have attended to. For example, a distressed husband may attend to instances in which his wife complains, ignoring all instances when she is considerate or affectionate.

Attributions

Attributions are explanations about the cause of events. Attributions have received the vast majority of attention in cognitive studies of marriage (see Bradbury and Fincham 1990 for an exhaustive review). Although a variety of dimensions of attributions have been studied, attributions can be described as *distress-maintaining* or *relationship-enhancing* (Holtzworth-Munroe and Jacobson 1987). These collapsed categories seem to be the most useful clinically.

Distress-maintaining attributions for a partner's negative behavior are those that hold the partner responsible or that attribute the causes for the behavior to the partner himself or herself (as opposed to outside circumstances), to the negative intentions of the partner, to the partner's personality, or to a stable pattern of behavior. An example is a husband who believes: "We don't have a problem. *She* has a problem. She always tries to control things; it's part of her personality." Relationship-enhancing attributions are the converse (i.e., partner is seen as not responsible or the causes attributed are external, unintentional, specific, or unstable). For example, a husband might think, "She's late. She's probably been held up in traffic."

Expectations

Expectancies form a category of cognition that, with only a few exceptions, has not been well researched (see Heyman 1992; Pretzer et al. 1992; Vanzetti and Notarius 1991; Vanzetti et al. 1992). Expectancies refer to both *efficacy* expectancies ("Can I do it?") and *outcome* expectancies ("Will it make any difference?"). It seems clear that distressed spouses who have low efficacy and low outcome expectancies would manifest resistance to changes suggested by a therapist.

Assumptions

Assumptions are cognitive structures about the roles spouses play or about the way spouses interact. Spousal roles are called *personae* (e.g., "The incompetent-at-child-care husband," "The nagging wife"). Patterns of interaction are called "scripts" (a husband might say "She'll tell me I'm not doing enough around the house, I'll tell her to get off my back, she'll keep complaining, I'll leave the house").

Standards

Standards are beliefs about the way relationships *should* be. A husband with a standard that "A good wife will have sex with her husband whenever he wants" will surely have difficulty living with a woman who holds a standard that "A woman should never have sex unless she's really in the mood."

Although critical to furthering the study of cognition in marriage, the descriptive focus of Baucom et al. does not provide a model for how cognitions function in marriage. Bradbury and Fincham have attempted to provide such a model (e.g., Bradbury and Fincham 1991; Fincham and Bradbury 1991). *The contextual model of marital interaction*, as Bradbury and Fincham have labeled their model, describes how these cognitions affect our perception of the world and thus our behavior. This cognitive processing happens automatically and can in turn be affected by our experiences. The model is complex and is only beginning to be explored empirically. Clinically, the framework is a useful heuristic tool for organizing assessment data and observations about the couple (see Fincham and Bradbury 1991 for greater detail).

Outcome Studies: Evaluating Cognitive Additions to BCT

Thus far, outcome research has found that cognitive treatment approaches have efficacy that is comparable to that of standard BCT treatment (Baucom and Lester 1986; Baucom et al. 1990; Emmelkamp et al. 1988; Huber and Milstein 1985; Margolin and Weiss 1978). However, investigations have not found significant increases in treatment success by adding cognitive components to BCT (i.e., BCT narrowly defined, such as communication training or contingency contracting). There are substantial problems with these studies (e.g., low power to detect differences among effective treatments, insufficient measurement of cognitions) (Fincham et al. 1990). Given that in most of these studies the couples were invariantly assigned to standard treatments without regard to assessment data, it is not surprising that no treatment won the *horse race*.

Thus, substantial amounts of work are needed before we can draw conclusions about the utility of *cognitive* elements of BCT. We see false comparisons being made, however, that make the whole cognitive-behavioral vs. behavioral BCT test unsavory. If BCT is based on social learning theory or more traditional forms of behaviorism (take your pick), and the core of each of these models is the reciprocal influence of cognitive, behavioral, and environmental factors, how can one test cognitive vs. behavioral methods?

How can any treatment, *behavioral* or *cognitive*, be BCT if the choice of treatments does not derive from a functional analysis? It is clear that research design demands from a nomothetic perspective (e.g., random assignment to treatment, use of standard protocols) do not fit well with those of an idiographic perspective (e.g., functional analysis). These are issues with which behaviorists in general (Houts and Follette 1992), and BCT researchers in particular, continue to struggle.

Emotion

BCT has always been concerned with increasing positive emotion and decreasing negative emotion. Indeed, the critical concepts of *conflict* and *marital satisfaction* are embedded in an emotional context. Procedures such as "love days" (Weiss et al. 1973), in which spouses increase their levels of positive behavior, have been incorporated from the beginning. Because descriptions of first-wave BCT were weighted toward social exchange and overt behavior, behavioral change was seen as the pathway to emotional change. In other words, change the behavior and the emotional responses will follow (e.g., Jacobson and Margolin 1979).

In the 1980s, research findings, clinical limitations and clinical outcome studies prompted both BCT proponents (Bradbury and Fincham 1987a, 1987b; Jacobson et al. 1989a; Margolin 1983, 1987) and critics (Greenberg and Johnson 1986a, 1986b, 1986c; Johnson 1986; Johnson and Greenberg 1985a) to champion the need for emotionally based treatment components in marital therapy.

Although BCT therapists were moving toward incorporating *affect* into their work (e.g., Jacobson et al. 1989a; Margolin 1987), Johnson and Greenberg's (1985b) outcome study showing that emotionally focused therapy was more effective than BCT caught researchers' attention. Although the study was seriously flawed (see Weiss and Heyman 1990a for a critique), it nevertheless was the first *horse race* that BCT lost.

Coincidence or not, the publication of the study's findings coincided with increased discussion among therapists about how BCT practitioners work on affective change *within* the therapy session. During sessions BCT therapists traditionally discouraged intense emotion because it was shown to be associated with distressed couples and because it was seen to be antithetical to the *constructive* style of problem discussion taught during communication skills training. Many master therapists began to rethink this position. Relatively independent of each other, several therapists (Baucom and Epstein 1990; Jacobson 1991b; Jacobson and Christensen 1996; Margolin 1987) developed very similar techniques for interrupting conflict within sessions and exploring with each partner his or her affective and cognitive reactions to the conflict (see Weiss and Heyman 1990a for a more detailed comparison of BCT and emotionally focused therapy).

Innovations of the 1990s

Two innovative therapies were added to traditional BCT in the 1990s: integrative couples therapy (ICT) (Jacobson and Christensen 1996) and self-regulatory couple therapy (SRCT) (Halford et al. 1994). As Halford (1998) says, these innovations were developed in part because of the growing concern that changes in communication directly influenced and guided by the therapist might not always produce the best results. More effective seemed to be therapy that encouraged partners to be more aware of and accepting of each others' interpersonal patterns, such as ICT, and therapy that promoted self-directed behavioral changes, such as SRCT.

Integrative Couples Therapy

Jacobson and Christensen's (1996) ICT builds on traditional BCT by using ways of promoting acceptance by couples of their problems, in addition to the often used behavioral change techniques developed in traditional BCT. They extend the emphasis that traditional BCT has on the therapist's functional analysis and formulation of the distressed couple's negative interaction style. In fact, the ability of the therapist to present this analysis convincingly is paramount in helping the couple to see their particular pattern, understand how each spouse contributes to it, and identify ways of decreasing its pernicious effects. For example, in ICT a *demand/withdraw* pattern of interaction might be confused with a *closeness/distance* relationship theme, which is a consequence of quite normal differences in spouses' preferences for emotional intimacy. Over time and after repeated conflicts over an issue, the spouses become *polarized*, and each becomes trapped in ever-escalating efforts to meet his or her needs for more closeness (or more distance). The role of the therapist is to help the spouses see how this pattern has developed, how it is repeated in the couple's current interactions on a daily basis, and what the feelings are that underlie each spouse's behavior. Clearly, the success of the approach lies in the ability of the therapist to develop an accurate and useful functional analysis of the couple's difficulties. Jacobson and Christensen describe several additional relationship themes, including *conventionality/unconventionality* and *control/responsibility*, but there are many possible similar themes and innumerable ways of communicating them to couples.

The primary interventions used in ICT illustrate the nature of assumptions about change through this form of therapy. *Empathic joining* is used to help couples gain some initial acceptance about their pattern, frequently through a refocus on softer emotions such as sadness or hurt feelings. Encouraging couples to recognize and discuss these emotions with each other leads to an increase in their empathy for and a decrease in their antagonism toward each other. Rather than depending on the therapist to convince them that their fate depends on their ability to pull together as a team, both spouses gradually become more cooperative as their empathy and understanding for their partner increases. Another intervention, *unified detachment*, involves giving their relationship theme a name, thereby objectifying and learning to identify the behavior each spouse is enacting when it occurs. Unlike empathic joining, unified detachment encourages the couple to intellectually examine their pattern of behavior, thereby decreasing the couple's tendency to become embroiled in conflict whenever spouses recognize the presence of pattern. Finally, in *tolerance building*, the therapist helps spouses to decrease their emotional reactions to their partner's behavior, a technique that epitomizes the *acceptance* aspect of ICT. Tolerance building involves pointing out the positive aspects of negative behavior, or asking the couple to reenact a problematic interaction in the therapy session. These techniques have the effect of changing the valence of the behavior, either through relabeling of the behavior or by disassociating the behavior from the emotional intensity of the conflict. In addition, enacting the negative behaviors during a session outside the context of an argument may lead to very mild shame (Jacobson and Christensen 1996), which may function as a mild punishment for the behavior. Finally, greater individual self-care is advocated when appropriate (e.g., maintain or improve relationships with friends), so that each spouse can better tolerate disappointments and stresses that every relationship may include.

Jacobson and Christensen argue that ICT is an extension of traditional BCT rather than a replacement for it. They still recommend the use of behavioral exchange methods with couples, as well as communication and problem-solving training. However, the techniques are seen as adjuncts to ICT that can be used after the couple has greatly decreased its level of conflict and has a sense of common purpose.

Self-Regulatory Couple Therapy

A key starting point for SRCT is that traditional BCT is focused on the therapist's direct change efforts and the efforts of one spouse to have an effect on the partner (as in, e.g., behavioral exchange procedures). Halford (1998) reasons that few spouses are empowered enough to feel confident that their change efforts will have the desired effect. Furthermore, the efforts of one spouse to change the behavior of the partner, albeit in a positive way, constitute a continuation of the struggle that many couples are engaged in at the start of therapy. SRCT is based on self-regulation theory (Karoly 1993) and involves encouraging each spouse to examine and change his or her own behavior, cognitions, and affects in order to improve mutual satisfaction with the marriage.

According to Halford et al. (1994), there are at least five types of individual responses to marital dissatisfaction. First, one can focus spouses on their own methods of communicating their dissatisfaction to their partners. Although this is similar to traditional BCT, the emphasis is on each spouse's evaluating and taking responsibility for his or her own efforts to effect change. Second, each spouse can alter his or her response to the conflict, either through cognitive change or through reducing the distress by exposing himself or herself to it. Third, each spouse can examine ways in which his or her needs might be met in another way, such as seeking the support of friends. Fourth, either spouse may decide to leave the relationship. Fifth, each spouse can decide to make no change and hope that the situation or the partner may eventually change in a desired way.

Initial Outcome Data for ICT and SRCT

Thorough tests of these innovations in BCT have not been conducted, but the initial empirical support for both ICT and SRCT is promising. The content of ICT sessions was shown to differ reliably from that of BCT sessions (Jacobson et al. 1996). Furthermore, ICT sessions yielded greater emotional expressiveness and less blaming than BCT sessions (Cordova 1996). A small pilot study provided evidence that ICT produces greater increases in relationship satisfaction than BCT (Jacobson et al. 1996).

Several initial studies of SRCT indicate that the approach can yield effects on satisfaction in three sessions comparable to the effects found in 15 sessions of BCT (Halford 1998). It should be noted, however, that the design used was quasi-experimental with no random assignment to treatment condition and no assessment of the maintenance of outcome. In another study, a psychoeducational approach based on SRCT was compared with a minimal intervention using a nondistressed population (Halford 1998). The SRCT intervention resulted in significant improvements in communication that were maintained over time.

When these recent developments in BCT are included, there are several basic components that constitute the behavioral approach. In the next several sections we will describe in more detail clinical assessment and the clinical application of BCT.

Clinical Assessment

The concept of a *behavioral* approach to couples therapy implies a thorough functional analysis of the couple's interaction; therefore, clinical assessment and treatment are intertwined. BCT traditionally allots the first several sessions to assessment to establish rapport, promote positive outcome expectancies, elicit a relationship history, and make a functional assessment of the affective, behavioral, and cognitive contributions to the couple's distress (e.g., Baucom and Epstein 1990). Typically the therapist concludes the formal assessment phase by presenting an individualized case conceptualization and treatment plan to the couple, who then decides whether or not to proceed with therapy (see O'Leary et al. 1998 for a collection of behaviorally oriented treatment plan templates for different presenting problems). Assessment continues during the *treatment* phase to judge the effectiveness of the intervention and make modifications, as required by the functional analysis.

A thorough discussion of BCT assessment theory, techniques, and tools is far beyond the scope of this chapter. Many excellent resources exist, including those by Baucom and Epstein (1990) and O'Leary (1987). We will, however, briefly mention some of the basic assessment measures used by behavior therapists.

Behavior

Direct Observation

Direct observation is based on the idea that to understand how a couple responds to problems and attempts to resolve conflict, one needs to observe an actual communication sample. It is necessary that the therapist have an in-depth understanding of functional and dysfunctional communication and be able to identify communication patterns as they are observed during sessions. To use direct observation at the beginning of the assessment, the therapist explains to the couple the importance of assessing communication patterns in a way that does not necessarily depend on the spouses' self-report. The therapist helps the couple identify a problem of moderate importance and asks them to spend up to 10 minutes in the session attempting to solve it. The clinician explains to the spouses that he or she wants to observe and not interrupt them while they do this. The therapist videotapes and/or observes the couple in the least obtrusive manner possible. While the couple discusses the problem, the clinician makes careful notes of the patterns displayed in their interaction, the activity level of each of the spouses, and the level of skill used by each. After the 10-minute period has elapsed, the therapist stops the spouses and asks them to describe their subjective experience as they performed the exercise and how it compared with their discussions at home. (See Gottman 1999 and Heyman 2001 for more detailed discussions of incorporating in-session observations into treatment planning.)

Spouse Observation Checklist

The Spouse Observation Checklist (SOC; Weiss and Perry 1983; Weiss et al. 1973) comprises 408 behaviors grouped into 12 content areas (e.g., affection, household management). Each day, typically for 2 weeks, spouses record whether their partners performed any of the behaviors and if the behavior was pleasing or displeasing. In addition, they rate their daily level of relationship satisfaction.

The purpose of the SOC is to enable the therapist to access behavioral performance in a natural setting. By examining reported behaviors and their effect on daily satisfaction, the therapist can attempt to identify behaviors in need of change. The SOC's length is its primary drawback, and reliability between spouses is low (Christensen 1987; Weiss and Perry 1983), even for discrete, presumably high-salience behaviors such as recent sexual intercourse. Broderick has developed an abbreviated version of the SOC, dubbed the Daily Checklist of Marital Activities (DCMA), which can be found in the O'Leary (1987) marital assessment book. Finally, Johnson and O'Leary (1996) present a method of individualizing DCMA/SOC to couples' needs, making it more efficient and more acceptable to clients while still retaining excellent psychometric properties.

Cost-Benefit Analysis

As its name implies, the Cost-Benefit Analysis (CB; Weiss and Perry 1983) is an operationalization of social exchange theory. The CB is a derivative of the SOC. Spouses rate the perceived benefit for each of the 400 behaviors were they to receive it; in addition, they rate the perceived cost were they to perform each behavior. A computer scoring program (available from Robert L. Weiss, University of Oregon) matches up the spouses' scores and provides the therapist with a list of good therapy items (i.e., high benefit for the receiving spouse and low cost for the giving spouse) and high-conflict items (i.e., high benefit for the receiving spouse and high cost for the giving spouse). The CB not only can be an aid in the functional analysis but also can help determine the order of behavioral interventions.

Inventory of Rewarding Activities

The Inventory of Rewarding Activities (IRA; Birchler and Weiss, in Weiss and Perry 1979) is an inventory of 100 recreational or pleasurable activities. For each activity, spouses answer if they have participated in that activity during the past month and with whom they did it or would like to do it (alone, with spouse alone, with spouse and family, with spouse and other adults, or with nonfamily members). For each activity, they choose from the following answers: 1) have not done activity and do not want to do it; 2) have not done it but would like to do it; 3) have done it but would like to do more of it; and 4) have done it but do not want to increase it. During therapy, the therapist can help the couple maintain activities they were already doing and increase those that they would like to try. Furthermore, problem areas (e.g., an activity that the wife wants to try with her husband but that the husband does not want to do) can be identified easily and can be put on hold until problem solving is taught.

Conflict Tactics Scale

The Conflict Tactics Scale (CTS; Straus 1979) assesses the frequency of 18 conflict behaviors, from constructive talk ("discussed issue calmly") to verbal abuse ("insulted or swore at partner") to physical abuse ("pushed, grabbed or shoved" through "used gun or knife"). Researchers have noted significant discrepancies between spouses' reports (e.g., Jouriles and O'Leary 1985). Jouriles and O'Leary (1985) recommend that both partners report on husband-wife and wife-husband violence and that when discrepancies occur, the report of more frequent violence be retained. This is the current standard clinical use of the CTS.

Although the CTS appears to be psychometrically sound, it has been criticized on several grounds: its list of abusive behaviors is by no means comprehensive, its 1-year time frame for reporting may result in retrospective biases (especially when frequency estimations are required), it does not measure the result of the behavior (e.g., *nonsevere* pushes can result in broken necks), and it ignores the context of behavior (e.g., was the violence in self-defense?) (Gelles 1990). The CTS has recently undergone a thorough revision (see Conflict Tactics Scale–2 [CTS-2; Straus et al. 1996]). The CTS-2, although longer, has improved scales for measuring verbal aggression, severe physical aggression, sexual aggression, and injury.

Research suggests that any aggression, including common, supposedly *mild* aggression, has deleterious effects and that clinicians will vastly underdetect aggression without systematic assessment (Gelles and Straus 1988; O'Leary et al. 1992; Straus et al. 1980). Thus, O'Leary and colleagues make several recommendations for clinical assessment of spouse abuse: First, clinicians should use both a questionnaire (such as the CTS-2) and a clinical interview to assess aggression. Second, because spouses underreport aggression as a presenting problem for a variety of reasons (Ehrensaft and Vivian 1996), assessment of spouse abuse should be done with all couples presenting for treatment. Third, clinical sensitivity to serious but underreported and minimized problems such as spouse abuse is necessary. For a discussion of clinical assessment of spouse abuse, see O'Leary and Murphy 1992; for a discussion of whether and how to treat aggressive couples in a couples' framework, see Vivian and Heyman 1996.

Cognition

Relationship Beliefs Inventory

The Relationship Beliefs Inventory (RBI; Eidelson and Epstein 1982) is a 40-item measure that taps five *dysfunctional* beliefs: *disagreement is destructive*; *mindreading is expected*; *partners cannot change*; *sex must be perfect*; and *the sexes are different*. Whether these beliefs are dysfunctional when taken out of context is arguable (e.g., an abused wife might rightly believe that in her relationship, disagreement is indeed destructive), but when taken in the context of a particular couple, the RBI can be useful in developing a cognitive-behavioral functional analysis.

Marital Attitude Survey

The Marital Attitude Survey (MAS; Pretzer et al. 1992) is a 74-item questionnaire that measures expectancies (efficacy and outcome) and attributions (causal attributions to own and partner's personality and to own and partner's behavior; attributions of spouses' malicious intent and lack of love). The subscales have been demonstrated to have adequate internal consistency and to be significantly correlated with the Dyadic Adjustment Scale (DAS; Spanier 1976) in the expected directions (Pretzer et al. 1992). For an attribution measure that uses more traditional dimensions, the Relationship Attribution Measure (Fincham and Bradbury 1992) is a good alternative.

Marital Agendas Protocol

The Marital Agendas Protocol (MAP; Notarius and Vanzetti 1983) has couples rate 10 causes of conflict in marriage (e.g., money, communication) using the following standards: 1) severity of problem, 2) estimation of spouse's rating of severity, 3) percentage of disagreements resolved, and 4) responsibility attributions. Notarius and Vanzetti (1983) discuss how the MAP can be used clinically and have described in more detail its use as a measure of efficacy (Vanzetti et al. 1992).

Adjustment and Desired Change

Areas of Change Questionnaire

The Areas of Change Questionnaire (AOC; Weiss and Perry 1979; Weiss et al. 1973) asks spouses to rate the amount of change they desire on 34 different behaviors (e.g., "I want my partner to participate in decisions about spending money") and how much change they think their partner desires on the same 34 behaviors. It is an excellent tool for determining both the extent of changes desired and the concordance between changes perceived and actual changes desired. A valuable computer program is available that not only scores the AOC but provides interpretive feedback written by Weiss.

Affect

Measures of Marital Adjustment and Marital Satisfaction

The most widely used measures of spouses' overall appraisal of their marital happiness are the Locke-Wallace Marital Adjustment Test (MAT; Locke and Wallace 1959) and its more contemporary update, the Dyadic Adjustment Scale. These measures are not without significant problems (see Eddy et al. 1991; Fincham and Bradbury 1987; Norton 1983) but are certainly acceptable as measures of overall adjustment in clinical uses. Measures of marital happiness, especially those that contain ratings of happiness with a variety of content areas (e.g., affection, finances), are also available. These measures (e.g., Marital Happiness Scale [Azrin et al. 1973]; Relationship Satisfaction Scale [Burns and Sayers 1992]) have been recommended on psychometric and theoretical grounds (Heyman et al. 1994). For a more detailed, multidimensional view of marriage that includes an overall satisfaction scale, see Snyder's 280-item Marital Satisfaction Inventory (Snyder 1983).

Finally, the Marital Status Inventory (MSI; Weiss and Cerreto 1980) is a Guttman-scaled, 14-item measure of steps taken to divorce. Because many couples come to therapy when one or both spouses have already essentially decided to leave the marriage, assessment of steps toward divorce is a useful pretherapy tool. Gottman and Levenson (1992) found that couples do indeed move toward divorce in a Guttman-scaled fashion, lending some support to the MSI's premise.

Positive Feelings Questionnaire

The Positive Feelings Questionnaire (O'Leary et al. 1983) is a 17-item measure of general positive affect within a marriage. Means and standard deviations for clinic and community couples are presented by O'Leary (1987).

Conceptualization From a Cognitive-Behavioral Perspective

Conceptualization using a cognitive-behavioral perspective (i.e., a behaviorally specific description of a couple's problems) is crucial to understanding and changing the spouses' functioning and current level of happiness. The hallmark of the behavioral approach is that there is no general description and etiology of marital difficulty for all couples. Thus, the therapist must take self-reports and observational and historical data from the assessment to explain current problematic transactions the spouses have from day to day. Several important questions must be answered:

- When does the couple have the most problem interactions?
- Are these events predictable in terms of the time or context in which they occur, or in reference to the marital issue involved? (One couple recently treated by us had repeated conflicts related to the husband's parents. It was quite predictable that a conflict would ensue whenever the husband spoke with his parents, when family gatherings were planned, or when his parents dropped by the house.)
- What is the sequence of events when the couple begins to fight?
- What circumstances or behaviors prevent the couple from being playful or enjoying pleasure with each other?

An important aspect of the conceptualization is the specification of how reinforcers, punishers, and communication processes are involved in maintenance of the problem. For example, escape conditioning may be operating in such a way as to lead to greater disengagement. In such a scenario, the husband may withdraw from incipient confrontations with his wife as a way of minimizing emotional upset. He is *negatively reinforced* for the withdrawal by the reduction of emotional arousal in the short term. What he does not realize is that although the strategy is effective for most of the individual conflicts, over time the discrete conflicts increase in frequency as his wife's anger and dissatisfaction increase. After this problem has continued for long enough, his own attempts to address their problems may in fact be punished because of the high level of negative affect expressed by the wife.

The therapist should be aware that many spouses may not actually have the appropriate communication skills to decrease the intensity of interpersonal conflicts when they occur or to solve overwhelming and complex problems that most couples face. Daily contact and greater familiarity may reduce the initial enthusiasm and excitement that the couple felt early in their relationship. Increased financial demands and the arrival of children may present problems that the couple is unprepared to solve. The therapist should use the assessment data to weigh the extent to which the couple's problems are due to their inability to work effectively as a problem-solving team or to their lack of attention to the positive aspects of their relationship. If skill deficits play an important part in the development and maintenance of the couple's problems, communication and problem-solving training may be indicated.

Cognitive factors may play an important role in the development and maintenance of relationship conflict. As noted earlier, there has been a great deal of support for the role of attributions in relationship marital discord, but it is far too early to state that attributions, or other types of cognitions, play an etiological role. We believe, however, that integrating cognitions into the conceptualization of the couple can greatly enhance the therapist's explanation of the couple's problems. For example, one couple had continual conflict about roles and responsibilities concerning the care of the children and the household as well as conflicts about decisions affecting where the family would live. This led to efforts to improve communication enough to introduce conflict resolution for these issues. On further exploration of the spouses' beliefs and expectations, it was found that they were in the process of reevaluating their long-standing standards about the husband's *protective* role. Both of the spouses had begun their relationship seeing the husband as a *knight in shining armor* and the wife as a *lady to be protected*. Moreover, the husband was expected by both partners to anticipate his wife's feelings and needs. Much of their conflict centered around their obvious failure in these unrealistic roles and their ambivalence about giving them up. Thus, intervention focused on renegotiating their expectations of each other and on acquiring the communication style needed to relate in an egalitarian fashion.

Historical information has a specific status in behavioral conceptions of marital discord. Historical data, the context out of which the current conflict arose, are unlike psychodynamic theories that ascribe some etiological importance to the spouses' individual or couple history. Moreover, the behavioral view is unlike family systems theories that use the idea of repetition of family relationship themes across multiple generations as an important force in the development of marital conflicts. Taking the history of couples or individuals is important in that it helps the therapist develop ideas about the development of specific behavioral patterns in the marriage. Historical data might be useful in identifying the determinants of behavior in problematic communication sequences that the couple presents to the therapist. At all times it is important to recognize that the problems brought to the therapist exist in the present rather than in the past.

Historical information can also help the therapist understand how the spouses think about their current problems. Thus, history is a contextual factor in that clients have specific beliefs about the past. The therapist must often struggle directly with the spouses' perceptions of the past because these beliefs may inhibit them from attempting some change for the future. An example is the wife who thought that her husband had always acted for his own benefit and did not want to express her needs to him because these needs would be frustrated. A major hurdle in therapy was to convince her to question this conclusion about the past and to learn to express her needs more directly and appropriately. A crucial aspect of the conceptualization of their problems consisted of historical information about her husband's intentions and behavior, and her beliefs about that. It is important to recognize that the past was relevant only to the extent that it was manifest in the wife's perceptions about it.

In summary, the clinician uses observational, self-report, and interview material to formulate the personal and environmental factors crucial to the maintenance of the couple's current problems. From a behavioral perspective, this formulation should be rooted in specific, observable phenomena and should describe and explain important transactions between marital partners. The most important sequences of communication should be understood and described using the concepts of reinforcement and punishment. The clinician should also attempt to understand the development of the problems as well as the couple's understanding and explanation of them. In what follows, we describe the procedures used to address these problems. It should be noted that although we present the intervention techniques here as a list of techniques, they should be selectively applied in a manner consistent with the therapist's formulation of the couple's behavior. We discuss this issue in a later section.

Specific Intervention Techniques

Increasing Positive Interaction

One of the first tasks of the behavioral marital therapist is to increase the number of pleasant events occurring between spouses. By the therapist's taking this as the first objective, the spouses can receive a small but relatively rapid benefit, which will encourage them to attempt even greater changes. It is a common belief that many spouses are unwilling to indulge in additional positive behavior toward their partner. We believe that with the proper preparation, couples will be willing to try to behave more positively at the therapist's request.

In this phase the therapist uses the information gained from the assessment to specify initial targets for intervention. For example, one husband had discovered that his wife was having an affair. Although the wife quickly ended the affair and the spouses pledged to commit themselves to the relationship, they had repeated angry exchanges about the affair in the months that followed. It was important that the couple begin the healing process. Part of that strategy involved helping the couple to increase positive interaction. This entailed *positive event scheduling*, which involves helping couples set aside time to do relaxing, pleasurable activities, such as walking or going to a movie together. The technique is most useful when care is taken to select an event with a high probability of success. In our clinical example, this consisted of having the couple decide when to spend time discussing their day together. Discussion of past events was *disallowed* by the therapist and *reserved* for the therapy sessions. With appropriate attention to the rationale behind the plan, the couple viewed the exercise as an investment in their relationship rather than a contrivance.

The "love days" (Weiss et al. 1973) or "caring days" (Stuart 1980) technique is also an effective way to help spouses increase positive exchanges. This exercise helps the couple plan to behave positively toward each other while still maintaining some spontaneity. To use this approach, the therapist explains to the spouses how they could experience more cooperation and affection from their partner by pleasing him or her. It is important to emphasize that when they are angry at each other, they may avoid positive behavior so as to express their anger. Behaving pleasantly may be seen as giving in. As an alternative, the spouses need to realize that they are working against their own interests by harboring their negative feelings and refusing to be positive. Together, they may be able to improve the atmosphere enough to promote some flexibility in each other's positions.

To start this exercise, the therapist identifies several positive behaviors in the form of *favors* that one spouse desires from the other. The behaviors should be simple and easy to perform, such as one spouse coming home early from work to take the children to their music lessons (in cases in which the other spouse typically performs this function), or one spouse bringing coffee to the other in bed. The therapist then works with the couple to select a day or days on which one spouse is to pick one or more of the caring behaviors to carry out. Great flexibility should be built into the selection of positive events so that the volitional aspect of the behavior is highlighted (i.e., the spouse must make a choice of which behavior to perform). The exercise should proceed on a parallel fashion for both spouses but without making one spouse's behavior contingent on the other. It is useful for the therapist to create and engender a playful atmosphere regarding this exercise.

Another way to increase the amount of positive interaction among spouses is the "Catch a Person Pleasing You" exercise (Falloon et al. 1984), which provides an opportunity for spouses to positively reinforce one another for pleasing behavior. The technique requires that the spouses begin to record each other's positive behavior on the "Catch a Person Pleasing You" recording form. Spouses are encouraged to write down seemingly inconsequential but meaningful behaviors, such as "Meg asked me how things were at the office" or "Bob offered to go to take the kids to their game (because I got busy) even though I had agreed to do it earlier." After spouses are able to record at least one positive behavior per day, three times a week, the therapist should ask them to respond out loud to the partner when he or she had just done something which pleased them. For example, the wife might say, "Bob, I *do* appreciate your taking the kids to the game for me; I said I would take them, but I wanted you to know I feel relieved that you offered to do it." Most spouses feel pleased just to know that their partner *actually noticed* the attempt to be helpful; thus, the exercise has the potential for reinforcing these types of positive behavior.

Decreasing Negative Interaction

Because the most consistent difference between happy and unhappy couples revolves around negative behavior, the crucial interventions are aimed at reducing negative, conflictual interactions and *teaching* spouses how to resolve the issues that underlie the conflict. This entails reducing negative escalation, teaching spouses how to express their feelings constructively, and teaching them the skills needed to resolve a problem effectively and efficiently.

In the beginning of treatment it is important to reduce rapidly the negative escalation that occurs when spouses start to discuss areas of disagreement. One couple we have worked with, for example, had a long history of fighting about plans for their house near the shore. Mere mention of the topic prompted angry and defensive responses from each of them. It was important that the couple learn how to cut short or exit these escalating interactions while still keeping open the possibility of discussing the issue in the future. Both spouses were taught anger management techniques, including how to recognize the situations that often led to arguments as well as the physical cues and cognitions that immediately preceded the escalation of the argument. Then each spouse was taught how to state politely that he or she needed "time-out to cool down" and to indicate the time he or she would return. Practicing this procedure during a therapy session was helpful in implementing this strategy at home.

Problem Solving/Communication Training

Problem solving/communication training is a method for teaching spouses specific strategies for resolving a variety of conflicts and relationship problems. For some couples this therapeutic approach constitutes learning new skills, whereas for others it will be a way to build a problem-solving focus into their interactional repertoire. First, couples are encouraged to work with the mindset of a team. Then, spouses are taught a set of specific problem-solving steps: 1) specific definition of the problem; 2) agreement to work on the problem; 3) generation of solutions; 4) selection of the specific solution and anticipation of problems with implementation; and 5) evaluation of the solution after a trial period.

The couple is taught the steps first by using a minor relationship difficulty that is easily solved (e.g., where to eat dinner after the session); more difficult and emotionally laden problems are tackled after the couple has greater facility with the approach. After the specific steps are described, the therapist introduces some guidelines to help the spouses use the most effective communication possible. The therapist should emphasize those aspects of communication that were deemed most problematic during the assessment. For example, the spouses might be encouraged to avoid *blaming* and *criticizing* statements, avoid *bringing up the past* and trying to *establish truth*, and expend the most effort on finding solutions (i.e., be *solution-oriented*). Each of these guidelines should be defined and illustrated with examples from the therapist. There are several excellent resources providing full descriptions of problem solving/communication training (e.g., Baucom and Epstein 1990; Jacobson and Margolin 1979; Lester et al. 1980).

Emotional Expressiveness Training

Emotional expressiveness training is a strategy that emphasizes communication of one's intimate feelings and thoughts. Described most fully by Guerney (1977), the essence of this technique is to teach empathic listening skills paired with subjective expression skills. Spouses are taught this communication style as a way of increasing intimacy and encouraging each spouse to be sensitive to the perspective of his or her partner. To teach emotional expressiveness, each spouse is taught to take turns expressing his or her feelings while the other spouse uses empathic listening skills. The guidelines involved in skillful expression of feelings include the following: 1) stay subjective (i.e., use "I feel . . ."); 2) refrain from blaming and referring to the partner using negative trait terms; and 3) be behaviorally specific in describing both the upsetting circumstances and the resulting emotion. Expressions are best when they are only a sentence or two long so as to keep from overwhelming the listener. For example, one spouse might say, "I was really livid when I heard you tell our friends about our disagreement last weekend; I felt exposed, vulnerable, and a little humiliated." Conspicuously absent from the expression is any blaming or reference to negative intentions of the partner whose behavior is being commented on.

The listener is coached to listen attentively with a non-negative facial expression. When the partner who is expressing feelings finishes, the listener paraphrases the feelings just expressed. The following empathic listening skills are emphasized: 1) concentrate on summarizing the feelings; 2) use empathic reflections that do not add to or contradict the feelings expressed in any way; and 3) maintain good eye contact while listening and speaking. The listener is discouraged from interrupting the speaker or actively trying to solve the problem. In this context, one transaction occurs when the speaker expresses his or her feelings and the listener has empathically summarized the feelings. Spouses are coached to take separate speaker and listener roles and to deliberately specify who "has the floor" or is the speaker during the transaction. This has the benefit of slowing the transactions down and preventing negative escalation.

Cognitive Interventions

The idea that people's happiness in marriage is substantially related to how they think about problems with their spouse may seem foreign to many couples. Thus, the groundwork for cognitive interventions in behavioral marital therapy should be laid down carefully and slowly over several sessions. First, the therapist should take the opportunity to introduce the idea that each person's interpretation of a situation differs from the next, using examples from the therapy. Most importantly, the therapist should convey the idea that our thoughts and beliefs about events occur to us automatically, usually without our evaluating whether they are reasonable, accurate, or supported by objective evidence. Second, the therapist explains how some thoughts and beliefs about conflicts can lead to extremely negative and angry feelings about the situation. For example, at this point the therapist can describe *overgeneralization* as a cognitive error often made by couples in conflict. When the couple has a fight, it is easy for each person to become pessimistic and believe that "we have no future." Both spouses may be overlooking or deemphasizing the significance of recent positive interactions. The therapist can emphasize that the spouses need to avoid overgeneralizations and focus only on resolving identifiable conflicts. Next, the therapist should describe types of cognitive distortions as identified by Ellis (1962, 1986), Beck et al. (1979), and Baucom and Epstein (1990). Using the material of these writers as resources, the therapist should use a didactic style in describing cognitive distortions such as *mindreading* ("He thinks I never do any work") or *catastrophic thinking* ("Because she showed no interest in sex *again*, our relationship is doomed"). The therapist should be careful to focus on the cognitive distortions that are most relevant to each specific couple in order to avoid overwhelming them.

The clinician can make quick inroads to the minimization of positive events (or selective attention to negative events) by having couples use the "Catch-a-Person Pleasing You" form described earlier. When spouses track positive events, their selective attention on conflicts can be reduced. Care must be taken to reassure the spouses that the problems they brought to therapy are important but that to overemphasize the negative aspects of their relationship makes both of them less willing to work together. As described earlier, the therapist works with the spouses to gradually increase the number of positive partner behaviors recorded on the form.

Another method of altering dysfunctional cognitions is to have each spouse use the Daily Record of Dysfunctional Thoughts (Beck et al. 1979) to capture their thoughts on paper. They are encouraged to think about *events* as being separate from their *thoughts* about the events. Most people need some help in making this distinction, so the therapist should be ready with examples from the couple's treatment. After collecting thoughts for upsetting events during the week, the therapist works with both spouses to learn to challenge their own thoughts, using their knowledge of cognitive distortions. Although this exercise can be done conjointly, the spouses should be encouraged to challenge only their own thoughts—not those of their partner.

As the clinician helps the couple collect cognitions about upsetting events, he or she will begin to notice themes in the thought records. The therapist can identify in these themes the *assumptions* and *standards* that each spouse has about the relationship. For example, as described earlier, spouses in one couple believed that the husband was *the knight in shining armor* or *protector* in the relationship and the wife was in the position of the *lady* who should be protected. The unrealistic nature of these beliefs was discussed with the couple, and they were encouraged to substitute new, more realistic and functional standards for the relationship.

Integrative Couples Therapy

Integrative couples therapy involves a much more intensive focus on helping couples identify their central relationship theme than traditional BCT. Having couples join around the problem and achieve unified detachment from the problem might extend many sessions into treatment before any traditional BCT interventions are attempted.

To help the spouses join around the problem, the therapist guides the spouse expressing a hard emotion such as anger to reveal feelings that display more vulnerability. For example, the therapist might ask a spouse who is expressing anger about her partner's lack of interest in sex, "Monica, I'm hearing that you are angry about Kevin's decreased interest in being 'physical' with you, but I'm also wondering whether you are sad or, perhaps, hurt about it. Can you say anything about those feelings too?" Within the framework of ICT, most hard emotions are assumed to have softer counterparts, as in the following pairs: anger-hurt, resentment-disappointment, aggression-insecurity (Jacobson and Christensen 1996). If the therapist has intervened in a key transaction that is part of the couple's primary theme, the partner often responds with a much softer approach, allowing for greater intimacy and caring regarding the problem.

Unified detachment can occur within the same therapeutic discussion, although the goal is different with empathic joining. The therapist might make reference to the couple's idiosyncratic term for their theme; the therapist and couple above might have described the arguments about the husband's avoidance of intimacy as their "I want you—you can't have me" routine. The couple is encouraged to discuss when and how this interaction unfolds, as if the interaction is a separate entity from the couple. In essence, the couple is helped to develop a functional analysis of the problem in layperson's language. This intervention is repeated throughout the bulk of the therapy in order to help the spouses gain the distance and objectivity from the problem that is necessary for a less intense (i.e., more accepting) reaction to it.

Helping couples build tolerance is attempted after each spouse has a clear idea of the behaviors involved in the couple's problematic interactions. Interaction behavior to which the spouses are still reacting strongly may be targeted for in-session role-playing. Unlike role-playing during skills training exercises, these exercises are meant to inure the spouses to the targeted behavior by making the behavior ritualized, without the same emotional intensity or momentum as their arguments at home. To accomplish this task, the therapist asks the couple the following question: "As you describe how your argument unfolded, I am wondering exactly what that looks like. Can you show me, right here? Try to get the routine right like you've described it to me, with everything including the faces you make at one another." As described above, the therapist may also point out positive aspects of the negative behavior. For example, in the example involving the husband's refusal of intimacy, the therapist might suggest that this has the positive effect of the couple's never injecting anger or conflict into their sexual interactions, thereby keeping that arena *pure*.

Self-Regulatory Couple Therapy

The primary task of SRCT is to help both spouses quickly examine their alternatives in the context of their most distressing conflicts. For example, a therapist might say, "Bob, Emily, let's review the types of choices that each of you have regarding your disagreement about whether to have another child. As we've discussed, you can each continue to try to change your partner's mind, but that stalemate is what led you to your current state of unhappiness. Let's broaden the discussion."

The therapist would then ask the spouses to review their choices, first by focusing on his or her communication behavior on the issue in order to minimize distress between them. Second, the therapist could work with each spouse on adjusting to the situation as if the issue were resolved contrary to his or her preference. This might take the form of assuming a particular outcome and teaching each spouse cognitive therapy approaches to minimize his or her distress about it. Third, each spouse could be asked to review ways to minimize his or her distress by taking some course of action; for example, the wife might generate ways to minimize the burden of having another child, such as hiring a nanny to help with childcare, or suggesting specific ways the husband could be more involved with the care of the children. Fourth, the couple might be asked to review the scenario of separating, primarily as one of the choices open to them rather than an inevitable outcome. Finally, the spouses could be reminded that they had the option to not decide anything at this point and could review the decision at a later time.

Clinical Issues in Conducting Behavioral Couples Therapy

Behavioral couples therapy is tailored to each couple, on the basis of the information gathered in the assessment. Unfortunately, because BCT has been widely investigated in therapy outcome studies, manualized versions of the approach have come to be regarded as prototypic forms of this marital treatment. One study that compared a structured, research-based BCT intervention with a clinically flexible variation of the same treatment suggested that not tailoring the therapy to the specific couple results in a worse outcome (Jacobson et al. 1989b). The structured and flexible forms of BCT proved to be equally effective at the conclusion of treatment; however, at 6-month follow-up, the relationship between couples in the structured version deteriorated while that of the couples in the clinically flexible version did not. Thus, the behavior therapist should use idiographic information to adapt the treatment to a specific couple in order to help the couple maintain their gains over time.

There are general principles that the therapist should keep in mind when deciding which interventions to apply and in what order. First, it is important to engender a *collaborative set* or *cooperative orientation* early in treatment (Jacobson and Margolin 1979). This can be accomplished by using exercises to alter the spouses' selective attention in favor of the positive aspects of the relationship. Also, using the concept of social exchange, the therapist might describe the advantages of working in a common direction. As discussed earlier, using empathic joining around the couple's problem can help the spouses develop the teamwork needed to confront their predicament. The therapist might also teach the couple problem solving in order to resolve concrete problems that they have brought to therapy. Another important task early in therapy is to reduce the degree of negative escalation. Again, refocusing the selective attention is an effective strategy. The therapist also might teach structured empathic listening skills or, in severe cases, teach the couple how to use the time-out procedure described above. As stated earlier, the therapist might need more time to introduce cognitive interventions to couples. This approach might be implemented later in treatment.

It is important to assess the existence of individual symptomatology (such as anxiety or depressive symptoms) and to know the degree to which these symptoms interfere with the spouse's functioning. The greater the interference, the greater role the therapist should take in defining this as a problem to be addressed by treatment. Although anxiety and depressive disorders almost always contribute to or are affected by marital conflict, the therapist works with the couple to avoid pointing to individual psychopathology as a sole cause of marital problems. Seeing the marital problems as a result of individual problems often leads to patterns of blame that rarely allow a collaborative set. However, if individual psychopathology is to be addressed through treatment, it is often most appropriate to begin treatment of it first so as to gain some immediate improvement in symptoms. The spouse with the most severe symptomatology will need to return to the highest level of functioning possible in order to participate fully in marital treatment.

One misconception of behavioral treatment is that it is a technology that is coldly *imposed* on a couple and that spouses' concerns are not validated. To the contrary, behavior therapists in general, and behavioral couples therapists in particular, strive to have empathy and attempt to convey this empathy to the couple. However, because behavior therapists recognize the need to be persuasive, many times a therapist's empathic statement followed by an attempt to persuade the spouse to change his or her behavior sounds a bit like "Yes, but . . ." To avoid this unfortunate perception, the therapist can present requests for behavior change in the following way:

> Bob, you have told me you are frustrated and angry when Cathy points out that you have not done yardwork without highlighting your progress on other parts of the house—in fact, I think you said "*really* pissed." Those are important feelings that need to be expressed. I will illustrate another way of expressing that frustration, because I believe that your point cannot get across when you raise your voice louder than Cathy is comfortable with. Let me demonstrate another way to get your feelings across but in a way that they can be received.

By recognizing Bob's feelings as legitimate and refocusing the goal of the interchange to be the *effective* expression of negative feelings, the therapist can engage him in the process of behavior change.

In the traditional approach to BCT, the therapist regulates the agenda and direction of the sessions (note the differences of this approach with the ICT and SRCT approaches). Traditional behavioral marital therapy involves direct attempts to change the spouses' behavior and attitudes. Thus, the therapist should feel comfortable establishing what characteristics of the couple's interaction are addressed in each individual session. However, it is useful to distinguish between the *process* of the couple's interaction and the *content* of the problems that they wish to discuss. That is, the therapist should focus on *how* the spouses talk to each other; the spouses can be given the freedom to define *what* problems they discuss. To make sure that the spouses do not feel the direction of the session was imposed on them, the therapist should address the agenda at the beginning of each session. For example, the therapist might say the following:

> Now that we've had a chance to review the week, did either of you have something you wanted to particularly discuss today? Or were there some issues that last week's session raised that got you thinking over the week? I was thinking we would pick up on the problem we were working on last week—namely, how to get your will resolved—but I wanted to make sure that that direction made sense for both of you.

By explicitly raising the issue of the agenda, the therapist ensures that he or she is not fighting some unspoken agenda of the spouses.

In a skills-oriented behavioral treatment such as BCT, it is necessary for changes gained in sessions to generalize to the home environment. Success in this goal is facilitated by the couple's willingness to do *homework* assignments. After teaching a communication skill, the therapist asks the couple to practice this skill at home at least three times during the week. Practice sessions should last no longer than 15 minutes. Clear expectations about what skill is to be enacted, as well as the goals of the exercise, must be discussed in detail with the couple. Any compliance with homework assignments, however minimal, should be applauded in order to *shape* the couple's compliance. Reviewing homework for the previous week at the beginning of each session also demonstrates its importance to the therapy.

Resistance to treatment has been discussed at length by writers with a psychodynamic orientation. Resistance is also of concern to the behavioral couples therapist, but the causes and cures of resistance are somewhat different in the behavioral perspective (Birchler 1988; Liberman 1981). The source of resistance can actually be as mundane as presenting too much information and making more interventions than can be reasonably understood and integrated by the couple. Other sources of resistance include 1) asking the spouses to make a drastic change in behavior without their understanding the relevance to their problems; 2) suggesting changes in the relationship that directly contradict their normative beliefs about marriage (without providing a rationale); and 3) understanding the perceived, high, personal costs of behavior change, relative to the perceived benefits. Thus, when confronted with resistance to behavioral interventions, the therapist should ask the following questions:

- Have I presented too many communication guidelines or too many concepts at one time?
- Have I used jargon or not adjusted my language to the spouses?
- Have I integrated the couple's conceptualization of their problems with my rationale and recommendations for change?
- What do I know about the family's *rules* for normative behavior, and do these interventions challenge these ideas too directly?
- Have I demonstrated the techniques or communication guidelines well enough?
- Does the couple know *what* to do and *why* to do homework?
- Have I helped the couple develop cues for remembering to do homework assignments?
- Have all obstacles to homework performance been addressed through troubleshooting?
- Have I reinforced compliance with the behavioral procedures at all times?

As one might note, there are many sources of resistance to behavioral procedures that a clinician might investigate before considering intrapsychic factors or hidden agendas. Although a clinician may find himself or herself wondering about these sources, more time can be spent on addressing these factors than is warranted. In most cases, resistance can be addressed by evaluating the questions listed above.

Conclusion

During recent years, behavioral couples therapy has gone through a painful re-examination of its roots, goals, and techniques. Reacting to BCT's *asymptote* of success, many therapists have, like troubled coaches, experimented with their line-up to come up with the magic combination. Some have lengthened treatment, some have incorporated new elements, and some have even studied factors that distinguish successful from unsuccessful cases.

If the late 1980s saw the *world champion* BCT team searching for that elusive right mix, 1991 ushered in the decade with a crushing loss on their home court. A well-conducted outcome study showed that BCT's divorce rate was substantially higher than that of the psychodynamic insight oriented marital therapy (IOMT) (Snyder et al. 1991). In a rejoinder, Jacobson (1991b) argued that the BCT administered in the study was overly regimented and lacked the therapeutic soft skills found in the IOMT manual. He concluded that considering the way the treatments were employed, IOMT was much closer to true BCT than was their version of BCT. Indeed, research from Jacobson's laboratory has found that five areas of clinical skills (which are probably used in IOMT) are necessary for optimal implementation of BCT: structuring skills, instigative skills, teaching skills, skills that lead to positive couple outcome expectancies, and emotional nurturance (Holtzworth-Munroe et al. 1989).

Baucom and Epstein (1991) have stressed other points of overlap between IOMT and BCT, while acknowledging the lack of true consensus among BCT theorists. They indicate that BCT and IOMT share insight as a common ingredient, "with the major divergence being the manner in which [BCT] trains clients to evaluate the validity and appropriateness of their assumptions and other cognitions." In reference to these observations, we believe that the current debate is an argument over picking the best paradigm from which to understand the changes within marriage, rather than focusing on what works. Perhaps it would be more constructive for investigators simply to operate from within their own paradigm and *explore it to its limits*. As indicated, despite BCT's heavy research tradition, BCT advocates have not done this to the full extent possible through either basic or applied research.

There are a number of new directions that do not fall clearly within the scope of this chapter. Marital dysfunction is certainly understood to develop over time, and, accordingly, marital discord has begun to be seen as more explicitly developmental (see Bradbury 1998 for an excellent volume on this topic). We hope that developmental thinking is hopefully part of any good behavioral conceptualization of a couple's current problems. However, in no way do the methods of BCT in past or current forms require certain interventions for couples at specific points in their relationship or in the development of their distress. Future innovations in BCT might take these factors into account and provide different interventions based on the couple's relationship at different developmental phases.

Regarding the direction of BCT in the future, we believe the debates over BCT have been highly instructive. BCT is not the caricature of first-wave BCT: an invariant *technology* that downplays the need for therapeutic skill (Greenberg and Johnson 1990). Even if non-BCT theorists viewed BCT this way, it is not, and for the most part never was, like that. BCT is the application of social learning principles, which has always included behavior, cognition, and affect. These principles include the use of functional analysis, the importance of operant conditioning, and the reciprocal influence of person (including affect and cognition), behavior, and environment. BCT is also practical in that it recognizes the wisdom of many strategic, insight-oriented, and emotionally focused interventions and may occasionally use similar techniques to the extent that they comfortably fit within the behavioral conceptualization of the case. We argue that the behavioral framework offers the greatest potential for understanding both the spouses' and the therapist's contributions to a well-functioning marriage.

The consensus from all within the BCT camp is that BCT will be reinvigorated only by reaffirming its philosophical stance as valuable. We already know that BCT helps many couples, much of the time. As behaviorists, we await the outcome data before judging whether the latest moves within BCT help more couples, more of the time.

Chapters on Related Topics

The following chapters describe concepts related to behavioral couples therapy:

- Chapter 7, "Behavioral Family Therapy"
- Chapter 20, "Couples Therapy: An Overview"
- Chapter 37, "Couples Therapy Research: Status and Directions"

23

The Divorcing Family

Characteristics and Interventions

G. Pirooz Sholevar, M.D.
Linda D. Schwoeri, Ph.D.

Introduction

Divorce and remarriage have dramatically changed the character and configuration of the contemporary family. The landscape of the American family that was once dominated by traditional two-parent households now features equally prominent peaks of divorced, single, and remarried families. These changes have made it even more necessary for mental health professionals to learn about the continuum of the divorce process—its normative or pathological nature and course and its psychological and economic impact. The term *binuclear* was coined by Ahrons (1979) to describe the postdivorce family structure consisting of two interrelated, separate nuclear divorced households that sequentially share the children. The shared children are usually affected by the events in each of the two nuclei of the binuclear family, even if one nucleus has less importance in the child's life. The term has much in common with the terms *remarried family* (Sager et al. 1983) and *stepfamily*.

The concept of divorce as a *normative process* has gained in importance. Initially, divorce was viewed as a pathological phenomenon and a sign of personality disorder or psychopathology in one or both of the spouses that limited their capacity for intimacy. The painful experiences of the divorcing families, particularly those of the children, were taken as evidence for the pathological nature of divorce. However, the large increase in the proportion of families who now choose to divorce can be taken as an indication that such a widespread phenomenon should not be viewed as pathological. A variety of recent theories, particularly those by Ahrons and Rodgers (1987), have suggested that divorce should be considered as a normative process in the course of family life rather than as an end point to the family unit. Most divorcing families continue with the fundamental task of a family—namely, rearing their children—within a binuclear family setting. This new perspective considers that divergent developmental courses by spouses may make divorce inevitable. The *normative* concept of marriage has been criticized by some for ignoring the possible interconnection between *spousal psychopathology*, family system dysfunction, and divorce. The phenomenon of *interlocking neuroses*, which is the extension of neurosis in the spouses in the marital relationship, is an example of the overlapping between psychopathology and possible divorce.

The phenomenon of *good divorce* (Ahrons 1994) has been described as the relatively prevalent form of divorce. In this type of divorce, couples part ways without damaging the lives of the children they love. They continue to make emotional, psychological, economical, and physical contributions to the lives of their children and continue to function as a larger family. The resulting family is a binuclear one, with each of the households headed by one of the parents. The family continues to remain a family, united by their bonds to their children rather than by their marital bonds.

Divorce Rate

The *crude* divorce rate for 1984 was 5.0, which means that 5 out of every 1,000 people (men, women, and children) in the United States divorced that year. This represents a 10-fold increase over the divorce rate of 0.5 around 1900. The *refined* divorce rate in 1984 was 22 (Piercy et al. 1986), which means that approximately 22 out of every 1,000 marriages in the United States ended in divorce. Demographers use the *cohort* approach, which tracks the marriages that begin each year, and compare the percentage of those that ended in divorce with those that remained intact. For example, of those marriages that began in 1969, 29.7% resulted in divorce by 1980. By combining demographic projection with the cohort approach, it is predicted that eventually 42.2% of the marriages that occurred in 1964 will end in divorce. Glick (1984) projects that 49% of those born between the years 1946 and 1955 will end their first marriage.

In 1986, about 159,000 divorces were registered in the United States, representing 7.8% of all those over 18 years old. Approximately 1.5% of the U.S. population is involved in divorce. The median duration of marriage is slightly less than 7 years, with the peak period of divorce being 2–5 years after marriage. Three out of five couples filing for divorce have at least one child younger than 18 years. One million children are affected by divorce each year, about one-half as many as adults. Sixteen percent of all family groups with children younger than 18 years are one-parent families due to separation and divorce. Many of the children in these families will experience more than one family transition because most divorced individuals remarry within an average of slightly more than 3 years.

In 1984, one partner had been previously married in 22.2% of all new marriages, while both partners had been married before in 23.4% of all new marriages. One-sixth of all children live in reconstituted families: about one-third of them are under the age of 5 years at the time of the remarriage. Sixty percent of all *second marriages* end in divorce. Therefore, many children go through the divorce cycle two or more times. Only about *one-half* of the children living in the United States will reach the age of 18 having lived *continuously with both biological parents*.

Younger couples divorce more readily than older couples and are more likely to have younger children. Therefore, children tend to be disturbed by divorce early in their lives. Men are consistently more likely to remarry than are women. Not only are they more apt to marry someone not previously married, they also tend to marry younger women and have a larger pool of potential partners than do divorced women. Divorced women with physical custody of the children have less of a chance to remarry.

From 1900 through the 1970s, the divorce rate continued to climb, until it reached 5.2 for every 1,000 marriages in 1980 and until the number of marriages beginning each year that ended in divorce reached 49%. However, the divorce rate began to decline in 1980, decreasing to 4.7 for every 1,000 marriages in 1990, and continued to decline in the 1990s (Ahrons 1994).

Divorce Process and the Stages of Divorce

Divorce does not constitute a single point but a process. Many theorists have proposed conceptualizing divorce as a series of overlapping stages, with psychological and emotional consequences related to each stage of separation and divorce (Raschke 1983). The divorce process (Ahrons and Rodgers 1987; Raschke 1983) is generally conceptualized as having four stages: 1) predivorce decision making; 2) divorce restructuring; 3) postdivorce recovery; and 4) remarriage (Sprenkle 1985). In the first stage, the couple considers divorce as one alternative to relationship problems while attempting to compare the consequences of remaining married with those of getting divorced. In the second stage, the spouses decide to end the marriage and prepare to make the necessary legal, emotional, financial, social, and parental arrangements and adjustments. In the third stage, the spouses attempt to establish themselves as autonomous individuals with stable lifestyles and social relationships independent of the former marriage (Sprenkle 1985) Difficulties with the parent-child relationship and problems with custody or visitation can constitute major points of stress during this period. Many theoreticians include a fourth stage, when one or both of the spouses marry others.

Divorce Process

The divorce process is set in motion when the couple and the family realize they do not have any constructive future together, a phenomenon entitled *emotional divorce* (Ahrons and Rodgers 1987). The couple proceeds through legal channels to arrive at an economic division of their assets and to decide on custody of the children. It is hoped at this point that the children will be offered the opportunity to maintain a relationship with both parents. The couple then begins the process of forging new and separate futures.

Transitional Stages

There are three major transitional stages during the divorce: 1) the separation transition, 2) the divorce transition, and 3) the remarriage transition.

Separation Transition

The separation transition consists of four stages: *pre-separation, early separation, mid-separation,* and *late separation*. During *pre-separation*, the idea of separation as a solution to marital conflicts emerges from a fleeting thought and becomes a more concrete coping strategy, while other forms of resolution and coping receive less energy. The private ideas of one or both partners slowly evolve into a shared idea between them and then into a public announcement and actual physical separation. During *early separation*, the couple physically separates and negotiates necessary decisions regarding children and residence. High ambivalence results in crises. During *mid-separation*, the spouses live separately and move toward making tentative decisions rather than being controlled by pure crisis situations. In *late separation*, the family begins to reorganize some of their needs as a separated family and lifestyle changes occur. Ahrons and Rodgers (1987) refer to this stage as one of *systemic separation*, when the spouses may rely on each other for certain family roles. Power struggles and conflict between the spouses may extend into many areas of family life.

Divorce Transition

At this stage the spouses go through the tasks of establishing separate and independent lives while simultaneously carrying out the obligations of the original family. Ahrons (1979) has introduced the concept and the term *binuclear family* to illustrate how in most divorced families there is some remaining positive involvement between the spouses.

Ahrons' cross-national study examined 98 families from Wisconsin over a period of 5 years and included the stepparents. She described 50% of the spouses as having an amicable relationship following the divorce and acting as cooperative colleagues, managing their conflicts well. As a result, their children were not caught in the parental disagreements. The amicable ex-spouses were happier in their remarriages.

The following typology describes the diversity in the ex-spouse relationship based on Ahrons' sample of national study. She divided the spouses into either the well-functioning categories of perfect pals or cooperative colleagues or the poorly functioning categories of angry associates or fiery foes. She added a fifth category of dissolved duos, in which one of the parents had very little relationship with the children following divorce.

Perfect pals, who constituted 12% of the population, were characterized by a high level of interactions and communications. The positive elements of long-standing relationships continued and they remained best friends and collaborated optimally on behalf of their children. They all had joint custody arrangements.

Cooperative colleagues, who constituted the largest percentage of post-divorce families (38%), were characterized by a moderate level of interaction and a high level of communication. They were able to compromise for the welfare of their children. Some cooperative colleagues had joint legal custody, and usually one parent's house was considered "home."

Angry associates, who accounted for 25% of the initial sample, were characterized by a moderate level of interactions and a low level of communication. They allowed their anger to spread into their relationships with the children. Angry associates had some form of sole custody arrangement, with the nonresidential parent spending a range of time with the children (about 2–3 days per week).

Fiery foes, who made up another 25% of the sample, were characterized by low interactions and low levels of communication. They were highly litigious and fought frequently. Two-thirds of the couples who were fiery foes at the initial interview continued to maintain that behavior, while the remaining ones became cooperative colleagues or divided duos.

Divided duos made up less than 1% (only two single-parent families) of the original 98 families. In these two families, one parent discontinued contact entirely with the children, and the noncustodial parents left the geographic area. Frequently, the noncustodial parents were not aware of the major events in the lives of their children.

Remarriage Transition

At this stage the remarried families represent a complex system with many potential configurations. The functional level of a remarried family is to a large degree dependent on the clarity of the boundaries between the two families, which defines the nature and extent of their interactions.

Divergent issues emerge at different stages of the divorce process. In the predivorce stage, high expectations and unfulfilled needs are common complaints. Prior to divorce, 56% of women are unsatisfied with their spouses' contribution to the household tasks, while 40% of women and 20% of men do not live up to their spouses' expectations as a parent. Fifty to sixty percent of predivorce spouses have extramarital sexual relationships.

Theories of Divorce

The function of marriage has changed significantly from an *institutional marriage* to a *companionate marriage*. In an institutional marriage, each member plays a socially determined role and remains married in order to meet the survival needs of the family members and to conform to societal expectations. Companionate marriages were promoted by industrialization and urbanization and are organized around meeting the requirements of the couple and family members for love and basic human emotional needs. In this type of marriage, the divorce is acceptable if it helps family members obtain greater emotional well-being.

Social learning theory, the most widely used theory for the psychological explanation of divorce, proposes that individuals evaluate the cost relative to rewards associated with staying married versus ending the relationship (Levinger 1976). People remain in relationships based on conscious and unconscious accounting of three factors: 1) their attraction to the relationship; 2) the barriers they perceive to divorce; and 3) their current relationship in comparison with available alternatives. The divorce occurs when their internal attraction to the marriage and the barriers to divorce become weaker than available alternatives. An individual partner's interests and values can mature at a different rate, or the couple may be unable to achieve intimacy to the point that divorce becomes inevitable.

Sociological theories of divorce attribute the increased divorce rate to a wide range of societal changes. The enhanced economic position of women, the weakening of taboos against divorce, the concept of no-fault divorce, the availability of birth control pills, and the new available options for women are all seen as major reasons for the increased divorce rate.

The *crisis theory* of divorce explains how a stressor event would result in family crisis and subsequent marital dissolution (Hill 1949). According to this theory, the stressor event is mediated by the resources of the family and the definition of crisis (Raschke 1983). For example, the parenting of a newborn infant can be a major stressor, and the way a family reacts to such an event can enable us to predict the relative level of stress necessary for a person in that family to abruptly abandon his or her spouse. Sholevar and Sholevar (1984) have proposed that the increased rate of divorce is intimately related to the *weakening of traditional American family structure* and to the isolation of the nuclear family from its extended family. As a result the nuclear family, with its limited resources, is not adequately prepared to successfully address the stressful events facing it that were once buffered by the extended family. Furthermore, the young and inexperienced spouses do not have the assistance of the extended family to help complete the maturational process needed to develop a reciprocal, cooperative, and intimate relationship with each other or to provide a satisfactory context for child rearing. Instead, the couple falls back on blaming each other.

The major clinical reasons given by couples for seeking divorce are ineffective communication, poor problem-solving skills, sexual incompatibility, difficulty with long-term commitment, few shared activities, infidelity, and lack of sensitivity to the partner's feelings or wishes. The major sources of conflict are related to control, finances, independence, changing family roles, child abuse, or physical abuse.

Reaction of the Children to Divorce

The extensive developmental research on children in divorced families has been summarized by Santrock and Sitterle (1985). They divide the studies of children of divorce into three groups: *family sociological studies, clinical studies*, and *quasi-experimental developmental studies*. The advantage of *sociological studies* is their ability to examine a large number of families in the larger social context. For example, only one out of eight African-American children, compared with four of seven white children, were in a stepfamily

5 years after the family disruption (Furstenberg and Nord 1985). African-American children were more likely to experience the divorce of their parents than were white children. Frequent contact with the noncustodial parent occurred in only 17% of the disrupted families, regardless of race. And child support payments were made in only 25% of the families.

In the *clinical studies* group, a series of well-known investigations was conducted by Judith Wallerstein and Joan Kelly (Wallerstein 1983; Wallerstein and Kelly 1974, 1975, 1979, 1980). The authors suggested that as adolescents and adults look back on their childhood and adolescence, their mood is somewhat sad and contains feelings of unfulfilled wishes of wanting to have lived in an intact family as they grew up (Wallerstein 1983; Wallerstein and Kelly 1974).

The best known of the *quasi-experimental developmental* group of studies on the mediating factor of the nature of postdivorce family functioning are the controlled studies of Mavis Hetherington and colleagues (Hetherington 1987, 1988, 1989; Hetherington and Anderson 1987; Hetherington et al. 1981, 1982, 1986, 1989). These studies exhibit the remarkable disequilibrium that occurs in families during the first year after separation and divorce, a time when many families are struggling unsuccessfully with new life circumstances. By the second year after divorce, however, patterns of equilibrium are established. In these studies, the effects of divorce seemed to be more damaging to boys than to girls.

Wallerstein's research with 60 families from Marin County, California, has been criticized for the bias of the sample and the lack of a control group. The sample was recruited by advertising for people who needed divorce counseling. The lack of a control group did not allow a comparison of the divorcing families with nondivorcing ones. Even in Wallerstein's samples, 45% of the children did not experience any long-term psychological damage. According to Wallerstein, "They emerged as competent, compassionate and courageous people." The study's figure of two-fifths (41%) of the children who did poorly cannot be interpreted readily because of the lack of a control group.

Development of Children in Divorced Families

The acute and temporary emotional reaction of children to divorce is followed by a long-term reaction associated with the child's postdivorce adjustment in a single-parent family. The first year following divorce is the most difficult one for the child. After 2 years, considerable improvement in the child's adjustment appears, particularly for girls. There is a tremendous variability in children's responses to divorce, and some of these responses may actually be related to relationship disturbances in the family *prior* to divorce.

All children initially experience divorce as highly stressful. However, some children emerge as competent, well-functioning individuals, while others exhibit severe or enduring disruptions during their development.

Impact of Divorce According to Children's Developmental Stage

Children's reaction to parental divorce varies according to the child's developmental status. During *infancy* (0–2 years), offspring of divorced families exhibit insecure attachments and socially incompetent behavior in preschool ages. The anxious/resistant infants are easily frustrated, whiny, and negativistic, even when faced with simple problems. They are not easily comforted by contact from the caregiver. The anxious/avoidant group withholds contact and avoids the caregiver. Subsequently, insecurely attached children of divorce exhibit more peer difficulties and are more dependent on their teachers. The disruption in attachment after divorce is particularly significant when there is a task overload that may make the custodial parent tense and inattentive toward the child. The child may respond with reduced responsiveness, hyperactivity, or insecurity. The aftermath of such experiences can later result in lower IQ and achievement test scores in school-age children.

In *early childhood* (3–5 years), preschoolers react to parental divorce with aggressive behavior, increased irritability, confusion, and anger. They may exhibit excessively dependent, clinging, demanding behavior or pervasive oppositional reaction. The initial reaction to divorce can be one of pervasive sadness, fear, anger, and feelings of guilt, helplessness, and anxiety. Boys tend to become more oppositional and aggressive, while girls are more likely to whine, complain, and sulk. Difficulties with peers in school can be observed. Because of the child's limited cognitive capacities, the tendency for self-blame and distorted perception of parental behavior is common. The regressive behavior may include separation anxiety, enuresis, and eating difficulties. Wallerstein's 10-year follow-up of preschool children (Wallerstein et al. 1988) found that the children had few memories of the intact phase of the family or of the family disruption. However, they felt they would have been happier if they had been raised by both parents, and they continued to harbor fantasies of reconciliation. Wallerstein (1983, 1987) concluded that when divorce occurs very early, children are less burdened and may carry fewer bad memories. She found that divorce in later years is more detrimental to the developmental course of the children than earlier divorce. When the divorce occurs during the first 2 years of the child's life, it has a more detrimental effect than when the divorce occurs in preschool years.

In *middle childhood* (6–8 years), children had the most intense reaction to divorce, including intense feelings of sadness and grief. They were frightened by the family instability and felt their entire world has been profoundly shaken. They became involved in intense fantasies of parental reconciliation. The boys in mother-custody families were particularly saddened and felt rejected by the departure of their fathers. They were generally unable to express their anger toward their fathers but had no difficulty expressing their anger openly toward their mothers and *safe* targets, such as teachers and friends, which created school and peer problems. They had behavioral difficulties and a prolonged decline in their academic performance. At this age, children had an increased awareness and express their feelings about the divorce and its implications. They experienced and openly expressed their feelings of sadness.

In *late childhood* (9–12 years), the children looked surprisingly different from the younger children. Underlying feelings of loss, rejection, and helplessness were not as immobilizing to them as to younger children. They actively struggled to master their painful feelings. Few children from this group expressed feeling responsible for their parents' divorce. They made particularly strong alignments with one parent and attacked the other parent. This age group's values of commitment, loyalty, steadfastness, and reliability as a friend and team member can be co-opted in the service of one parent to continue his or her postmarriage power struggle against the other parent.

Children fare better when they are in a custodial relationship with a parent of the same sex. Boys show more socially competent behaviors in father-custody families and girls are more socially competent in mother-custody homes. Authoritative parenting, as exhibited by warmth, clear setting of rules and regulations, and extensive verbal give-and-take (Baumrind 1973), is significantly related to increased self-esteem, maturity, sociability, social conformity, decreased anger, and fewer demands on the part of the child. Additional caregivers are a significant resource for single parents and enhance a healthy development. Custodial fathers use these support systems twice as much as custodial mothers. Father-custody children have more frequent contacts with the noncustodial mothers than mother-custody children have with their fathers. The amount of contact with noncustodial parents and other nonparental caregivers is positively related to the child's warmth, sociability, and social conformity. Mothers with custody report deterioration in the father-child relationship, whereas fathers with custody report an improvement in the mother-child relationship.

In *adolescence* (13–18 years), divorce may increase the level of parent-adolescent conflict. The studies of Hetherington (1988, 1989) have shown that female children of divorced families get involved at an earlier age in heterosexual behavior, are more open and responsive, and seek attention from men. They tend to marry earlier than girls in intact families and are more likely to choose men who have drug problems and erratic work histories. The daughters from intact families, on the other hand, report fewer sexual and marital adjustment problems. They seem to be more relaxed and competent as wives, indicating that they have worked through their relationship issues with their fathers and feel free to succeed in relationships with men. The adolescents perceive their parental divorce as a painful family event. They feel vulnerable about their own future marriages and question their competence as sexual partners. Some adolescents experience major setbacks in response to parental divorce and exhibit regressive and immature behavior, delinquency, sexual promiscuity, and severe depression.

The behavioral configuration exhibited by children at the time of parental divorce may actually be related to relationship disturbances in the family prior to divorce. Families that are eventually disrupted by divorce are less stable, less peaceful, and less child-centered. The mothers of boys from divorced families impose strict disciplinary control while de-emphasizing warm and intimate interaction with their children. Each child's individual characteristics and availability of resources will determine whether, in the long run, the child will be a survivor, loser, or winner of the parents' divorce and remarriage (Hetherington 1988, 1989).

In summary, children in some developmental stages (such as preschool) are particularly vulnerable to the impact of divorce, whereas children in other stages show more resilience.

The Social World of Divorced Adults

Hetherington described one phenomenon of the social world of divorced adults as *task overload* in single parents (Hetherington et al. 1982). The single-family home exhibits greater chaos and disorganization, particularly during the first year after divorce. There are financial hardships, erratic meals and bedtimes, frequent school lateness, and a decrease in enjoyable parent-child activities. Some parents assign excessive tasks to children, which makes children feel grossly overburdened or incompetent. Some parents sleep less and eat meals on the run. Men frequently receive help from female friends.

During the first year after the divorce, mothers are frequently depressed due to inadequate childcare, constriction of social network, and other pressures. This frequently results in ineffective parenting practices, which in turn escalates oppositional behavior, especially in sons. The mothers respond by feeling more incompetent and helpless and employ even less effective parenting practices. Divorced parents of both sexes report feeling more anxious, depressed, angry, rejected, and incompetent. Very often the social network they enjoyed in the past drops away and they must begin to establish a new set of friends.

One year postdivorce marks the beginning of a gradual emotional upswing. The divorced parents begin to date, socialize with friends, attend social gatherings and parties, and exhibit an enhanced interest in self-improvement. At the 2-year mark, the frenzy of social activity and self-improvement gradually begins to wind down (Hetherington et al. 1982). This ushers in the third issue for the divorced adults, which is the establishment of intimate interpersonal relationships. Most of the divorced parents enter a close relationship by this time, and many move toward remarriage. The syndrome of *displaced homemaker* is particularly difficult for women who have assumed a long-term homemaker identity.

The economic situation of the family declines following the divorce in 30% of cases (Weitzman 1985). However, many of the divorced parents do not complain of the economic situation because they felt they now had more control over the finances.

Special Syndromes in Divorced Parents

- *Part-time parent and part-time child.* In this relationship, which has no prior counterpart in the predivorce period, there is no daily routine or responsibility, and many feelings are expressed within the narrow confines of a visit.
- *Feeling trapped.* Divorced mothers complain of feeling *trapped in* and the noncustodial fathers complain about being *shut out* (Hetherington and Clingempeel 1992).
- *Santa Claus syndrome.* Many divorced fathers resort to extravagant gifts to make visits more fun for the children, which enrages the ex-wife.
- *Feelings of loss.* Children often feel the loss of their individual time with the parent, time that now has to be shared with the lover when the parent forms a new relationship.
- *Acrimonious visits.* The visits can become a major acrimonious battleground for divorced spouses.
- *Attachment to ex-spouse.* Some parents continue to remain attached to the ex-spouse. Hetherington (1988, 1989) reports that 6 out of 48 couples have sexual intercourse with their ex-spouse during the first 2 years after divorce, indicating that the prior attachments are hard to break. Two years after divorce, the intensity of the anger between divorced people has generally subsided.

Family Process in Divorcing Families

Conflict and Stress

Conflict and acrimony accompany most divorces and often escalate following the divorce (Hetherington et al. 1982; Wallerstein and Kelly 1980). The relationship between family conflict, divorce, and maladjustment in children is complex. Initially, family conflict may be more harmful to children living in divorced families than to children living in nondivorced families (Hetherington 1988). However, the differences between the two groups change markedly over the course of 2 years following the divorce. Furthermore, boys appear to be more vulnerable to the effects of both marital conflict and divorce than girls (Hetherington et al. 1982). Two years following divorce, the pattern is reversed and the children from conflicted nuclear families exhibit more aggressive and less prosocial behavior than children from low-conflict divorced families. Therefore, the old concept of *staying together for the sake of the children* does not hold true. In the long run, marital discord may be associated with more adverse outcomes for children than divorce itself (Hetherington et al. 1982). Children residing in stable, conflict-free single-parent families are able to recover from the hostility associated with the separation and divorce of their parents in approximately 2 years. A clearly defined and consistently enforced roster of rules, responsibility, and a nurturing environment can buffer the ill effects of divorce and enhance the child's adjustment to a single-parent family (Hetherington and Anderson 1987).

Multiple phases of divorce require a significant level of adjustment on behalf of the children. The impact of divorce on children varies significantly to the point that Hetherington (1989) has divided the children of divorce into *winners*, *losers*, and *survivors*. The child's developmental stage, temperament, family relations, and extramarital resources influence the outcome. Some of the children in divorcing families show remarkable resiliency. There is a great diversity in the response of parents and children to divorce and remarriage. Most family members recover within a 2–3 year period. Some parents and children may show no significant immediate reaction to divorce but may exhibit delayed effects. The children in divorced families generally grow up faster (Weiss and Perry 1979).

Rutter (1983) has suggested that the factors of temperament, family relations, and extramarital resources are largely *inert* on their own but can serve as catalysts when they are combined with stressful events. Rutter (1987) later proposed that protective factors make available potentially supportive resources and the children's characteristics may allow them to use such factors to a higher or lower degree. *Vulnerability* factors refer to variables that increase the effects of stressors, while *protective* factors refer to the factors that diminish the effects of stressors. Garmezy (1983) has referred to a *triad of protective factors* that repeatedly emerges in the research on children of divorce: the personality and disposition of the parents, a supportive family medium, and an external societal system that includes social agencies serving as a support system.

Hetherington's study of a 6-year follow-up of well-educated middle-class parents of divorced children in mother custody families has revealed a variety of factors. The children in this study were 4 years old at the beginning of the study. During the first 2 years following divorce, most children and many parents experienced emotional distress. By 2 years following the divorce, the majority of parents and children had adapted reasonably well. However, in comparison to control groups, boys from divorced families showed more academic underachievement and antisocial, noncompliant, and coercive behavior at home, at school, and with peers. The divorced mothers monitored their children less closely in contrast to the mothers in undivorced families and knew less about where the children were. Boys showed more behavioral problems at the younger age in contrast to the girls, who showed difficulties at the time of entering early adolescence. Boys were more adversely affected by divorce and life in a mother-custody one-parent household. Girls had more long-term difficulties than boys did in adjusting to the introduction of a stepfather (Hetherington et al. 1981, 1982, 1986).

The Hetherington studies have supported the work of Baumrind (1973), who suggested that disengaged and permissive parenting styles are more likely than authoritative parenting to be associated with the development of behavior problems and low social and cognitive competence in children. Temperament and personality of the children played a role in their reaction and adjustment to divorce. Intelligence, age, and sex are also important factors. The more intelligent children were more resilient. Older children were more affected than younger children by extrafamilial factors. Temperamentally difficult children have been found to be less adaptable to change and more vulnerable to adversity than temperamentally easy children. Temperamental factors of irritability, unsoothability, fearfulness, activity, sociability, and irregularity in basic biological functions such as sleep and eating predicted later child behavioral problems.

Personality problems of a parent, including depression, irritability, and anxiety, in combination with difficult temperament in the children correlated with a higher rate of negative stressful life events and behavioral problems in the children.

Adjustment After Divorce

The stressful period of adjustment after divorce was generally 2 years, after which family relationships general stabilized. The remarriages introduced another period of instability requiring another 2 years for their stabilization. Divorced and unmarried mothers continued to exhibit many of the same unadaptive behaviors with their sons 6 years after divorce that they did in the initial stressful period. They were generally ineffectual in their control attempts and gave many instructions with little follow-through. Their interaction with their children was characterized by nagging, "nattering," and complaining, with many periods of negative "start-ups." The relationships between the mothers and their early adolescent boys can be best described as intense and ambivalent rather than hostile and rejecting.

Reaction of Children

Children's reaction to divorce can often be described in terms of coping. Weiss and Perry (1979) and Wallerstein and Kelly (1980) report that one way children cope with their parents' divorce is by becoming disengaged from the family, spending significantly less time in the home and staying alone or with peers. Early-maturing daughters create a higher level of conflict in divorced, nondivorced, and remarried family types in comparison to late-maturing girls. The mothers and daughters may experience problems as the daughters become pubescent and enter into heterosexual activities (Hetherington 1987, 1989).

Stepfathers generally exhibit a low level of affection for their stepchildren in the first 2 years of remarriage. They remain generally less authoritative and much more disengaged than fathers in nondivorced families. The family interaction sequence of "Mother commands/child is noncompliant/father intervenes" was less common in remarried families than in nondivorced families (Hetherington 1989).

Any kind of active control by the stepfather is initially perceived by the stepchild as coercive. After 2 years, authoritative parenting by stepparents resulted in fewer behavior problems and greater acceptance of the stepparent by stepsons than before. By the time the children were 10 years old, maternal behavior had more impact on the antisocial and prosocial behavior, as well as the self-esteem, of girls than of boys in all family types. Biological fathers in nondivorced families had more impact on such behaviors in boys.

Sibling relationships were generally adversely affected by divorce, as siblings became increasingly rivalrous and hostile while competing for the scarce resources of parental love and attention. Sibling relationships in the stepfamily improved over time but remained more disturbed than those in nondivorced or divorced families.

The presence of the grandparent in African-American families who lived at the same home with the children was associated with better adjustment in the children in contrast to the families in which the children lived with the mother alone (Kellam et al. 1982). Grandparents did not play a potent role in the social, emotional, and cognitive development of their grandchildren unless they lived in the home. Conflict between divorced mothers and residential grandmothers was associated with increased destructive behaviors in boys.

Schools and Peers

Schools and peer relationships can help stabilize divorced families. Authoritative teachers and an authoritative school environment attenuated adverse outcomes for children of divorced families, remarried families, and nondivorced families with high conflict. The protective effect of an authoritative school is most marked for boys with difficult temperaments. Peer relationship became more influential with age. The supportive relationship with a single friend could moderate the adverse consequences of marital transition.

Three clusters were noticed in the Hetherington study. One cluster involved *aggressive, insecure* children. They were sullen and brooding and exhibited periods of withdrawal. They were unpopular with peers and the majority of them did not have a close friend. The style of parenting in this group of families involved verbal or physical attacks, power plays, or withdrawal rather than compromise. The second cluster represented *opportunistic-competent* children, and the third group was one of *caring-competent* children. Children in both of these clusters were high in self-esteem, popular with their peers and teachers, and low in behavior problems. They were curious, energetic, assertive, self-sufficient, and exhibited a wide range of interests. They were competent, flexible, and persistent in dealing with demanding or stressful situations. The conflict level in these families was higher for the girls than for the boys. The children in the caring-competent cluster were similar to the second group but were less manipulative and less concerned with prestige and power in their relationships. They were less striving in their attempts to gain the attention and approbation of adults. They befriended neglected or even rejected children. They were more sharing than children in any other group. The caring-competent cluster comprised almost totally girls from divorced, nonremarried, mother-headed families.

Divorce and Child Custody

In the past two decades, issues of divorce and child custody have been increasingly addressed by the legal system. Legislation regarding legal and residential joint custody has been effected throughout most of the states. Legal joint custody enables both parents to have a significant role in major life decisions for their children. The many forms of joint residential custody allow the children to share a substantial amount of time with both parents, which simultaneously reduces the burden of childcare on one parent. The configurations for residential joint custody are quite varied. In the 5-year follow-up study by Furstenberg and Nord (1985) that examined the long-term effects of divorce, it was noted that the children were significantly and mentally affected by the marital dissolution. Differences were observed in the variables of sex, race, age, and marital education. One significant and perhaps unexpected finding was that the relationship between the noncustodial parent and child became one of "pals" rather than of the parent as disciplinarian and teacher. Co-parenting was viewed as more of a myth than a reality, since primary discipline and responsibility for the child rested with the custodial parent (Furstenberg and Nord 1985). Furstenberg and Nord concluded that children who had not seen their fathers during this 5-year span actually did better because of inconsistencies and problems during visitation. Furthermore, they concluded that no evidence was shown of benefits to the child by legislative or judicial interventions designed to promote paternal participation beyond financial support (Furstenberg et al. 1987).

There is still a significant social bias that children are primarily the responsibility of the mother. Mothers gain sole residential custody of their children in more than 90% of the cases of divorce, particularly in the less educationally and economically privileged groups. However, there is an increasing trend for the fathers, particularly the better educated ones with a secure financial status, to seek a more active participation in the lives of their children following divorce.

Divorce Phenomena and Psychopathology

The interrelationship between divorce phenomena and individual and family systems psychopathology should not be undermined by the extant clinical investigation on divorce as a normative process for a substantial number of families. Generally, the normative divorce phenomenon occurs between couples with satisfactory premarital adjustment whose functioning has generally deteriorated following their marriage due to either the incompatibility of their personality structures or value systems or a divergent course of development, which may have created more disparity in their interests and values.

A high rate of divorce has been recognized in a variety of psychiatric disorders, particularly in depression, alcohol or substance abuse, and severe personality disorders. The interference of depression with the development of marital intimacy makes the marriage particularly vulnerable to divorce. The preponderance of psychopathology in the children in a divorcing family, as well as in the spouses of depressed patients, adds further vulnerability to such marriages (see Chapter 19, "Parent Management Training," and Chapter 28, "Depression and the Family: Interpersonal Context and Family Functioning"). Alcoholism and substance abuse burden the family and the marriage with a multitude of problems, increasing its vulnerability (see Chapter 31, "Alcoholic and Substance-Abusing Families"). Certain personality disorders are major contributors to divorce. Paramount among such disorders are narcissistic and antisocial personality disorders (see Chapter 33, "Family Therapy With Personality Disorders"). Antisocial persons function exploitatively and irresponsibly within a conflictual marriage and family. This enhances the likelihood of a marital breakup. Spouses with narcissistic personality disorder fail to develop a cooperative marital relationship, and their relationship is characterized by extensive mutual blaming. Other personality disorders such as obsessional disorder and histrionic personality disorder limit the functioning of the person within an interpersonal context, making the marriage vulnerable to divorce.

Children in divorcing families are more vulnerable to a range of disorders, including conduct disorders, depression, and somatization. The more recent clinical research findings place the origin of many of such disorders in the conflictual predivorce stage of the marriage. Additional pathogenic factors following divorce include the lack of social, financial, and personality resources in the parent following the divorce.

Divorce Therapy and Divorce Mediation

New clinical practices (such as divorce therapy and divorce mediation) are designed to assist divorcing families in achieving satisfactory postdivorce adjustment through a less acrimonious divorce (see Chapter 20, "Couples Therapy: An Overview").

Interventions

Children do best with continued involvement of both parents following divorce. Frequent contacts with the noncustodial parent are associated with positive development, social adjustment, and peer relationships, particularly for boys (Hetherington and Anderson 1987; Wallerstein and Kelly 1979). The extrafamilial support system is important for divorced families, particularly those with low incomes (Colletta 1978). Divorced parents can be more socially isolated than parents in intact families. They work longer hours and receive less emotional support from friends and from their own parents, and their support system tends to be less stable (Weinraub and Wolf 1983).

Infants from divorced families exhibit less secure attachment and do not exhibit socially competent behavior in preschool ages. Insecurely attached children of divorce experience more peer difficulties, are more dependent on their teachers, and exhibit more anxious/resistant and anxious/avoidant behavior. The anxious/resistant infants are easily frustrated, whiny, and negativistic, even when faced with simple problems. They are not easily comforted by contact with the caregiver.

Clinical Implications

Many families experiencing divorce require assistance from mental health professionals to "put their lives back together." They require help particularly in the crisis period following the divorce and when they decide to remarry. The knowledge of expectable "norms" for children of divorce can be helpful toward recognizing when a realistic timetable for the duration of this process is exceeded. A range of community services are available to divorced families and their children, but these services frequently remain unused.

The services for divorced families should address a number of their needs. These needs include assistance with the initial period of stress following divorce, improvement in parenting skills, and primary prevention through providing information, education, and resources to reduce the rate of subsequent and more damaging emotional disorders. Some of the well-known groups that provide such extensive services include Parents without Partners; Marin County Divorce and Mourning Project, Marin County, California; the Children of Divorce group, South Orange, New Jersey; the Center for Children in Family Crisis, Pittsburgh, Pennsylvania; and the Family Change Project, Minneapolis, Minnesota.

Co-Parenting Relationship

A constructive co-parenting relationship can be of great assistance in the post-divorce period. *Co-parenting* refers to the relationship between both parents that permits them to continue their child-rearing obligations and responsibilities after divorce (Ahrons 1994). It is necessary to provide measures to reduce hostility and animosity between former spouses. Significant principles of co-parenting include continuing contact with the noncustodial parent, providing a predictable and stable home environment, improving parent management skills of the custodial parent, and disciplining the children for unacceptable behavior.

Need for Treatment

The need for treatment becomes apparent when the symptomatic behavior of the child continues beyond the expected time limits. There is usually a span of 2 years necessary for completion of this process, with an all-time low around the end of the first year postdivorce. The following conditions are indications for consideration of treatment:

- Persistence of adjustment problems beyond the 1.5- to 2-year mark
- Severe initial reaction to parental divorce by behaviors such as suicidal attempts and running away from home
- Long-standing problems either at home or at school coupled with serious deterioration in academic performance or classroom behavior

Therapeutic options are multiple and include individual and group psychotherapy with children and parents and family-based treatment. The major goal of treatment is to establish a secure and loving environment for the child to enhance his or her feelings of security. Initially, the children need to be reassured that the divorce will not take away the basic items that make them feel secure, such as food, clothes, and shelter (Gardner 1977).

Conclusion

The increasing rate of divorce has changed the landscape of the American family, with divorced, remarried, and single families now assuming the prominent peaks once held by traditional two-parent families. Increasingly, the divorce process is recognized as a normative one necessitated by the divergent developmental course of the two spouses. The new emphasis on *companionate marriages*, in addition to multiple sociological and psychological factors, is a significant contributor to the increasing divorce rate.

The increasing rate of divorce is a significant contemporary challenge, as is the impact of the divorce process on the children according to the stage of divorce process and the developmental phase of the children. Divorce therapy and divorce mediation have emerged as two major intervention methods that address divorce as a point and process in the family development cycle requiring extensive negotiation between the divorcing spouses. The successful divorce therapy course would assist the families in establishing a functional *binuclear family*, which would in turn continue with the most important task of the family—namely, the socialization of their children. The recent emphasis on joint legal and residential custody can provide the parents with novel and creative ways of maximizing both parents' access to their children while equalizing the significant burden of childrearing and divorce. Functional solutions to the divorce and the sharing of the children could enable the parents to proceed with their next developmental stage, be it single parenthood or remarriage.

Chapters on Related Topics

The following chapters describe concepts related to divorcing families:

- Chapter 20, "Couples Therapy: An Overview"
- Chapter 24, "The Remarried Family: Characteristics and Interventions"
- Chapter 28: "Depression and the Family: Interpersonal Context and Family Functioning"
- Chapter 31, "Alcoholic and Substance-Abusing Families"
- Chapter 33, "Family Therapy With Personality Disorders"

24

The Remarried Family

Characteristics and Interventions

Emily B. Visher, Ph.D.
John S. Visher, M.D.

Introduction

Recently, the structure of the family has undergone a revolution in the United States. Until a few years ago the predominant family was the first-marriage family (original husband and wife and their biological children). This model continues to be presented as the *ideal family*, to the detriment of other kinds of families. Stepfamilies and stepchildren, in particular, are often the targets of negative stereotyping (Coleman and Ganong 1987), and the general public can be actively hostile toward stepparents.

Recent statistics document the changes that are taking place (Glick 1989). Today, approximately 50% of first marriages end in divorce, and half of all marriages are remarriages for at least one of the adults. Eighty-five percent of men whose marriages end in death or divorce remarry, the majority within 3 years. Women remarry in about 65% of the cases, unless they are over 40. A woman's ex-husband will probably marry a younger person, who is not likely to remarry. Sixty percent of the adults who do remarry have children from previous relationships. It is estimated that by the year 2007, there will be more stepfamilies than any other type of family. Because of the number of terminated first marriages, children who were born in the 1980s have a 45% chance of experiencing the divorce of their parents before they are 18 and a 35% chance of living with at least one stepparent before that age. In some areas of the country one child in four in the public schools is a stepchild.

For research and census purposes stepfamily households are defined differently than first-marriage households. We define a stepfamily as a household in which there is an adult couple, at least one of whom has a child from a previous relationship. As therapists we consider that a broad stepfamily definition is psychologically realistic because similar basic dynamics are present in all types of stepfamily households. If each of a child's two biological parents have remarried, both households are stepfamilies according to our definition. The U.S. census, on the other hand, uses a narow definition of a stepfamily because a child cannot be counted twice, and therefore only the household that is a *primary residence* of the child is counted.

There are also many households containing an adult couple with children from previous relationships in which the adults have a committed relationship but are not legally married. In such households, basic stepfamily characteristics and dynamics exist, and the household must meet the usual stepfamily challenges.

It is easy to apply old values and ideas to these stepfamilies, often with disastrous results. A stepfamily has important structural differences from the traditional model that need to be understood. These differences are not often consciously recognized. This nonrecognition can result in stepfamily adults experiencing high levels of stress and loss of self-esteem as they attempt to deal with situations that they do not anticipate and are not prepared for. Stepparents especially tend to blame themselves for difficulties, seeing them as a result of personal failures and inadequacies. Remarried parents tend to deny responsibility for family difficulties, and children often experience severe emotional conflicts. Thus, members of stepfamilies frequently come to therapy in crisis, convinced that there is something very wrong. They are not aware that stepfamilies are families in transition with characteristics that usually make integration a lengthy process with many predictable challenges along the way.

Stepfamily Characteristics

There are a number of major ways in which stepfamilies differ from first-marriage families, and each of these characteristics or differences carries with it a set of tasks that need to be accomplished if the family is to move toward successful integration. Frequently, therapeutic help is sought because the integration process is not progressing satisfactorily.

Integration

Integration is difficult in stepfamilies because individuals come together after experiencing many important losses. Parent-child relationships have been disrupted by death or divorce, and previous marriage relationships have ended. Adults who have not been married before may have to give up some earlier hope they had of settling down with the man or woman of their dreams (and no marital past) and having children with him or her. (This dream family also does not include instant children—no little girl playing at being a mother imagines that she will grow up to be a stepmother.) In a remarriage, children now need to share their parent with a new partner and perhaps with instant stepsiblings, and they may have lost their ordinal position in the family and moved to a new home far away from friends and relatives.

Remarried adults may not be aware of their losses and depression because these are masked by the euphoria of a new relationship. Transported by their happy feelings, they are only hopeful about having another chance with a new person whom they believe their children will welcome and appreciate. Very often they are not aware of, nor can they understand, the depression that their children may feel.

Therapists can help individuals to mourn their losses. Sometimes it is enough to bring the losses to the attention of the people concerned, since talking about depressive feelings and having them accepted can be very helpful. In some cases, therapists may see the couple together, but in other cases they may need to see one or both in individual therapy to give each an opportunity to talk about their disillusionment, the result of lost dreams and failed hopes in previous relationships.

Children can be helped by having their feelings accepted by the adults, and by contacts with other children who have been through divorce and remarriage experiences. Bibliotherapy can be especially useful, and support groups for children and for adults can be a valuable adjunct to therapy. There are now many good books that provide information and opportunities for identification with those who have successfully dealt with their stepfamily situations (Visher and Visher 1982) These books may be ordered from Stepfamily Association of America (650 J Street, Lincoln, Nebraska 68508; telephone: 800-735-0329) if they are unavailable in local book stores or libraries.

Incongruent Cycles

In stepfamilies there are incongruent individual, marital, and family life cycles. One of the adults may be a parent with older children, the other an adult who has never had children or whose children are younger. One issue that can cause great psychological disturbance is the question of whether to have a child, especially when one partner has never had children and the other does not wish to become a parent again.

Teenagers in a new stepfamily are at a developmental stage in which they are trying to become independent, and their primary orientation is to their peers. They may have little interest in investing much time and energy in helping the *remarriage family* or participating in its activities, and this usually is upsetting to the couple who is in a new *nesting stage*. Although the adults need to let go of their teenagers, they also need to leave the door open for them to participate as much as they are willing. Reminding the adults of their own needs when they were adolescents can be helpful. At times, there may be partial *cut-offs*, which can be painful for everyone, as adolescents try to deal with their ambivalent feelings about being independent, at the same time they want to continue enjoying the comfort of having their needs taken care of by adults. Later on, when they become young adults, the young people in stepfamilies often wish to *rejoin* the family.

Previous Experiences and Expectations

Children as well as adults come together with previous family experiences and expectations that derive from their families of origin, previous marriage families, and single-parent households. They all know how the spaghetti should be cooked and where the dog should sleep.

Most daily routines involve actions that have become primarily unconscious. Then suddenly someone is watching too much TV, setting the table incorrectly, or not observing the anticipated holiday rituals. Differences of opinion about what is right and what is wrong arise frequently, accompanied by considerable emotion. Family members need to share their expectations, move past arguments over right and wrong to view behaviors as simply *different*, and negotiate what they would like to have happen in this new family unit. Considerable therapeutic time may be needed to help stepfamily members become tolerant and flexible so that they can accomplish this task.

Family meetings can be productive in this regard. At times the family needs coaching during the therapy sessions regarding ways of handling this type of family communication. One couple reported that their children did not care for such *councils*, so whenever a meeting was scheduled to deal with specific difficulties, the children made certain their behavior changed in a positive direction. Thus, the family discussion became unnecessary! Having two containers, one for notes mentioning difficulties and the other for notes calling attention to events or behaviors that have been appreciated, is another way to acknowledge positive as well as troublesome elements. Families that cannot manage full family councils can often alter a negative household ambience by utilizing the *appreciation* container.

Parent-Child Relationships

In a stepfamily, unlike a first-marriage family, there are parent-child relationships that have preceded the new couple relationship. This reversal of the familiar family pattern tends to create significant difficulties for stepfamilies, difficulties that often last for a number of years. Instead of the adults becoming parents after they have developed a strong bond as a couple, the parent-child bonds are the prior attachments.

Unfortunately, many parents who remarry do not realize the importance to the entire family of giving priority to the couple relationship, so that the two adults can work together as a team (as is also the case in functional first-marriage families) to pay attention to the needs of the children in the family and do what they can to meet the needs of everyone in the household.

At times remarried parents seem to need a therapist's *permission* to form a strong adult attachment, often because they fear that valuing this adult-adult relationship is somehow a betrayal of their parent-child relationships. Understanding the importance to the children that the parental relationship be a good couple relationship can serve to decrease the remarried parent's guilt.

Because they have witnessed the dissolution of their parents' marriage, children in stepfamilies often fear that the new couple will break up. They are usually better able to form new attachments and to *settle down* if they perceive that there is a warm and solid relationship between the two adults. In addition, the model of a good couple relationship will benefit the children when they mature and form their own couple relationships.

The stages of stepfamily integration have been studied extensively by Patricia Papernow (1993), and it seems clear that the adults in stepfamilies go through predictable stages in developing new bonding patterns. We believe that it is important to the development of the new couple relationship to work therapeutically with the adults alone without including the children in the sessions, until the couple has reached the stage in which parent and stepparent are able to work together as a team. In a study of therapeutic interventions, Elion (1990) found that the stepfamily couples who participated considered help in consolidating their relationship as one of the most helpful interventions in their therapeutic experience.

With stepfamilies, however, forming a close couple relationship does not ensure good stepfamily functioning (Crosbie-Burnett 1984). Parent-child relationships need to be maintained, and the new steprelationships need to be developed. Encouraging dyadic interactions is an important intervention, since children feel the loss of exclusive time with their parent who has remarried. New relationships benefit from the nourishment of *one-on-one* encounters, and making plans for these special interactive occasions helps children anticipate and look forward to their turn. Planned occasions for larger groups help members of the family feel more included; thus they experience more overall family satisfaction.

Absent Biological Parents

In stepfamilies there is a biological parent elsewhere in actuality or in memory, a parent who is not part of the immediate household unit but who exerts considerable influence on what happens there, even after a death. Although many adults would prefer that these other parents no longer existed, there is considerable research that suggests advantages to the children in having contact with both of their original parents (Kelly 1988). It is often those children who are cut off from a parent who exhibit the most psychological disturbance and who refuse to accept a stepparent.

Since there are adults who remain important to the children, if a *parenting coalition* (Hetherington et al. 1989; Visher and Visher 1989) can be formed between the adults in the children's two households, things go better for all the individuals involved. Children are less torn by conflicting loyalties when their parents and stepparents can permit them to enjoy both households and do not expect them to be messengers or pawns in an ongoing adult struggle. Also, it is helpful for the adults to have time for themselves when the children are at the other household.

It is generally unrealistic to expect that this cooperative arrangement can be worked out in the first months after a remarriage. During the early months, when the stepfamily couple has not yet had enough time to feel comfortable working across the households, therapists can assist in helping the couple to plan ways to deal with family events such as graduations, weddings, and special holidays, which fortunately are time constrained. Later on, when it is clear that there is a psychological as well as a physical separation between the former spouses, a cooperative arrangement can often be negotiated. Nodal family events (i.e., those of great significance such as weddings and birthdays) frequently take place at times when stepfamilies are more receptive to making changes in interhousehold relationship patterns.

Therapists are powerful persons whose recommendations carry considerable weight. They can be very helpful in educating parents about the importance of developing a parenting coalition and about the techniques for accomplishing this shift. Often an ex-spouse is responding with anger to mask the pain of loss or fear of further losses. Understanding this dynamic frequently enables a parent and stepparent to reach out and try to break a vicious cycle of retaliation and reaction.

Migration Between Family Cultures

Often children are members of two households as they go back and forth between their parents, probably experiencing two quite different family cultures. As one teenager poignantly remarked after his father's remarriage, "I feel as though I've been plucked out of one family and dropped into a completely new one."

As a rule the adults are eager for a sense of *family* to develop quickly, and they tend to push for relationships to form between individuals who feel like strangers living together under the same roof. Therapists can help the adults relax and allow relationships to develop at a comfortable pace. The adults can be *fair* to the children, even though stepparents and stepchildren may not have developed a positive bond yet.

Parents disappear from their children's lives for many reasons. While at times this happens because of lack of interest, at other times it is for the opposite reason: it is very painful for the nonresidential parent to be separated from his or her children and to feel powerless with respect to their lives. At times therapists are in a position to advise parents who are contemplating withdrawing from contacts with their children that continuing to be in touch can mean a great deal to the children and also to the parent as time alleviates the pain of the separations. Children whose parents have disappeared generally feel that there is something lacking in them. If they had been loveable, their parent would have remained in their lives. The therapeutic task becomes one of helping restore the child's self-esteem and helping him or her accept that the parent's abandonment was not due to some personal failure of the child's but to the adult's emotions and decisions.

Even when there is considerable difference in lifestyles, values, and behavior patterns between households, children can usually adapt readily if the adults make their expectations clear and not criticize the other household. Being part of two households can even be beneficial. Exposed to more diversity, children may experience more ways of thinking and doing things. This can provide them with more choices as they mature and develop their own ideas.

Social and Institutional Support

Stepfamilies lack social and institutional supports. For example, there is little or no legal relationship between stepparents and stepchildren. Stepparents cannot give permission for medical treatment. Conciliation court staffs may exclude the stepparent from negotiation sessions, even when the stepchild will be part of his or her household. If there is another divorce, the stepparent-stepchild bond may be abruptly broken with no option for continued contact or an opportunity to mourn the loss. Schools often fail to acknowledge the existence of different types of families, and a number of churches do not make stepfamilies feel accepted or supported.

In our experience this lack of cultural acceptance is an important factor in deep feelings of being *second class* that many stepfamily members experience. No wonder they are reluctant to acknowledge their family type, even in therapy. Validating the worth of this family form is certainly a major key to therapeutic success.

Contextual Considerations

Because of the characteristics just discussed, living in a stepfamily differs contextually from living in a nuclear family. Understandably, the psychological response generally is more complex and more acute than in first-marriage families. The stepfamily context also impacts the therapeutic process in the following ways.

Supra-Family System

There is a *supra-family system* (Sager et al. 1983) that can involve several households that are connected through the children. This system includes more than two parents, so that therapists are required to broaden their concept of family far beyond the ideal of a tightly knit, nuclear family household.

Family Cohesiveness

Prior to satisfactory integration there is little family loyalty or cohesiveness (Chollak 1985). In fact, research reveals that there is often little agreement between household members even regarding who is part of the family (Pasley 1987). Because of the lack of family loyalty, therapists need to see the two adults without the children until the couple has reached the stage when the adults have formed a team that can work together reasonably well. Before this has occurred, biological groups tend to become adversarial, and the therapy process can become divisive rather than helpful. Therapy sessions are often the first time the couple has worked on stepfamily challenges alone. If indicated, the children can be seen apart from the adults.

Steprelationships

Even when there is a close working relationship between the adult couple, it does not necessarily lead to good steprelationships. Such relationships will need to be created separately. When the individuals in a remarriage family come together, they share no history and there are preexisting coalitions. The therapist's task may be to help the family change previous alliances so that individuals go from feeling disconnected to feeling they belong to the family unit.

Power Issues

There are complex power issues in stepfamilies. A new stepparent initially does not have a relationship with his or her stepchildren and is therefore not in a position of authority as far as the children are concerned. The biological parent needs to take the leading role with the children, in so far as disciplinary issues are concerned, until a relationship between stepparent and stepchildren has been established. If the biological parent is to be away, he or she needs to make a clear delegation of power to the stepparent in the presence of the children, and both adults need to support each other.

Many stepparents are expected by their spouse and also by themselves to become an instant parent. A more acceptable alternative for both the stepparent and the stepchildren may be becoming an *adult friend* or a *parental helper*. What usually works best is to develop whatever is most satisfying for those concerned (Crosbie-Burnett 1984). When only the stepparent will be present, the biological parent needs to delegate his or her authority to the stepparent in front of the child or children.

Attempting to put a stepparent *in charge* of the family before a relationship has developed is a major pitfall for many stepfamilies. It is helpful to encourage the parent who has remarried to remain in an executive role with his or her children, or to reclaim it if it has been relinquished. When this is an area of concern, we find that the adults may be willing to change if they have answered "no" to the question "Is the present approach working in your household?"

Therapeutic Interventions

There are a number of interventions that are particularly valuable with stepfamilies or individuals in stepfamilies (Visher and Visher 1988). In our experience they are useful treatment considerations whatever may be the basic theoretical approach of the therapist. In this section we comment briefly on all of them and discuss important ones we have not spoken about previously.

Enhance self-esteem. It is important for therapists to accept and validate stepfamily situations. Increased self-esteem allows individuals to cope better with challenges.

Assist with recognition and acceptances of losses. Stepfamilies are families born of loss, and therapists often need to help with the mourning process. Adults may need individual help to be able to let go of their disappointment about the failure of their previous marriage or their feelings of loss about giving up the dream of a so-called ideal first marriage.

Children often express their depression and anger in the form of withdrawal, poor school grades and conduct, poor social relationships, and acting-out behavior (Bray and Kelly 1998). Therapists can help them by

- Validating and normalizing their feelings
- Helping them to stay out of the middle of hostile parents
- Encouraging them to express feelings in words rather than in behavior
- Giving them a sense of control in their lives, and helping them to understand that there are things that they cannot control (e.g., they can control what they do in school; they cannot control whether their parents divorce or remarry)

Clarify realistic expectations. Three important, unrealistic expectations hinder rather than facilitate the integration process in stepfamilies: 1) expecting that stepfamilies are the same as first-marriage families; 2) expecting relatively quick adjustment and instant love; and 3) being unaware of the length of time the integration process usually takes (Papernow 1993).

Make educational comments. Familiarity with stepfamily issues helps therapists make valuable educational comments. Three basic areas that have already been discussed are of primary concern: 1) the need for a strong couple relationship; 2) the acceptability of many different roles for stepparents; and 3) the process of developing successful disciplinary roles in stepfamilies. Stepcouples in treatment have considered education to be one of the most valuable aspects of their therapy, according to research by Elion (1990) and Visher et al. (1997).

One other important aspect of stepfamily life is the need of many divorced parents to share children with another household. This may be difficult during the single-parent-household phase, and it tends to become even more problematic after a remarriage. Couples need help in understanding the value for their children, and also for themselves, of working on forming a *parenting coalition*, a working relationship between the adults in the children's two households (Visher and Visher 1989). When cooperation rather than competition can be negotiated, children have fewer loyalty conflicts and do not get *caught* in *the middle*. Also, adults can share the responsibility of parenting.

Reduce a sense of helplessness. Stepfamily adults report this intervention to be very helpful to them. As a rule, individuals in stepfamilies have less control than those in first-marriage families because there is a parent of the children in another household who can and often does exert considerable influence on the stepfamily household. Stepfamily adults may relinquish more control than is necessary, and they need to find ways to achieve greater mastery over their situation. The following case illustrates the beginning of such a process:

> Delia and Jim had been married for 3 years. Jim's two sons lived with the couple most of the time, but spent several weekends a month with their mother, Gladys. When Gladys came to pick up her sons, she frequently would walk into Delia and Jim's house, use the telephone or the bathroom, and rummage in the refrigerator for a cold drink. Delia and Jim were extremely upset with this behavior but felt helpless to handle the situation. Gladys had been unwilling or unable to respect their request to change her behavior. In therapy Delia and Jim were able to solve the problem in a way that would place them back in charge of their own household, so they felt more comfortable.
>
> They decided to have the boys ready to leave when their mother came, with their knapsack by the door containing what the boys would need for the weekend. The couple watched to see when Gladys arrived, and when she did they immediately called the boys, who would run to the door to greet their mother. There was little opportunity for Gladys to behave as she had previously. If she requested a drink or asked to use the telephone, Delia and Jim had prepared a ready response for her (they would say they were on their way out, or that the boys would like to stop somewhere and have a drink too). As other situations arose that left the couple feeling powerless, they used their success with this model to work out ways they could have more control. Their increased sense of mastery resulted in their being able to relax and enjoy their life together rather than dreading the days when Gladys would appear.

Use genograms. Drawing a genogram of a stepfamily's supra-family system may require more time and paper than a similar recording of a nuclear family. It is worth it. We use the standard system of drawing genograms discussed by McGoldrick and Gerson (1985), with one addition of our own: a method of indicating on the genogram where the children in the stepfamily reside, and for what amounts of time. This information is important when assessing stepfamily situations (Visher and Visher 1988). In addition, the therapist becomes less confused about all the people involved, and stepfamily members often see much more clearly why they feel overwhelmed or upset by feelings about the apparent complexity of their stepfamily life. One family discovered when their genogram was completed that the anxious and depressed 12-year-old member of the family was expected to relate to 70–75 different individuals. Talking about the impossibility of this task helped everyone to understand and to move the therapy forward.

The words of one remarried mother give a clear expression of the feelings of many stepfamily adults:

> The genogram is extremely helpful. I think anyone who is even remotely thinking of becoming part of a stepfamily should go through the genogram experience, and I think it would provide a lot of information. It would show you where you're at, and the whole scheme. That part of the therapy was what was really, really helpful in seeing the dynamics of the whole thing. It puts it into a nutshell and makes it more real and precise. It gives you the big picture.

Fill in past histories. It has been said that a stepfamily is a family with no history. In the process of becoming closer to each other, the adults have shared their past histories with each other. The children and adults have usually not done so. One therapist helped a teenage girl and her father to share with each other, and also with the other family members who were present at the session, what the 3 years of separation had been like for both of them when she went to live with relatives following her mother's death.

Another type of sharing occurred when three stepchildren believed they were responsible for their stepmother's periodic depression. She reassured them by saying, "It has nothing to do with you. I was depressed long before I met your dad." The stepparent and stepchildren did not know each other very well, and the children's relief was evident when they learned about her previous experiences with depression. Helping stepfamily members communicate with each other about their likes and dislikes, their interests, and the things that have happened to them in their previous family experiences can lead everyone in the family to feel more familiar and comfortable with one another.

Relate past family experiences to present situations. When stepfamilies get *stuck* after learning what to expect and having the opportunity to understand the dynamics of their family, an exploration of individual experiences in former family situations becomes important. Relating these to present difficulties, where applicable, can help clarify the emotions that are creating problems in the present.

For adults, the relationships they perceived in their family of origin can be of primary importance. For example, remarried parents who remember the principal emotional bonding when they were growing up as being between parent(s) and child(ren) and not between their mother and father frequently find it difficult to form a bond with their new partner. To them the parent-child relationship is primary. Two other examples illustrate different types of dilemmas:

> Debbie, a stepmother with one son from a previous marriage, remained conflicted over her role with a stepdaughter. In therapy the couple worked hard to alter many unhappy situations, but this part of Debbie's life did not change despite numerous shifts made by her husband. In an individual therapy session, Debbie sobbed, "Not knowing what my role with my stepdaughter is gets worse the more I like her."
>
> Debbie had an older sister who she believed had always been her parents' favorite child. Debbie's husband also spoke about the parents' unfair treatment of Debbie in comparison to their treatment of Debbie's sister. Exploration of this aspect of her life touched her deeply, and as she shed many tears she came to recognize that she was afraid that she might grow to love her stepdaughter as much as she loved her son. She had not experienced a parent who loved more than one child, and she had unconsciously felt that she could not love her stepdaughter *and* her son.
>
> Children in stepfamilies also have experienced previous family constellations. In Rhonda's case, her father had disappeared from her life. Her mother Louise had been remarried for 2 years and things had been going well. Then suddenly, when Louise, her husband David, and 14-year-old Rhonda were going out for dinner, Rhonda became hysterical. She threw things around her room, broke glass on the floor, and cried unceasingly. She refused to talk to the adults. David sat quietly in Rhonda's room, and his stepdaughter began to regain her composure. Louise joined them and they were able to talk together.
>
> Rhonda cried and said that she wanted to be so awful that David would go away and leave her as her father had done. She wanted to get it over with. As she began to understand that David was not going to leave, even if she acted badly, she slowly developed trust that the two adults were going to remain together.

Encourage dyadic relationships. Remarried parents feel pulled in many directions by the needs of their new spouse and those of their children. One way to help balance these needs is by planning one-on-one times for parent and children. Usually it is not possible for everyone to have all the time and attention they might wish, but even so, knowing there will be exclusive time at a definite point in the future can be very helpful. Stepparents and stepchildren also need one-on-one times together, to build their relationships. Valuable information and helpful steps that can assist stepfamily adults with building dyadic relationships are outlined in many publications, such as *Stepfamilies Stepping Ahead* and *Stepping Together: Creating Strong Stepfamilies*, published by the Stepfamily Association of America.

Make specific suggestions. There can be considerable anxiety in stepfamilies. Because anxiety reduces the ability to find solutions to problematic situations, specific suggestions can often be helpful. In one family, for example, accepting the therapist's suggestion to ask a friend of the younger child to come with him when he was spending weekends with his father, stepmother, and stepsiblings almost eliminated the tensions that had existed previously between the younger child and his older stepbrothers during the weekend.

Suggest helpful rituals. A sense of familiarity and knowing what to expect make up one element of feeling connected to a group. Knowing you will be the one to choose the game for the family to play on Friday nights, going out for pizza once a week, looking forward to familiar birthday celebrations—all help stepfamily members feel more relaxed and connected to one another.

Separate feelings and behavior. Members of stepfamilies are often supersensitive to, maybe even superconscious about, the feelings they have for each other. They see that stepparents and parents feel differently about his, her, and their children, and that children care more about parents than about stepparents. However, this does not necessarily mean that family members will be treated badly—people can control what they do about their feelings. The adults can be fair to all the children, and children can be civil to both adults. Sometimes adults feel it is hypocritical to behave in a way that does not mirror inner feelings. Perhaps they need to be reminded that people don't reveal the *whole truth* all of the time; it may even be a prerequisite to getting along with others to be less than open about many emotions. And sometimes when parents act as though they like a stepchild that they have trouble feeling affection for, they work wonders in improving a tentative relationship.

Teach negotiation. Because children as well as adults come into a stepfamily with expectations and ways of behaving that have developed in former families, much needs to be worked out. Modeling the negotiation process and helping stepfamily members with this important skill can be crucial to helping them acquire the ability to live together. At times, deep-seated intrapsychic blocks may make negotiation difficult for one or more of the individuals and will need to be the focus of therapy.

Restructure and reframe. This can be especially important in stepfamilies, in which there is an acute awareness of interpersonal interchanges and actions. Sixteen-year-old Clara began to see that her stepfather was caring rather than domineering as she believed, after the therapist reinterpreted his wanting her to be home by 10 P.M. on school nights as his wish for her to be safe and healthy and to have a good school experience.

Use accurate language. Referring to a stepparent as a parent or expecting a child to call a stepparent by a relationship term suggests that the therapist does not understand the nuances of stepfamily living. Following the lead of family members is a safe rule most of the time, although sometimes using an accurate, but unfamiliar, descriptive term not usually used by the family may be therapeutically important in beginning to deal with unrealistic expectations.

Reduce therapeutic tensions. As a rule, stepfamilies enter therapy with considerable turmoil in their lives. They do not need to be energized by therapeutic comments that jostle them emotionally and produce strong reactions. Usually emotions need to be diminished rather than heightened. It may help to have the interchanges go through the therapist rather than directly to family members. One therapist also found that using a tape recorder helped to keep chaotic families under control during the sessions.

Conclusion

Stepfamilies coming for therapy may appear chaotic and experience difficulties that suggest they are highly dysfunctional or even pathological. However, these families in transition probably just have adjustment problems, so stepfamily changes become the first focus of therapeutic attention. Subsequently, and at times concomitantly, deeper intrapsychic aspects may need attention. Remarried families often make changes relatively quickly because their difficulties are transitional in nature and they are strongly motivated to find solutions for the stressful events and feelings that can occur during the long process of integration.

Following positive therapeutic outcomes, many individuals in stepfamilies speak appreciatively of all they have learned in therapy that helps their households function more satisfactorily. In addition, they claim they have developed greater understanding of others, are more flexible in meeting day-to-day situations, and have learned to not take interpersonal relationships for granted. These positive outcomes also can make working with stepfamily members stimulating and worthwhile for the therapist.

Although current stepfamily research has been helpful to therapists, clinicians could benefit greatly from certain types of studies that have not yet been undertaken. While there has been a dramatic increase in stepfamily research in the last 7 or 8 years, most of this research has been quantitative in nature and has focused on stepfamilies from a problem-oriented perspective. Much of this research has been based on the assumption that stepfamilies are, by definition, pathological because they differ in a number of important ways from the idealized nuclear family. More qualitative research is needed, as well as more research studies that compare stepfamilies with each other (Coleman and Ganong 1990a) with the goal of determining the characteristics of successful functioning in stepfamilies.

Another important area of research concerns custody issues. To date, research projects concerned with custody fail to distinguish single-parent households from stephouseholds; thus, there is no way to determine whether the same or different custody arrangements are beneficial after a divorce and after a remarriage. Other research focused on the effects of cultural pressures on the success of remarriage is also important. There are different emotional stages that occur in remarriage families as they move toward integration (Papernow 1993). What is seen during the first 1–2 years of a remarriage can look quite different 5 years later. These changes are clear indications that more longitudinal research is necessary.

The information provided by the types of research just suggested would be most useful to therapists and counsellors, who are often unable to respond helpfully to questions from the families they are trying to assist, who need more normative information than is now available. It is fortunate for therapists and for stepfamilies that the stepfamily research of the 1990s appears to be taking these directions.

Chapters on Related Topics

The following chapter describes concepts related to remarried families:

- Chapter 23, "The Divorcing Family: Characteristics and Interventions"

25

Marital Enrichment in Clinical Practice

Paul Giblin, Ph.D.
Mark P. Combs, Ph.D.

Introduction

Recently deceased scholar, educator, and clinician David Mace wrote and spoke tirelessly in his final decade of the value of marriage enrichment, particularly with couples beginning marriage. Continuing in the spirit of Mace's work, the authors of this chapter seek to provide resources for therapists who want to add enrichment offerings to their practice. Areas covered by this chapter include: definition and background; the value of enrichment; an overview of programs for which either national training or package materials are available; implementation considerations; cautions and limitations; and finally, outcome research.

Definition and Background

A great deal of professional, popular, and media attention is currently focused on marital dissolution and other family-related crises. Indeed, the most popular academy award movie for the new millenium was about a highly dysfunctional couple captured in the film *American Beauty*. Concurrent with these warnings and troubled portrayals is an emphasis on addressing and fixing the problems that are apparently threatening the venerable institution of marriage.

This upsurge of attention on marital issues has produced popular gender dichotomizations (Fisher 1992; Gray 1989); scientifically based accounts of how to fight for one's marriage (Markman et al. 1994); identifying indices that predict divorce (Gottman 1994b; Gottman and Levenson 1981); and studies of the corrosive societal impact of divorce on health (Burman and Margolin 1992) and on children (Hetherington and Clingempeel 1992). As the national media continue to run banner headlines on troubled families and wayward, violent youths, interest in clinical marital enrichment and other psychoeducational approaches aimed at minimizing conflicts and strengthening marriages has reemerged.

Marriage enrichment, by definition, is psychoeducational group work, with relatively well-functioning couples in structured contexts, to improve marital functioning and satisfaction. Enrichment focuses on the present and future more than the past and attends especially to strengths and resources of the couple. It emphasizes affective, behavioral, and experiential learning in addition to cognitive learning and information transfer. The similarities and differences between marital enrichment, therapy, and education—"three ways to help married couples" as Mace (1987) would say—are well described by Hoopes et al. (1984) and Mace (1987).

Various assumptions guide enrichment work. For example, it is thought that many couples function at a fraction of their potential and can benefit from an "energizer," conscious-raising, or a "check-up" on a regular basis. At the same time enrichment does *not* espouse a model of marriage that consists only of peak experiences and is free of dormancy or "plateau times." Marriage is a dynamic process, and while change is a given, growth needs to be intentional. Early in their marriage, couples can benefit from preventive, skill-building work, especially with regard to communication, conflict resolution, and anger management. For couples beyond the newlywed stage, the giving and receiving of support and altruistic acts enhances marital growth. In particular, intercouple observational learning can help to normalize struggle and overcome emotional isolation in the couple. Given high divorce rates, increased expectations for marriage, lack of consensus for marital and gender roles, equity issues regarding division of childcare and housework as women increasingly join the labor force, and economic and cultural pressures of careerism and materialism, marital enrichment offers a timely, cost-efficient, highly relevant intervention strategy.

Marital enrichment is a relatively young movement begun in the 1960s. Simultaneously in 1962, David and Vera Mace, Father Gabriel Calvo, and Leon and Antoinette Smith began offering marriage enrichment programs primarily through religious institutions—Quaker, Catholic, and Methodist, respectively. In the 1970s programs emerged from university settings. Sherod Miller and associates developed the popular and subsequently heavily researched Couple Communication Program (CCP) for premarital and marital couples. Bernard Guerney and associates at Penn State University developed marital and family enrichment programs, Relationship Enhancement (RE) and Parent Adolescent Relationship Development (PARD), again with extensive research following. Programs begun in the 1980s include Training in Marriage Enrichment (TIME) (Don Dinkmeyer and Jon Carlson); Listening and Loving (Gleam Powell); Practical Application of Intimate Relationship Skills (PAIRS) (Lori Gordon); Prevention and Relationship Enhancement Program (PREP) (Howard Markman); and Growth in Marriage for Newlyweds (Phyllis Michael). Programs begun in the 1990s include Growing Together (Preston and Jeannie Dyer) and Relationship Enrichment Facilitating Open Communication, Understanding, and Study (REFOCUS) (Barbara Markey). Most of the pioneers behind these programs, as well as many program designers and current facilitators, gathered in Atlanta in 1988 for the First International Marriage Enrichment Conference. The conference remembered the beginnings of marriage enrichment, celebrated its achievements, and strategized for the future in an informative, collective manner.

A number of other marital enrichment programs exist besides those listed above. However, the focus of this chapter is on those programs accessible to a clinician by virtue of their relatively easy replication. There are a dozen or more well developed, researched programs that currently exist as reasonably priced "packages" (i.e., providing a detailed leader manual, participant books, and audio tapes), and for which there is often leadership training on a regular basis across the country. Table 25–1 compares these programs across several dimensions and provides information for further contact. The Association for Couples in Marriage Enrichment (ACME), founded by David and Vera Mace, has become the major clearinghouse for marital enrichment programs, materials, and leadership training.

Focus of Enrichment

What is the focus of enrichment, and how do programs seek to "enrich" marriages? David Mace contrasts two approaches to enriching relationships: *inductive*, drawing from resources from within a couple that are currently untapped, and *deductive*, which seeks to add something to the relationship (Mace 1979). We propose instead to contrast the process and content dimensions of enrichment. At the *process* level, enrichment generally targets skill building, specifically communication, conflict resolution, and decision making; in addition, group development and a sense of community among

Table 25–1. Marital enrichment programs in brief

Program	Group	Program length	Type of marriage	Degree of structure	Theory	Author/address
Association for Couples in Marriage Enrichment (ACME)	4–8 couples	Weekend and support groups	Healthy	Low	Systems Social learning	D. and V. Mace ACME P.O. 10596 Winston-Salem, NC 27108 Tel: (800) 634-8325 www.bettermarriages.org
Couple Communication Program (CCP)	4–8 couples	4×3 hours	Healthy or troubled	High	Systems Communication	S. Miller 30752 Southview Drive Suite 200 Evergreen, CO 80439 Tel: (800) 328-5099 www.couplecommunication.com
Growing Together	4–8 couples	8×2.5 hours or weekend	Healthy	High	Systems Communication	P. and G. Dyer PREPARE/ENRICH Minneapolis, MN Tel: (800) 331-1661
Growth in Marriage for Newlyweds	4–8 couples	6×2.5 hours	Healthy	High	Systems	P. Michael ACME P.O. 10596 Winston-Salem, NC 27108 Tel: (800) 634-8325 www.bettermarriages.org

Table 25–1. Marital enrichment programs in brief *(continued)*

Program	Group	Program length	Type of marriage	Degree of structure	Theory	Author/address
Listening and Loving	12–18 women or couples	5 × 2.75 hours	Healthy	High	Rogerian Adlerian Systems	G. Powell 112 Stafford Drive Athens, GA Tel: (404) 546-6014
Marriage Encounter (ME)	18–20 couples	Weekend and follow-up	Healthy	High	Communication Religious	Marriage Encounter 47104 Jamerson Orlando, FL 32806
Practical Application of Intimate Relationship Skills (PAIRS)	30–36 individual couples	16 × 3 hours and 4 weekends	Healthy or troubled	High	Systems Psychodynamic Social learning	L. Gordon 9400 North Central Expressway Suite 310 Dallas, TX 75231 Tel: (888) PAIRS-4U www.pairsfoundation.com
Prevention and Relationship Enhancement Program (PREP)	3–5 couples	6 × 1.5/2 hours or weekend	Healthy or troubled	High	Systems Communication	H. Markman P. O. Box 102530 Denver, CO 80250 Tel: (800) 366-0166 www.prepinc.com
Relationship Enrichment Facilitating Open Communication, Understanding and Study (REFOCUS)	4–8 couples	5 × 2.5 hours or weekend	Healthy	High	Systems Religious	B. Markey Omaha, NE 68104 Tel: (401) 551-9003

Table 25–1. Marital enrichment programs in brief *(continued)*

Program	Group	Program length	Type of marriage	Degree of structure	Theory	Author/address
Recovery of Hope	3–12 couples	1×3 hours and follow-up	Troubled	Low	Religious	S. Wilke Wichita, KS Tel: (800) 327–2590
Relationship Enhancement (RE)	Flexible	12×1.5 hours	Healthy or troubled	High	Psychodynamic Systems Communication	B. Guerney Jr. 17 West State Street Doylestown, PA 18901 Tel: (814) 237–4805 www.relationshipenhancement.com
Structured Enrichment (SE)	1 or more couples	6×1 hour	Healthy or troubled	High	Systems Eclectic	L. L'Abate Georgia State University Atlanta, GA 30345
Training in Marriage Enrichment (TIME)	8–10 couples	10×2 hours or weekend	Healthy	High	Adlerian Social psychology Educational psychology	D. Dinkmeyer and J. Carlson American Guidance Tel: (800) 247–5053

couples is an important process dynamic. At the *content* level, enrichment facilitates the sharing by couples of values, visions, expectations, and hopes for each other and for the relationship. Also at a content level, couples seek insight into differences such as personality, gender, and family of origin; they also examine the developmental nature of marriage, particularly with a preventative eye to understanding developmental life stages, tasks, and issues. Below, we examine in more detail the process dimensions.

Community

Couples are provided with the opportunity to become part of something bigger than themselves in joining a group of 6–12 couples. A couple entering the group observes other couples interacting, identifies with them, and learns that they are not alone in their struggles. They experience themselves as known, belonging, supported, and challenged. In commitment to the group they experience the interdependence of need and giftedness. The couple has something to offer, as well being a recipient of the support and gifts of others. Enrichment groups are countercultural in that they emphasize interdependence versus independence, cooperation versus competition, responsibility versus blaming and scapegoating, shared vulnerability versus persona of strength, and commitment versus no liability. In the group context, intermarital "taboos" of privatism and naturalism are challenged (Mace 1976). That is, groups help overcome the beliefs that marriage is private and not to be shared with others, that success in marriage is a given for "normal" adults, and that difficulties or the need to work at the relationship implies inadequacies of the individuals involved.

Community is about caring for and being cared for, knowing and being known, altruism and being vulnerable. All of these dimensions contribute to a healthy sense of individual and marital identity. Research clearly indicates that social support is an important asset in moderating stress. Given mobile modern America, many couples lack the social supports of both extended family and/or neighborhood, a lack that enrichment groups may begin to fill. Marital programs that by design are long term and/or have a follow-up component emphasize more of this dimension of community. Such programs include Marriage Encounter, ACME, and REFOCUS; they all emphasize the communal dimensions through support groups. However, most other program designs could be extended to include more of the communal dimension. Some enrichment program groups have met weekly or monthly for 15–20 years—ACME and Marriage Encounter groups in particular—and are clearly meeting an important need in couples' lives.

Values and Strengths

Values and strengths are some of the raw materials of enrichment. Enrichment is aimed at increasing couples' awareness of the strengths of their marriage, as well as each individual's good feelings, positive regard, respect for each other. Many couples lose sight of the hopes and vision with which they began, because the marriage bends to demands of family and work but lacks inner direction or purpose. While disillusionment and the moderation of unrealistic expectations are natural to healthy marital development, for many other couples what is unhealthy is the failure to make their relationship a priority, or the tendency to "coast" and exchange very few positive behaviors (Margolin 1981).

Enrichment programs provide the opportunity to rekindle strengths in a marriage. In the PREP design, Markman addresses the importance of the "spiritual values" of honor, respect, forgiveness, and intimacy. The Maces and the Dyers in the ACME designs focus on increasing the attitude and behavior of thankfulness. An exercise of the ACME approach asks couples to write about and then share 3–5 things they like about the relationship and for which they are thankful. Dinkmeyer and Carlson in TIME ask couples to ritualize "encouragement meetings or days," much as in Stuart's "Caring Days," aimed at learning about each other and exchanging increased caring, (i.e., "pleasers"). Bassoff (1985) developed a similar enrichment intervention called the "Memory Board," which is simply a bulletin board on which couples post memorabilia, ticket stubs from the theater, cards, playbills, and so forth. The board serves to keep positive dimensions of the marriage in mind and counters the tendency of couples in conflict to distort the past and to forget the good. Enrichment then provides a time and structure for couples to reevaluate their relationship and to set directions and priorities for the marriage.

Communication Skills Building

Communication skills building is the entire focus of some programs and the subject of at least one session in other programs. The specific skills taught therefore vary across programs. Speaking skills taught typically include increasing self-awareness (see especially Miller's CCP framework, the "Awareness Wheel"), making "I" statements, sharing feelings, and being specific. Listening skills taught typically include active listening, hearing both content and feelings, seeking clarification, conveying acceptance and positive feelings as well as regard and empathy, distinguishing between acceptance versus agreement, and giving feedback. Markman et al. (1994) instruct couples on how to make the impact of communication match intent; about the interference of content, emotion, and family-of-origin "filters"; and about the need for "leveling and editing." Communication styles and nonverbal communication are addressed in several programs.

Communication principles and skills are generally taught with short lectures, followed by couple practice and feedback from the facilitator and/or group. All programs emphasize the volunteer dimension of participation. Skills are taught in hierarchical fashion; that is, communication before conflict resolution, with more focus on skills than on content. Couples are encouraged to practice well the skills before applying them to difficult relational issues. Some programs (e.g., PREP, Marriage Encounter) do not include couple practice in the group context and instead offer the individual couple feedback from a professional (the practice in PREP) or utilize written dialogue between partners. For example, Marriage Encounter uses the "ten and ten," in which partners reflect and then write on a theme and share the results with each other. The reader is referred to L'Abate (1992) for an extensive description of writing interventions for both marriage enrichment and therapy. Gottman et al. (1976a) and Satir (1972) are used extensively as communication resources.

In his seminal research on marriage, Gottman (1999) notes that one goal of communication skills training is not to prevent couples from fighting but to maintain communication. Specifically, both members of the couple should be helped to

1. Process issues following an argument
2. Express themselves in a collaborative fashion without excessive levels of defensiveness or criticisms
3. Improve their ability to make amends for negative feelings expressed during the argument

What is crucial is the establishment of a continual dialogue through thick and thin; that is, through the acute and chronic issues that persist in all marriages. The Gottman Institute (founded by Gottman and his wife Julie) continues to use the principles listed above to help strengthen marriages.

Problem-Solving Skills

Problem-solving skills are another staple of marital enrichment. Skill building focuses on the discrete steps of 1) problem identification and discussion and 2) problem and solution exploration versus problem solving. Generally, step one, *skills building*, helps couples to show mutual respect, pinpoint the real issue in arguments, explore feelings and thoughts on issues and problems, and identify areas of agreement. Step two, *problem and solution exploration*, helps couples learn to maintain a present and future focus, brainstorm alternatives, identify areas of agreement, mutually participate in decision making, seek mutual gains, decide on courses of action, and then evaluate decisions.

Markman (1991) noted that in his experience of training couples in PREP, 80% of the time couples solve their problems with thorough work at step one—sharing feelings and perceptions, conveying respect, feeling listened to and validated—and never need to move on to problem solution steps. Markman's observation appears well supported by research on marital conflict.

Notarius and Pellegrini (1987) indicate that in distressed couples, *wives* report many more negative behaviors than husbands (i.e., criticism, rejection, or attack), view their husbands' behaviors more negatively, and attribute their husband's lack of responsiveness to unemotionality. *Husbands* appear to behave in ways that reflect insensitivity to their wives' behavior, inaccurately decode or receive wives' nonverbal behavior (but not that of other women), and attribute wives' emotionality to "irrationality." In this context, the goal of both enrichment and therapy with couples is helping partners change their attributions, realize that they both want the same things in the end (i.e., validation and affirmation), and understand the ineffectiveness of their current behavioral repertoire. "At the interactional level, husbands and wives must come to understand the impact of their behaviors on each other. A wife's negativity appears to promote her husband's withdrawal…and the husband's withdrawal promotes his wife's increased negativity.…This dysfunctional cycle without clear cause and effect must be disrupted" (Gottman 1999; Notarius and Pellegrini 1987).

In most enrichment programs, there is increased acceptance of conflict as a normal process in close relationships. Couples are helped to master the ability to manage and contain anger; to understand the notion of anger as a secondary emotion triggered by primary emotions of guilt, sadness, shame, and so forth; and to understand the need to become comfortable dealing with difficult issues. These issues are dealt with didactically (by principles and rules for managing anger and conflict) and experientially (by couple practice with feedback). Frequently used resources are Mace (1983), Fisher and Ury (1981), and Gottman (1999).

Couples that appear to benefit most from the conflict resolution dimensions of programs present with problems of a fairly high degree of severity. If the problems are deep seated, they are usually better addressed with therapy than with marital enrichment.

Expectations

Expectations, whether too low or too high, are often addressed by the cognitive methods of marital enrichment. Cognitive dimensions of a couple's health and well-being are discussed in the literature under the categories of cognitive distortions (Beck 1988), unrealistic expectations and faulty attributions (Epstein 1982; Schnarch 1998), and conscious and unconscious individual and marital contracts (Sager 1976).

Another category of expectations concerns individual and collective goals. Gary Bowen's (1991) book *Navigating the Marital Journey* uses the metaphor of the MAP program to guide couples and is based on the Value-Behavior Congruency Model. This approach is unique in that it ties together trends from corporate America and was field-tested with samples from Fortune 500 corporations. Again, this model explores marital ambition as the value inherent in the expectations of couples.

Markman's PREP program helps couples to clarify expectations about communications, ideal relationships, and relationship rules and to write about them and share them with each other. Couples are made aware of possible family-of-origin influences on expectations. A homework assignment asks couples to "talk about expectations that you may never have talked about before." Gordon, in PAIRS, also helps to explore a couple's unrealistic expectations of marriage or possible hidden agendas by addressing them in a playful and nondefensive fashion. Helpful resources include Gordon's "Laundry List of Marital Knots" (Gordon 1981) and the lists of "marital myths" by Lazarus (1985) and Lederer and Jackson (1968a). To recap, marital enrichment provides couples the opportunity to address and modify the cognitive dimensions of their relationship.

The role of expectations is variously addressed in marital enrichment programs. David Olson has produced a number of widely used instruments, such as PREPARE (for premarital couples), ENRICH (married couples), PREPARE-MC (premarital couples with children), and MATE (couples over 50). These instruments are used in programs (e.g., Growing Together and TIME) to help couples clarify realistic expectations in general, and particular expectations regarding personality issues, communication, conflict resolution, financial management, leisure activities, sexual relationship, children and parenting, family and friends, equalitarian roles, religious orientation, family or marital adaptability, and cohesion.

Dealing With Differences

An acceptance of differences—and the movement from stark judgments of right and wrong or good and bad—is the beginning of marital peacemaking and perhaps marital satisfaction as well. Enrichment programs can help couples to understand and deal with differences. This goal is achieved through design of the program, as well as from the activity of observational learning; that is, couples simply watching other couples deal with their issues and/or differences.

With some variety across programs, attention to differences focuses on one or more of the following: family-of-origin influences, sibling positions, gender, and personality. (Ethnic influences are insufficiently examined within enrichment contexts.) Gender differences interact with communication and conflict resolution styles (Beck 1988; Tannen 1990). Couples may benefit from exploring their communication styles and should be receptive to the possibility of, if not the need to, change or be flexible with styles as they seek to get more of their needs met

Personality assessment tools can provide an expanded context for understanding a couple's differences without making them defensive. Typical of these tools are the Myers-Briggs Type Indicator (Briggs-Myers and McCauley 1985) and the Lazarus's (1981) Structural Profile based on the BASIC-ID. The genogram (McGoldrick and Gerson 1985) and the Circumplex Model/Family Adaptability and Cohesion Evaluation Scales III (FACES III) (Olson et al. 1985) are used to assess family-of-origin differences. (For more discussion of the Circumplex Model and FACES III, see Chapter 13, "Family Assessment.") Another personality metric was designed by Cook et al. (1995), who identified three different types of stable couples: 1) volatile couples who try strongly to influence each other in their interactions; 2) validating couples who emphasize collaboration; and 3) couples who avoid conflict, seek acceptance, and agree to disagree.

Life-Cycle Issues

Life-cycle issues are central to some enrichment programs. Growth in Marriage for Newlyweds, Growing Together, and PREP are all designed specifically for premarital couples or couples early in marriage but also welcome other couples. Ongoing research shows that Relationship Enhancement and the Couple Communication Program, while designed for "healthy" couples, have demonstrated increased effectiveness with distressed couples, a finding cautiously put forward by Brock and Joanning (1983) and Giblin et al. (1985). PREP and PAIRS are also designed to include couples struggling with life-cycle issues.

Marital enrichment for groups that provide long-term support (e.g., ACME or Marriage Encounter), and perhaps some of the other programs, is about collective, supportive storytelling. In more homogeneous groups, couples give and receive support for similar life issues; in groups with members at more diverse life stages, couples both impart experience of and learn about stages and tasks yet to come. Although not listed in Table 25–1, various marital programs were designed for parents of college freshmen for orientation weekend (Dyer 1988), retirement couples (Johnston 1990), dual-career couples (Avis 1986), and college and graduate student couples (Amatea and Clark 1986; McLaughlin 1985). L'Abate and Weinstein (1987) and Hoopes et al. (1984) offer a broad range of marital enrichment programs addressing development for the entire life cycle.

Table 25–2 compares six marital enrichment programs according to the focus or theme of each session. Note the similarity of focus.

Implementation Considerations

Implementation considerations for marital enrichment programs are discussed in this section. Above, we identified specific programs and common themes and foci across programs; here, we address various design and implementation considerations, including size, composition of the group, structure and length of program, leadership, and learning theory.

Size

Groups range in size from one or two couples (Structured Enrichment, Relationship Enhancement) to two dozen couples (Marriage Encounter). Obviously, the more the program emphasizes skill building, couple practice, and facilitator observation and feedback, the smaller the group needs to be (4–6 couples is ideal for small-group programs). Group size influences group trust, the ability to connect with other couples, and comfort levels with self-disclosure.

Composition

The composition of group populations, as mentioned above, ranges from homogeneous to heterogeneous. Unless groups are targeted at development specific to a certain life stage, leaders should anticipate that advertising a program in the media or through a church setting will draw in couples at various life stages and from diverse economic and educational backgrounds. However, two other aspects of group composition should be noted. First, research on participants in marital enrichment indicates that couples report below the statistical norm of pretreatment levels of marital satisfaction. These reported levels are not low enough to warrant therapy, but they also do not correspond to the assumption of "healthy, well functioning cou-

Table 25–2. Six enrichment programs compared by session

Couple Communication Program (CCP)	Growing Together	Training in Marriage Enrichment (TIME)	Listening and Loving	Prevention and Relationship Enhancement Program (PREP)	REFOCUS
Tuning into self; awareness; disclosure	Relationship assessment; PREPARE/ENRICH	Accepting responsibility; marriage goals	Accepting differences; listening	Gender differences; communications skills	Marriage as process; change
Tuning into partner; listen, share meaning	Family of origin; relationship expectations	Encouragement; skills	Encouragement; empathy	Destructive communications; expectations	Twelve facets of intimacy; sexuality
Four communication styles; behaviors and intentions	Strengths; growth areas; differences	Priorities; values; power	Conflict resolution; anger	Hidden agendas; strengths; priorities	Compatibility; personality; family of origin; expectations
Shared meaning; enhancing esteem; attitudes; spirit	Communication; principles and skills	Congruent communication awareness; affect; intentions	Affection; sexuality	Problem solving; commitment	Communication; conflict resolution
	Managing anger and conflict	Listening and responding	Future plan for growth	Spiritual values; sexuality	Commitment; values; priorities
	Intimacy and sexuality	Communication skills; nonverbals			
	Financial management	Choice-making skills			
	Plan for growth	Conflict-resolution skills			
		Equal marriage goals			

ples" (Powell and Wampler 1982). Second, enrichment programs do not attract a high proportion of lower-income, less educated, ethnically diverse populations (Giblin et al. 1985).

Russell et al. (1984), following their research with Couple Communication Program and Structured Behavioral Exchange contracting (SBE), recommend matching couples and programs according to couple goals. Couples looking to increase understanding would appear to do best with CCP, whereas couples who want to solve problems would do better with a behavioral exchange program such as SBE or Relationship Enhancement. Additional research should also address the question of a match between couple, program, and perhaps setting. Screening issues will be addressed in a later section of this chapter.

Structure and Length

We discuss below the structure and length of marital enrichment. Enrichment by definition is structured intervention. However, the degree of structure varies widely. "Packaged programs" such as Couple Communication Program, Training in Marriage Enrichment, and Growing Together all provide detailed information in leader and participant manuals. Other programs, such as ACME, Relationship Enhancement, PAIRS, and PREP, require and provide leader training. Structured programs are intentionally easy to replicate; they can be adapted for use with an existing, intact group; a marital support group; an adult church group; or a neighborhood group. The drawback of "packaged" programs is the imposition of structure at the expense of initiative or creativity.

Less structured programs such as ACME and marital support groups emphasize community building, mutual responsibility for process and success, and leadership that resides in the group rather than with the "expert." A downside of the less structured groups is the loss of participants who benefit from and perhaps need structure. We conjecture that men are more often lost to less structured groups than women.

Length of programs has been related to successful outcomes, with longer and more structured programs demonstrating greater efficacy. Programs typically total 12–14 hours distributed across 4–6 sessions. Program format is typically either a weekend design or successive weekly sessions. Most packaged programs present both formats. Research indicates no significant differences in outcome by format. The number of sessions and the length of programs are listed in Table 25–1.

More time-limited programs offer the "security" of known parameters and are more compatible with couples' busy schedules. However, time may be a critical factor in developing group trust and openness, a sense of community, and social support, and this may be gained only in long-term group enrichment. A related observation by many researchers is that program effects diminish over time, although problems never return to pretreatment levels. Such research repeatedly argues for follow-up or "booster sessions" to maintain therapeutic gains.

Leadership

Programs such as Couple Communication Program, TIME, Growing Together, and Listening and Loving, among others, contain extensive written guidelines for leadership skills and tasks. Other programs such as PAIRS, PREP, Relationship Enhancement, and REFOCUS (as well as CCP) provide leadership training nationally at regular intervals. ACME provides frequent beginning and advanced-level training across the United States.

Two facilitation concerns frequently surface: individual versus co-leadership of groups, and professional versus lay leadership. Male-female co-facilitation is the clear approach of choice, and some experts maintain that individual leadership of marital enrichment is a contradiction of terms. However, less-than-ideal circumstances may necessitate individual leadership, and leader manuals frequently provide suggestions to deal with this contingency. The second concern, lay versus professional leadership, is not addressed in this chapter as the reader is assumed to be a professional. However, clinicians may wish to train laypersons to lead enrichment programs, and research makes a good case for the effectiveness of this approach (Most and Guerney 1983; Olson 1982a, 1982b).

What leadership skills and theoretical knowledge are required for marital enrichment leadership? Typically skills include the ability to do the following:

- Teach via brief presentations or "lecturettes"
- Model and role-play
- Self-disclose and communicate a warm and caring attitude
- Observe, coach, and provide feedback that is both descriptive and process-oriented
- Set and maintain structure
- Facilitate inclusiveness and expressiveness

Group theory and skills—for example, summarizing, evaluating, diagnosing, and group building—are also valuable.

Learning Theory

The learning theory of marital enrichment emphasizes a holistic approach to education, inclusive of affective, cognitive, and behavioral elements of couples' lives. The model is that of *andragogy* (the art and science of helping adults learn) rather than pedagogy. Andragogy assumes that adults are active, self-directed learners who bring considerable experience to a learning context that emphasizes mutuality, respect, and collaboration (Knowles 1978).

Learning is hierarchically organized proceeding from low-order to high-order skills, allowing a gradual introduction to more challenging material as the program evolves. Communication skills precede conflict resolution skills. Directing couples *not* to deal with troublesome content early on emphasizes skill development. To that same end, individuals may practice skills with nonpartners at the beginning of a session and later work with the partners. It is the leader's task to create and maintain a safe environment, minimizing anxiety, fear of self-disclosure, and shame.

Cautions and Limitations

Marital enrichment is not a panacea. While it provides a cost-efficient, time-effective alternative to therapy, it is not the best treatment for all couples. Well-functioning couples who are committed to working on their marriage and have a good support system will likely find that enrichment has little to offer them. Heavily conflicted couples can obstruct the enrichment group process and would do better in marital therapy.

A happy marriage does not automatically follow from good communication and skillful problem solving. In fact, improved communication may allow for sharing difficult information that becomes problematic for the relationship. Screening couples is important to maximize positive outcome. What are the couple's expectations? Do they seek intimacy at the expense of healthy autonomy? If there is conflict in the relationship, can it be contained so as to benefit from and not obstruct the group process? Is the couple in fact looking for therapy? How realistic and patient is the couple in seeking change in the relationship? L'Abate (1981) urges particular caution with couples who have experienced a recent, major loss; expect magical results; are planning separation or divorce; show considerable disorganization and chaos; or are uncooperative and hostile, with heavy blaming and projective identification.

Enrichment leaders should also be aware of the need to present programs to the public in ethical fashion. Leaders should provide a clear explanation of program processes, goals, benefits, and liabilities (i.e., as in the therapy process, "things often get worse before they get better"). Enrichment participants also need to be "debriefed" following a positive weekend retreat, and they need to normalize their struggles and become aware of plateau times and nonpeak times (Doherty et al. 1978; Leigh et al. 1986; Smith 1979).

Outcome Research

A thorough review of the outcome research on marriage enrichment is beyond the scope of this chapter. Interested readers are referred to Giblin et al. (1985) for a meta-analytic review of 85 premarital, marital, and family enrichment programs; Zimpfer (1988), Guerney and Maxson (1990), and Silliman and Schumm (2000) provide reviews. *Marriage Enrichment: Preparation, Mentoring and Outreach* (Hunt et al. 1998) also reviews marital enrichment programs and research. While many research questions are as yet unanswered, there is some convergence of findings, which is summarized briefly as follows:

- Marital enrichment programs do work. The clear majority of participants were better off on some measure of relationship skill or satisfaction than nonparticipants.
- Longer, more structured programs showed better outcome than shorter programs.
- When programs were compared, Relationship Enhancement scored significantly higher than Couple Communication Program or Marriage Encounter (Giblin et al. 1985; Brock and Joanning 1983). We are unaware of comparisons between other marital enrichment programs.
- Younger, less-educated participants with shorter marriages showed greater gains. In terms of socioeconomic status, enrichment has been offered to middle- and upper-middle-class populations, with little extension to more diverse populations. There are no consistent differences in outcomes between sexes. However, enrichment group leaders frequently note that men need more coaxing to become engaged in the process.
- Enrichment-induced change takes time. Mace (1979) hypothesized that it takes at least a year for a couple to incorporate significant cognitive, behavioral, and affective dimensions of change. A second finding regarding time is that program effects diminish over time, although problems never return to pretreatment levels. Many researchers advocate "booster" or follow-up sessions.

Conclusion

This chapter is meant to encourage clinicians to commit time and professional expertise to the important endeavor of marriage enrichment. Given high divorce rates, diminishing social supports, changing gender and social roles, and increasing societal competitiveness for couples' time and energy, the need to help couples find marital resources is enormous and immediate. Marriage enrichment offers an important, additional, rewarding intervention approach for clinicians to help couples. The growth of these programs has expanded into both secular and religious contexts. Additionally, the Internet has introduced new support mechanisms. In closing, we note that much attention is now focused on how divorce and relationship dissatisfaction affects couple development and the development of their children. What truly remains to be seen is how widespread the use of these measures will become as additional research reviews the effectiveness of the various marital enrichment programs.

Chapters on Related Topics

The following chapters describe concepts related to marital enrichment in clinical practice:

- Chapter 14, "The Family Life Cycle: A Framework for Understanding Family Development"
- Chapter 15, "Functional and Dysfunctional Families"
- Chapter 26, "Sex Therapy at the Turn of the Century: New Awareness and Response"

26

Sex Therapy at the Turn of the Century

New Awareness and Response

Linda D. Schwoeri, Ph.D.
G. Pirooz Sholevar, M.D.
Mark P. Combs, Ph.D.

Introduction

The treatment of sexual problems was an integral part of the changing sexual atmosphere of the 1970s, and the publication of *Human Sexual Inadequacy* by Masters and Johnson (1970) represented a radical change in the treatment of sexual dysfunction. There was a new and growing appreciation that sexual problems could be modified through more immediate and short-term interventions than psychoanalysis. The invention of safe and reliable birth control methods, the legalization of abortion, and the more open expression and discussion of sexual matters paralleled the enthusiasm in the research of sexual physiology and sexual dysfunction (Sadock 1991). Invisible but nevertheless insidious in the whole sexual culture was the spread of AIDS, in addition to a variety of other illnesses including venereal diseases and hepatitis.

The possibility of improving sexual functioning, overcoming sexual anxiety, and further enjoying relationships through sexual fulfillment created a renaissance in the field of psychiatry. Kaplan's *The New Sex Therapy* (1974) broadened the understanding of the many intrapsychic as well as the many learned or conditioned causes of sexual dysfunction. Couples could be treated together for all aspects of their marital relationship, including the most intimate of all—their sexual difficulties. The field of sex therapy was new and challenging and offered couples the opportunity for rapid cures to persistent problems. There was optimism and enthusiasm visible in the development of new treatments for a range of sexual symptoms. Sensate focus exercises became a well-known and accepted treatment for a range of sexual difficulties. Interest was also apparent in the outpouring of material from different disciplines—urology, family psychiatry, psychology, and feminist and marital therapy. Publications by the popular press kept pace with the wave of academic research.

Research has shown that the treatment of sexual dysfunction is far more complex than may have been indicated, and this has created many changes in the field of sex therapy. Individuals seeking treatment have more than sexual difficulties to address, and this necessitates a broader and more comprehensive approach than some of the early behavioral approaches offered. Although Masters and Johnson initially dealt with specific physical symptoms such as erectile, ejaculatory, and inorgasmia problems, Kaplan's (1974) addition of *desire* to aspects of sexuality that could be treated added a strong psychological component to sex therapy. This greater attention to desire disorders and sexual inhibition influenced changes in the classification and treatment of sexual dysfunction and sexual disorders. Treatment therefore shifted from more behavioral and cognitive perspectives to more interpersonal and systems-oriented models.

This chapter addresses the need for a multidisciplinary approach that utilizes the expertise of urologists, gynecologists, geneticists, and endocrinologists, as well as psychiatrists, sex therapists, and marital therapists, in the treatment of sexual dysfunction. Cases are presented reflecting different approaches.

Changing Views in the Treatment of Sexual Dysfunction

There have been significant changes in the approaches taken to the treatment of sexual dysfunction in the past two decades. Historically, treating a couple meant long-term *individual* treatment, essentially psychoanalytic psychotherapy. This approach was due to the pioneering work of Havelock Ellis (1906) and later Freud (1905/1953). Masters and Johnson's publications in the 1970s changed the focus from essentially individual psychodynamic treatment to short-term behavioral interventions with the couple. The focus became more directly behavioral and educational in nature. There was also a new and growing concern for anxiety in the etiology of sexual dysfunction. The use of systematic desensitization and other behavioral techniques such as relaxation interventions in the treatment of sexual dysfunction (Lazarus 1965; Salter 1949; Wolpe 1958) influenced the treatment of anxiety-driven, conditioned responses together with a fear of failure. New behavioral approaches such as *sensate focus exercises* and the *squeeze technique* for premature ejaculation were practiced by couples in their own homes with support and instruction from the clinician. These direct behavioral techniques were successful without attention to etiological factors.

Education and Its Role in Treatment

The ordinary process of socialization can result in lack of information or misinformation about sexuality and sexual relationships. This situation is quite different from a neurotic conflict but can impair the individual's capacity to perform adequately in sexual situations. Provision of simple information such as the need for interpersonal attention, stimulation, and the use of different methods during the course of foreplay can result in remediation of many sexual dysfunctions. Some common misconceptions that require correction include the bias toward superiority of achieving orgasm through vaginal intercourse alone rather than through clitoral stimulation; the importance of having a large penis in order to satisfy a woman; the need for men to ejaculate every time there is sexual intercourse; or the need for men to have and maintain erections as a way of showing their attraction to a woman. Other factors also contribute to sexual dysfunction, such as communication issues, insufficient education about sexual problems, marital conflict, and family-of-origin issues.

Integration

A more current view of sex therapy is one that integrates sex therapy with marital therapy. The patient's complaints and symptoms represent only a small portion of the total problem. Because of multiple factors involved in the etiology of sexual dysfunction, anything less than a multidimensional perspective would fall quite short of addressing the problems. Currently, the treatment of sexual problems has both biological-medical and insight-relational focused approaches, a duality that highlights the many factors involved in sexual dysfunctions. Treatment now aims to identify family as well as couple issues; it often takes longer, is more diverse, and includes multiple indices for assessment and interventions. Comprehensive treatment considers the issues discussed below.

Relationship Issues

The dynamics of control, power, entitlement to pleasure, and the ability to share and trust can all interfere with sexual functioning. These issues create major interpersonal problems for couples because they are usually below awareness or unspoken (Scarf 1987, 1995) and can hinder successful treatment (Sager 1976). When taking the history of a sexual relationship, such issues as body image, the meaning of sexuality, shame and guilt, family or cultural views of sexuality, and the nature of the relationship should be addressed. The roles played by the sexual dysfunction and the impact of improvement are also vitally important dimensions in treatment. There has been a corresponding shift of emphasis in professional literature and treatment from phasic, performance-oriented interventions toward experiential and qualitative indices (Atwood and Dershowitz 1992; Burg and Sprenkle 1996; Rosen and Lieblum 1995; Schnarch 1991, 1998; Sternberg 1986; Weeks and Hof 1987). These approaches are frequently employed with traditional approaches but pursue sexual-meaning systems.

Health and Developmental Factors

Illness, weight, aging, nervous system problems, spinal cord injury, or a disease such as diabetes and genital abnormalities and cancer can all affect sexual behavior, resulting in sexual dysfunction. Knowledge of, having, or living with a person with a chronic illness can create a range of emotional responses, including sadness, discouragement, and depression, and can impair the ability to enjoy life to the fullest. Four physical illnesses are discussed as examples below:

1. *Diabetes.* Masters et al. (1986) noted that 50% of diabetic men have organically based erectile dysfunction. Women are often diagnosed with secondary anorgasmia 4–6 years following the diagnosis of diabetes (Masters et al. 1986). Over time, diabetes damages every organ of the body and places the individual at risk for neuropathy and macroangiopathy and microangiopathy (diseases of the large and small blood vessels). Women report difficulties with sexual arousal, especially lubrication (Jensen 1981, 1986; Schreiner-Engel et al. 1987).
2. *Prostatitis.* Prostatitis causes painful urination and back pain and can interfere with sexual functioning, in particular creating painful ejaculation. The risk of prostatitis and prostate cancer increases with age.

3. *Cancer.* Recent studies estimate that one in five women will develop breast cancer. Removal of the breast results in dramatic changes in a woman's self-concept. Not feeling "womanly," a female often loses interest in sex. Cancer of the uterus and cervix places great emotional stress on a couple's sexual relationship. The treatment for prostatic cancer can likewise diminish sexual interest because the male feels "less like a man."
4. *Severe injuries.* Spinal cord injuries causing paraplegia or quadriplegia result in loss of bodily sensations below the level of injury. Loss of bladder and bowel control, normal erectile dysfunction, ejaculation difficulties, and loss of fertility are commonly experienced.

Sexually Transmitted Diseases

The fear of sexually transmitted diseases (STDs) obviously presents obstacles to the sexual functioning and satisfaction of the couple. Syphilis and gonorrhea are highly contagious and can be transmitted through many types of sexual contact. Chlamydia, a bacterial-like STD infection, and herpes, another highly contagious and chronic STD, can be transmitted through nonsexual contact. Above all, the fear of HIV, which can be transmitted through sharing intravenous needles or through blood transfusions, psychologically impairs functioning; AIDS causes some people to avoid sexual contact, or at least decreases their interest in sexual activity (Wincze and Carey 1991).

Life-Cycle Issues

Different life-cycle issues influence the sexual needs of couples (Carter and McGoldrick 1980a). *Infertility*, which is defined as the inability to conceive a child after 1 year of regular unprotected coitus, or the inability to carry a pregnancy to live birth (Scher and Dix 1990), may present as a major crisis in the life of the couple. The need to have sex at specific "fertile" times can lead to anxiety, depression, disturbance in desire, and feelings of sexual inadequacy and can make the couple's sexual life quite problematic. The *climacteric*, which is the period before and immediately following menopause, may last up to 15 years. During this time, as Masters et al. (1986) noted, 8% of women suffer hormonal changes that vary in intensity due to estrogen deficiency. Some problems include loss of or decrease in vaginal lubrication during intercourse, loss of tissue elasticity, and hot flashes. Sexually active postmenopausal women are known to have less shrinkage of the vagina (Leiblum 1992); however, many women suffer discomfort and pain during intercourse and find it an unpleasant experience. *Menopause* and the existential problems of this phase of life create great emotional difficulty for a woman and have an impact on her self-esteem as well as her sexual relationships. Women face depression and loss resulting from children leaving home and often lose interest in sex as a result. The male correlate of climacteric is not equivalent, since there is no major shift in hormonal levels. Testosterone production does, however, diminish between ages 55 and 60 (Mason 1991). Kolodny (1979) and Masters et al. (1986) noted a reduction of potency, some depression, and decreased sexual desire due to the lowering of testosterone. Men over 55 commonly need more protracted time and stimulation to achieve erection. They experience a decrease in the intensity of orgasm and report less physical need to ejaculate.

Medications

Different medications can affect sexual response, such as antihypertensive medications, antiparkinsonian agents, propranolol, and benzodiazepines, as well as psychiatric medications such as antidepressants, monoamine oxidase (MAO) inhibitors, and major tranquilizers. Antidepressant drugs have been associated with orgasmic dysfunction, decreased libido, and erectile failure. Because of these known side effects, psychiatrists and primary care physicians need to evaluate and manage sexual dysfunction in patients with an affective disorder (Segraves 1992). The establishment of a baseline for sexual function in these patients is difficult, yet needed.

Assessment, Classification, and Treatment of Sexual Dysfunction

Sexual dysfunction may be a manifestation of biological, interpersonal-relational, situational, or intrapsychic problems and therefore requires a comprehensive, multidisciplinary approach for diagnosis and treatment. As discussed by Schiavi (1992a, 1992b), the assessment of sexual dysfunction must include a thorough sexual history of both partners. The interview should assess the following:

1. Is this a sexual dysfunction, or is it mislabeled?
2. What is the dysfunction?
3. Is dysfunction situational or generalized?
4. Is it lifelong or acquired?
5. What is the reaction of both patient and partner to the dysfunction?

Sexual dysfunction is classified broadly in relation to the sexual response cycle, comprising desire, arousal, release, and resolution phases (Kaplan

1974). DSM-IV-TR (American Psychiatric Association 2000) separates sexual dysfunctions into four categories: sexual desire disorders; sexual arousal disorders; orgasmic disorders; and sexual pain disorders. The major diagnostic criterion is that the sexual dysfunction is an interruption at any of the phases in the sexual response cycle (Sadock 1991). The dysfunction may be lifelong or acquired, generalized or situational. The criteria for a diagnosis of sexual dysfunction include organic causes and the use of medication, as well as functional problems.

Rarely are sexual dysfunctions separate from other psychiatric syndromes; however, comorbidity is in fact quite common. Sexual dysfunctions are associated with a range of personality disorders, neurotic disorders, affective disorders, and substance abuse and use disorders, as well as relational impasses. Comprehensive psychiatric evaluation of existing depression, anxiety, and panic disorders can enhance treatment because medication for the primary disorder may effect rapid change in the sexual problems.

In addition to psychiatric and medically informed models, there are newer approaches and assessments that address contextual issues instead of "resolving" sexual dysfunction. Newer approaches stress the idea that the etiology of sexual dysfunction is multifaceted and subsumed within relationship and meaning systems (Piercy et al. 1996; Schnarch 1998; Weeks and Hof 1987). The hegemony of a universal sexual response cycle has been predicated on orgasmic functioning and defined biologically and genitally (Tiefer 1995); hence, the increased emphasis on observing and addressing ecosystemic indices.

In addition to the initial interview, there are a number of psychometric measures that can be administered to differentiate psychogenic and psychiatric symptoms from situational and relational sexual problems. These measures are as follows:

- Beck Depression Inventory (BDI)
- Hamilton Rating Scale for Depression (Ham-D)
- Minnesota Multiphasic Personality Inventory (MMPI)
- Taylor-Johnson Temperament Analysis (T-JTA)
- Symptom Checklist–90—Revised (SCL-90-R)
- Substance Abuse Subtle Screening Inventory (SASSI)

Furthermore, the assessment of the sexual and marital relationship can be aided by the use of measures of the couples' relationship:

- *Spanier Dyadic Adjustment Scale* (Spanier 1976). This device offers an assessment of the couple's consensus, satisfaction, expression of affect, and cohesion in the relationship.

- *Sexual Interaction Inventory* (LoPiccolo and Steger 1974). This measure gives information on frequency, pleasure, and perception of the sex.
- *Sexual genogram* (Hof and Berman 1986). This measure combines information gathered traditionally in a sexual history with information on the functioning of the family and marital systems. It can include data on marriage, divorce, death, and birth similar to that obtained in a family genogram, with an added focus on issues of sexuality and intimacy in the family system.
- *Sexual status examination* (Kaplan 1983, 1995). This measure is part of the self-reported psychosexual evaluation and elicits both subjective and cognitive-relational descriptions and attributions.
- *Derogatis Sexual Functioning Inventory* (Derogatis and Melisaratos 1983). This measure inventories 10 areas of functioning collated from a 245-item questionnaire.
- *Prepare-Enrich* (Olson 1982a, 1982b). This measure is a general assessment of couple functioning including a subset scale of sexual satisfaction.

Sexual Desire Disorders

Hypoactive Sexual Desire Disorder

Hypoactive sexual desire disorder is described by DSM-IV-TR criteria (American Psychiatric Association 2000) as deficient or absent sexual fantasies or desire for sexual activity. Persons with this disorder—both men and women—are known to fantasize less than control subjects. Factors that affect sexual functioning such as age, sex, culture, and life-event contexts are taken into account. Having intercourse in response to a partner's demands or because of feelings of obligation in the relationship does not invalidate the diagnosis of hypoactive sexual desire. In making a diagnosis, the lack of actual interest in sexual activities that the patient admits to should be ascertained.

Etiology. Studies indicate different factors in the etiology of this disorder.

Biological. Although the differences between low and normal desire subjects were modest, Schiavi et al. (1988, 1990) reported lower plasma testosterone levels in patients with hypoactive sexual desire. Certain medications have also been shown to cause hypoactive sexual desire, including drugs for treating hypertension, such as diuretics; adrenergic-inhibiting agents; psychiatric medications, such as antidepressants, MAO inhibitors, and lithium; anticonvulsants; and chemotherapy (Segraves 1988). A premorbid history of depression (Schreiner-Engel and Schiavi 1986) has been found in these patients, and this further complicates treatment decisions.

Individual and relationship issues. LoPiccolo and Friedman (1988) found many individual and relationship factors in hypoactive sexual desire disorder, including gender identity problems, fear of pregnancy, fear of STDs and AIDS, history of sexual trauma, unresolved death of a spouse, aging, and concerns about appearance. These multiple factors influence the development and persistence of sexual dysfunctions.

Treatment. In all cases treatment must take into consideration the underlying cause for the problem, including the individual's attitude toward sex, the sexual history, and his or her relationship with family and spouse. Treatment must be sensitive to real issues. For example, lubricants may be prescribed for vaginal dryness and discomfort during intercourse. However, if the woman is not aroused because her relationship with her partner is unsatisfying and unrewarding in both sexual and nonsexual ways, the prescription is not helpful. Schnarch (1998) clearly advocates for making the relational distinction between the arousal and orgasmic thresholds and argues that sexual desires reflect context and couple communication. Schnarch's popularity in treatment stems from his use of intimacy building, communication tolerance, and self-validation versus validation of the partner. Other relational approaches, such as structured sexual tasks (SIGS) (see Kaplan 1979), are concurrently assigned to the couple in an effort to modify underlying dysfunctions.

Sexual Arousal Disorders

Male Erectile Disorder

Male erectile disorder is estimated to be the most common presenting problem in sexual treatment for males. Occurrence is reported in approximately 36%–53% of all cases seen in sex therapy clinics (Hawton 1982). It is possible that the number of cases is even higher than the figures obtained. The DSM-IV definition of male erectile disorder involves not only the physiological achievement of erection but also a sense of pleasure and excitement in sexual activity. Erectile dysfunction may be organic or psychogenic. It is estimated that in 20%–50% of cases, there is an organic basis (Sadock 1991).

Evaluation. Emphasis on male sexual adequacy has increased in relation to a growing appreciation of changes in women's attitudes toward sexual behavior. Women's sexual desires and preferences are more openly discussed, and this may increase anxiety in many men. Physicians and other clinicians are becoming more sensitive to the devastating effect of male erectile disorder in terms of the male gender role (Zilbergeld 1992a, 1992b).

The anxiety and shame attached to erectile disorder is a commonly admitted symptom and highlights the psychological and physiological implications of power and control in the couple's relationship. An examination of the couple's relational contract can shed light on underlying issues. Many physicians now request a psychological evaluation of both patient and partner to better assess interrelated factors. Psychological conflicts over sexual impulses often create fear, anxiety, or inhibition in the patient. The failure to maintain an erection further contributes to the patient's difficulty in attaining sexual pleasure and this reinforces the dysfunction. In a comprehensive assessment, Tiefer (1995) recommends a discussion of the patient's sexual history and problem, including a description of sexual difficulties as well as frequency, quality, and conduct of sexual activity, including masturbation, fantasy, desire, and so forth. Wise (1992) also recommends a model for the assessment of sexual dysfunction that emphasizes *etiology*. His model suggests: 1) diagnosing the sexual disorder and comorbid affective and/or medical disorder; 2) identifying individual personality traits and their relationship to the dysfunction; 3) taking a complete life history of an individual or couple; and 4) determining the goal-directed activities of the partners.

The spread of AIDS and the many illnesses that accompany the disease has made physicians more aware of the role played by medical illnesses in sexual dysfunction (Schover and Jensen 1988). The evaluation of erectile disorder now includes a series of medical tests (Tiefer 1995), including

- Hormone assays
- Glucose tolerance tests
- Pelvic arterial and venous function tests
- Pelvic sensory-motor function tests
- Nocturnal penile monitoring and visual sexual stimulation, as well as an initial interview, history, and examination by the urologist that includes reviews of all medications used

The emphasis of Tiefer and Melman is on the role of vascular, neurological, and endocrinological factors in erectile problems. Many psychiatric drugs, including tricyclic antidepressants (Tofranil, Elavil, Vivactil); major tranquilizers such as Prolixin, Mellaril and Haldol; and alcohol, barbiturates, cocaine, and other commonly abused drugs can play a role in erectile dysfunction. The key to evaluation is an integration of psychosocial, psychiatric, and medical history and examination.

Treatment. In addition to the appreciation of biological factors in sexual dysfunction over the past 10–15 years, there has been an increasing use of pharmacological interventions, such as injections of papaverine or papaverine plus phentolamine. Penile injection treatment is very common; however, it carries the risk of permanent penile scarring, reaction to the drug or needle, infection, and liver damage.

Another pharmacological treatment is the use of Yocon (yohimbine), an alpha-adrenoreceptor blocker. It increases blood flow into the penis and decreases outflow (Meyer 1988). Modest improvements in sexual functioning were noted through the use of this medication (Sussett et al. 1989). However, a side effect of the use of injections is reported distress in the partner, who may begin to feel unattractive and unable to arouse the partner being treated without the injection (Wincze and Carey 1991). It is therefore important to educate partners on the importance of *communicating* their attraction to each other in other ways. If partners do not focus as much on the act of intercourse and attend more to the sexual play, the distress accompanying treatment will be lessened.

Several antidepressants and antianxiety drugs are now also being used for men with psychogenic as well as organogenic erectile dysfunction.

Physiological methods for treating erectile disorder include a vacuum device that draws blood into the penis; a constricting band placed around the base of the penis then traps this blood.

In conjunction with this method, there are surgical treatments for erectile disorder that have proven to be effective options for couples. Prosthetic penile implants, once used exclusively for impotence with organic etiology, are being used for psychogenic problems. It is estimated that 25,000 prostheses are implanted annually (McCarthy 1989). Both semirigid and multicomponent, hydraulic, inflatable devices are being used (Beutler et al. 1993).

Female Sexual Arousal Disorder

Female sexual arousal disorder, or the occurrence of arousal phase disorders in women, occurs in 11%–50% of women in the general population (Spector and Carey 1990). Although women's arousal difficulties are usually attributed to psychological causes, including anxiety, depression, or a history of relationship conflict, women may also lack information about appropriate stimulation needed for the arousal phase. Women who are lactating or menopausal may also have difficulty lubricating as a result of diminished estrogen or, in the case of lactation, elevated prolactin level. This hormonal imbalance may cause painful or uncomfortable intercourse because the vagina becomes thin and fragile. The clinician should assess the environment in which the sexual intercourse occurs.

Orgasmic Disorders

Female Orgasmic Disorder (Inhibited Female Orgasm)

Eight percent to ten percent of women never experience orgasm under any circumstances, and perhaps 50% do not experience orgasm in coitus without additional stimulation. Therefore, the lack of orgasm during coitus is not necessarily a dysfunction.

Treatment. Treatments successfully used include

- Directed masturbation training followed by partner training (LoPiccolo and Lobitz 1972)
- Instruction in Kegel exercises, which increase orgasmic potential, in conjunction with directed masturbation
- Encouragement for role playing of orgasms
- Progressive movement of sexual activities toward being more sexual (Masters and Johnson 1970)

These progressive activities are meant to expand the couple's comfort level as well as increase mutual stimulation. Diagnosis and treatment of orgasmic disorders should determine how active the woman is during sexual activities, since it is known that active women are more likely to receive the stimulation needed for orgasm (Leiblum 1992). Some women may need to vary positions, relax their bodies, and alter breathing. Masturbation exercises are utilized to encourage self-stimulation and to determine what is effective in increasing arousal in orgasm. Each woman needs to learn what works for her sexually. Since 30%–40% of women are known to have arousal difficulties, the history of individuals seeking treatment helps to isolate each patient's problems and determine the best course of treatment.

Cognitive-behavioral approaches. Cognitive-behavioral approaches are useful for treating inhibited female orgasm when it is thought to be a conditioned fear reaction or a learned phobia. According to cognitive-behavioral therapists, treatment requires overcoming the fear of penetration (Leiblum and Rosen 1989). Masters and Johnson approach treatment by explaining to partners the involuntary nature of the vaginal spasm or contraction. Treatment consists of the use of the Hegger dilator in graduated sizes to enable the woman to accept penetration by an object comparable in size to a penis. One form of desensitization training is use of imagery in which a 21-item hierarchy is generated. The couple moves through these items to images of intercourse (the final item on this hierarchy). Therapy also engages the patient in deep muscle relaxation together with this desensitization procedure.

Multimodal therapy. Lazarus (1981) developed a behavioral approach that he named "multimodal" or "multidimensional." This approach assesses the couple's sexual behavior, deficits in their sexual techniques, and their expressed feelings of physical attraction. His technique looks at the location, type, frequency, intensity, and duration of the woman's pain. Techniques utilized in treatment include Kegel exercises, progressive relaxation training, fantasy exercises, finger insertion, films, and sensate focus exercises. Lazarus emphasizes the importance of the patient-therapist relationship in sex therapy to enhance patient cooperation and treatment success.

Inhibited Male Orgasm

Inhibited male orgasm, or retarded ejaculation, is defined as the achievement of climax during coitus but with great difficulty (Sadock 1991). The man's erectile functioning remains intact, but ejaculation is impaired. This disorder may be classified as primary if the man has never been able to ejaculate during coitus, but it may be situational and occur after a time of normal coital functioning. Retarded ejaculation differs from retrograde ejaculation, in which the seminal fluid passes back into the bladder. Inhibited male orgasm may not have a solely organic cause. The occurrence of primary ejaculatory dysfunction is part of a larger, more complex psychiatric profile requiring extensive evaluation of the couple's relationship.

Premature Ejaculation

Premature ejaculation refers to the achievement of orgasm before or immediately after intromission or stimulation. This dysfunction is usually associated with anxiety about performance, issues in the relationship, or the orgasmic response of the partner. Benzodiazepines continue to be prescribed for anxiety. In cases of premature ejaculation, these medications help suppress P-J ejaculatory sensations during the period of high sexual excitement (Kaplan 1983). Anti-anxiety medication is usually necessary because panic disorders are not amenable to psychological therapies alone (Kaplan 1983, pp. 266–267). The absence of organic factors is one of the criteria for diagnosis. Sexual tasks in treatment are focused on helping the man attend to the sensations of his impending orgasm while making love (Kaplan 1974), and Seman's "stop-start" technique is also integral to treatment. The new selective serotonin reuptake inhibitors (SSRIs) have been used successfully in treating premature ejaculation in males and premature orgasm in females.

Inhibited Female Orgasm

Inhibited female orgasm is classified as a *primary* orgasmic dysfunction when the woman suffers with persistent inhibition of orgasm regardless of stimulation. This dysfunction is considered *secondary* when orgasm has occurred in the past either through masturbation, while asleep, or by other means of stimulation. This is a commonly reported sexual dysfunction, with an overall prevalence rate estimated at 30% (Sadock 1991).

There are many psychological factors to consider in making the diagnosis of inhibited female orgasm, including fear of pregnancy; issues concerning loss of control; damage to the body (specifically the vagina); or feelings of guilt over sexual impulses seen as an expression of aggression, destructive behavior, or violence. Diseases related to the endocrine system (e.g., hypothyroidism and diabetes) can affect the ability to reach orgasm. The role of medications is not as well studied in females as in males; however, it is known that certain antidepressants (imipramine and nortriptyline) and major tranquilizers such as thioridazine and trifluoperazine affect orgasm in women.

Sexual Pain Disorders

Dyspareunia

Dyspareunia refers to the pain associated with intercourse. It can occur in both men and women; however, it is more common in women. Men rarely experience pain on ejaculation; however, vasocongestion during sexual activity without orgasm can result in discomfort. Dyspareunia is commonly experienced in postmenopausal women. The thinning of the vaginal mucosa and lessened lubrication are significant factors in this condition. There may also be organic abnormalities such as scarring from surgery, endometriosis, or pelvic disorders, including irritations and infections. Dyspareunia is often difficult to diagnose unless the pain is localized and described. The patient also needs to describe the nature of the stimulation and lubrication that she experiences that make penetration comfortable (Leiblum 1992).

The psychological manifestations of this very real pain can make sex unbearable and result in complete avoidance. Dyspareunia rates are reported at an estimated 3% (Hawton 1982) to 5.1% (Renshaw 1988). These figures may not reflect true prevalence, since many women, due to embarrassment or anxiety, may report this condition to gynecologists or general practitioners but not obtain a psychiatric consultation or sexual therapy.

Vaginismus

Vaginismus is involuntary vaginal constriction that prevents intercourse and vaginal entrance during sex (Carey et al. 1996; Laumann et al. 1994; Teitelbaum and Carey 1996). Muscle spasms occur in anticipation of intercourse. Women with this disorder may be capable of sexual arousal, may lubricate, and experience orgasms, yet cannot have intercourse. Estimates of prevalence range from 5% to 42% of sex therapy patients. The psychological considerations of this diagnosis include the woman's anxiety; her ability for arousal; a past history of sexual abuse or trauma; and the nature of her present relationship. Historically, psychoanalytic explanations focused on the woman's rejection of her feminine role or a defense against incestuous fantasies. Masters and Johnson (1970, p. 250) described the phenomenon as a psychosomatic illness and one that is "due to imagined, anticipated, or real attempt at vaginal penetration." A more contemporary view considers the illness as a conditioned sexual response associated with painful or aversive sexual stimulus (Kaplan 1974).

Treatment

Treatment must be approached with the aim of making the woman feel comfortable and in control. She can begin to gradually adjust to the insertion of a dilator or her finger while in bed or relaxing on her back. Her partner is included once this level of comfort is attained. Leiblum and Rosen (1989) suggest that the most important factor in determining success or failure of treatment is the nature of support for change. This necessitates an understanding of each partner's history and how it perpetuates the sexual difficulty, in addition to a range of exercises. There is discussion of the couple's attitudes about sex, their feelings and thoughts about the fantasy exercises, and the need for fewer sexual demands from the spouse. As the partner becomes more sensitive to the woman's fears and adjusts to the gradual and fear-reducing elements of the sexual experience, the woman progresses to the point where she feels more in control and is able to become aroused and enjoy intercourse.

Treatment

Models of Intervention

Preferred models of intervention for the treatment of sexual disorders have mostly vacillated between behavioral and psychodynamic approaches. There has been a parallel vacillation between addressing psychological issues and investigating physiological and organic ones.

When psychogenically based sexual disorders are being treated, data emerging from clinics and clinical research fields indicate a hierarchy of psychotherapeutic interventions that should be instituted. This hierarchy includes educational, behavioral, interpersonal, and individual psychotherapeutic interventions.

When "organically based" factors play an important part in the genesis of sexual disorders, the use of mechanical interventions may become necessary. Kaplan (1974, 1995) proposes a technique by which, following initial assessment, she introduces behavioral interventions such as sensate focus. As the treatment progresses, she helps the patient become aware of the immediate cause of the problem and the relationship patterns that affect or are affected by the problem. It may then become necessary to explore more serious or remote causes of sexual dysfunction. Kaplan's eclectic blend of techniques combines the strategies of Masters and Johnson, family systems interventions, various behavioral prescriptions, and psychodynamic psychotherapy.

Solution-oriented approaches are more systemic and try to increase the differentiation of self, which minimizes narratives of failure. Such approaches also help to maximize skills that promote relational stability (e.g., Schnarch 1998).

Direct Behavioral Techniques

We previously discussed behavioral techniques in relation to specific sexual dysfunctions. Even in the absence of attention to etiological factors, behavioral techniques can be very effective. Masters and Johnson (1970) have emphasized the significant role of *performance anxiety* in sexual dysfunctions. Performance anxiety leads to *spectatoring*—that is, watching oneself "perform," with great anxiety, during sex.

The Squeeze Technique

The *squeeze technique* developed by Masters and Johnson (1970) is an effective treatment for premature ejaculation. The patient's partner is asked to stimulate his penis until he begins to feel preliminary sensations of orgasm. He then cues the partner to grasp his penis with the thumb and first finger of both hands and to squeeze the shaft just below the corona ridge for about 3–4 seconds. The squeeze technique works rapidly to diminish erections, and from this point of view is superior to the more frequently used *stop-start* technique.

The Stop-Start Technique

With the *stop-start* technique, the patient's partner is asked to stimulate his penis until he begins to feel premonitory sensations of orgasm. He learns to instruct the partner to "stop" and the cycle is repeated. This method encourages *concentration* on preorgasmic sensations, rather than suppressing them (Kaplan 1974).

Sensate Focus

Sensate focus is a procedure developed by Masters and Johnson (1970) in order to reduce performance anxiety and spectatoring during intercourse. The couple is encouraged to be sensual rather than sexual through body exploration and physical touching. The partners receive and provide feedback to each other about the activities that feel good. Both the "giver" and the "receiver" are encouraged to be aware of their own sensations. This process is designed to interrupt the disabling effect of anxiety during sexual activities by reducing performance pressure and expectation. The couple is instructed to initially refrain from caressing genitals or breasts in sensate focus, phase I. In sensate focus, phase II, partners may pleasure each other's primary erotic areas but not to the point of orgasm. In sensate focus, phase III, orgasm can be included. By focusing treatment on the couple, the relational component of dysfunction can be addressed as well as mechanical aspects of sex. It is hard to consider treating an individual's sexual dysfunction without involving a partner in some form of conjunct treatment.

Eyes-Open Orgasm

Eyes-open orgasm is a process that helps couples explore, master, and then enhance sexual responses and behaviors that formerly provoked anxiety. This relational approach is taught by Schnarch (1991, 1998) as a way to transcend the "doing" and mechanics so often prescribed in sexual activities. Schnarch's approach builds on Tantric practices of sexual enlightenment.

Guidelines for Treatment

Decisions about treatment depend on the nature and severity of the sexual dysfunction in one or both partners and the therapeutic orientation of the therapist. In treating couples, relational and psychodynamic considerations should be raised. For example, how does the couple manage conflict and stress in their present relationship? How is conflict, anger, or retaliation involved in sex? How do conflicts relate to earlier life conflicts that created failure along certain developmental lines? Depending on the ego development of the couple, sexual intimacy can create discordant functional responses. The partner may be viewed as threatening or dangerous by the patient with sexual dysfunction, which increases the patient's feelings of vulnerability and deactivates attachment responses in favor of defending one's self (Scarf 1987; Scharf and Scharf 1987; West and Sheldon-Keller 1994).

When interracial and intercultural couples present with dysfunctions, a wide and diverse context must be applied to their sexual difficulties. Only such a context will allow therapists to appreciate the sources of sexually discordant views that lead to self- and emotional preservation, coping behaviors, and intrusive defense mechanisms.

A frequent defense mechanism utilized by couples is attempted control—of a partner, of one's own reactions, or of other situations that trigger defensive reactions, including sexual encounters. Reciprocal attempts by the partners to control each other can make sexual situations a battleground for self-object differentiation. A frequent scenario in the struggle for differentiation involves one partner demanding sex more frequently and the other refusing it as a way to extend control or self-protection. Mutual attempts at control can also result in sexual avoidance.

Treatment of sexual dysfunction generally entails multiple stages:

1. Delineation of both partners' sexual behavior
2. Recognition of broader patterns of behavior and personality in both partners that were the foundation of the current behavioral pattern in sexual situations
3. Reconstruction of early relationship patterns between partners, when children, with their parents and the contribution of the child-parent relationship on dysfunctional interpersonal patterns and personality traits
4. Recognition of the partner's shared defensive patterns against shared neurotic conflicts that perpetuate developmental failures in early life
5. Evaluation or presence of other psychiatric disorders, including depression, anxiety, and phobias

The phobic avoidance of sex is a common contemporary problem and distinct from disorders of desire, excitement, or orgasm. If panic accompanies the phobia, 80%–85% of such patients will improve with the addition of antipanic medications (Kaplan 1983, p. 35). However, it may be quite difficult to distinguish between true inhibited sexual desire and the phobic avoidance of sex.

The following treatment guideline emphasizes the use of intervention methodologies in a hierarchical fashion (Kaplan 1983). The goal is to employ the less rigorous, short-term, and educational-behavioral interventions prior to employing the more extensive psychological, interpersonal, and mechanical interventions:

1. Education
2. Relaxation interventions
3. Relaxation and relationship-enhancing interventions with the couple

4. Sensate focus intervention
5. Couple therapy
6. Individual psychotherapy
7. Use of medication and mechanical devices

Shared defenses, neurotic conflicts, and mutual developmental failures are addressed in the context of combined, conjoint, or individual psychotherapy. Our hierarchical technique resembles Kaplan's as "psychosexual therapy," by which she addresses the behavioral, psychodynamic, and interpersonal processes involved in psychosexual dysfunction. Kaplan's approach—and our hierarchical treatment guideline—is based on the view that sexual disorder occurs on "multicausal levels." In addition to the goal of relieving sexual disorder, sexual and communicational tasks are utilized to enhance relationship and sexual interactions.

Case Examples

The first case below illustrates the complex relational and psychological factors contributing to sexual disorders:

> John and Marlene had a sexual relationship that had begun 5 years previously when John was married to another woman. He found Marlene very attractive, and their sexual relationship was highly satisfactory. Marlene was separated from her husband and raising two young children. Approximately a year before therapy, John's wife found out about the affair and asked him to leave. Simultaneously, Marlene's husband sued for the custody of the children, charging her with child neglect. Marlene became highly distracted, exhibited some financial discrepancy in her account at work, and lost her job of 9 years. At the same time, she lost legal and residential custody of her children to her husband. When John consulted a urologist because of premature loss of erection (partial erectile incompetence), none of the above factors were revealed to the examining physician. In a referral to a psychiatrist John complained of Marlene's coldness and lack of emotional responsiveness. John perceived Marlene as being highly critical of him while remaining silent. He felt like "less of a man" because he could not satisfy her. An attempt at the sensate focus technique had failed previously due to the predominance of emotional and relational difficulties. Marlene had lost her apartment following the loss of her job, was working at a lower-paying job in less satisfactory working conditions, and did not seem to enjoy many activities. When the partners argued, John would ask Marlene to leave his apartment, which made her feel very rejected.
>
> The treatment plan consisted of enhancing communication between John and Marlene with the goal of identifying everyday problems and resolving them through more effective methods. Marlene was encouraged to speak about the loss of custody, her plans to obtain better employment, and

regain more substantial access to her children. The sensate focus techniques were reintroduced within this new context. Both partners were encouraged to gain more awareness of their own feelings rather than concentrating on sexual performance to satisfy the other partner. The treatment result was quite satisfactory after a few months.

Brad was seen for a urological consultation following a car accident because of persistent premature ejaculation, as well as loss of erection during intercourse without ejaculation. Brad and his wife Janet had been engaged for 2 years and married for 5 months. They both felt inadequate and incompetent sexually, although Brad's feelings of inadequacy surpassed those of his wife. The couple had relatively satisfactory sexual encounters during the first year of their relationship when they were involved in heavy petting and genital touching while still dressed. They were less successful sexually in the second year of their relationship when they were undressed and focused on each other's genital area. Sexual difficulties increased when they became involved in sexual intercourse a few months before their marriage. Brad felt great pressure to succeed at sexual intercourse but encountered repeated and worsening failures. Janet complained of the shortness of the foreplay and felt highly dissatisfied because she had never experienced an orgasm with Brad or other partners.

The treatment plan was established by asking the couple to value feedback from each other rather than fearing control by each other. They were asked to totally refrain from intercourse for two weeks and return to heavy petting with their clothes on to reintroduce the earlier, more satisfactory phase of their sexual encounters. They were also encouraged to get involved in playful activities centering on physical and bodily touching prior to sexual encounters. The goal of reducing the emphasis and obsession with performance and choosing playfulness was gradually accomplished. The couple matured in their overall interactions and relationship.

Sara and Robert were an attractive middle-aged couple (ages 48 and 55, respectively). Both had been married before and both experienced sexual dissatisfaction in their first marriage. Sara described her first husband as aggressive, sexually unfaithful, and unable to consider her needs. She had a history of sexual repression and emotional constriction and had a severe eating disorder. She had been bulimic for over 25 years. Her first memory of the disorder was at the time of her first period. Robert's first marriage ended after the couple tried living an "open marriage." He could not handle his wife sleeping with other partners. Robert was overweight, was diabetic, had had bypass surgery, was on medication for high blood pressure, suffered from prostate and erectile problems, and had low sexual desire.

A detailed history, including the use of a sexual genogram (Hof and Berman 1986), identified relevant family dynamics. It became apparent that the couple was still in the throes of differentiating from their families of origin. Sara thoroughly maintained her family concern for keeping up appearances and controlling her emotions. Robert was still mourning the loss of his father (through parental divorce) and rejection by his biological mother.

During the marital therapy sessions, both Sara and Robert clearly regarded their respective family's views of sex and intimacy as sacred and not to be questioned. Sara's conflicts over growing up, leaving home, becoming sexual, and becoming a mother were explored and treated in individual sessions. Her eating disorder and the sexual relationship were treated in concurrent marital therapy. Robert's sexual problems, as well as his weight and his lack of direction in life, were worked out in a separate program that included group and marital therapy focusing on control issues. He was being treated by a urologist for his prostatic problem, and options were explored concerning noninvasive penile devices for his erectile problems. Sara and Robert's relationship was suffering because neither could express anger or disappointment over failures in life. Their sexual problems were treated by sensate focus combined with education on the squeeze technique and more activities involving playfulness while in the shower. They were both comfortable sexually expressing themselves in this setting so it was encouraged.

Richard and Mary asked for marital and sex therapy. This request followed an initial evaluation for sex therapy that resulted in intensive individual psychotherapy for each spouse for many years. When they entered marital therapy, they were both around 48 years of age; had 5 children, who all had exceptional educational achievements; and had a reasonably comfortable economic life (following one or two periods of financial difficulty because of Dick's, and subsequently Mary's, job difficulties). Dick was considered aloof, self-centered, highly intellectualized, quiet, and ungiving to his wife in particular and to his children to a lesser degree. Mary was considered very controlling inside of the family, a behavior that extended into her relationships at work and her family of origin. Both spouses closely involved with their families of origin due to the substantial financial assets of their parents.

Dick had premature ejaculations throughout his marital life, a problem partly concealed by Mary's need for extensive foreplay in order to relax and be aroused. Dick considered Mary's preference for certain types of foreplay as very messy, and she considered him to be overly clean, to the point that it interfered with the sexual relationship.

During the course of marital therapy, it became clear that Dick and Mary both had very conflicted relationships with their parents, particularly their fathers. Dick considered his father to be a brilliant and successful businessman who constantly contrived to make his children appear ignorant during family interactions. Early in life, Dick adopted a defensive pattern of remaining uninvolved with another person while appearing compliant. This pattern allowed him to laugh internally for having defeated his father in their interpersonal games, while his brothers became embroiled in conflictual and heated interactions. Dick carried the same pattern into his relationships with coworkers (resulting in two business failures), his wife, and his individual therapist throughout the many years of individual psychotherapy.

Mary felt that her father, who had lost his father early in life, could not allow himself to enjoy life in spite of his significant economic and social successes. His major mission in life was to turn any opportunity for enjoyment into one of suffering and misery. She repeatedly remembered incidents where her father had squeezed her arm to remind her that she should "get tough" and become capable of enduring pain. Her personality showed a pattern of doing a lot for others and expecting satisfaction in return. However, she was constantly miserable because others were failing her and did not like her.

The extension of Dick and Mary's problematic interpersonal patterns in their sex life was revealed in therapy. For example, Mary demanded optimal sexual satisfaction during foreplay and sexual encounters, and Dick attempted to defeat her by not becoming involved and let her sink under the weight of her own expectations. Both partners exhibited their characteristic way of interacting with others during the treatment sessions. Mary brought in a single agenda item about Dick's failure, spent the whole session talking about it, and left the session disappointed that treatment was not changing Dick's behavior. Dick characteristically remained uninvolved and managed to say nothing throughout many sessions while dutifully driving in for treatment and paying the therapy bills on time.

Dick and Mary had received little warmth or affection from their mothers, although they never complained about it. It appeared that the relative emotional neglect by the two mothers made them turn, early on, to their fathers for affection. Dick and Mary were very disappointed that their relationships with their fathers were rather impersonal and lacked sensitivity and tenderness. The relative emotional neglect by the mothers also left them vulnerable to any stressors in the relationship with the fathers.

Addressing the early relationship patterns of Dick and Mary as the source of marital transference was the centerpiece of the treatment. The triadic transference toward the therapist was seldom used as a basis for interpretation. The treatment was long but successful due to the strong relationship between Dick, Mary, and the therapist.

Conclusion

Given the complex interaction between biological, psychological, and interpersonal aspects of sexual dysfunction, its diagnosis and treatment requires close attention to the assessment and individual dynamics of a couple's relationship, as well as medical and developmental issues. Wider ranges of treatment options are now available for both male and female arousal and orgasmic disorders. Clinicians with relational, behavioral, and psychodynamic orientations are integrating sex therapy approaches with marital and couples therapy. Pharmacological intervention plays a more important role today in the treatment of sexual aversion, phobias, and severe anxiety, especially when combined with sex therapy. Furthermore, given the crisis nature of the AIDS epidemic, sexual treatment is an adaptive and judicious decision for couples who wish to strengthen and enhance their relationship.

Sexuality needs to be addressed in intra- and interfamilial contexts, and not just as the problem of an individual. Issues of intimacy, affection, and communication of feelings about sexuality are part of family life. This necessitates communicating to families a view of sexuality as a moral and expected part of a person's development. Treatment of sexual dysfunction cannot be separated from the treatment of the total family context, although in the past clinicians may have operated as separate entities depending on their various professional orientations. To enhance the total treatment possibilities, sex therapy must be integrated with marital and family therapy. Unless the therapist looks for the meaning of the couple's communication about their sexual problem—be it continual anger, emptiness, or some other pattern of behavior or affect—treatment cannot adequately address the sexual as well as the relational context of the problem.

Chapters on Related Topics

The following chapters describe concepts related to sex therapy:

- Chapter 20, "Couples Therapy: An Overview"
- Chapter 25, "Marital Enrichment in Clinical Practice"

VI

Family Therapy With Different Disorders

27

Family Variables and Interventions in Schizophrenia

David J. Miklowitz, Ph.D.
Martha C. Tompson, Ph.D.

Introduction

Several family variables have been found to distinguish families of patients with schizophrenia from those of nonschizophrenic individuals, to predict the onset of schizophrenia and related disorders, and to predict the course of schizophrenia once it is manifest. These family variables are all potential targets of inquiry in family or individual interventions, and knowledge of these variables is therefore valuable to clinicians who work with schizophrenic patients. In this chapter we review what is known about three family *risk indicators*, all measured in the relatives (usually the parents) of schizophrenic or preschizophrenic offspring:

- Communication deviance (CD; lack of communication clarity)
- Expressed emotion (EE; negative emotional attitudes)

Preparation of this chapter was supported in part by NIMH Grants MH43931, MH42556, and MH55101.

- Affective style (AS; negative emotional-verbal behavior in family interactions)[1]

We will also review controlled studies of the efficacy of family intervention in schizophrenic disorders, especially as applied to attempted modifications of the three family risk indicators. Table 27–1 describes the CD, EE, and AS constructs and their methods of measurement.

Table 27–1. Definition and measurement of family stress measures

Construct	Definition	Measurement method
Communication clarity		
Communication deviance (high vs. low)	Unclear, amorphous, or fragmented communication in relatives	Responses of relative to projective tests such as the Rorschach or TAT
Affective climate		
Expressed emotion (high vs. low)	Negative emotional attitudes of criticism, hostility, and/or emotional overinvolvement in relatives	Camberwell Family Interview, a 1.5-hour interview conducted with relatives during inpatient period
Affective style (benign vs. negative)	Emotional-verbal behavior of relatives during family discussions with patient; number of criticisms, guilt inductions, intrusions, and support statements	Verbatim transcripts of 10-minute interaction between relative and patient, assessed during postdischarge phase.

The Vulnerability-Stress Model

When investigating the role of family variables in schizophrenia, one must think of them as occurring within a network of genetic, biological, psychological, and environmental stress variables (as well as coping mechanisms).

---

[1] In studies of schizophrenia, the relatives assessed for these attributes have usually been biological parents. However, because some studies have included stepparents, spouses, and siblings, the more general term *relative* will be used throughout this chapter in lieu of *parent*.

This network and the family variables interact in a recursive fashion. It is no longer commonplace to think of family influences as an isolated variable in the study of schizophrenia. Rather, these influences are seen as linked to the pathogenesis of schizophrenia in terms of a vulnerability-stress model (Nuechterlein and Dawson 1984; Zubin and Spring 1977). In this model, a biological predisposition in an at-risk person is presumed to be present. Environmental stress serves to evoke or "kindle" this predisposition, which is expressed as episodes of schizophrenic disorder. These episodes in turn fuel family communication disturbances or conflict.

When a strong biological predisposition is present (i.e., the family pedigree is heavily loaded for schizophrenia), a minimal amount of stress may exceed existing individual or family coping mechanisms and precipitate an episode. When the predisposition is minimal, the stress must exceed a certain threshold (and coping must be inadequate) before an episode will occur. However, minimizing the predisposition through medication or other biological treatments, or minimizing stress and enhancing coping through psychosocial intervention or direct environmental manipulation, should reduce the synergistic impact of these factors and thereby reduce morbidity. Studies of CD, EE, and AS seek to clarify the nature of specific stressors in this equation, and determine whether modifying these stressors reduces their impact.

Communication Deviance

Studies of Diagnostic Discrimination

Perhaps the best-studied family variable in schizophrenia research is communication deviance. Although families of schizophrenic individuals have long been thought to be characterized by unclear communication (e.g., Bateson et al. 1956), Wynne and Singer (1963) are to be credited with the first operational and empirically based definitions of deviant communication styles. CD, also originally referred to as "transactional style deviance," denotes unclear, amorphous, or fragmented communication styles in families that disrupt the development of attention and logical thought in a developing child. Wynne and Singer (1963) measured CD through the responses of family members to the Rorschach exam and classified responses into three major categories: 1) closure problems, 2) disruptive communication behavior, and 3) peculiar language or logic. Although CD was thought to characterize the interactions of the whole family, it was typically the CD scores of parents that received the most attention in Wynne and Singer's empirical work.

Singer and Wynne (1963, 1965a, 1965b) found that parents of schizophrenic patients could be distinguished from parents of nonschizophrenic patients (i.e., families with autistic, withdrawn, borderline, neurotic, or normally developing offspring) on the basis of high scores on CD. Later studies have replicated this basic result, with 12 published studies indicating that levels of CD are higher for parents of schizophrenic patients than for parents of non-schizophrenic patients (for a review, see Miklowitz and Stackman 1992). This finding has been replicated in studies using both recent-onset and chronic patients, as well as remitted and acutely ill patients. It has also been replicated in studies employing different CD coding systems, including the original Rorschach system and a related system based on the Thematic Apperception Test (TAT; Jones 1977). However, studies subsequent to the Wynne-Singer work did not always find the degree of group differentiation in levels of parental CD that were found in the original studies.

There is some evidence that CD is more related to the level of offspring dysfunction than to the offspring's actual diagnosis. High levels of CD occur with equal frequency in parents of schizophrenic and bipolar-manic patients (Miklowitz et al. 1991) and increase as a direct function of the severity of the offspring's diagnosis (i.e., from normal to neurotic to borderline to schizophrenic) (Wynne et al. 1977). Levels of parental CD may also characterize the family environments of only certain subtypes of schizophrenic patients, particularly those considered to be highly thought-disordered (Sass et al. 1984).

What Role Does Communication Deviance Play in Schizophrenia?

Consistent with the vulnerability-stress model, early family researchers assumed that family factors correlated with the diagnosis of schizophrenia are also associated with, and causally related to, the onset of schizophrenia. Of course, family variables could also present as the result of reactions on the part of family members to disorders within the offspring. It is also possible that family variables such as CD only appear to have an environmental impact. These variables may actually be genetically based measures of vulnerability to schizophrenia that reflect heritable psychopathology in the parent or genetically transmissible disorders of attention or information processing. Each of these views will be considered and the supporting evidence examined.

Psychosocial Transmission Model

The first view, which will be referred to as the psychosocial transmission hypothesis, states that CD in parents develops well before any psychopathology in the child and directly affects the child's ability to reason, attend, and interpret stimuli within the environment. In this model, CD is believed to be a direct environmental contributor to vulnerability to schizophrenia, separate from but possibly interacting with other preexisting vulnerabilities (i.e., genetic or biological factors). It is presumed that the child internalizes the parents' deviant ways of thinking, processing information, deriving meaning, and interpreting reality. When the child is under stress in later life, these vulnerabilities of attention and logical thought become manifest as episodes of schizophrenic disorder (Woodward and Goldstein 1977; Wynne and Singer 1963).

There is evidence that CD tends to be highly stable over a period of at least a year (Velligan et al. 1995). CD also appears to be resistant to change even in the face of family interventions aimed at teaching communication skills (Nugter et al. 1997; Rund et al. 1995). Thus, among patients with high-CD family members, exposure to disordered communication may persist over time.

All of the diagnostic discrimination studies cited above were cross-sectional in design and employed samples of already diagnosed schizophrenic patients. The only direct evidence for the psychosocial transmission hypothesis comes from a longitudinal study of adolescents at high risk for schizophrenia, reported in a 5-year (Doane et al. 1981) and 15-year follow-up (Goldstein 1987). In this longitudinal study, four groups of disturbed but nonpsychotic adolescents were administered a series of behavioral and family assessments, including a TAT for each parent and family interaction tasks. Nearly all adolescents who developed schizophrenia spectrum disorders by the 15-year follow-up were from families that, at baseline, scored high on CD (based on the TAT assessments) and/or negative in AS (based on the interaction assessment). (Note that schizophrenia spectrum disorders are defined by DSM-III [American Psychiatric Association 1987] as a schizophrenic disorder or a schizotypal, paranoid, schizoid, or borderline personality disorder.) That is, those adolescents from families in which the parents communicated unclearly and/or were highly critical or intrusive in interactions with the adolescent (e.g., parents that indulge in "mind reading") were more likely than adolescents from families without these attributes to show disturbance within the psychotic spectrum in adulthood.

The relationships between family variables and longitudinal outcomes could not be fully explained by the adolescents' initial levels of behavioral disturbance or by psychopathology within the relative (Goldstein 1987). However, an interesting interaction emerged between CD and family history of severe psychiatric disorder in first- and second-degree relatives. Eighty-six percent of adolescents from families with high CD and a family history that was positive for severe psychopathology had developed spectrum disorders at follow-up, whereas only 20% of adolescents from families with high CD and no family history had developed these disorders (Goldstein 1987).

Using data from the Finnish Family Study that studied adoption in relation to schizophrenia, Wahlberg et al. (1997) examined genetic risk (defined as having a schizophrenic biological parent) and environmental risk (defined as having an adoptive parent high in CD) in the development of subsyndromal thought disorder. Findings revealed a highly significant interaction between genetic and environmental risk factors. Those offspring with both risk factors showed the highest level of thought disorder. Offspring with high genetic risk but low-CD adoptive parents showed the lowest level of thought disorder, suggesting that exposure to parental CD may place the vulnerable individual at risk for the development of disturbed thinking, even without shared genetic predispositions. These findings are consistent with Wynne and Singer's (1963) initial claims, as well as the vulnerability-stress model: family stress (as measured by CD) may only predict the development of schizophrenia or other severe psychiatric disorders in an adolescent if a genetic vulnerability to these disorders is already present.

In patients with manifest schizophrenic disorder, there is emerging evidence that parental CD may also be an ongoing stressor associated with higher risk of psychotic relapse following discharge from psychiatric hospitalization. Observing 20 male patients with schizophrenia, Velligan et al. (1996) evaluated parental CD during a family problem-solving task completed immediately before hospital discharge. Follow-up evaluations were then conducted at 3-month intervals. At 1 year after discharge there was a moderate association between CD and patient relapse.

Reactivity Model

In the reactivity model, CD is thought to come about in parents as a result of interacting with a disturbed child who has a thought disorder, delusions, hallucinations, or other forms of behavioral disturbance. Goldstein's (1987) finding that parental CD still predicted schizophrenia spectrum outcomes when the adolescents' initial levels of behavioral disturbance were covaried argues against this view. However, even in Goldstein's study, there may have been subtle aspects of the clinical profiles of the adolescents that affected parents' communication styles and that also explained the later appearance in these adolescents of schizophrenia spectrum disorders.

If CD is indeed a reaction to offspring disturbance, one would expect to find that 1) parents only express CD to their schizophrenic offspring and not to other persons, and 2) patients have levels of communication disturbance that equal or most likely exceed those of their parents. Data on these issues generally do not support a reactivity model. First, most of the existing studies have shown CD to have diagnostic discriminatory power even when CD scores were based on Rorschach or TAT examinations done individually with parents, rather than with the patient or offspring present. Glaser (1976) found that levels of parental CD on the Rorschach, when measured in an individual, a spousal (other parent present), and a family setting, were actually lowest when the parent was interacting with the target patient. Second, in a sample of 114 offspring with conditions ranging from normal to severely schizophrenic, Wynne et al. (1977) found that parents of schizophrenic patients had higher CD scores than the patients themselves (both assessed using individual Rorschach methodology). Wynne and colleagues also found that parent CD scores were more closely associated with the diagnosis of schizophrenia in offspring than were offspring CD scores. Finally, Johnston and Holzman (1979) did find that levels of parental CD were correlated with levels of CD in schizophrenic offspring, but the association was weak.

It appears that parental CD is not simply a reaction to offspring communication disturbance. However, other attributes of schizophrenic patients, such as irritability, negative symptoms, and psychotic behavior, might disrupt the communication styles of parents. Thus, the reactivity model has not been adequately explored.

Shared Vulnerability Model

The shared vulnerability model suggests the possibility that parents and schizophrenic or preschizophrenic offspring share a genetically (or psychosocially) transmitted vulnerability in cognitive processing. This model reflects the finding that CD in parents is both cross-sectionally and prospectively associated with offspring schizophrenia, in addition to the well-documented finding that schizophrenic patients have information processing deficits (Nuechterlein and Dawson 1984). Certain CD codes in the Rorschach and TAT systems (i.e., misperceptions, inability to integrate stimuli into a coherent whole) resemble attentional or perceptual anomalies, whereas other codes appear to represent linguistic or verbal reasoning disturbances (i.e., sentence fragments, unintelligible phrases). Thus, one might expect to find that scores on the Rorschach and TAT CD codes would be highest among parents whose schizophrenic offspring have pronounced attentional disturbances.

In a sample of 25 chronic schizophrenic patients, Wagener et al. (1986) found that high maternal scores on two TAT-based CD substyles—"Misperceptions" and "Failure to Integrate Closure Problems"—were associated with poor performance by these mothers and by their schizophrenic offspring on measures of attentional vigilance (the Continuous Performance Test, or CPT) and guided visual search (the Span of Apprehension Test, or SPAN). Similar cross-generational associations between CD in mothers (most consistently the Misperceptions CD factor) and offspring attentional performance were found in a sample of patients with recent-onset schizophrenia (Nuechterlein et al. 1989) and in a sample of schizophrenic and schizotypal school-aged children (Asarnow et al. 1988).

These linkages between CD in mothers, their own information-processing deficits, and the information-processing deficits of their diagnosed offspring lend credence to the view that certain forms of CD may reflect broader, cross-generational vulnerabilities in perceptual-cognitive functioning. Because attentional test performance in schizophrenic patients appears to be at least in part genetically mediated (Holzman 1987; Nuechterlein and Dawson 1984), the possibility arises that CD in itself reflects an inherited attribute. Of course, these findings could also be construed as consistent with a psychosocial model that postulates an internalization of deviant styles of attending or interpreting reality by an at-risk child. In addition, not all forms of CD necessarily reflect attentional disturbances. Those forms of CD that reflect disturbances in linguistic-verbal reasoning (e.g., odd word usage) may come about through different etiological mechanisms.

Parental Psychopathology Model

The parental psychopathology model states that CD is an indirect measure of psychopathology in parents. Parents with high CD generally have not been found to have more severe psychopathology than parents with low CD (Goldstein 1987; Goldstein et al. 1992; Wynne et al. 1976, 1977). Most of these studies, however, defined psychopathology rather broadly (i.e., mild versus moderate versus severe disorders) rather than focusing on specific disorders or considering psychopathology on a continuum that includes subsyndromal disorders. Thus, this model deserves further exploration.

Communication Deviance: Summary of Findings

Several conclusions can be drawn about the communication deviance research:

- CD occurs at greater levels among parents of schizophrenic patients than among parents of nonpsychotic patients, but the levels are not necessarily greater than among parents of patients with other forms of psy-

chosis. Perhaps most parsimonious is the conclusion that levels of CD are correlated with the severity of offspring psychopathology.
- High CD, along with negative AS, may be a risk marker for the development of schizophrenia spectrum disorders among vulnerable adolescents, particularly if a genetic predisposition is also present.
- CD in parents may be associated with schizophrenia in offspring via vulnerabilities in attending, perceiving, or processing information that are shared across generations.
- Much remains to be learned about CD, including 1) whether this attribute is related to the distress caused by interacting with a schizophrenic offspring; 2) whether CD in any way reflects subtle forms of psychopathology in the index parent; and 3) whether CD's association with long-term outcomes in at-risk children is a function of shared genetic vulnerabilities, psychosocial mechanisms, or both.

Negative Affective Communication Variables: Expressed Emotion and Affective Style

Whereas studies of CD concern communication clarity, studies of EE and AS concern the affective tone of family attitudes or interactional behaviors. Also, whereas CD studies generally concern diagnostic discrimination or prediction of the onset of schizophrenia, studies of family affective variables focus on predicting the course of schizophrenic disorder once it is manifest. Identification of family risk indicators in the course of schizophrenia has been useful in generating psychosocial intervention strategies that appear to reduce the morbidity of schizophrenia in otherwise relapse-prone patients.

Negative Affective Communication as a Predictive Index

As indicated in Table 27–1, EE and AS differ in two important ways. First, EE is a measure of emotional attitudes (i.e., criticism, hostility, and/or emotional overinvolvement [EOI]) among relatives, whereas AS is a measure of a relative's emotional-verbal behavior toward the patient during interactions (i.e., critical, guilt-inducing, intrusive, or supportive statements). Second, EE is typically measured during the patient's hospital stay, whereas AS is typically measured once the patient has returned to the community and achieved a degree of remission.

As of this writing, there are 27 published studies of the predictive validity of family EE attitudes in schizophrenic patients (Table 27–2).

Table 27–2. Expressed emotion and schizophrenic relapse

				Relapse rate (%)	
Study	N	Duration	Location/population	High EE	Low EE
Brown et al. 1962	97	1 year	Great Britain	56	21
Brown et al. 1972	101	9 months	Great Britain	58	16
Vaughn and Leff 1976	37	9 months	Great Britain	48	6
Vaughn et al. 1984	54	9 months	Great Britain	56	17
Kottgen et al. 1984	34	9 months	Germany	50	55[a]
Moline et al. 1985	24	2 years	United States[b]	71	29
Nuechterlein et al. 1986	26	1 year	United States	37	0
MacMillan et al. 1987	77	2 years	United States	63	39
Karno et al. 1985	44	9 months	United States[c]	59	26
Leff et al. 1987	49	1 year	India	33	14
Rostworowska et al. 1987	36	9 months	Poland	60	9
Hogarty et al. 1988	70	1 year	United States	19	15[a]
Tarrier et al. 1988b	48	9 months	Great Britain	48	21
Parker et al. 1988	57	9 months	Australia	48	60[a]
Arevalo and Vizcarro 1989	31	9 months	Spain	44	38
Barrelet at al. 1990	36	9 months	Switzerland	33	0
Stirling et al. 1991	33	1 year	Great Britain	31	47[a]
Bertrando et al. 1992	42	9 months	Italy	58	22
Montero et al. 1992	59	2 years	Spain	29	23[a]
Mozny and Votypkova 1992	125	1 year	Czech Republic	59	23
Niedermeier et al. 1992	49	1 year	Germany	57	29

Table 27–2. Expressed emotion and schizophrenic relapse (*continued*)

Study	N	Duration	Location/population	Relapse rate (%)	
				High EE	Low EE
Nuechterlein et al. 1992	43	1 year	United States	39	0
Vaughan et al. 1992	88	9 months	Australia	53	24
Ito and Oshima 1995	72	9 months	Japan	48	8
Phillips and Xiong 1995	49	3 years	China	72	66[a]
Linszen et al. 1996	39	15 months	Netherlands	23	0
Mino et al. 1997	52	2 years	Japan	58	21

[a]Indicates nonreplication.
[b]Mostly African Americans with low socioeconomic status.
[c]Spanish-speaking Mexican Americans.
Source.   Butzlaff and Hooley 1998; Koenigsberg and Handley 1986; Parker and Hadzi-Pavlovic 1990.

Of these 27 studies, 21 have shown that patients returning to high-EE families (those in which at least one key relative is highly critical, hostile, and/or emotionally overinvolved) relapse at two to three times the rate of those returning to low-EE (not critical or overinvolved) homes (see reviews by Butzlaff and Hooley 1998; Goldstein et al. 1997; Koenigsberg and Handley 1986; Kuipers and Bebbington 1988; Parker and Hadzi-Pavlovic 1990). This rather robust result has been replicated across different cultures and languages, across recent-onset and chronic patients, and across patients maintained on standardized neuroleptic medications and those for whom medication regimens and compliance have varied. Finally, the EE-relapse association has been extended to samples of unipolar depressive (Hooley et al. 1986; Vaughn and Leff 1976), bipolar affective (Miklowitz et al. 1988), alcoholic (O'Farrell et al. 1998), eating-disordered (Hodes and Le Grange 1993), and obese patients (Fischmann-Havstad and Marston 1984). Thus, EE may function as a more general risk factor associated with poor outcome among individuals with psychiatric disorders.

As indicated in Table 27–2, knowing that a patient is returning from hospital to a low-EE home yields more reliable prognostic information than does knowing that a patient is returning to a high-EE home (Goldstein et al. 1992). Specifically, one can be relatively confident of a nonrelapsing outcome in a patient from a low-EE home (77% will stay well), but forecasting relapse in a patient from a high-EE home would be wrong about half of the time. This pattern of results has led some (e.g., Mintz et al. 1987) to suggest that EE is best conceptualized as a protective rather than a risk factor in the vulnerability-stress equation.

Less is known about the prognostic utility of AS. The utility of AS in predicting schizophrenia spectrum outcomes among vulnerable adolescents has already been discussed (Goldstein 1987). Only one study (Doane et al. 1985) has examined the prognostic utility of AS in diagnosed schizophrenic patients. Among patients receiving individual, supportive therapy with neuroleptic medication (the Falloon et al. [1984] treatment-outcome study), relapses at 9-month follow-ups were more frequent if, at 3 months after the patient's hospital discharge, the family had been rated negative in AS (at least one relative was harshly critical or excessively intrusive) rather than benign in AS (no relatives were harshly critical or excessively intrusive). A similar result was documented in a 9-month naturalistic follow-up of bipolar, manic patients (Miklowitz et al. 1988).

Negativity within the family milieu, expressed either as an attitude or as an interactional behavior, appears to represent a risk marker for subsequent relapse among schizophrenic and other psychiatric patients. It may be that EE and AS are generic stress variables that interact with illness-specific vulnerabilities in bringing about episodes of psychiatric disorder.

What is less clear is what is actually measured by these variables: which aspects of the intrafamilial milieu these variables describe, whether they are reactive to attributes of the patient or instead measure processes "located" within the relative, whether they are state or trait, and whether they can be said to have a causal influence on patient outcomes. These questions will be addressed below.

Expressed Emotion and Affective Style as Clinical Constructs

What are the origins of expressed emotion and affective style? As was the case for CD, several models of the genesis of EE attitudes or AS behaviors have been proposed. A *reactivity* model views family affective variables as responses to attributes of the patient—attributes that have their own prognostic utility (e.g., symptom severity, premorbid adjustment). A *within-relative* model views these attributes as directly arising from relatives' attributes (e.g., levels of psychopathology). A *transactional* model views family variables as reflecting both relative and patient attributes. In this view, relatives and patients are locked into interaction patterns that are mutually produced but that in some cases have negative consequences for the course of the patient's illness. The existing research literature will be evaluated in light of these models.

Expressed Emotion and Affective Style

Are EE and AS correlated with symptomatic or illness attributes of patients? The reactivity model postulates that the disruptiveness of some forms of schizophrenic disorder engenders critical and/or overprotective attitudes or behaviors in relatives. Are patients from high-EE or negative-AS families indeed "sicker" to begin with, and therefore more relapse-prone?

In general, no relation has been found between the level of patient symptom severity during or following the acute episode and the family's EE status (Brown et al. 1972; Miklowitz et al. 1983; Nuechterlein et al. 1986; Vaughn and Leff 1976). Whereas earlier studies did find relations between EE and the patient's previous level of work impairment or disturbed behavior during the 3 months prior to admission (Brown et al. 1972; Vaughn and Leff 1976), these factors apparently did not account for the longitudinal-predictive value of EE.

Perhaps more valid tests of the relation between EE, AS, and patient illness status are provided by studies that assess family variables during the baseline hospitalization and again after a 9-month or 1-year interval. The purpose of these studies was to determine if changes over time in family variables are correlated with changes in patient state. Several studies (Brown et al. 1972; Dulz and Hand 1986; Hogarty et al. 1986; Tarrier et al. 1988b) have found that 25%–50% of initially high-EE critical parents are low-EE by follow-up. In several of these studies, the degree of reduction in relatives' criticisms paralleled improvements in the patient's clinical state. Indeed, EE may be more likely to go from high to low over time when, due to the patient's improved social functioning, relatives experience a reduction in their burden of care (Scazufca and Kuipers 1998). Levels of EOI appear less likely than criticism to change in concert with patient improvement.

It does appear that EE criticism is to some extent state-dependent, although only a proportion of high-EE relatives show these state-based changes. Hooley (1989) was able to show that even though high-EE-critical parents of schizophrenic patients showed mean reductions in EE criticisms from an inpatient assessment to a 3-month outpatient assessment, these parents preserved their sample rank order (in terms of number of EE criticisms) at the 3-month follow-up. Despite the restricted range of scores at follow-up, the most critical parents were still the most critical when the patient was in remission.

Equally notable is Hooley and Richters' (1985) observation that the frequency of critical comments among parents of schizophrenic patients increases monotonically with the duration of the patient's illness. Relatives who had been coping with the illness for 3–5 years showed an average of 15 critical comments on the Camberwell Interview, whereas those coping with the illness for less than 1 year averaged 4.2 critical comments. Hooley and Richters (1985, p. 145) explain their results as follows:

> Coping with a chronic psychiatric illness in a close relative strains the financial, physical, and emotional resources of the best of families....Despite intentions to the contrary, initially supportive attitudes may become replaced by feelings of frustration, intolerance, and lack of patience for the symptoms and behavioral impairments that typically accompany severe psychiatric conditions.

There is some evidence that the EE attitudinal subtypes criticism and EOI are differentially associated with patient attributes. Miklowitz et al. (1983) found that schizophrenic patients from emotionally overinvolved, high-EE homes had poorer premorbid psychosocial adjustment and higher levels of residual symptoms postdischarge than did patients from high-EE critical or low-EE homes. Nuechterlein et al. (1986) found that over-involvement was far less frequent an attitude than criticism among parents of schizophrenic patients who had been ill for less than 2 years. In contrast to criticism, overinvolvement may come about in part as a reaction among relatives to patients with a poor-prognosis subtype of schizophrenia.

Fewer data exist on these questions for AS. In two samples of schizophrenic patients, AS scores were not related to patient symptomatology scores, demographic variables, illness history variables, or premorbid ratings (Miklowitz et al. 1984, 1989). In a controlled family treatment study (Falloon et al. 1984), AS scores became more negative from a postdischarge assessment to a 3-month follow-up among untreated families, even though patients improved over this same time interval (Doane et al. 1986). Thus, AS is not clearly driven by global features of the patient's illness, although this issue deserves more consideration.

Is EE or AS associated with physiological changes in the patient? Data on patient symptomatic states, illness history, and premorbid variables reveal only a certain amount about the viability of the reactivity model. For example, do patients change on a physiological level when interacting with a high- or a low-EE relative, and do relatives detect these changes and react with negativity? Can a bridge be drawn between the neurophysiological vulnerabilities characteristic of schizophrenia and family environmental factors that may impact or be affected by these vulnerabilities?

Tarrier et al. (1979) devised a paradigm in which remitted schizophrenic outpatients were interviewed by a clinician while being assessed for skin conductance fluctuation rate (SCR, a measure of arousal), after which the patients' high- or low-EE parents entered the room. Patients whose low-EE parents entered showed a habituation of SCRs, indicating decreased physiological arousal, whereas patients whose high-EE parents entered did not habituate. Tarrier et al. (1988a) replicated this result in acutely ill schizophrenic patients but also found that there were overall mean differences between high- and low-EE patient groups in skin conductance level (a more stable measure of tonic physiological arousal), independent of the presence or absence of patients' relatives. Finally, among acutely ill schizophrenic patients from high- and low-EE families, Sturgeon et al. (1984) did not replicate the findings of Tarrier et al. (1979, 1988a) in the relative-absent/relative-present paradigm but did find group differences in SCRs in the resting (baseline) state.

Two of these three studies suggest that patients are generally more aroused by high-EE than by low-EE parents. Resting differences in arousal, however, have only been found during the acutely ill state. When patients from high- and low-EE families are in remission, differences in physiological arousal may only become evident when an environmental challenge (i.e., entry of the relative or other stimulation) is introduced.

Future studies should examine whether these patient differences in physiological reactivity are in any way indicative of proclivity for relapse, independent of family variables. Perhaps measures like SCR reflect disorders in neurotransmitter systems that may in themselves bode poorly for outcome. Also, examining whether physiological state changes occur in a predictable sequence among schizophrenic patients participating in family interactions (e.g., do changes in SCR occur immediately prior to or following a relative's AS criticism or intrusive statement?) would help to determine whether 1) patients are indeed affected by their relatives on a physiological level or 2) whether relatives, on interacting with the patient, somehow sense changes in the patient's physiological state, code these changes as interpersonal defensiveness, and react with negativity.

Is EE or AS associated with factors within the relative? Are relatives who are high-EE (or negative-AS) at higher risk for schizophrenia or other forms of severe psychopathology than are low-EE (or benign-AS) relatives? Goldstein et al. (1992) reported no association between parental EE attitudes (assessed during an inpatient period with the Camberwell Interview) and independently obtained diagnostic data on these parents. However, when they considered ratings of EE obtained during the outpatient period—based on a brief measure of EE known as the *five-minute speech sample* (FMSS; Magana et al. 1986)[2]—an interesting interaction emerged. Parents who were rated high-EE on *both* the Camberwell and FMSS measures were more likely to have psychiatric diagnoses (7 of 7, or 100%) than those who were high-EE on one measure and not the other (11 of 22, or 50%) or who were low-EE on both measures (12 of 27, or 44%).

The correspondence between Camberwell- and FMSS-rated EE is less than perfect (Miklowitz and Goldstein 1993). Thus, it is unclear whether to attribute the association between the two measures of EE and parental psychopathology to time or method variance. That is, parents who are high-EE on both measures (assessed at two different time points) may have stable, traitlike EE attitudes that do not vary with changes in patient state. It may also be that these parents have lower thresholds for expressing negative attitudes, such that these attitudes are as easily identified by a brief probe like the FMSS as by the longer Camberwell measure, regardless of the time of administration. Thus, psychopathology in a relative may predict the stability of

---

[2]Magana et al. (1986) devised a system for coding EE from a 5-minute speech sample (FMSS), which requires the respondent to talk about another family member and describe "what kind of person he/she is and how the two of you get along together." Rates of correspondence between Camberwell and FMSS ratings of EE status (low versus high) averaged 72% over four studies (sensitivity, 0.60; specificity, 0.89) (Miklowitz and Goldstein 1993). The most frequent errors of classification by the FMSS are false negatives: a number of relatives rated high-EE on the Camberwell are classified as low-EE by the FMSS.

EE attitudes over time or the threshold for their expression.

Hooley (1987) took a cognitive-attributional perspective on the internal processes occurring within a key relative who is high- or low-EE. According to her model, critical relatives are those who make "internal," "personal," or "controllable" attributions about the patient (e.g., that the patient is actually able to control his or her symptoms but is refusing to do so). In contrast, low-EE relatives are those who adopt an illness or other "external" model in explaining their son or daughter's behavior, viewing this behavior as at least to some degree out of the patient's control. Several investigators have provided evidence in support of this view. First, Berkowitz et al. (1984) found that high-EE parents of schizophrenic patients were more likely to believe that the patient's disturbed behavior was not due to an illness, whereas low-EE parents more readily accepted the illness notion. Second, Weisman et al. (1998) conducted content analysis of CFI protocols and revealed that relatives were more likely to criticize "deficit" symptoms, which may be interpreted as controllable by the patient, than symptoms reflecting psychotic processes, which can easily be understood as uncontrollable. Third, higher CFI criticism has been found to be associated with more attributions of controllability (Lopez et al. 1999). Finally, among relatives participating in psychoeducational programs targeted at reducing EE, changes in EE were paralleled by increases in universal attributions and attributions to the illness, suggesting a link between EE and attributions (Brewin 1994).

Hooley (1998) has showed that high-EE relatives of schizophrenic patients are themselves more likely than low-EE relatives to themselves have an internal locus of control. It may be that relatives who view events, problems, successes, and failures as largely under a person's control are more likely to be intolerant of a patient-relative who may appear to be doing very little to improve his or her situation.

Putting Hooley's model together with the data from Goldstein et al. (1992), it could be argued that a prior history of psychiatric problems in an index parent, problems that the parent largely succeeded in overcoming, may generate an attributional style about psychiatric disorder that says, "I handled my situation through hard work and effort. Why can't others?" Indeed, most of the diagnosable psychopathology that Goldstein et al. (1992) found among relatives occurred in the past rather than being present at the time of the EE interviews. Thus, high-EE critical attitudes may in some relatives reflect the endpoint of a pathway from prior psychopathology to specific attributional patterns. If the patient, in turn, views his or her only hope as coming from the outside (e.g., through finding the best doctor), a fundamental difference in opinion about treatment and recovery may develop between the patient and relative. This difference of opinion may in turn be reflected in their reciprocal interactional behavior (see discussion of transactional model, below).

Emotional overinvolvement, on the other hand, may involve somewhat different processes. Bentsen et al. (1998) showed that guilt-proneness in family members is highly associated with EOI and negatively associated with criticism. Thus, family members who feel particularly guilty about the patient's symptoms may be inclined to take extraordinary measures to help the patient overcome his or her difficulties.

There are no published data on the relations between AS and diagnosable psychopathology or specific attributional processes in relatives. These issues deserve exploration, as the affective qualities of transactions within the family milieu may be explainable in part by the phenomenon of *interlocking psychopathologies.*

Do relatives express EE? The transactional model states that EE and AS both reflect ongoing interactional processes in the family that are mutually and reciprocally produced by relatives and patients. If so, one should see a relatively high correspondence between the two measures. Does a dichotomous variable like EE in any way characterize the way a family behaves once the patient has returned home from the hospital?

Several studies have investigated whether EE, measured during the inpatient phase, is associated with AS interactional behavior during the outpatient phase (Miklowitz et al. 1984, 1989; Strachan et al. 1986a, 1986b). In each of these studies, high-EE relatives of schizophrenic patients were found to be more negative in AS interactional behavior (i.e., more critical and/or intrusive) than were low-EE relatives. There were also parallels between the specific EE attitude manifested by relatives and their specific AS behavior during the interaction task. Miklowitz et al. (1984) and Strachan et al. (1986) both found that high-EE, primarily critical parents of schizophrenic patients were most frequently AS-critical in family interactions, whereas high-EE parents who were primarily emotionally overinvolved tended to be more AS-intrusive (i.e., using many "mind-reading," boundary-crossing statements).

In one of our studies of the EE/AS relationship (Miklowitz et al. 1989), we found that high-EE critical attitudes measured during the inpatient phase (by the Camberwell Interview) were associated with AS-critical behavior during the outpatient phase only if parents were also rated high-EE critical on the brief FMSS measure of EE administered during this same outpatient session. Families who were initially high-EE on the Camberwell and later were low-EE on the FMSS were no more critical in direct interaction than were consistently low-EE relatives. These different results may reflect that patients in this sample, as contrasted with earlier samples, were drawn from an ongoing study of recent-onset schizophrenia (Nuechterlein et al.

1986) and achieved more complete remissions once discharged to the home. Perhaps as a result, the EE attitudes expressed by relatives during the height of the psychotic episode were less predictive of their interactional behavior during the aftercare period than were the EE attitudes they conveyed during this same aftercare period.

Do patients reciprocate these attitudes or behaviors? There is a related question raised by the transactional model: do patients reciprocate high-EE attitudes or negative-AS behaviors? That is, do family variables like EE or AS tap a system of transactional processes, or are they best viewed as emanating from the relative?

Miklowitz and Goldstein (1993) found that in a pilot sample of 20 schizophrenic and bipolar patients, EE attitudes in mothers (as measured by the FMSS) were reciprocated by patients (also on the FMSS) about 75% of the time. However, the form of the patient's high-EE attitude toward the mother (i.e., critical versus overinvolved) as expressed on the FMSS did not always match that of the corresponding mother.

Strachan et al. (1989), working within the Nuechterlein et al. (1986) recent-onset schizophrenic sample, found that schizophrenic patients from high-EE critical and/or negative-AS homes were likely to behave in direct interaction in one of two ways: by emitting "counter-criticisms" of the parent (a *symmetrical* interaction pattern) or by internalizing criticisms through making "self-denigrating" statements (a *complementary* pattern). In contrast, patients from low-EE homes were more likely to emit *strong autonomy* statements when interacting with their low-EE parents (i.e., statements indicating self-sufficiency and goal-directedness).

In this same sample, Hahlweg et al. (1989) observed that long chains of "negative reciprocity" occurred in high-EE families, interchanges that were equally likely to be initiated by parent or patient. In some high-EE families, volleys of criticism followed by countercriticism occurred as many as 10 consecutive times in a single 10-minute parent-patient interaction. In contrast, when negative interchanges occurred in low-EE families, the parent or patient was likely to interrupt these processes before the interaction spiraled out of control (Hahlweg et al. 1989).

In a series of studies of families with a schizophrenic member, investigators at the University of California at Los Angeles coded both verbal and nonverbal subclinical symptomatic behaviors of patients during laboratory-based family interaction tasks (Rosenfarb et al. 1995; Woo et al. 1997). Patients with high-EE relatives were more odd and disruptive and displayed more hostile and unusual nonverbal behavior during the family interactions than did patients with low-EE relatives, who demonstrated more anxious nonverbal behavior. Furthermore, high-EE relatives were more likely than low-EE relatives to respond with criticisms to unusual verbalizations made by the patients, which in turn increased the likelihood of subsequent unusual verbalizations from the patient. Thus, high-EE relatives were more likely to be exposed to odd and difficult behavior in the patient and to respond critically; patients seemed to increase their symptomatic behaviors in response to these criticisms. These data support the notion that transactional processes in the families of high-EE patients may lead to increasingly symptomatic patient behavior.

Together, these data suggest that patients are aware of high-EE attitudes and behaviors on the part of their relatives and respond in a symmetrical or complementary manner. Thus, EE and AS may be indicative of ongoing, mutually produced transactional processes within the family.

Affective Communication Variables: Summary of Findings

Several overall conclusions can be drawn from the existing literature on EE and AS in families of patients with schizophrenia:

- EE and AS are two related but not isomorphic measures of family functioning. EE attitudes are reliable predictors of relapse in schizophrenia over 9-month to 1-year periods of follow-up. The data on the predictive value of AS are sparse but speak to the potential of this construct as a prognostic indicator.
- Although overall levels of EE and AS are not strongly correlated with patient illness attributes when evaluated cross-sectionally (reactivity model), there is evidence from longitudinal studies that as patients improve, levels of EE criticism drop. In contrast, levels of EE emotional overinvolvement are less reactive to changes in patient state. Over-involvement may be cross-sectionally associated with poor prognostic patient attributes.
- Patients from high- and low-EE families differ in levels of physiological arousal, with the difference becoming most evident when the patient encounters the key relative.
- Levels of EE criticism may to some extent reflect internal attributes of relatives such as prior psychopathology or specific behaviors attributed to the patient (the within-relative model).
- EE and AS in part reflect ongoing, bidirectional interaction patterns within the family, in which the patient is an active participant (transactional model).
- Identification of the determinants of high-EE attitudes and negative-AS behaviors, and the protective factors that operate in low-EE and/or benign-AS families, are important goals for future research.

Family Intervention Studies

Family intervention studies can help clarify cause-and-effect relationships between family variables and patient outcomes. None of the studies reviewed above can fully resolve the cause-effect association between family variables and patient outcomes, because a virtually unlimited number of third variables could explain these predictive relationships. A more convincing test of the causal-reactive question is to attempt to modify levels of EE, AS, or CD via family intervention and then determine whether making these modifications leads to reductions in the short-term morbidity of schizophrenia. Of course, controlled family intervention studies are also of interest because they may 1) provide evidence for the utility of adjunctive psychosocial treatments for relapse-prone schizophrenic patients, and 2) lead to the identification of previously unobserved aspects of family functioning that serve as risk or protective factors in the vulnerability-stress equation.

A number of studies have examined the use of family-based treatments. Goldstein and Miklowitz (1995) distinguished between "first generation" and "second generation" family studies. First-generation studies focus on establishing the efficacy of family interventions as adjuncts to psychotropic medications during the stabilization and maintenance phases of treatment for schizophrenia. They answer the question "Do family treatments improve the course of the illness?" First-generation studies have generally compared family intervention with either medication only or medication plus individual therapy conditions. Second-generation studies attempt to answer the question "Is one form of family treatment superior to other forms?" These studies have compared different models of family treatment with each other.

First-Generation Family Intervention Studies

Several controlled family intervention studies have been conducted (Tables 27–3 and 27–4), and most have attempted to reduce existing levels of negative affective communication and morbidity. None to date has attempted to modify levels of CD.

The Goldstein Crisis Intervention Model

The first study (Goldstein et al. 1978) was an implementation of the Goldstein crisis intervention model. The study occurred before the research on EE and AS was fully developed and therefore did not include assessments of these variables. In this study, 96 hospitalized, acutely ill schizophrenic pa-

Table 27–3. Family intervention studies: first-generation studies

Study	Follow-up period	Family group: % relapsed	Comparison group: % relapsed	Nature of comparison group
Goldstein et al. 1978	6 months	0	17	Moderate neuroleptic dose; no therapy
Leff et al. 1982[a]	9 months	8	50	Routine treatment
Falloon et al. 1984[b]	9 months	6	44	Family education
Hogarty et al. 1986[c]	1 year	19	20	Individual skills training
Tarrier et al. 1988b	9 months	12[d]	53	Routine treatment
Leff et al. 1989	9 months	8	36	Education; relatives groups
Xiong et al. 1994	1 year	33	61	Routine treatment
Randolph et al. 1994	1 year	14	55	Routine treatment

[a]Two-year relapse rates: family, 33%; comparison, 75%.
[b]Two-year relapse rates: family, 17%; comparison, 83%.
[c]Two-year relapse rates: family, 29%; comparison, 50%.
[d]Relapse rate is a mean for two behavioral family treatments.

Table 27–4. Family intervention studies: second-generation studies

Study	Follow-up period	Family group: % relapsed/rehospitalized	Comparison group: % relapsed/rehospitalized	Nature of comparison treatment
Schooler et al. 1997	2 years	29% (hospitalized)	35% (hospitalized)	Psychoeducational workshop; monthly family group meetings
McFarlane et al. 1995a, 1995b	2 years	27%	16%	Psychoeducational sessions (three or four) with individual family plus multiple family groups
Linszen et al. 1997	15 months	16%	15%	Family sessions (three or four) plus individual treatment

tients participated in a study with a 2 × 2 factorial design, in which neuroleptic dosage (low vs. moderate) was crossed with family therapy versus no family therapy. The family therapy was a six-session outpatient crisis treatment in which patients and their family members attempted to understand the events and precipitants surrounding the current psychotic episode and plan for possible future episodes by identifying stressors and developing coping strategies.

Relapse rates at 6-month follow-up were as follows: no therapy, low-dose neuroleptics, 48%; no therapy, moderate-dose, 17%; family therapy, low-dose, 22%; and family therapy, moderate-dose, 0%. Thus, there was an additive effect of family therapy and neuroleptic dosage in delaying psychotic relapses, as would be predicted by the vulnerability-stress model.

Leff's Social Intervention Program

The first study by Leff et al. (1982) compared a social intervention ($n=12$)—consisting of an educational program about schizophrenia, a relatives support group, and in-home family treatment sessions that included the patient—with routine outpatient care ($n=12$). All patients began in an acute phase of illness and were maintained as outpatients on neuroleptics. Patients were selected to be at high risk for relapse based on having high face-to-face contact (over 35 hours per week) with a high-EE parent or spouse. The goals of the social intervention were to reduce face-to-face contact and EE, which the investigators had found in earlier work to be conjoint predictors of relapses of schizophrenia (Leff and Vaughn 1985; Vaughn and Leff 1976).

Relapses at 9-month follow-up were 8% for patients whose families received the social intervention and 50% for those in routine care. Furthermore, when EE and/or face-to-face contact were successfully reduced in treated families, no patient relapsed. Reductions in EE and contact were also observed in the control families, but less frequently. Results were weakened over a 2-year follow-up (Leff et al. 1985).

The second study (Leff et al. 1989) selected schizophrenic patients on the basis of similar high-risk inclusion criteria. In this study, however, Leff and colleagues attempted to determine which aspects of the social intervention from the first study were most potent in bringing about reductions in EE, contact, and relapse. They compared a 9-month relatives group ($n=11$) with a home-based family therapy ($n=12$). Patients once again received maintenance medication. Families also received two sessions of education about schizophrenia.

Relapses occurred in 8% of the patients in the family therapy condition, and in 36% of those in the relatives group condition, a nonsignificant difference. Reductions in EE and amount of contact were achieved in 73% of the family therapy cases and in 71% of the relatives group cases. However, the relatives groups were attended by only 6 of the 11 assigned families, and the relapse rate among patients from families not compliant with the relatives groups was 60%, versus 17% among patients from compliant families. Thus, the two treatments were comparable in efficacy when relatives actually attended, but the family therapy, perhaps because it was held in the home, was more readily accepted by families.

Falloon's Behavioral Family Management

Falloon et al. (1984), working within a behavioral family management (BFM) model that emphasized the protective effects of skill acquisition in high-risk family situations, compared a 9-month trial of home-based BFM ($n=18$) to a 9-month supportive individual therapy regimen for the patient ($n=18$). Both the BFM trial and the individual therapy regimen were of equal frequency and administered with maintenance medication. Families in both conditions received two sessions of education immediately following the patient's hospital discharge. The BFM consisted of two additional components: training in communication skills, and problem solving. After 9 months, only 1 of the 18 BFM patients (6%) had relapsed, whereas 8 of 18 (44%) of the individually treated patients had relapsed. After 2 years, patients in the family condition had spent less time in the hospital, had shown less behavioral disturbance, had more friends and better occupational adjustment, and reported better intrafamilial relations.

Ratings of EE were not available after treatment as they had been in the Leff studies discussed in the previous section. However, Falloon's group did conduct family interaction assessments prior to treatment and again 3 months into the treatment, allowing a comparison of pretreatment versus follow-up AS scores (Doane et al. 1986). They found that 69% of the families of patients who were in individual treatment showed increases in overall levels of AS from the pretreatment to the 3-month follow-up assessments, whereas only 29% of the families in BFM showed increases in AS. Relapses in the individual treatment condition were most likely to occur by the 9-month follow-up if the family showed increases in AS over the first 3 months of treatment. Doane and colleagues (1986) also showed that decreases in AS for families in BFM were accompanied by corresponding increases in "problem-solving statements." Thus, the interactions of families in BFM became less affectively charged and more goal-directed.

Although this treatment was clearly effective, its home-based format made it unwieldy in many regular outpatient treatment settings. Randolph et al. (1994) completed a study examining the utility of a clinic-based version of Falloon and colleagues' BFM (Falloon et al. 1984). Patients were seen at a Veterans Administration outpatient clinic and were randomly assigned to BFM and customary care or to customary care only. Families in treatment attended an average of 21 sessions over the 12-month intervention period. Whereas only 15% of patients (3 of 20) receiving the BFM treatment had an exacerbation of symptoms during the intervention, fully 52% of those in customary care (11 of 21) experienced an exacerbation of symptoms. Thus, the BFM model appears efficacious in both home- and clinic-based settings. Randolph and colleagues found that the BFM was equally effective in both high- and low-EE families (Randolph et al. 1994); however, this study was not able to examine change in EE as a possible mediator of treatment effects.

Hogarty and Anderson's Psychoeducational Family Model

Hogarty et al.'s (1986) psychoeducational family model study provided further data on the prophylactic utility of family treatment. Neither the Falloon nor the Leff studies addressed the question of whether involvement of the family in treatment is necessary in order to reduce EE, AS, or relapse or whether an individual program for the patient with goals similar to family treatment could accomplish the same results. Although the Falloon et al. study included an individual treatment condition, its focus (as contrasted with the BFM) was on support rather than on skills training.

Hogarty et al. (1986) reported the results of a 1-year follow-up of hospitalized schizophrenic patients who, on discharge, participated in one of four conditions: psychoeducational family treatment plus medication ($n=21$); individual social skills training plus medication ($n=20$); family treatment and individual skills training with medication ($n=20$); or medication alone ($n=29$). All patients had at least one high-EE relative. The psychoeducational family treatment consisted of developing a therapeutic alliance with the family, a "survival skills" educational workshop for relatives (1 session), and a 6-month phase of biweekly sessions in which the patient's reintegration into familial and societal roles was emphasized. The individual skills training focused on the patient's social interactions with and social perceptions of other family members and later emphasized extrafamilial relationships. Thus, the individual treatment had goals that were similar to those of the family treatment. Psychosocial treatments continued for 1 year and often longer.

Relapses at 1-year follow-up in the four conditions were as follows: family treatment, 19%; individual social skills, 20%; family and individual treatment, 0%; and medication alone, 41%. Thus, the prophylactic effects of family and individual treatment were both equivalent and additive.

However, results at a 2-year follow-up were more complex (Hogarty et al. 1991). At 2 years, Hogarty and associates reported the following relapse rates: family treatment, 29%; social skills training, 50%; combination, 25%; and medication only, 62%. These figures suggest an advantage for family intervention over medication alone or social skills training plus medication, but no additive effect of the two psychosocial treatments. Thus, adding individual social skills training to family intervention (with medication) provides an advantage over either psychosocial treatment (with medication) over 1 but not 2 years of follow-up.

Expressed emotion ratings were obtained at index hospitalization and at 1-year follow-up or at the time of a symptomatic exacerbation. Over the first follow-up year, no relapses occurred among patients from families that changed from high to low EE over the year, whereas 36% of the patients from families that remained high in EE relapsed. However, there were differences between the treatments in their ability to reduce EE: 39% of the families in family intervention changed from high- to low-EE over the first year, whereas only 25% of the families who did not receive family treatment showed this shift. Interestingly, among those patients whose families remained high-EE over 1 year, only the combination of family and individual skills treatment was effective (0% relapsed).

Hogarty and colleagues' well-designed, large-sample study provides further data on the prophylactic utility of family treatment and, again, suggests that the efficacy of this treatment is at least in part based on its ability to reduce EE. However, their results also suggest that, at least during the first year after an index psychotic episode, reductions in morbidity can be accomplished "from the patient up" by changing the ways in which the patient interacts with or perceives his or her family.

Tarrier's Behavioral-Enactive and Symbolic Family Models

Tarrier et al.'s (1988b) controlled treatment trial differed from the other trials in several important ways. First, they compared two 9-month behavioral family treatments for acutely ill schizophrenic patients from high-EE families. In one treatment, coping skills were taught via discussion and instruction (symbolic, $n=16$); in the other treatment regimen, coping skills were taught via role-playing, behavioral rehearsal, and guided practice (enactive, $n=16$). Like the Hogarty and Leff models, these interventions were aimed at reducing EE and enhancing the patient's functioning in the community. Second, Tarrier et al. included comparison conditions in which high-EE families received two sessions of education only ($n=16$) or routine outpatient treatment ($n=16$) for the patient, to determine whether the goals of the longer family treatments could be met with a short-term, focused family intervention. Third, they included comparative samples of patients from low-EE families, who received education only ($n = 9$) or routine treatment ($n = 10$).

The relapse rates at 9 months were comparable for the family symbolic (8%) and family enactive (17%) treatments (all involving only high-EE families), with rates below those of the high-EE/education only (43%) and the high-EE/routine treatment (53%) groups. The relapse rates for the two behavioral family interventions were comparable to the rates found in the low-EE/education (22%) and low-EE/routine treatment (20%) conditions. Education by itself was not particularly effective in preventing or delaying relapse.

Tarrier and associates also found that over the 9-month follow-up, the greatest reductions in initial EE levels occurred among the high-EE families treated with either of the two family interventions, although reductions of lesser magnitude occurred in the control conditions. Generally, reductions in criticism were easier to achieve in family treatment than reductions in emotional overinvolvement, as found by Leff et al. (1982, 1989).

Cross-Cultural Adaptations of Family-Based Treatment

Family-based interventions for schizophrenia have been developed primarily in the United States and British Commonwealth countries. These interventions are now being "translated" for patients in a variety of countries. For example, Xiong et al. (1994) adapted family treatments to the cultural needs and mental health system in China. This intervention includes a 2- to 3-month introductory phase in which medications are discussed and education is provided. This introduction is followed by a 1- to 2-year treatment phase in which families are taught to spot signs of impending relapse, understand mental health laws and needs, and cope with exacerbations of the patient's symptoms. Finally, a maintenance phase begins in which families are seen every 2–3 months for group meetings, monitoring of symptoms, and ongoing communication. Sixty-three patients were randomly assigned to either this experimental family-based treatment or to standard care consisting primarily of irregular follow-up visits for prescription renewal. Those in the experimental treatment had significantly fewer hospitalizations and more months of employment at both 12- and 18-month follow-up and fewer relapses at 12 months. Studies of the cross-cultural applicability of family psychoeducation (and mediators of its effects in different cultures) will be quite important as this research progresses.

Second-Generation Family Intervention Studies

Second-generation family intervention studies have compared different models for family treatment with one another and, in some cases, examined the role of intensive family treatment within a comprehensive treatment package.

McFarlane's Multiple-Family Education Groups

McFarlane et al.'s (1995a, 1995b) study using multiple-family education groups compared two forms of family-based treatment: behavioral family treatment conducted with individual family units and a psychoeducationally focused group conducted with multiple families. This study differed from most others, which contrasted family intervention with a nonfamily-based alternative or to routine treatment. In McFarlane et al.'s study, treatment began following hospital discharge and continued for approximately 2 years. Prior to entry into the multiple-family group format, families were provided three or four individual psychoeducation sessions. The multiple family group approach was more efficacious than behavioral family treatment with individual family units in reducing relapse and improving psychosocial functioning. McFarlane and associates studied primarily patients with chronic schizophrenia, and the multiple-family group format may have provided a unique opportunity for family members to share experiences, model coping strategies for one another, and reduce social isolation. Interestingly, superiority of the multiple family groups was apparent only among those patients who showed positive symptoms at the beginning of the intervention.

Treatment Strategies in Schizophrenia Study

The Treatment Strategies in Schizophrenia study (TSS) was a large multisite investigation ($n=313$) that examined family intervention among schizophrenic patients who were receiving one of three dosing regimens of fluphenazine (Schooler et al. 1997). All families were invited to participate in an intensive psychoeducational family workshop. Families were then assigned to either the *supportive family intervention*, consisting of monthly family group meetings, or the *applied family intervention*, consisting of monthly group meetings plus in-home family skill-building sessions. There were no differences between the two family treatment groups and no family treatment–by–medication dose interactions. The authors of TSS have speculated that in both family treatment conditions the family was engaged in the treatment process and the more intensive engagement of the applied condition did not add to this treatment effect. The lack of a no–family treatment comparison group makes it impossible to evaluate the relative merits of family treatment as an adjunct to phenothiazine treatment for schizophrenic patients.

Amsterdam Family Intervention Study

An intervention study conducted at the Amsterdam Medical Center examined the impact of behavioral family treatment among 52 patients with recent-onset schizophrenic disorders (Linszen et al. 1996). All subjects participated in a comprehensive intervention program in which patients received a rich, 3-month inpatient treatment and families received three or four sessions of education and intervention. Patients were then discharged to day-hospital treatment for an additional 3 months. Throughout the 15-month intervention patients participated in an individually tailored psychoeducational treatment aimed at improving understanding of the disorder, acceptance of the role of medication in treatment, and developing coping skills and relapse-prevention strategies. Following this 6-month psychoeducational period, patients were randomly assigned to clinic-based behavioral family management (Falloon et al. 1984) or no additional psychosocial treatment conditions for a 9-month period. Overall, the relapse rate for the entire sample by the 15-month follow-up was quite low, only 16%, and there was no treatment group effect. The additional family-based intervention may have added little to an already rich, responsive program of intervention. This speculation is supported by data indicating that in the 17-to-55-month follow-up period after the 15-month comprehensive program had been withdrawn, 64% of the patients relapsed. EE was measured at both the outset and conclusion of treatment using the FMSS, and changes in FMSS-EE across the course of treatment were not associated with outcome (Nugter et al. 1997).

General Conclusions: Family Intervention Studies

- Family interventions that focus on educating the family about schizophrenia; reducing intrafamilial tension, guilt, or anxiety; easing the patient's return to the family and social community; and teaching communication and problem-solving skills lead to reductions in relapse rates among relapse-prone schizophrenic patients.
- The efficacy of these interventions in delaying relapse appears to be in part based on their ability to modify baseline levels of EE and/or AS, but the role of other mediating variables (e.g., improving medication adherence, increasing patients' cooperativeness, and engagement with family members) has not been adequately explored.

- There is not yet convincing evidence that one type of family intervention is clearly superior to any other, nor is it clear which components of these programs are the most efficacious. Future research should address these issues as well as the question of whether similar results can be obtained via individual psychosocial treatments with goals that center on improving the patient's family relationships.

Future Directions

This chapter has been oriented around the assumption that episodes of schizophrenia are a product of interactions between individual vulnerabilities and environmental stressors. The particular stressors identified—family communication deviance (CD), negative affective attitudes (EE) and behaviors (AS)—may affect and be affected by existing genetic and/or biological vulnerabilities in the target person, who may be at greater or lesser risk for episodes of schizophrenia depending on the nature of this vulnerability-stress interface.

Research Issues

Much has yet to be learned about how family variables interact with individual vulnerabilities. First, what are the acting mechanisms of family risk indicators? Are these variables themselves indirect indices of familial vulnerabilities to schizophrenia (i.e., products of attentional dysfunction or subsyndromal psychosis)? If so, why do these variables predict outcome in disorders other than schizophrenia? What disordered neurophysiological processes in patients might be affected by family variables? To what degree do variables such as EE, AS, and CD reflect attributes of the patient, the relative, or their mutually produced interactions?

Second, the cause-effect relationship between family variables and the onset or course of schizophrenia has never been resolved. Studies of high-risk offspring have the potential to clarify a great deal about the role of the family in the etiology of schizophrenia. However, these studies must demonstrate that family variables are present before the onset of schizophrenic disorder and are not driven by early, prodromal "soft signs" of the disorder in at-risk children.

As concerns the course of schizophrenia, the intervention studies perhaps provide the most convincing evidence that the family plays a role in bringing about or protecting against relapses of schizophrenia. However, even controlled intervention studies can never fully demonstrate causal relationships. Studies that use the traditional ABAB reversal methodology, in which treatments are administered, withdrawn, administered, and withdrawn (with levels of EE, AS, and patient relapse obtained during each treatment and nontreatment segment), would provide more convincing data about family causality, but such studies are very difficult to do.

Third, future studies should attempt to clarify what aspects of family interventions are the most powerful in preventing or delaying relapses of schizophrenia. What are the necessary ingredients of successful family treatment? What are the optimal durations of these treatments? What can be accomplished with the parents alone versus the patient alone?

Finally, any nonspecific factors that make these treatments efficacious should be identified. Is it really the learning of skills that leads to reductions in EE, AS, and relapse rates, or are factors such as breaking family taboos against talking about the illness, the development of new alliance patterns, and relations with the therapist equally important?

Clinical Issues

For the practicing clinician, two major issues are raised by family research. First, can the clinician learn to recognize family variables, such as high-EE attitudes, in the relatives of the patients they treat? This is much harder than it sounds: Coding of EE takes a great deal of training, and the actual determinations of EE status are based on detailed and careful judgments of the content and voice tone of relatives' statements. Alternative ways of measuring EE and AS have been developed that are potentially more "user-friendly" to the clinician (i.e., the FMSS-EE system [Magana et al. 1986] and perceived criticism patient self-report rating [Hooley and Teasdale 1989]). However, the prognostic validity of these systems in samples of schizophrenic patients has yet to be demonstrated, and use of these scales as substitutes for the traditional EE method must await this validation.

A second issue concerns the disseminability to clinicians of family treatment techniques. How can researchers encourage clinicians in mental health centers to administer behavioral family management or other psychoeducational family interventions? Will clinicians obtain family assessments in order to determine whether such treatments are indicated? Will mental health centers reimburse costs incurred by clinicians such as driving to and from patients' homes? If not, can these psychosocial treatments be redesigned to fit the needs of the particular mental health setting?

Although much needs to be learned about family variables and interventions in schizophrenia, it is time to move toward building two bridges simultaneously. The first will link what we know about the genetics and neurobiology of schizophrenia with family environmental factors that are of prognostic importance; the second will link research findings with what clinicians do in practice. Without these linkages, family research will remain in the realm of the academic. With these linkages, our understanding of patients with schizophrenia may become more complete, and our treatments may become more successful.

Chapters on Related Topics

The following chapters describe concepts related to family variables and interventions in schizophrenia:

- Chapter 7, "Behavioral Family Therapy"
- Chapter 30, "National Alliance for the Mentally Ill (NAMI) and Family Psychiatry: Working Toward a Collaborative Model"

28

Depression and the Family

Interpersonal Context and Family Functioning

G. Pirooz Sholevar, M.D.
Linda D. Schwoeri, Ph.D.
Howard Jarden, Ph.D.

Introduction

Depression is a disturbance of three distinct but interrelated areas—mood, cognition, and interpersonal relationships. Despite the parallel advances in the knowledge of the biochemical (mood) and cognitive dimensions of depression, the interpersonal disturbances that affect marriage, childrearing, and all other facets of family life have *not* been widely recognized. A large number of depressed patients remain undiagnosed or receive erroneous diagnoses because depression may be masked and therefore go unrecognized. Furthermore, the interpersonal aspects of depression frequently do not respond to antidepressants and psychotherapy.

According to the American Psychiatric Association (1993b, 1994, 2000a), the lifetime risk of depression is between 8% and 11% for men and 18% and 23% for women. The National Comorbidity Survey, the first national probability sample in the United States (1990–1992), found that a major depressive episode was the single most common disorder. Of the 8,098 persons surveyed, approximately 20% (about 1,619 people) reported a history of the disorder during their lifetime. However, of those with lifetime histories of one or more depressive episodes, only 42% received any professional care.

Depression and depressive symptomatology constitute a complex phenomenon that requires attention to the biological, psychological, and cognitive as well as interpersonal factors in order to enhance treatment outcome. Interpersonal relationships have been shown to create stress for the depression-prone person. Haas et al. (1985) showed a relationship between the individual's symptoms and the psychosocial environment. Chronic stressors become part of the everyday interactions with family and friends. Patients often attempt unsuccessfully to handle and reduce anxiety and tension through eating, smoking, sleeping, crying, and/or complaining, which only adds further to their interactional problems. The patient's symptoms become manifest in family and marital relationships, in child rearing, and in other interpersonal relations, which creates extreme hardships for all concerned. Furthermore, the depressed person's pessimistic attitudes toward self and the environment become reciprocally distressing experiences for family members and loved ones. Depression impairs the person's ability to work, and the relapse rate significantly erodes occupational outcomes (Mintz et al. 1992), further disrupting the family's functioning as well as inducing stress on the family. Depression affects all ages and involves varying degrees of debilitation. According to Eaton et al. (1997, 2000, 2001), the lifetime risk for a major depressive disorder is between 7% and 12% for men and 20% and 23% for women. Comorbidity for major depressive disorder can be as high as 43% (Coyne et al. 1994).

This chapter reviews the interpersonal context of depression and discusses a comprehensive model both to enhance the diagnostic and therapeutic effectiveness with this disorder and to reduce the pathogenic impact of depression on the offspring of depressed patients.

Vulnerability: Biology, Early Attachments, and Loss

Vulnerability to depression can have genetic, environmental, interpersonal, and traumatic roots. Early losses or exposure to a neglectful or depriving situation provide a common path to future depression. Some pathogenic aspects of early losses may be related to inadequate or inappropriate functional replacements for a lost love object. Selection of a depressed, depression-prone, or depriving person as a marital partner in assortative mating has always been suspected and is currently an established mechanism in depressed couples. In this manner, the person who has been traumatized by a depriving situation puts herself or himself again at risk in a similar environment. The combination of genetic factors, early losses or depriving experiences, and the repetition of the depression and depriving situations in adult life are potent factors for the family transmission of depression to the offspring of depressed parents.

Biological Factors

The importance of biological factors was examined in retrospective cross-sectional studies based on clinical evidence. These studies demonstrated that children and adolescent offspring of depressed parents are at a significant risk for depression (Beardslee et al. 1985, 1987a, 1987b, 1988; Orvaschel et al. 1988; Weissman et al. 1987). Downey and Coyne (1990) also documented this risk with an extensive review of available research. The rate of depression in children of parents with bipolar or unipolar disorders is several times higher than in the control group. The risk of depression is intensified if there is a family history of psychiatric disorders, including alcoholism, schizophrenia, and unipolar or bipolar disorders. Furthermore, the family history of affective disorder strongly contributes to the transmission of depression in childhood, especially when parental depression is chronic without a clear-cut psychosocial precipitant (Klerman et al. 1984; Warner et al. 1992). The studies of depression do not present a clear route of causality; however, both biological and psychological factors play a role in etiology.

Early Attachments and Loss

The loss of an early attachment can lead to depression. The significance of the individual's relationship context, his or her relational needs, and the effects on his or her personality were discussed by Sullivan (1953) and Fromm-Reichmann (1948) and provided a background for the understanding of the interpersonal therapy of Klerman et al. (1984). Bowlby (1969) contributed a significant understanding of the human need for attachment and its influence on personality development. These attachments enhance the quality of the individual's life by providing experiences for nourishment, protection, and love. In the absence of attachment the individual is intensely vulnerable to depression (Bowlby 1969, 1977). The work of Ainsworth on attachment (Ainsworth 1972; Ainsworth and Bell 1974; Ainsworth et al. 1978, 1979) and the longitudinal studies of Sroufe (1977, 1986) and Main and Weston

(1985) all support the role of attachment bonds in the development of psychosocial adaptation over time. These early relationships provide an initial organizing context for children (Zeanah et al. 1989). If they are secure (Ainsworth et al. 1978), as adults they will be capable of withstanding imperfection in themselves and others, more self-reliant, and less dependent on others to meet their emotional needs. They will be, in effect, more ego resilient in that they can use their cognitive, social, and affective skills to manage the hardships they will encounter.

In a most profound way, the death of a loved one is an irreversible disruption in the attachment bond and produces the equivalent of a clinically depressed state. Weller et al. (1994) researched children's reactions to parental death and the relationship between bereavement and subsequent psychopathology. They concluded that following the death of a parent, children developed the clinical symptoms of major depression, including appetite disturbance, sleep disturbance, psychomotor agitation and retardation, and morbid or suicidal ideations, as well as feelings of guilt and worthlessness. Both the child and surviving parent are at great risk because the grieving process itself can severely jeopardize the relationship with the child in terms of parental care and nurturing. It is not necessarily the loss of the attachment that creates the clinical depression, but the absence of other attachments.

Interpersonal responses to loss are also part of the child's experience with parental divorce and separation. Availability of a social support network as well as a close relationship with the custodial parent at this time has been shown to be a significant factor in the child's overall well-being (Furstenberg et al. 1987). The mother-child relationship is a central factor in the child's emotional well-being during the 10-year postdivorce period. This relationship, together with the child's inner resources and resiliency, helps him or her through the difficult experience of losing the security provided by the parents' marriage (Wallerstein 1983, 1985, 1986, 1987, 1990; Wallerstein and Kelly 1980). An assessment of the interaction between the child and custodial parent is paramount to treating the depression.

Marital and Family Characteristics of Depression

Depression has a pervasive effect on multiple aspects of family and marital functioning. Communication becomes defensive and irritable; problem solving is reduced, tasks are left unattended, and a pervasive negative affect with reduced initiative adds to the tension in relationships.

Role of Relationships

Social support through close relationships provides a sense of intimacy and social and psychological well-being, which are all important protective factors against depression. The protective quality of an intimate and supportive relationship is the most helpful factor in defending against development of depression in women (Brown et al. 1977).

When intimacy is missing in a marital relationship, the course of depression is worsened. It is a well-known clinical observation that the threatened disruption of a marital attachment through separation, divorce, or abandonment is very often related to the onset of adult depression. Birtchnell (1988), Gotlib and Whiffen (1989), and Johnson and Talitman (1997) studied the effects of the lack of intimacy and social support and reported that marriages of depressed women were significantly more problematic than those of control subjects. Depression is two to three times higher in women than in men. It interferes with their roles as wives and mothers and interrupts all aspects of interpersonal functioning. Brown and Harris (1978) found that severe life events, including the loss of a significant close relationship, predated the onset of depression in 83% of the women they studied. Involvement in an intimate relationship was found to be a successful buffer against depression in 96% of the cases studied (Brown and Harris 1978).

Depressed women are more likely than nondepressed women to be seen as dependent, dominated by their husbands, and unable to make their own decisions (Hoover and Fitzgerald 1981; Horowitz et al. 1979). Fadden et al. (1987a, 1987b), Cohan and Bradbury (1997), and Culp and Beach (1998) all found that depressed women tend to be aversive to others and have control and power issues that dominate their interactions. These issues create more of a burden and hardship for spouses than the woman's vegetative signs.

Assortative mating is evidenced in the selection of similarly disposed mates; the consequence of this is further marital dysfunction (Merikangas et al. 1983). Coyne (1990) reported that 40% of adults living with a patient with depressive episodes were distressed themselves to the point of meeting the criteria for needing therapeutic interventions. This distress is yet another indicator of the type of emotional atmosphere in the home.

Interactions with depressed spouses are difficult because of the patients' withdrawal, irritability, and preoccupation, which add to any preexisting marital problems (Bebbington 1987a, 1987b). Crowther (1985) noted that patients with major depression report more difficulty in their marriages than do patients who have schizophrenia, anxiety disorder, or other disorders. In studying interactions, it has been found that subjects were less willing to give positive responses to depressed persons, and in turn depressed subjects reported receiving fewer positive responses. This observation reinforced the Weissman and Paykel (1974) finding that depressed persons have relatively few social contacts. Hooper et al. (1977) and Hinchliffe (1975, 1977, 1978a, 1978b) found that depressed persons are less responsive to partners, more preoccupied with themselves, and more hostile. These behaviors seemed to generate the spouse's withdrawal, which in turn led to more anger and demanding behavior, and fewer positive exchanges with family members. As suggested by Coyne (1990), depressed persons are depressing to have around. Depression exaggerates the person's underlying personality disorder and intensifies narcissistic vulnerabilities.

Depression reduces the ability to be an effective disciplinarian, negotiator, and emotional caregiver, which are all part of competent and caring parenting (Schwoeri and Sholevar 1994). Depressed mothers become overprotective, irritable, preoccupied, and emotionally distant (Klerman et al. 1984; Weissman and Paykel 1974). The depressive symptoms in one parent may potentiate existing conflict or tension in the family, thus interfering further with effective parenting. Angry competition and retributive behavior often result from this interaction over parenting. Keitner and Miller (1990) reported that 75% of the depressed families in their study identified family impairment. They reported significantly more marital maladjustment and a desire for significant changes in their marriages.

Family Dysfunction

Family dysfunction was examined in a longitudinal study by Warner et al. (1992) that provided insight into the nature, course, and persistence of depression and supported the earlier work of Orvaschel (1990) on risk factors for depression in children (Hammen et al. 1990; Keller et al. 1988; Weissman et al. 1987). The Warner study indicated that five family risk factors—poor marital adjustment, divorce, parent-child discord, affectionless control, and low family cohesion—all contribute to the incidence rates; however, only divorce accounts for a protracted time for recovery. A family history of depression and poor marriage before the onset of depression is associated with the emergence of both endogenous and nonendogenous depression. The bulk of evidence suggests that disturbed marriages and a disturbed family environment serve a facilitating role for the emergence of depressive symptoms, particularly in those individuals already vulnerable to developing a major depression. Even more relevant is the "attributable" risk factor of prior depressive symptoms. This indicates that depression is part of a long process that can be gathering momentum slowly over time. Depression is not merely an enemy to middle age but an illness that manifests itself as early as childhood. The symptoms may appear to be less threatening to the overall functioning of the child but if left unchecked will manifest in more severity by adolescence, when interpersonal factors requiring action and thought are crucial to the adjustment of the individual.

Families with depressed members experience more problem-solving difficulties than families of patients with either schizophrenia or bipolar illness. They complain of difficulties maintaining emotional stability, handling day-to-day problems, acting on decisions, addressing problems, and dealing with problems that involve feelings. These families are less able to show love and affection. Establishing and maintaining family rules and regulations are also problematic, and the families are unclear about what to do in various situations, particularly emergencies.

Certain factors play an interactive role in the family pathology when a mental disorder such as depression is present. Keitner and Miller (1990) recommended attention to the following when assessing the family's ability to handle the difficult problems associated with depression:

- Premorbid functioning of the family
- Family's financial and social situation
- Family and social supports that bear on the family's ability to cope with crisis
- Developmental stage of the family
- Mental health of all family members, especially in the presence of illness in one or more members

Parent-Child Relationships

Depressed parents have impaired relationships with their children, and these impairments have been studied at different developmental levels and among different age groups. There is an interactive effect created by the experience of living with the depressed parent's helplessness and fatigue that makes the children exquisitely sensitive to the parent's illness. This sensitivity increases around adolescence. Seligman (1975) noted that a negative attributional style in these adolescents predicted depressive symptoms 6 months later. The implications were that over time children who become overly involved in the parent's problems develop a protective or distancing mechanism that may hinder the quality of later relationships and place them at risk for later depression. Depressive symptoms in parents expose the child to an impoverished interpersonal environment as evidenced by the family's impaired social and leisure activities and extended family relationships. There is increased hostility in the family interactions, and children, especially adolescents, learn to exploit this. Interpersonal functioning around problem solving, discipline, communication, and the expression of affect is inevitably reduced.

Risks Associated with the Parent-Child Interaction

The psychiatric literature has produced substantial evidence that children whose parents have an affective disorder run the risk of multiple problems in their social and emotional development. They run a 65% to 75% risk of any DSM-III-R diagnosis (Keller et al. 1986; Weissman et al. 1987). Depressive illness interferes with family relationships. It also interferes with relationships with peers, which is where the capacity for mutuality and collaboration develops (Beardslee et al. 1987a, 1987b), and limits exposure to other possible relationships. These social and supportive relationships are a crucial protective factor against the many hardships of living with a depressed parent or coping with any related mental illness.

Each situation is different and is influenced by the duration of the illness, by the child's capacity to understand the illness and maintain his or her autonomy, and by his or her individual temperament and style. However, the longer the parent is depressed, the longer the child is deprived of the needed family relationships, and so the greater the risk. Furthermore, both vulnerability to depression and the behavior characteristics of depression increase over time. Disruptive behavior, depression, and anxiety-related problems increase substantially in children over age 5 as they begin to move into other social relationships at school.

There are many interacting stresses in a child's life when he or she is faced with parental depression. Goodman et al. (1993) studied the effects of the mother's recurring major depression on the development of positive self-concept, self-control, and peer relation skills of 5- to 10-year-olds. They found that the children were faced with multiple problems since they lived in family environments in which marital discord was very common. For example, their mothers were often married to men who probably had a psychiatric disorder, perhaps depression, and the children were subject to the stress resulting from the poor marital relationships. Goodman was looking at how the children's social skills and popularity with peers were affected. He found that children who were exposed to hostile and critical mothers were prone to lower self-concept. If this carried into their social exchanges, they would present a wary outlook in their relationships and encounter corresponding hostility. They would likewise misread gestures or looks in the absence of actual intent and would then present a defensive, equally hostile stance. This made them less accepted and less popular with peers, thereby interrupting the development of an important adaptive skill. What these studies most vividly revealed was the importance of understanding the social context and the interpersonal process experienced by the child and his or her family during the depressive illness. Beardslee et al. (1998a, 1998b) developed a theoretically sound and empirically validated psychoeducationally based program for intervention with children of parents with affective disorder. His model was tested throughout the 1990s, with very promising results. Brent (1997) applied the psychoeducational approach to intervention with depressed children and adolescents.

Family Functioning in the Course of Depressive Episodes

Acute Phase

The acute phase was the first of three phases in the course of a depressive episode as described by Keitner et al. (1986). Using the Family Assessment Device (FAD; Epstein et al. 1983) Keitner found that family functioning in the areas of communication, problem solving, and affective responsiveness was significantly impaired. During the acute episode, the depressive illness was associated with more distress than were other disorders, including schizophrenia, bipolar disorders, alcohol and substance abuse, and significant medical conditions (Keitner and Miller 1990; Miller et al. 1986). This distress was observed by looking at the interactional and communicational styles of the family members. As noted by Coyne (Coyne 1976; Coyne et al. 1994), when individuals have depression, they shift the interactional burden to others. Communication becomes more constricted due to the patient's withdrawing and nagging behavior. There is a reciprocal withdrawal of affection, which intensifies the loss for the depressed person. Keitner et al. (1987a) found that during the acute phase of depression, families were especially unclear about rules and could not discuss their problems or fears, which led to further misunderstanding among members. Because families often lacked the skills needed to stop the poor communication pattern, a mutually reinforcing, aversive, and dysfunctional style persisted and led to repercussions that were felt in interactions with children and social friends.

Remission

When compared with the acute phase, communication improves slightly during remission (Keitner et al. 1987a). However, depressed patients continue to exhibit greater dissatisfaction when compared with nondepressed groups of women (Hinchliffe et al. 1977; Merikangas et al. 1988). Marital difficulties continue, and adolescents experience significant psychosocial problems with peer relationships. There are negative mother-child relations, and school performance difficulties continue (Puig-Antich et al.

1993). These multiple domains, which were also discussed in studies by Merikangas et al. (1985), Puig-Antich et al. (1985a, 1985b), and McGee et al. (1990), are indicative of the risks to which children are exposed. Adolescents in particular have been shown to be at high risk for recurrent episodes of major depressive disorder (Harrington et al. 1986; Keller et al. 1988).

Recovery

Keller et al. (1988) found a high rate of chronicity in young adult patients. Twelve percent of these patients did *not* recover during the 5-year period in which they were followed. Those who did recover did so during the first 6 months of the study, and recovery was related to the severity of problems at onset. Social adjustment improved slowly but was not complete. Keitner et al. (1987a) reported that families who improved their general functioning had a shorter recovery time (4.1 months) compared with nonimprovers (8.1 months). Impairments in peer relations persisted following recovery, and depressed children continued to view themselves as more isolated and less liked (Puig-Antich and Chambers 1978; Puig-Antich et al. 1985a, 1985b, 1993).

The Warner et al. (1992) study of the offspring of depressed parents indicated that 13% of the children studied had *not* recovered in the 2-year period and that children diagnosed with major depressive disorder *prior* to age 13 took a longer time for recovery—74 weeks—than those diagnosed after age 13. They also found that dysthymia *predicts* recurrence. The 2-year period replicated Keller et al.'s findings (Keller et al. 1992). An average episode of major depression in childhood lasts about 10 months (Puig-Antich 1987). The greatest recovery is in the first 6 months, in which approximately 61% of the study group recovered, while a total of 74% recovered after a year. The recovery rate may be high, but the recurrence rate is also high. The family history data indicated that first onset of major depression, as well as earlier age at onset, predicted a more protracted course for the illness (Klerman and Weissman 1992).

Relapse

Family functioning has been shown to affect the course of the illness. Families with high levels of critical comments have a threefold greater rate of increase for relapse within 9 months after recovery (Vaughn and Leff 1976). In an 18-month naturalistic follow-up study of depressive symptoms, Shea et al. (1992) showed that 19%–30% of patients recovered during an acute period. The relapse rate for those who recovered was 30%–50%. The Shea et al. (1992) study showed a reduction in depressive symptoms with a course of antidepressants (with and without psychotherapy). A supportive, nonstressful environment with more open discussion of family feelings may actually predict lower rates of relapse or hospitalization, as was previously noted by Keitner and Miller (1990).

Suicidality

Keitner et al. (1987b) studied the relationship between family functioning and suicidality and found that depressed suicidal patients held a more negative view of their family functioning than that held by other family members. One possible explanation given was that the patient's cognitive distortions create a demonstrated sense of hopelessness and negativity. Patients lose their sense of agency and coherence. This was especially pronounced in the interpersonal sphere, wherein depressive cognitions and attributions create the self-fulfilling prophecies of rejection and abandonment.

Measurement of Family and Marital Functioning

Clinical evaluations of depressed patients and their families include assessments of the many interpersonal aspects of this disorder. The family can readily describe the clinical picture of the patient's symptoms; however, the clinician is best prepared to help the family by observing the interactions and understanding the pathological family process. The following measurements are adjuncts to assessments. They enhance the value of *individual* differential diagnosis of the patient through the use of such tests as the Beck Depression Inventory (Beck et al. 1961) and the Hamilton Rating Scale for Depression (Hamilton 1960, 1968) and clinical evaluations based on DSM-IV criteria.

Family Assessment Device

One of the family instruments used extensively for the assessment of depression is the Family Assessment Device by Epstein et al. (1983). This instrument is based on the McMaster model of family functioning. It examines six dimensions of family functioning: problem solving, communication, family roles, affective responsiveness, affective involvement, and behavioral control. Two of those dimensions—affective responsiveness and affective involvement—are sensitive to the assessment of depressed families.

Family Environment Scale

The Family Environment Scale (FES) by Moos and Moos (1981) assesses the social climate of the family. It focuses on the interpersonal relationships among family members. The scale identifies the following: cohesion, expressiveness, conflict, independence, achievement orientation, intellectual-cultural orientation, active recreational orientation, moral or religious emphasis, organization, and control. This measure is sensitive to the hypothesis that women are vulnerable to depression and experience their environment as nonsupportive. The significant variables that predate the onset of depression include dependence on the family, lack of family support, and lack of control. As emphasized in the chapter, family support through the family environment is an important factor in the course of depressive illness.

Dyadic Adjustment Scale

The Dyadic Adjustment Scale (DAS) by Spanier (1976) is a 32-item, Likert-style, self-report questionnaire. The scale has been designed to assess the quality of dyadic relationships. The DAS includes subscales of satisfaction, consensus, cohesion, and affectional expression. It is compatible with a variety of therapeutic frameworks and is useful in identifying the severity of the problem and making an assessment of the effectiveness of treatment. It can be used in combination with individual measures of depression such as the Beck Depression Inventory.

Treatment

Interpersonal Therapy

Basic Concepts

In the treatment of depression, the combination of individual and family therapy with medication is the preferred intervention. Interpersonal therapy addresses many of the areas of concern in treating depression. The clinical research efforts that focus on interpersonal psychotherapy for depression (Klerman and Weissman 1987; Weissman et al. 1984) provide a foundation for understanding the particular problem areas encountered by depressed patients. These problem areas include role conflicts and disputes, stressful life events, and interpersonal deficits. An interpersonal approach looks at the etiology of depression from different vantage points, stressing the view that there is no one single factor that explains depression. This approach is rooted in the work of Harry Stack Sullivan (1953), who viewed psychiatry as the study of the *interactions* between individuals. He emphasized social and family factors such as love relationships, friendships, and patterns in adolescence and young adulthood (Klerman et al. 1984) that contribute to different mental disorders.

Social Stress and Stressful Life Events

Social stress, stressful life events, and interactional and interpersonal problems that arise while establishing and maintaining different relationships are viewed as both antecedents and consequences of clinical depression.

Role Conflicts

Depression leads to conflict in the depressed person's different social and family roles. It also has an impact on a person's social and leisure activities and relationships. Impairments involve low expectations and functioning.

Interpersonal Deficits

Some of the interpersonal deficits experienced by depressed persons include withdrawal from family interactions and increased hostility toward husband, children, friends, and work associates. The problems are amplified because of the combination of these factors and their exaggeration through depressive cognitions, bodily symptoms, and complaints.

Multimodal Therapy

The multimodal therapy approach developed by Arnold Lazarus (1992) has two main objectives: the rapid *remission* of depressive symptoms and the *prevention* of relapse. This approach is based on the assumption that an effective way of assessing and treating the patient is by addressing the following seven areas of functioning:

1. *Behavior.* The relationship between affect and activity level is targeted by emphasizing the value of rewarding activities, making checklists of pleasant events, and establishing behaviors, images, and places that the patient finds rewarding. This list of activities enables the therapist to start prescribing potentially therapeutic changes.
2. *Affect.* Depressed persons experience anxiety as well as anger. Relaxation and meditation combined with a program of exercise to promote muscle tone are interventions aimed at both the anxiety and the anger.
3. *Sensation.* A list of pleasant auditory, visual, tactile, and olfactory stimuli is added to the patient's list of other pleasant events and activities.

4. *Imagery.* Recalling past successes and picturing small but positive steps helps the patient to move into more positive and pleasurable activities.
5. *Cognition.* Ellis's rational and emotive therapy technique called *cognitive education* is utilized.
6. *Interpersonal relationships.* Social skills deficits are addressed by helping patients deal with their social network. Role playing, saying no, and expressing positive feelings as well as disapproval are part of the training.
7. *Neurophysiology.* When the diagnosis is major depression, psychotherapy and psychopharmacology are combined. This approach offers a comprehensive approach that addresses the sensory, cognitive, and interpersonal aspects of depressive illness.

Marital dissatisfaction is associated with higher rates of relapse (Rounsaville et al. 1979). Interpersonal psychotherapy has been shown to be effective in improving marital satisfaction when the couple is also treated in marital therapy (Haley 1976). It is also effective in reducing depression both with and without spouse involvement.

Strategic Therapy

Strategic therapy is an approach that provides pragmatic, goal-oriented, and relatively short-term interventions to individuals, families, and couples. The goal of strategic family and marital therapy in cases of depression is to modify what people do in their everyday lives. Therefore, it relies heavily on making direct and indirect suggestions and assigning of extra therapy tasks. In keeping with the interpersonal model, the interventions of the therapist are focused on attempting to provide *solutions* rather than returning to past history and elaboration of past events. The critical task is to help the depressed person and the family to feel empowered rather than to continue feeling cut off and neglected. This emphasizes helping the person view his or her situation in terms of something that is manageable and for which he or she has the necessary resources to promote a positive outcome. Some of the standard strategic techniques include reframing, paradoxical intervention, disengaging, and redirecting efforts (Coyne et al. 1994). Strategic therapy of depressed persons is based on the assumption that interactions are relevant to both the continuation and resolution of the depressive episode. Treatment does not search for reasons but rather imposes solutions.

Psychodynamic Family Therapy

Psychodynamic family therapy helps the couple to recognize their distant and covertly punitive interactions and move toward the establishment of an empathic relationship in which listening, understanding, and satisfaction of the partner's needs are of paramount value (Bemporad et al. 1994). The couple's mutually irritating and provocative relationship frequently needs to be brought to their attention and necessary corrective measures instituted. The delineation and reconstruction of early patterns of relationships helps the family recognize the powerful hold these early relationships have on current marital and parental interactions. The empathic response of the therapist can serve to establish a therapeutic frame and encourage the couple to change their relationship into a rewarding and nondepressive one. The therapist must not, however, become *inducted* into the family system and viewed as a rewarding alternative to the nonrewarding and distant spouse, which can further undermine family relationships.

The provision of a satisfactory environment for the development of the children is a significant goal of the psychodynamic family therapist. The establishment of this capacity can ensure the resumption and continuation of a healthy developmental course in the children and prevent the transmission of a depressive and pessimistic perspective across the generations.

Behavioral Family Therapy

The principles of behavioral family therapy can be beneficially combined with other types of family treatment approaches such as psychodynamic, strategic, structural, and intergenerational therapy. Behavioral family therapy concentrates on the enhancement of the reinforcement system to encourage a high level of rewards and pleasing interactions and to undermine the avoidance and punishing behaviors typical of depressed families. The high level of rewarding interaction in turn encourages the family to become more involved with one another in a pleasing fashion. Institution of affectionate exchanges, "caring days," and "loving days" are highly effective in buffering the persistent negative affect that is the hallmark of depressed families.

Combining Family and Marital Treatment With Pharmacology

In contrast to the 1950s, today the combined use of pharmacotherapy and psychotherapy or family therapy is readily accepted. Initially, it was feared that the patient's resistance would be increased through a combined approach. When the treatment of choice is family therapy, the issue becomes even more complex. However, clinicians from different orientations are increasingly treating depressed patients with this combined approach as a way of stabilizing them by reducing relapse rates and improving their concentration, energy, and affect.

There is an additive effect of combining family therapy with pharmacotherapy. Medication can effect improvement in the depressive symptoms, which can help the individual to look at family related problems. When family psychoeducation is combined with family therapy and pharmacotherapy, the family can begin to address the many interrelated aspects of the patient's depression while being supported in their understanding of the illness. It appears from the literature that the pharmacotherapy improves libido and vegetative signs while the family treatment improves the social functioning of the patients.

Epstein et al. (1988) have reported four broad groups of *family types* with respect to the clearing of depressive symptoms through a combined treatment of family therapy and pharmacotherapy:

- *Group 1:* In this group there is a rapid clearing of symptoms of depression once the problematic family issues are delineated.
- *Group 2:* In this group there is minimal, if any, family pathology even during the acute phase of the illness of the identified patient.
- *Group 3:* In this group there is a wide spectrum of family pathology and the patients and their families all respond very well to the combination of pharmacotherapy and family therapy. In these families, the proper pharmacological treatment improves the affective episode while the family works on their family problems.
- *Group 4:* In this group there is severe depressive symptomatology and the patients prove difficult to engage in any type of therapy. Once the patients are involved in combined family therapy and pharmacotherapy, their depressive symptomatology disappears only to reveal severe underlying character pathology and/or severe dysthymia. However, very often this group benefits most by freeing the other family members from the interpersonal problems caused by the patient's depression.

Inpatient Family Intervention

Inpatient family intervention (IFI) for affective disorder is a model of intervention developed by Glick et al. (1990, 1991, 1993) (see Chapter 19, "Parent Management Training"). Identification and measurement of mediating goals include assessment of key family members' attitudes toward the patient, the illness, the family's burden with the illness, and the need for future treatment. IFI aims to help the family and patient understand the nature and course of the illness and develop the most appropriate strategies for dealing with the problems involved. Investigators who followed the course of IFI reported a shortened average hospital stay for patients who received it when compared with those in the control group. IFI promotes a positive treatment effect, especially for female patients. The family's attitude toward treatment was significantly better than that of the families in the control groups, particularly with male patients.

Psychoeducation

Another technique that is incorporated into many inpatient and aftercare programs is the utilization of a psychoeducational family approach. This educational approach was highly effective with schizophrenic patients and has since been applied to depressed patients and their families. It is based on the psychoeducational model of Holder and Anderson (1990), which presents an outline that includes a *definition* and *description* of the interpersonal environment of depression. The outline covers such crucial issues as oversensitivity, self-protection, unresponsiveness to reassurance, support, feedback, empathy, and negative interactional sequences. The *treatment phase* includes an outline of how to cope with depression and describes what to avoid, such as too rapid assurance, taking comments literally, attempting to be constantly available and positive, and allowing the disorder to dominate family life. The *coping mechanisms* that are stressed include creating a balanced response that is neither over- nor underresponsive, taking care of self and of family members other than the patient, developing skills for self-preservation, and coping with special problems such as suicide threats and attempts.

Conclusion

The significant advances in the fields of biological psychiatry and cognitive psychotherapy in understanding the biological and cognitive dysfunctions in depression have been supplemented in the past two decades by the recognition of interpersonal deficits in depressed patients. The investigations into the interpersonal dimension of the lives of depressed patients have uncovered a variety of deficits in the marital, parental, and overall family functioning that make people of different ages significantly vulnerable to depression and its recurrence. The interpersonal conflicts emerge early in the course of childhood and may be ultimately interrelated to later evidenced biological and cognitive dysfunctions.

The major deficiency in the marital dimension is the selection of a depressed or depression-prone mate by a depressed patient, which results in a marital relationship lacking in intimacy. The lack of intimacy in turn leaves the couple vulnerable to depression in stressful situations. The children raised within this context do not experience a secure attachment to their parents and are further traumatized when one parent becomes clinically depressed, particularly if the second parent fails to compensate for the emotional absence of the first one or joins or recruits the child in attacking the depressed parent.

Interpersonal therapy combined with family psychotherapy works synergistically with the biological, cognitive, psychodynamic, and behavioral treatment of depression. Such a comprehensive model results in a more optimal treatment outcome and a lower rate of recurrence of illness. The development of depressive disorder and psychopathology in the offspring of the depressed patients can also be prevented through the use of this intervention model. Because the family environment is so important for the support of the patient's remission, family and individual therapy is the preferred treatment combination.

In all cases the type of family structure and strengths available for the patient will determine the best strategy. For example, a family that is flexible and allows some differences among members will be better able to work with the therapist to keep the patient actively involved in treatment and recovery. Relapses will not be as traumatic because the family will have the skills to understand and support the patient. Behavioral approaches as well as psychoeducation can be most helpful with the family while the individual is being seen for individual issues, including medication follow-up.

The future directions in the investigation of the interpersonal dimension of depression should enable us to recognize the biological, psychological, and interpersonal correlates of depression proneness and depression in depressed patients, their mates, and their offspring. The preventive measures should then be directed toward the correction of such dysfunction and the prevention of a clinical depression.

Chapters on Related Topics

The following chapters describe concepts related to depression and the family:

- Chapter 8, "Psychoeducational Family Intervention"
- Chapter 27, "Family Variables and Interventions in Schizophrenia"
- Chapter 29, "Family Intervention and Psychiatric Hospitalization"

29

Family Intervention and Psychiatric Hospitalization

G. Pirooz Sholevar, M.D.
Ira D. Glick, M.D.
Ellen Harris Sholevar, M.D.

Introduction

Diagnostic and therapeutic intervention with families in the psychiatric hospital has been attempted throughout most of the history of inpatient treatment. However, development of a theoretical system to integrate the two modes of therapy—namely, inpatient treatment and family intervention—has been limited and delayed. There are multiple reasons for the relative failure to integrate these two treatment modalities. Paramount is the divergence in the prevailing theoretical orientations. Inpatient treatment has generally been guided by an individual and biological orientation, whereas family theory has adhered exclusively to an interactional perspective and has downplayed the importance of individual psychopathology, biological factors, and management problems with seriously and acutely ill patients. A second factor is the lack of attention to the long periods of hospitalization that facilities were allowed to keep patients for in the past. They would *adopt* people with disorders rather than seek effective ways of recognizing and addressing familial variables, which theoretically could shorten the length of the hospital stay, reduce relapse rate, and enhance the individual's level of functioning after discharge from the hospital. Against this background, recent literature has emphasized the complementary roles of family intervention and hospitalization, defining not only the importance of including and allying with families for effective short- and long-term care of individuals, but also recognizing the limits of hospital practice in addressing the multiple stages of a person's psychopathology.

Inpatient family intervention has emerged as a major challenge to family therapists to integrate the biological, individual psychopathological, and familial variables and combine the multiple treatment modalities available in the psychiatric hospital setting to address the range of etiological factors. The specific objectives of family intervention in a psychiatric hospital system are to 1) understand the role of the family in the psychiatric hospitalization of one of its members, 2) involve the family in the goal of preventing rehospitalization, 3) reach the highest functional level for the identified patient and family, and 4) recognize and use the family approaches and other alternatives to hospitalization (Glick et al. 1987).

History

Family therapy in its early stage opposed psychiatric hospitalization even though supportive and therapeutic relationships between the hospital staff and families of the mentally ill patients were common, at least during short-term hospitalization, and particularly in general hospitals. The relationship between staff and families of the chronically mentally ill in state hospitals was somewhat different because these hospitals essentially *adopted* individuals and the families were not involved in their treatment. Early family theory regarded hospitalization as detrimental to the wholeness and functioning of the family and therefore encouraged families to bring home hospitalized members as soon as therapeutically possible. This move was expected to reestablish family integrity and restore its functioning.

A major initial development in the application of family theory to psychiatric hospitalization was the Treatment of Families in Crisis project initiated in Denver, Colorado, in the early 1960s (Langsley and Kaplan 1968). The individuals participating in the project, who were judged in need of psychiatric hospitalization, were randomly assigned to hospital admission or crisis intervention by a family treatment team consisting of a psychiatrist, a social worker, and a psychiatric nurse. The lives of these families were followed for up to 18 months to evaluate any relapse of the crisis situation and readmission to psychiatric hospitals. The rate of rehospitalization proved lower and the level of functioning higher throughout the course of follow-up for the group treated with brief, outpatient, family-crisis treatment in contrast to the hospitalized group. Although this study did not have a far-reaching impact on the field of inpatient treatment or family therapy in general, it established that both families and psychiatric hospitals are called on to deal with the crisis and decompensation involving individuals and families. Further, both hospitals and the family have a common function of reestablishing a supportive environment to contain an individual's illness and assist with his or her recovery.

At present, family intervention with hospitalized members includes the more modest goals of reducing the rate of relapse and rehospitalization and shortening the length of the hospital stay by enhancing the reentry of the individual into the family. Family intervention has also entered a synergistic relationship with pharmacotherapy and crisis intervention, rather than presenting itself as a competing and preferred treatment modality. Family intervention, in particular psychoeducational intervention, has been added to traditional psychodynamic psychotherapy in conjunction with psychotropic agents, crisis intervention, and *milieu therapy* to restabilize the patient and his or her family in a more efficient manner. This approach has enabled family treatment to gain a respected position among the range of psychotherapeutic interventions rather than remain a sole, competing orientation to the treatment of acute emotional disorders.

Definition

Inpatient family intervention refers to a specialized application of family theory developed by Glick et al. (1987) in conjunction with the multiple therapeutic modalities available in a modern psychiatric hospital. It attempts to understand the patient's psychopathology through examination of the level of vulnerability and heightened environmental stress, both of which result in an acute exacerbation of the individual's condition and require his or her hospitalization. The patient's vulnerability can be related to biological, genetic, and personality factors on the one hand and ineffective or inadequate family resources on the other. The stressful situation is generally related to the external sources of stress impinging on one or multiple family members in such a way as to reverberate throughout the system and activate and mobilize stressful family interactional patterns.

The Group for Advancement of Psychiatry (GAP; 1985) report states that IFI does not assume that the etiology of major psychiatric disorders lies in family functioning and communication. However, it does assert that the contemporary family interactions of the patient can be a major source of stress or support.

Theoretical Background

IFI is the culmination of many theoretical positions. Recent developments in the field of family therapy have expanded the application of family theory by combining it with other therapeutic modalities such as medication and hospitalization. Family interaction still remains a very sensitive indicator of the ability of the individual and the family to cope with stress. However, the new expansion allows a more sensitive selection of loci for intervention in an inpatient unit or at alternative sites.

The diathesis stress theory of illness and its treatment (Falloon and McGill 1985; Rosenthal 1970; Zubin and Spring 1977) is a major theoretical perspective in IFI. According to this model, the emergence of emotional decompensation is related to two factors of patient vulnerability as well as the level of stress on the patient and the family. Reducing the level of stress on vulnerable people and their families can prevent illness. An alternative method is to decrease the patient's vulnerability so he or she can deal with a higher level of stress. With the wide acceptance of the stress-diathesis model of illness, attention has been focused on the role of two factors: the use of *medication* and the management of *expressed emotion* (EE) in the patients.

Psychotropic medication is considered an ally of family treatment, as it reduces vulnerability in the person being treated and enables him or her to cope with a higher level of stress tolerance in everyday living. The medication has proven particularly helpful in the treatment of schizophrenic and depressed individuals. This alliance between medication and family theory is in clear contrast to the early days of the family therapy movement, when the use of medication was avoided because of the fear it would increase the resistance of the family to changing their behaviors.

The positive response of a family member to psychotropic or antidepressant medication frequently makes the family more hopeful and enhances their problem-solving and interactional progression. At the same time, the judicious and effective use of medication enhances the therapeutic relationship between the psychiatrist and the family. The use of medication also reduces the grave effect of severely dysfunctional behavior, such as psychosis in one family member, on the rest of the family. The easing of this burden further reduces the negative and angry responses from other family members toward the identified patient and helps them to move forward productively.

Family Systems Theory

Inpatient family therapists share the view of family theorists about the family unit. The family unit is considered a social subsystem consisting of individuals interacting with one another according to certain rules (Glick et al. 1987; Shapiro 1980; Sholevar 1980; Stanton 1980). The family is seen as having homeostatic properties that attempt to balance its interacting parts. It uses a variety of negative and positive feedback to regulate the basic, adaptive, and defensive needs of different family members. The *family of procreation* is psychologically bound to the extended families (families of origin), and the behavior and interactions of the different family members have homeostatic and loyalty implications on the nuclear and extended family levels.

Specifically in regard to hospitalization, Sholevar (1980) has described the dynamics and patterns of families who institutionalize one of their members in a psychiatric hospital or residential treatment center. He defines *institutionalization* as the by-product of long-standing family dysfunctions in which the family attempts to reestablish homeostasis by extruding a member. The extrusion of a member is expected to bring harmony and stability to a family threatened by a serious imbalance caused by the increasing ineffectiveness of long-standing, defensive family patterns. Most of these dysfunctional and defensive patterns have been present in three generations. This length of time has often allowed them to attain sufficient intensity, chronicity, and lack of perspective to facilitate, rationalize, and justify a dramatic action such as the extrusion of a member from the family unit. The presence of similar relational and behavioral patterns in previous generations allows the family to feel, in an "ego syntonic" way, justified about extruding a member as the endpoint of the long-standing family conflicts.

GAP Report of Inpatient Family Intervention

Spencer and Glick have described the components of IFI in a 1985 GAP monograph:[1]

Description of Inpatient Family Intervention

I. Assumptions
   1. IFI does not assume that the etiology of the major psychotic disorders lies in family functioning or communication.

---

[1] The material in this section was taken in part from the study "Inpatient Family Intervention: A Controlled Study," funded in part by a NIMH grant (MH 34466), and was drafted by Drs. J. Spencer and I. Glick.

2. It does assume that the present-day functioning of a family with which the patient is living or is in frequent contact can be a major source of stress or support.

II. Aims

1. IFI aims to help the family to understand, live with, and deal with the patient and his or her illness; to develop the most appropriate possible ways of addressing the problems presented by the illness and its effects on the patient; and to understand and support both the necessary hospital treatment and long-range treatment plans.
2. It aims to help the patient to understand his or her family's actions and reactions and to develop the most appropriate possible intrafamily behavior on his or her part, in order to decrease his or her vulnerability to family stress and decrease the likelihood that his or her behavior will provoke it.

III. Strategy and Techniques

A. Evaluation

1. Evaluation is accomplished in one or more initial sessions with the family, with the patient present when conditions permit. Information gained from other sources is also used.
2. The patient's illness and its potential course are evaluated.
3. The present effect and the possible future effect on the family are determined.
4. The family's effect on the patient is evaluated, with particular reference to the stress caused by expressed emotion and criticism.
5. Family structure and interaction and the present point in the family life cycle are evaluated in order to determine whether particular aspects of the patient's role in the family are contributing to exacerbations of illness or to the maintenance of illness and/or impairment.

B. Techniques

1. The family and patient are usually seen together.
2. Early in the hospitalization an attempt is made to form an alliance with the family that gives them a sense of support and understanding.
3. Psychoeducation: (a) The family is provided with information about the illness, its likely course, and its treatment; questions are answered. (b) The idea that stress from and in

Family Intervention and Psychiatric Hospitalization

the family can cause exacerbation of the illness is discussed. (c) The ways in which conflicts and stress arise within each family are discussed, and a problem-solving approach is taken in planning ways to decrease such stress in the future. (d) The ways in which the illness and the patient's impaired functioning have burdened the family are discussed, and plans are made to decrease such burden.

4. In some cases, the initial evaluation of subsequent sessions suggests that there are particular resistances due to aspects of family structure or family dynamics that interfere with the accomplishment of (2) and (3) above. If it is judged necessary and possible, there may be attempts in one or a series of family sessions to explore such resistances and make changes in family dynamics. Such attempts may use some traditional family therapy techniques. Such families may be encouraged to seek family therapy after the patient's discharge.

Goals of Inpatient Family Intervention

Glick et al (1985a) have described a psychoeducationally oriented model of IFI as having multiple goals.

Acceptance of Illness by the Family

Early in the process of hospitalization, the therapist helps the family accept the illness—its seriousness, etiology, and ramifications—while beginning to formulate the emotional and cognitive understanding of the current episode. The family therapist has a great deal of latitude in choosing the technical methods that are most appropriate to the particular situation. Glick et al. (1985a) term the key family tasks of this first goal as accepting the reality of the illness and developing an understanding of the current episode. This work can begin during the acute, early phase of hospitalization when the family is most accepting of the expertise and authority of the hospital staff.

Identification of Stressors

The family often will require assistance from the staff in identifying the key stressors both within and external to the family. The family needs to both understand the variety of stressors that may have precipitated the current episode of hospitalization and rank them by degree of importance so that this brief therapeutic approach can be better focused.

Anticipation of Future Stressors

The family is helped to anticipate future stressors that will impinge on the patient. Again, as in the previous steps, stressors from within as well as outside the family are to be considered.

Recognition of Stressful Family Patterns

The pursuit of this goal requires the greatest therapeutic tact and skill on the part of the therapist. The family learns to identify the family interaction patterns that produce stress on the identified patient. It is essential that the family develop emotional insight into the interactional patterns that trigger the individual's symptoms without feeling blamed or developing the false idea that these stressful interactions are the *cause* of the problem of the hospitalized family member. This learning usually occurs when patterns are pointed out in a family session or sessions with the patient present. A variety of theoretical models may be used. It is felt that this goal most closely approximates traditional family therapy models.

Planning to Meet Future Stressors

Planning strategies for managing and/or minimizing future stresses usually come toward the end of the hospital stay when the patient and family are relieved that the acute phase of symptoms and distress has passed. At this point, the family may be more comfortable denying the possibility that this could happen again. The therapist needs to help the family adjust post-discharge expectations either up or down, as needed, to allow for adequate and appropriate planning. Role-playing is a suggested technique.

Relapse Prevention by Continued Treatment

This concluding part of IFI comes at a time when the sense of crisis is greatly diminished. The family must accept the need for appropriate continued treatment that takes into account the possibility of a repeat hospitalization and yet extends hope and encouragement to prevent this possibility. This latter can be accomplished with careful planning and effective ongoing treatment that may include pharmacotherapy. The family may need to be walked through possible future scenarios and the optimal reactions. Further education on pathogenesis and prognosis may be indicated. Families will vary widely on how much mastery is possible, but understanding even a few basic concepts may help prevent rehospitalization or give the family a greater sense of understanding, hope, and control.

Strategies and Techniques

The strategies and techniques of family therapy have been shown to reduce the length of hospitalization for psychiatric inpatients, even when the therapists have been relatively inexperienced trainees. The following are particularly applicable to IFI.

Timing

The first contact with the family takes place during the decision-making process leading to hospitalization (Glick et al. 1985a, 1985b). Early in the course of the hospital stay, the therapist begins to undertake several tasks. First, he or she becomes an ally in finding coping mechanisms that will prove useful later in the course of hospitalization. Second, by sharing in the experiences of the family with the acutely disorganized, hospitalized family member, the staff members underscore their empathic stance. Third, the therapist joins with the family at the time the patient's distress is most acute and thus helps define the familial variable of the problem rather than providing a predominantly individual perspective on the issues. The involvement of the hospitalized family member is adjusted during this time based on his or her ability to contribute to a family treatment plan.

Some family therapists disagree about when in the psychotic process it is appropriate to include the hospitalized member in the family sessions. Because of the possibility of disorganization under family stress, some feel the individual with the disorder should not be included until the acute phase has begun to abate. Glick et al. (1985a) notes that some psychotic patients become more coherent during focused and well-planned family sessions. He feels that the concern about including the psychotic individual may be a rationalization to avoid starting the family treatment, although it is not uncommon for the ill family member to be too psychotic to benefit from a family session.

Staffing

The hospital staff member designated as the family therapist may have been trained in a variety of disciplines—psychiatry, social work, nursing, psychology—or may be a trainee in one of these or allied fields. All of these professions can help families change their interaction patterns. The preferred model is the family therapist and also the designated primary hospital therapist, as this individual has the best grasp of the case. This combination may not always be possible and other arrangements may need to be made, depending on time constraints and other variables.

The family therapist has several functions. He or she may

- Work individually with the designated patient, work with the entire family, or work with selected family members
- Be available for personal meetings and phone contacts
- Gather information about the family from other hospital personnel
- Participate in overall management
- Coordinate discharge planning

Nurses designated as family therapists can meet with families during visiting hours, and occupational and recreational therapists can prescribe concrete activities for the family, such as preparing meals, helping the patient to wash his or her own clothes, or going on a picnic together.

Co-therapy may be especially helpful, as some therapists feel that work with certain very disturbed families who have a member in the hospital may be a very demanding type of psychotherapy. A co-therapist can also increase availability to the family and may help the therapist maintain objectivity and share the emotional burden.

The hospital milieu becomes a rich and varied source of information about a family and its functioning. On-the-spot observation of family functioning may provide explanations that otherwise would not have been available as clues to the patient's perceptions or behavior. The adolescent who is paranoid about the nursing staff may also be observed relating to his mother in the same way. Pointing out this similarity in patterns may be very helpful to him (although very short stays make this intervention difficult). Hospital staff, particularly line staff, who often do not attend team meetings or clinical case conferences, must be taught to report significant family information. If care is not taken, the family therapist may inadvertently diminish the importance of the information of other hospital staff members and thus discourage the reporting of crucial information. For example, Sholevar (1983) reported the situation of the reluctant father who never attended a family therapy session but appeared in the hospital drunk and abused his son. This significant information about the current functioning of the family can be reported to the family therapist by the staff.

Other Techniques

The issue of patient-therapist confidentiality may conflict with the need for optimal communication among staff in the hospital. It is necessary for hospital staff to communicate with one another in order to achieve the greatest treatment effectiveness. The family may be told that the family therapist will use all the material that is available in both family and individual contacts to improve family functioning.

It is important to encourage all family members to participate in problem solving and not to shift the entire problem to the identified patient to work through. Likewise, the family should not be allowed to blame the hospitalized person for all the family's problems. Rather than focusing on the patient's problematic behaviors, the family therapist should focus on the problems encountered by the family in the management of the patient's behavior and help encourage the family to join in the problem management (Anderson 1976). This strategy may help delineate the familial role conflicts and restructure the family system. For example, scapegoating may be reduced and cooperative problem solving enhanced by reducing tension in the family system.

Decompensation and disintegration often characterize the family of the hospitalized person. Family members may avoid contact with one another. Family members may refuse to attend family therapy sessions. A similar phenomenon has been termed the "absent member maneuver" by Sonne et al. (1962). Sometimes significant members may not attend sessions when certain other family members are expected. The family therapist should not be surprised if the family tries to misrepresent the views of the absent members.

Destructive family roles may perpetuate unresolved and long-standing family conflicts. These patterns may have their genesis in transgenerational patterns of inadequate parenting that can be effectively addressed by psychodynamic therapists. When the patterns are processed in family sessions, dramatic changes may take place that establish new, healthier family patterns in just a few sessions. For this phenomenon to happen, the therapist needs to establish an empathic atmosphere in which emotions can be identified, understood, and accepted. Paul and Grosser (1965) described a similar phenomenon, which they termed *corrective* or *operational mourning*, that can happen in single- or multiple-family sessions. The parents—who may have felt deprived and desperate and may have been uncooperative with the family therapist and hospital staff—may now develop insight into the genetic roots of the problems that allows them to follow therapist's directions and to take action to improve their parenting skills. The importance of this type of psychodynamic intervention has not been fully realized by some of the *communicational* family therapists when they use the label *historically* oriented family therapies.

The *enactive* style of giving concrete directions may be preferable to a more abstract level of exploration for certain severely disturbed families. The therapist may need to make suggestions such as "Talk to your son now" or "Go fishing with him this weekend." In this situation, an abstract discussion and a historical exploration of the father-son distance may be less helpful. When there are factions at war within the family system, a family member can be selected to be the family representative in the sessions for the absent and opposing members. Hospital staff members can also make themselves available to any family member at mutually convenient times, such as evenings and weekends.

Sholevar (1983) recommends that "the family therapist in the hospital setting be viewed as the final conduit for familial information rather than its sole repository." The family therapist in turn digests the information gathered and reported by multiple staff members, formulates it into a conceptual framework using a variety of different theoretical models, and communicates a plan of intervention that may be included as part of the treatment plan. This plan may then be implemented by different members of the treatment team, with the family therapist in formal family sessions, with the patient individually, with the family when they come for visits, during ancillary therapy sessions, or by almost any team member during interactions with the family or patient. This plan informs the treatment staff about what behavior may be expected from various family members and how to deal effectively with such behaviors. All members of the treatment team then participate in the planned interventions, a process by which the diagnostic and therapeutic reach of the family therapist is extended.

Family Intervention With Acute, Recurrent, and Chronic Disorders

Family theory has contributed significantly to the understanding of psychiatric patients in acute, recurrent, or chronic crises.

Acute Disorder

The acute psychiatric disorder represents not only an individual in crisis but usually a family that is decompensating under stress. This stress can affect any member of the nuclear or extended family. When the father loses his job, for example, tension and despair may spread throughout the family. Or serious illness in the mother can result in family tension and the psychotic breakdown of an offspring, who may be unaware of the mother's physical symptoms but is affected secondarily by the anxiety emerging in the relationship of the parents. Such stresses can be more easily recognized and treated by working with nuclear and extended family units than by focusing on the hospitalized person alone. Family theory can help the clinician to identify single or multiple points of stress affecting the nuclear or extended family.

Recurrent Disorder

Family studies in the past two decades have significantly enhanced our understanding of the phenomenon of recurrent psychiatric hospitalization, particularly in patients with schizophrenia and depression. The study of EE has revealed that families with a high level of criticism and overinvolvement with their psychiatrically ill members are faced with frequent hospitalizations. EE is characterized by a high level of tension-producing verbal output in a critical and hostile fashion by other family members toward the member with the disorder. *Overinvolvement* refers to face-to-face contact exceeding 35 hours per week with psychiatrically ill persons. In families with a high rate of EE and a history of overinvolvement, psychiatrically ill family members are at increased risk for frequent hospitalization. In families with a low level of EE and face-to-face contact, the rate of rehospitalization is significantly reduced. The investigations of a number of family researchers have indicated that interventions that succeed in the reduction of EE and overinvolvement with family members can result in reduction or prevention of rehospitalization. The studies on EE have been summarized by Sholevar (see Chapter 1, "Family Theory and Therapy: An Overview") and by Miklowitz and Tompson (see Chapter 27, "Family Variables and Interventions in Schizophrenia").

Chronic Disorders

Speck and Attneave (1973) point out that the social network of severely and chronically ill patients is significantly constricted in comparison to that of moderately or acutely disturbed people. This impoverishment of the social network limits the family's external support and input, making the family even more vulnerable to breakdown and disintegration in stressful situations. It is important to reestablish the family's relational ties and social network as a primary goal of the therapeutic intervention.

The following case reported by Sholevar (1983) illustrates the role of an impoverished social network in recurring psychiatric hospitalization:

Mrs. L is a 40-year-old divorced woman who was hospitalized because of anxiety, depression, a suicide attempt, and excessive drinking. The hospitalization occurred after her father rejected her endeavor to reestablish ties with him. Mrs. L's mother and grandmother died when she was in her early and late adolescence, respectively.

In the hospital, Mrs. L appeared to be a pleasant and attractive woman exhibiting extreme self-centeredness and very low self-esteem. An exploration of the composition of her family and social network revealed that her total social support system consisted of her father, with whom she had had no contact in the past several years because of his disapproval of her drinking. She viewed him as critical and rejecting. The other members of Mrs. L's network included her boyfriend, K, an alcoholic man whose brief encounters with Mrs. L had been followed by severe fights and prolonged periods of avoidance. The other two members of Mrs. L's network were an ex-patient from her previous hospitalization and an old co-worker. However, she avoided seeing them at times of stress, because she did not want them to see her in a stage of decompensation. Although a competent worker, Mrs. L arranged to work in her home, therefore depriving herself of the opportunity to develop a social network. She longed to reestablish a relationship with her father, although she felt pessimistic about it. She blamed her father's stubbornness for their relational breakup and took no responsibility for her role in it. She also wanted to see her only son, who lived with her ex-husband, having seen him on only one occasion in the recent past.

Families of Chronically Ill Patients

Talbott (1987) noted that 70% of chronically and seriously ill, hospitalized psychiatric patients have families willing to be involved with them after discharge. These families represent a very important resource that has not been appropriately used in some cases.

Innovative research done by Lefley (1985) studied clinicians with a close relative who had severe long-term disorders. Members of this group did not fault their parents for their sibling's illness but did note the burden the illness placed on the family and recognized the efforts parents made in the rehabilitation of the ill family member. Anderson (1986) found that families were more likely to be aggravated by the skill deficits and difficulties associated with the activities of daily living exhibited in the persons with the disorders. The families who were more actively involved in the care of the individuals were the ones who were more stressed. An inverse relationship was noted between the length of the illness and the degree to which it concerned the family.

The families of chronically mentally ill patients carry a heavy burden. Hatfield (1979, 1981, 1991) documents the emotional burdens the families bear. Stress, anxiety, and grief associated with the relative's illness were noted, as well as hardship on siblings and spouses. In addition to the grieving process and the ongoing needs for the care of the ill family member, there is often guilt, which unfortunately has been enhanced by professionals in some cases.

The National Alliance for the Mentally Ill, a rapidly expanding advocacy group for families of the mentally ill, points out the strong stigma that has come in part from pejorative language used by mental health professionals and theories that emphasize family interactions or early parent-child interactions as causative of serious mental illness. Hatfield (1986a) espouses the formation of a "new theory and language" of mental illness. The cornerstone of this new formulation is that the *family is the most important resource* and thus deserves support and respect.

An effective and appropriate professional stance has been one of a psychoeducational model. The family is provided with information about the expected course of illness, its causes, its treatment, and the role of stress and conflict on relapse into illness. Promotion of family problem solving, reduction of family guilt, and examination of the burden on the family are also necessary. Talbott (1987) emphasizes the need of the family of the mentally ill for 1) information about mental illness, its manifestations, and course; 2) help in handling the patient's behavior; and 3) knowledge of resources, respite care and services, economic relief, crisis care, and rehabilitation services.

Glick et al. (1985b) recommends a number of excellent books for the families of the mentally ill: Wasow's 1982 book, *Coping With Schizophrenia: A Survival Manual for Parents, Relatives and Friends* and a book by Bernheim (1982) entitled *The Caring Family: Living With Chronic Mental Illness*.

Inpatient Family Intervention With Children and Adolescents

The family literature in this area tends to be psychodynamically oriented and examines the family patterns of families who institutionalize and hospitalize their children.

The "institutionalization phenomenon" (Sholevar 1980, 1983) refers to the special processes in the family that attempt to reestablish family homeostasis by the hospitalization or institutionalization of a child. The families generally contact a professional person or agency when this process is highly advanced and the family is unwilling or unable to consider alternative courses. When the institutionalization of the child cannot be prevented, the family therapist has multiple crucial tasks to contribute to the treatment plan, including helping the family to use the hospital in a productive manner and urging them to refrain from signing the family member out of the hospital prematurely. The latter phenomenon is common in dysfunctional families who wish to reengage the child in the ongoing family conflicts.

In many of the families who hospitalize and institutionalize their children, one of the parents has been hospitalized as an adult or as a child had been placed in a foster home (Sholevar 1980). In one of the cases reported, the exploration of the roots of the decision for psychiatric hospitalization of a child revealed that the mother was repeating her early life experience when she was extruded from her family of origin. The mother was identifying with the aggressor (her own mother), projecting guilt on her own child, and extruding him from the nuclear family. The mother stubbornly adhered to the decision for hospitalization until she was made to realize the impact of her own foster-home placement and extrusion from her family of origin. She then reversed her decision to hospitalize her son, reduced her covert rejection of him, and searched for more adaptive solutions. The above changes were achieved in two intense family sessions with dramatic behavioral changes in the mother and the child (Sholevar 1980).

> Jim, a 15-year-old African American who was the oldest of five children in a divorced family, was admitted to the psychiatric inpatient unit for "explosive behavior" that exhibited itself by the destruction of furniture and significant damage to his household. He remained belligerent and aloof in the unit, forming no meaningful relationship with his peers or the staff. The three traditional family therapy sessions, which included the mother and the other children, who ranged in age between 6 and 13, generally focused on the description of the periodic explosive behavior of Jim and the mother's feeling overwhelmed. The mother was quite isolated socially. The review of the case with the senior family psychiatrist did not reveal any explanation for Jim's highly explosive behavior, the difference between his behavior and the quiet and submissive attitude of his siblings, or any explanation for the recent onset of the presenting problem. Therefore, the senior consultant was asked to meet with the family to explore the above issues.
>
> The family exhibited their traditional interactive pattern, while Jim acted belligerently toward the mother and called her "crazy." Fifteen minutes into the session, the consultant observed that the mother seemed to be very aware of the passage of time and inquired about when the session would end, an unusual sensitivity toward the passage of time for a highly dysfunctional family. The exploration of the nature of the mother's concern revealed that her older sister, who drove the family to their appointment and had encouraged them to participate in family treatment, was sitting in the parking lot with the car engine running waiting to give them a ride back home. The sister was invited to attend the session. It was then discovered that the sister was a *go-between*, connecting the family with the oldest sister, who had ceased to have any direct contact with the mother or the children. The oldest sister considered the mother "crazy" because she regularly told her chil-

dren that her estranged husband was entering her house at night and injecting some toxic substance under the scalp of the children and the mother. The mother and the children all claimed that they suffered from headaches on this basis. The oldest maternal sister would send messages through the middle sister to Jim telling him that his mother was "crazy" and he should not listen to her. It was then discovered that Jim's explosive behavior had always emerged following the mother's statement about their estranged father's visits. At such moments, Jim would shout that the mother was "crazy" while breaking the furniture. This explanation shed light on why Jim called his mother "crazy" in the family sessions and on the unit. The episodes had started shortly after the oldest maternal sister had ceased direct contact with the family, although she has been sending messages to Jim through the middle sister, with whom she lived.

The therapeutic strategy was to invite the oldest and middle maternal sisters to attend the family sessions and bring about an open discussion of the estranged father and the actual nature of his relationship with the children and his ex-wife. The heightened support from the two sisters and the open discussion of the relationship with the father/husband and the circumstances of his departure resulted in a rapid decrease in Jim's angry and explosive behavior, enhanced Jim's relationship with the hospital staff and peers, and led to a quick discharge from the unit. The mother's headaches disappeared subsequent to the reestablishment of the relationship with the oldest sister. The headaches of the mother had started approximately at the time of the breakup of the relationship between the mother and her oldest sister and were followed by the claims to headaches in the younger children. The outpatient family treatment continued with the goal of enhancement of the relationship between the mother and her older sisters, as well as the relationship between the aunts and the children, and decrease in the mother's social isolation. The relationship between the family and the father could not be reestablished by the end of the family treatment.

Hospitalization and Children of Divorce

An emerging new phenomenon is the interface between the psychiatric hospitalization of children and parental divorce. While the parents are still married, each parent tends to blame the child's problems on the shortcomings of the other parent and to overestimate his or her own ability to contain the child's behavior. A divorce often intensifies the conflict between the child and one parent and creates a pattern of rapid negative escalation, resulting in extreme behaviors such as suicide threats on the part of the child and depression in the parent at the height of an escalated crisis. At some point, the child and one parent—usually the parent who was overinvolved before the divorce—reach an impasse. As the result of years of blaming the other parent as inadequate and as the cause of the child's difficulties, the custodial parent cannot consider the option of sending the child to the noncustodial parent at the time of extreme crisis. Therefore, hospitalization is called on to resolve the situation. The frequent outcome is that the child enters the hospital following a crisis with the custodial parent and is discharged to the house of the noncustodial parent following the hospital course. Although there are no definite statistics available for this phenomenon, probably somewhere between 10% and 20% of hospitalized conduct-disordered children of divorced parents end up returning to the second parent following the hospitalization course. Here, the hospital seems to serve the function of introducing and opening an alternative residential custody option. Hospitalization can be made more efficient if hospital staff recognize their limited and specific role at this point rather than attempting to pursue a more ambitious course.

The phenomenon of *child switching* or *child keeping* has occurred historically but with less frequency in nondivorcing families. In such circumstances, the nuclear and extended families have arranged to shift the children back and forth at the time of crisis in order to diffuse the tension.

Results of Inpatient Family Intervention

Glick et al. (1991, 1993) have studied the impact of IFI by comparing the results of two kinds of treatment of individuals with schizophrenic and affective disorders: 1) treatment using a psychoeducational model in an inpatient setting and 2) standard hospitalization without family intervention. In this comparison, 169 patients and their families were assigned to one of the two treatments on a random basis. Assessments were made at admission, at discharge, and 6 and 18 months following discharge from the hospital. The assessment included both individual and family measures on multiple dimensions.

Results suggested significant effects favoring IFI for patients and their families. The treatment effects were limited to females and two diagnostic groups: chronic schizophrenia patients and persons with affective disorders of the bipolar subgroup. Using analysis of variance and correlational analyses, we examined three variables that mediate between family treatment and outcome: 1) posthospital medication compliance, 2) posthospital psychosocial treatment compliance, and 3) patient rejection by the family. Results showed robust correlations between these variables and outcomes for all diagnostic subgroups. The pattern of associations between the mediating variables and outcome was more prominent for patients treated with IFI. These results were seen most clearly in the total sample, and for the subgroups of "all females" and "poor pre-hospital functioning females with schizophrenia." Finally, family achievement of the goals of the family intervention was positively associated with better patient outcome, while increased family burden at discharge was associated with shorter length of time before rehospitalization.

Conclusion

Family intervention, even with briefly hospitalized patients, represents an important development in family psychiatry that combines family intervention with other treatment modalities and selects the psychiatric hospital as the locus of intervention for acutely and severely disturbed psychiatric patients. In addition to family theory, it uses diathesis-stress theory to address the vulnerability of the patient to the mounting stress both outside and within the family. Psychotropic medications are considered a major ally of family therapists, as they can reduce the patient's vulnerability to stress. The family interventions are generally psychoeducational in their orientation and address multiple sources of stress and vulnerability within and outside the family.

Family intervention with hospitalized adolescents and children recognizes the multiple factors contributing to psychiatric disability of these youngsters. It is often the state of decompensation in the family and the patient that precipitates the hospitalization of a young person. The role of the assessment is to recognize the contributing factors, which include the family burden, psychopathology in the parents, interpersonal conflicts of the parents, and use of the mechanism of extrusion of the child from the family to establish equilibrium in a dysfunctional family. Family intervention in turn attempts to reverse the decompensated state of the family and resolve the sources of stress that have given rise to it.

Chapters on Related Topics

The following chapters describe concepts related to family intervention and psychiatric hospitalization:

- Chapter 8, "Psychoeducational Family Intervention"
- Chapter 17, "Family Therapy With Children and Adolescents: An Overview"
- Chapter 27, "Family Variables and Interventions in Schizophrenia"
- Chapter 28, "Depression and the Family: Interpersonal Context and Family Functioning"
- Chapter 30, "National Alliance for the Mentally Ill (NAMI) and Family Psychiatry: Working Toward a Collaborative Model"

30

National Alliance for the Mentally Ill (NAMI) and Family Psychiatry

Working Toward a Collaborative Model

G. Pirooz Sholevar, M.D.
Linda D. Schwoeri, Ph.D.

Introduction

The deinstitutionalization of the mentally ill in the past three decades dramatically changed the locus for their care by shifting back to the family the primary caregiving responsibility. When institutionalization was the predominant model of intervention, the mental health professionals served as the "experts" and the family assumed the position of the interested but relatively passive support system. The hospital staff determined the symptomatology, chose the focus of intervention, developed and rendered the treatment plan, and assessed the therapeutic progression. For example, the family may have been told that the patient was exhibiting psychotic and erratic behavior and so was isolated from other patients. The progress of the patient in overcoming such symptoms with the assistance of the hospital staff was reported to the family. The family remained ready to receive the patient for home visits in order to strengthen the family ties, determine his or her adjustment at home, and ultimately help facilitate the discharge. Deinstitutionalization created a dramatic shift in the nature of care and treatment. The family was placed in the position of observing the entire range of the patient's behavior, determining the behaviors most problematic to the patient's adjustment, taking over the management problems of the patient, searching for effective intervention techniques, and asking for the assistance of the mental health professionals when they were overwhelmed by the patient's illness and symptomatology. The lack of effective management and intervention techniques with the chronically ill and the lack of a new model of collaboration then emerged as new obstacles and probably served as the basis for the misunderstandings that emerged between the families of mentally ill patients and mental health professionals. The schism between the two groups has been further fueled by a range of issues, some of them substantial in nature, and many of them the products of imprecise terminology and conceptualization complicated by limited knowledge about the nature and management of chronic mental illness.

The National Alliance for the Mentally Ill (NAMI) was formed against this background to enhance the treatment of mental illness, particularly schizophrenia, and to forge a productive relationship between the families of mentally ill patients and mental health professionals. Despite some misunderstandings, the collaboration has proceeded along converging and productive paths, and the two groups have become increasingly respectful and appreciative of each other's contributions to the welfare of the mentally ill. However, some of the old misunderstandings prevail.

In this chapter we describe the organization of NAMI, its belief system, and the substantial and insubstantial differences of opinion between NAMI and the field of psychiatry. We then propose an effective model for collaboration. We expect that the discussion of the training requirements of mental health professionals in collaboration with the family as discussed in this chapter will enhance the progression of this collaborative model.

History of the National Alliance for the Mentally Ill

The National Alliance for the Mentally Ill is a volunteer grassroots organization of families and friends of the mentally ill. Many groups are primarily composed of parents of adult patients, but there are separate groups for parents of children and adolescents with emotional disorders. NAMI was founded in 1979 in Madison, Wisconsin, by a group of 254 people who through public notice, phone calls, and determination joined in their common purpose of helping their severely ill family members and friends. As an organization, NAMI is both an advocacy and support group. Today, there are more than 1,000 local support groups or "affiliates." Each of the 50 states plus the District of Columbia has its own NAMI affiliate. The national headquarters in Arlington, Virginia, serves as the base and clearinghouse for its many educational, advocacy, and research-directed activities. NAMI represented 140,000 family members in 1997, and this number is growing rapidly (Hall et al. 1997). The (800) 950-NAMI help line is available to consumers and professionals alike. The formation of a local affiliate requires a minimum five-person membership and agreement with NAMI's goals.

According to its Public Policy Platform of 1992, NAMI's primary functions and goals are directed toward support, advocacy for research, and education of all professionals, providers, and the general public. The local affiliates maintain essentially a self-help philosophy and a self-reliant approach. They are encouraged to establish their autonomy by remaining independent of other mental health agencies and, through their tax-exempt status, to build an organization that relies on itself for mailings, meetings, and other related support. The state organizations, as well as the national organization, are made up of boards limited to persons with mental illness and their relatives. The reform of mental health care funding to achieve parity with all other health care services, and the support for biological research in the treatment of mental illness, are two very current legislative issues.

NAMI essentially came into existence as a response to the needs created by the deinstitutionalization of the severely mentally ill in the United States and the aftermath of long-term institutionalization and custodial care of the mentally ill. The establishment of NAMI is often seen in contraposition to the developments in the field of psychiatry and mental health during the three decades prior to its founding. During the 1960s and 1970s, with the continuous support of the National Institute of Mental Health (NIMH), there was a growth in investigation and treatment of schizophrenia and its biological and interactional processes.

In 1961, despite the use of medications and new approaches to treatment, the number of psychiatric patients overwhelmed the state hospitals, and the Joint Commission on Mental Illness and Health advocated deinstitutionalization. In 1963 Congress passed the Community Mental Health Centers Act to promote community placement. In theory, deinstitutionalization was an attempt to keep the mentally ill closer to family and neighborhood. This had been implemented with returning World War II veterans, some of whom experienced mental illness. The families of schizophrenic patients now reported their feeling of not understanding the complex phenomenon of collaboration with professionals that disregarded their perceived needs.

Founding Principles of NAMI

NAMI as an organization is built upon four principles:

1. *Mental illness as a brain disease.* The organization is committed to neurobiological research and the importance of psychotropic medication in the treatment of mental illness, especially schizophrenia. NAMI maintains that prevention is possible only through an understanding of brain neurochemistry, not alteration of psychological family communication and interactional patterns.
2. *Self-help.* As a volunteer association, NAMI offers mutual aid and assistance toward emotional support and education to members in order to better serve the needs of both the patients and their families.
3. *Consumer action and responsibilities.* NAMI assumes that as consumers of mental health services, patients and their families are responsible for taking action to meet their goals. NAMI has taken action to access and disseminate information about chronic mental illness and has produced literature expressly for that purpose. Many of the branches have lay referral groups. Others exert a great deal of pressure on institutions by joining advisory groups to ensure that the appropriate and most relevant information needed to provide service to the patient is disseminated.
4. *Families as advocates for the mentally ill.* Through collaboration and active legislative participation, NAMI has worked toward the following goals: finding appropriate housing for the mentally ill; securing mandatory insurance coverage for the chronically and severely mentally ill—coverage comparable to that for medical illness; supporting research into the etiology and treatment of mental illness; addressing the criminal justice system's treatment of individuals with mental illness; challenging commitment laws and procedures; and educating the community at large on mental illness through national weekly campaigns, educational material, and newsletters.

Sources of Disagreements Between NAMI and Mental Health Professionals

There are multiple sources for the differences of opinion between NAMI and providers of psychiatric care to mentally ill patients. Some differences of opinion or misunderstandings are related to perceived attitudes, while some concerns refer to substantial issues. These differences and misunderstandings collectively undermine the relationship between the psychiatric care provider and the family.

The nature of the relationship between the family of a mentally ill patient and the clinician is confusing and may at times resemble a doctor-patient relationship, with the family in the position of patient vis-à-vis the practitioner. The family's request may be subjected to clinical scrutiny rather than responded to in a satisfactory manner. For example, the family might ask for an increase in the amount of medication for the patient so he or she can sleep at night and not disturb the sleep of other family members. The family would like this to be taken literally and in a straightforward manner rather than have the clinician advise them to be more tolerant of the patient's nightly disturbances. The symptomatic lack of self-care by the patient can be particularly bothersome to the family, and they might frequently insist on effective measures for its correction. The practitioner, on the other hand, may take the position that the family should reduce its level of expectation of the patient.

The differences based on *form* include the use of certain terminology that was common several decades ago. The most offensive term to the family was that of *schizophrenogenic mother*, which attributed the genetic role in schizophrenia to the behavior of the mother and her methods of child-rearing. The term, coined by Freida Fromm-Reichmann (1948), became popular in the 1950s, and its use continued into the 1960s. It did not achieve the type of widespread recognition necessary to become a significant element in treatment planning for schizophrenic patients. The concept of *double-bind* proposed by Bateson et al. (1956) was more popularly used but also had a questionable impact on the actual treatment planning for schizophrenic patients. Neither of the above concepts constitutes an important facet in the psychiatric treatment of mentally ill patients today, and neither was supported by subsequent research. In fact, the limited investigation of both concepts tended to refute the concepts rather than confirm them.

In the attitudinal area, it has been difficult to treat families of schizophrenic patients as equal collaborators in treatment as one may do with a medical consultant on a case or an attorney and judge representing the patient's rights. It is a true test of professionalism and maturity to treat a disheveled, poorly dressed, and overweight mother of a schizophrenic patient, whose speech about her child has acquired the quality of a rambling, repetitive, and disorganized monologue, as an equal collaborator and colleague who shares your goal of stabilizing a psychotic patient. It is easy to ignore the fact that she actually has more power than the practitioner to bring about improvement in the patient's condition, provide guidelines for the use of pharmacotherapeutic or psychotherapeutic agents, assist in the administration of the therapeutic agents, and provide sensible feedback on the effectiveness of treatment. The task of collaboration with families also suffers because clinicians are taught primarily to evaluate, diagnose, plan, and render treatment. Such skills and approaches are more central to the role of a clinician than that of a consultant; the latter group attempts to contribute to the treatment approach while being mindful of the person who actually controls the clinical situation.

Another area of substantial difference between families of mentally ill patients and clinical practitioners has been the low level of importance assigned to biological and psychopharmacological research in contrast to that assigned to psychological and childrearing factors. In the past, the attempts of some practitioners to assign a high level of importance to questionable family or psychological factors may have directly or indirectly undermined sufficient emphasis on biological research. The need for extensive research into the biological nature of schizophrenia, depression, and alcoholism is currently well accepted by both clinician and NAMI. Indeed, the family researchers have been close allies of biological psychiatrists in emphasizing the need for examination of both the biological and interpersonal context of major mental illnesses and the interaction of the above factors with one another.

Significant Issues in the Care of Mentally Ill Patients

The following issues are strongly emphasized by NAMI.

Families as Caregivers

It is well documented that the deinstitutionalization of chronically mentally ill patients and their treatment in the community placed the burden and responsibility for monitoring their treatment on families (Brown et al. 1972; Falloon et al. 1978; Lefley 1998a, 1998b; Vaughn 1982; Vaughn and Leff 1981). It is estimated that 4.5% of the U.S. population (about 12 million Americans) have a serious mental illness. Studies estimate that more than 55% of these patients return to their families following discharge from the hospital (Goldman 1982). This is a burden on those families that becomes even graver when the issue of possible violence is considered. The actual incidence of violence in mentally ill relatives is between 5% and 38% (Hatfield 1992a, 1997).

Family Involvement in Discharge Planning

Frequently, families are inadequately involved with the discharge planning for their family members. This significant omission has a far-reaching negative impact on the course of illness in the patient.

Dissonance Between Family and Staff

There is consensus that mental health professionals need to respond to requests of the families of seriously mentally ill patients in a more helpful manner in order to reduce friction (Anderson et al. 1980; McElroy 1985). Studies of professionals who are also family members of mentally ill individuals indicate that some mental health professionals actually increased the burden of the illness during the time of crisis through a variety of deleterious transactions that were psychologically distressing (McElroy 1985; Waslow and Wikler 1983).

Members as Learners

Family members should be viewed as adults with different cognitive styles who are capable and interested in learning. They should be viewed as mature, self-directed, problem-focused, and practical people who are capable of being managers and decision-makers. (McElroy 1985). There is a great level of diversity in families of mentally ill persons (Hatfield 1997), and these families have demonstrated a high level of resilience (Lefley 1998a, 1998b; Marsh 1996).

The Family–Mental Health Professional Relationship

The relationship between families and mental health professionals passes through at least two stages. In the initial stage of *naive trusting*, the family accepts the lack of guidance or practical advice for the care of their mentally ill member. There is frequently a disparity between the treatment goals held by the family and those espoused by professionals (Hatfield 1981). However, despite dissatisfaction with services rendered, families appear to recognize the importance of professional help (Holden and Lewine 1982). This recognition results in the family's entering the stage of *guarded alliance* with the professionals (Robinson and Thorne 1984). Mental health professionals frequently underestimate the significance of the grieving process when the grief (or mourning) experienced by the family of the mentally ill person emerges periodically. The memories of the past deepen the family grief.

Educational Needs and Bothersome Behaviors

McElroy (1985) conducted a descriptive study to identify the educational needs of families of seriously ill patients and the bothersome behavior of mentally ill persons. In the study, nurses and families identified areas in which they required more information. The nurses assigned high priority to the management of suicidal behavior, drinking, physical aggression, confusion, and so forth. The families assigned priority to information about psychotropic medication, independence, self-esteem, housing, research on mental illness, and burnout among relatives.

The comparison of *bothersome behavior* as identified by the family members and the nurses revealed the following differences. The nurses were highly bothered by suicidal, homicidal, aggressive, socially embarrassing, and strange behaviors. The family was highly concerned about the lack of achievement of potential, the lack of motivation, and the inability to work or gain vocational training. Some discrepancies between priorities for the groups are obvious. The families focused on the social and everyday problems of living, while the concerns of the mental health professionals were more narrowly clinical. In the continuing efforts to gain information on the treatment options for chronically ill patients, a survey was conducted by NAMI, the American Psychiatric Association, and Columbia University. This coalition conducted a national telephone survey that included 112 caregivers, 80 patients, and 101 psychiatrists who treated four or more schizophrenic patients weekly. The coalition found that the illness had a negative effect on the quality of life of both patients and caregivers.

The patients continued to have difficulty maintaining a positive relationship with the caregivers and treatment facilities and maintaining a job. Community programs were unavailable, and the public opinion toward mentally ill people was negative (Psychiatric News 1994). While the actual incidence of violence in mentally ill relatives who live at home is between 5% and 38% (Hatfield 1992b), there is often fear, anxiety, and tension surrounding family life in many cases. Psychoeducational programs offered in different mental health settings teach families that violent behavior must *never* be tolerated and that they must stand their ground on the do's and don'ts rather than to permit ambiguity.

Family Intervention and the Nature of Treatment

Historically, the literature on the role of the family in major mental illness has been largely negative. The focus has been on pathogenesis resulting from what has been labeled "communication deviance" (CD) within the family (Wynne and Singer 1963; Wynne et al. 1977). As noted by Falloon et al. (1984), this has resulted in the de-emphasis of the more constructive and positive support that a family can offer to its severely mentally ill members. More recently, psychosocial programs have been developed that aim to mobilize the *rehabilitative* focus within the family through family education and psychoeducational family therapy. These programs are sensitive to the stress that arises from both the patient's illness and events within and without the family itself. A review of the literature indicates that psychosocial interventions aimed at strengthening both the patient's coping skills and the family's supportive efforts have been successful in reducing relapse and in improving communication skills within the family (Liberman et al. 1986).

The *psychoeducational family intervention* described by C.M. Anderson et al. (1980, 1986) has been successful in the management of long-term stressful factors with mentally ill family members. A comprehensive summary of this family approach is described in Chapter 20. Programs combining antipsychotic medication and brief family crisis treatment immediately after hospital discharge have been highly effective in preventing relapse of major mental disorders (Goldstein 1980; Hogarty et al. 1986). Falloon et al. (1993) has developed a complete program-training module using a cognitive-behavioral approach that can be followed by the family. The module enhances problem-solving and communication skills in the family. Communication skills training provides the family with exercises to express both genuine pleasant and unpleasant feelings. In problem-solving training, the family is instructed to follow certain steps when they are discussing problems: 1) pinpoint the problem, 2) list all possible solutions, 3) evaluate the pros and cons for each possible solution, 4) choose the optimal solution, and 5) review the results of the efforts.

A New Collaborative Model With Families

The following model is proposed to enhance collaboration between the psychiatrist and families of chronically mentally ill persons. In this model the psychiatric care provider refrains from assuming a diagnostic or therapeutic role toward the families of mentally ill persons. As a result the family is not intimidated by the psychiatric caregiver, which in turn enhances collaborative efforts toward the rehabilitation of the patient (Frese 1998; Hatfield 1992b; Sholevar 1983; Wynne et al. 1977).

The collaborative model is patterned on a consultation rather than a therapeutic model. The family is considered the major caregiving resource to the mentally ill. The psychiatric care provider recognizes that his or her assistance is requested because the caregiving and rehabilitative capacity of the family is rendered ineffective by the development of particular disturbances in the patient. The care provider enters the system being very aware that the family is a powerful resource and has at least as much claim to the patient's emotional state and welfare as the psychiatric caregiver. He or she exercises the *power of expertise* rather than the *power of authority*.

The psychiatric caregiver remains aware of the following factors:

- Any possible shortcomings of the family are *not* a subject for diagnostic scrutiny and corrective measures unless their negative impact on the patient's status can be concretely and immediately demonstrated. The recognition of high expressed emotion (EE) would be a good example of a permissible recommendation for intervention.
- The effectiveness of the psychiatric caregiver as a consultant is primarily dependent on his or her ability to gain the confidence of the family with his or her expertise. Without confidence in the recommendations, the family would be reluctant to carry them out.
- The caregiver remains cognizant that the current understanding and treatment of chronic mental illness is far from being definitive, as demonstrated by the high rate of chronicity or relapse. Therefore, the psychiatric caregiver attempts to assist with the "management" of the patient's behavior rather than its "cure," which may not be possible at the present state of our knowledge. Closely related to the assumption of the position of *power of expertise* is the role of the psychiatric caregiver as the provider of information rather than an agent of behavioral change toward the other party.
- The collaborative model encourages the family and the psychiatric caregiver to work as members of the same team. It is based primarily on the family and the psychiatric caregiver's recognition and utilization of mutual assets. Any attempts on the part of the caregivers and the families to scrutinize each other's behavior for shortcomings should be considered destructive and out of order.

A collaborative model recognizes the following:

- The mental health treatment system is not comprehensive for the care of the multiple needs of chronic schizophrenic patients and their families.
- Working with chronic schizophrenic patients is a demanding task, and most mental health professionals prefer to avoid it.
- Many mental health professionals do not fully understand the problems of the families of those who are chronically mentally ill.

- Many mental health workers do not believe that schizophrenic patients have a disease process similar to other disabling neurobiological illnesses.
- Some psychosocial treatment modalities can be highly stimulating to the schizophrenic patient and therefore can be harmful to him or her.

Training Requirements for Mental Health Professionals

The following principles are considered the necessary elements for the training of mental health professionals in working with chronically mentally ill patients:

1. Chronic mental illness is most likely a disease of the brain and its functioning rather than a by-product of faulty childrearing practices or family dysfunction. The childrearing practices and disturbances of the family are expected to play a secondary role, particularly by augmenting the risk factors in biologically vulnerable individuals.
2. The treatment models for chronic mental illness are based on the diathesis-stress model, which helps to recognize those variables that positively affect treatment course and outcome (Wahlberg et al. 1997).
3. One should be aware that the resources for the management of mentally ill persons in the community are dramatically inadequate or nonexistent.
4. There is a scarcity of research knowledge about effective management strategies to help chronically mentally ill patients. The high expressed emotion is a welcome departure from the prevailing practices and knowledge base.
5. There is significant ignorance of brain functioning and biological factors as they relate to mental illness. There is a need for increased funding of research that can further the biological and biopsychological understanding of the roots of mental illness.
6. An overly exclusive focus on biological factors such as genetic and neurotransmitter systems may impede the understanding of the nature and origin of mental illness. A meta-analysis of the research on biological and psychological origins of mental illness strongly suggests a combined role of biological and psychosocial factors working in tandem to create and maintain chronic mental illness. A genetically and biologically vulnerable individual may be placed at further risk by being reared in a dysfunctional family. Conversely, biologically vulnerable infants may be protected from becoming mentally ill by being reared in optimally func-

tioning families. The Finnish Adoptive Study (Tienari et al. 1987) supports such a combined model.
7. There should be clear knowledge of the difference between a consultative versus a therapeutic model for collaboration between the psychiatric caregiver and families of mentally ill persons.
8. Outreach activities from the professional community must address the need for ongoing and active case management services that are geared toward long-term involvement with the patient and family following discharge.

Treatment Skills Needed for Trainees

- Full grounding in the neurosciences, psychophysiology, psychopharmacology, and human genetics, as well as cognitive and behavioral psychology
- Extensive skills in making an accurate diagnosis, prescribing medication, conducting psychoeducational programs and therapy, acting as case managers, enhancing the patient's cognitive and behavioral skills, and assisting family members to modify their attitude toward the patient
- Familiarity with model training programs for effective treatment of the chronically mentally ill
- A light enough caseload to permit the *intensive* study of a few patients

In addition to teaching trainees these critical treatment skills, it is also very important to have clinical supervision of trainees by highly skilled professionals and to have affiliations with general hospitals or medical school departments of psychiatry in order to enhance a scholarly clinical approach.

Conclusion

Deinstitutionalization of mentally ill patients changed the locus of treatment and placed the responsibility and burden of caregiving on the families. The families were continuously made aware of the tremendous cost of the mental illness on their ill family members while recognizing the inadequacy of the community resources for the care of chronically mentally ill patients and the lack of effective guidelines for and methods to deal with the significant management problems with this population. Against this background, the National Alliance for the Mentally Ill, a grassroots organization of relatives of the mentally ill, was established to enhance the treatment of mental illness and form a productive partnership between the families of mentally ill patients and mental health professionals. The organization was formed, on the basis of clear and practical principles, to address the significant aspects of mental illness. Prominent among these principles is the necessity for paying more attention to the biological nature of schizophrenia as a "brain disease."

NAMI has been an effective force in establishing leverage to gain parity for the coverage of mental disorders comparable to that of physical ones. Their positive contributions have been increasingly recognized, and the families of mentally ill persons are currently viewed as the major resource for the patient rather than as a pathogenic or destabilizing factor. The new definition of the nature of the family's contribution to the treatment of mental illness has made it necessary to develop a new and collaborative model by which mental health professionals and families together can take part in the treatment of chronically mentally ill persons as the two major resources for this group of patients.

Chapters on Related Topics

The following chapters describe concepts related to NAMI and family psychiatry:

- Chapter 8, "Psychoeducational Family Intervention"
- Chapter 27, "Family Variables and Interventions in Schizophrenia"
- Chapter 28, "Depression and the Family: Interpersonal Context and Family Functioning"
- Chapter 29, "Family Intervention and Psychiatric Hospitalization"

31

Alcoholic and Substance-Abusing Families

G. Pirooz Sholevar, M.D.
Linda D. Schwoeri, Ph.D.

Introduction

Substance abuse problems affect 20% of the U.S. population and have far-reaching and devastating effects on families (Helzer and Pryzbeck 1988). Some 13 million Americans have been diagnosed as alcoholic, while another 14.5 million have used illegal drugs (U.S. Executive Office of the President 1989). Approximately 30% of all families include at least one alcohol- or drug-abusing member (National Institute on Drug Abuse 1991). It is often difficult to make clear distinctions between drug and alcohol dependence, because simultaneous and concurrent use of multiple drugs, including cocaine, and alcohol is common. The Epidemiologic Catchment Area (ECA) program reports that as many as 30% of alcoholic individuals qualify for (another) drug dependence diagnosis (Robins and Regier 1990).

Alcoholism is a significant medical, psychological, and social problem that affects the quality and integrity of the patient's life and that of his or her family. Alcoholism alone is still the most common pattern of abuse in the United States, despite the frequency of polydrug abuse (National Institute on Drug Abuse 1991). The National Comorbidity Survey (Psychiatric News 1994) reports a lifetime history of alcohol dependence among 14.1% of the 8,098 respondents in the U.S. survey. Current estimates suggest that more than 10 million Americans experience problems due to their drinking. Of this group, approximately 6 million are probably alcoholic. It is further noted that among the 6 million Americans who abuse alcohol, only 3% fit the stereotype of the "skid-row drunk." The remainder are found among every race, age group, and social class. Twenty to thirty percent of (treated) substance abusers have made suicide attempts in their lifetime, and the incidence of completed suicide is three to four times greater in this group than in the general population. Alcohol is implicated in 70% of drownings and 30% of reported suicides.

Prevalence figures released in 1984 by the National Institute of Mental Health (NIMH) reported that alcohol abuse and/or dependence is the most common psychiatric disorder found in adult males in the United States. More than 50% of all patients undergoing psychiatric treatment in this country are alcohol abusers or have mental disorders that are significantly complicated by their use of alcohol. Alcohol-related disorders account for 14.8% (the third-largest category) of admissions to inpatient units. Women usually develop alcoholism secondary to depression, whereas men have elevated rates of alcoholism and substance abuse in relation to antisocial personality disorders. Helzer and Pryzbeck (1988) (analyzing the ECA data) and Hesselbrock et al. (1985) identified major depression as the primary psychiatric diagnosis of female alcoholics. Major depression was frequently identified in female opiate addicts (Khantzian and Treece 1985), but antisocial personality disorder was primary in males. Ross et al. (1988) found an equal prevalence of affective disorder in male and female subjects. It has been observed that depressive symptoms persist after withdrawal and detoxification, which further suggests the possibility of concurrent affective disorder. Fifty percent of physically and sexually abused children come from substance-abusing families (Wertz 1986).

Fewer than 10% of addicted persons receive professional treatment or are involved in self-help groups, and very few ever receive psychiatric evaluation (Frances et al. 1989). The National Comorbidity Survey (Psychiatric News 1994) attempted to identify those individuals at risk due to a combination of two or more disorders. It found that only one in four substance abusers ever obtained treatment in a mental health facility; even more disturbing, only 8.4% of substance abusers were treated in substance abuse facilities. All undiagnosed and untreated persons with serious substance abuse problems create significant family problems, since substance abuse interferes with all aspects of family life. Intervention must address the comorbidity and risk factors involved.

Cadoret et al. (1980, 1986) uncovered the existence of a genetic factor in the transmission of alcoholism. The extensive research of Steinglass, Wolin, and their colleagues from the Family Research Center of George Washington University in Washington, DC, have contributed significantly to study of the degradation of the family environment when alcohol becomes the central and the organizing principle of family life (see Bennett and Wolin 1987; Jacobs and Wolin 1989; Steinglass 1979, 1980, 1981; Steinglass et al. 1977, 1987; Wolin and Bennett 1984; Wolin et al. 1988). Family research has investigated the relationship between family variables and the transmission of alcoholism and describes the family environment when alcohol invades and functions as a stabilizer of the family system.

Background and Rationale for Family Intervention With Substance Abuse and Alcoholism

Family factors in the etiology of substance abuse and alcoholism were reported in an early paper by Robert Knight (1937). Knight described the passivity of fathers and domineering quality of mothers in such families. A growing interest in the dynamics of the marital relationship of alcoholic spouses emerged during the 1940s and 1950s, especially when the male spouse was diagnosed with alcoholism. Including the wife of the alcoholic patient in treatment changed the focus of intervention (Gleidman et al. 1956), and abstinence became a treatment goal for both the alcoholic husband and his wife. Jackson's concept of "quid pro quo" (D. Jackson 1957) contributed to the idea of a homeostatic mechanism operating in marriages in which one or both spouses had alcoholism.

The growing interest in the family structure and dynamics of mental disorders in the 1950s and 1960s was gradually applied to alcoholism and substance abuse. The resulting research made clear that in treating alcoholism, it was necessary to target the entire family unit (Stanton 1979), which helped therapists to address the broad range of factors affecting different family members and subsystems. The use of family therapy expanded with the growing drug abuse epidemics of the 1960s. There was an outpouring of research interest in drug abuse treatment as part of the federal "War on Drugs" in the 1970s. The work of Stanton (1977, 1979; Stanton and Shadish 1997; Stanton et al. 1982), Kaufman (1984, 1994), and Steinglass (Steinglass et al. 1987) in the 1970s and 1980s paved the way for subsequent research into the treatment of adolescent substance abuse. The work of Liddle (Liddle and Dakof 1995b) and his colleagues, Friedman (1990), and Henggeler (1997) brought family therapy into wider use with adolescent populations.

Kaufman (1984, 1994) reviewed and described the general principles of family patterns and characteristics and observed common features among addicts and their families. He noted that addicts

- Had the role of symptom bearer for the family
- Maintained family homeostasis through their symptoms
- Kept their parents functioning in the parental role through their addictive behavior
- Were the scapegoat and displacement object for their parents' battles
- Were the recipients of the parent's (or parents') own drug and alcohol abuse
- Experienced diffuse generational boundaries with parents who competed with each other
- Experienced cross-generational alliances that further maintained parental separation

Kaufman sensitized family therapists to the importance of adapting treatment approaches to the severity of the pathology, the patient's ethnicity, his or her life-cycle phase, and the duration of the abuse.

The addiction literature describes codependency as a state in which the enmeshed and undifferentiated addicted person continues to receive "support" from the family for the unwanted behavior (which becomes part of his or her self-identity). Cognitive distortions that accompany this codependent behavior include feelings of helplessness. It is as if the family cannot exist without the addicted person, yet feels responsible and guilty if they cannot change the abusing person's behavior. Bowen's description of the family projection process has been aptly applied to addictions (see Chapter 5, "Multigenerational Family Systems Theory of Bowen and Its Application").

Stanton (1980), in his comprehensive literature review, suggested that addicts became locked into a particular family pattern due to the function of the symptom in maintaining homeostasis in the family. The homeostatic nature of addiction clearly indicated the need for family involvement if drug abuse was to be interrupted and siblings prevented from continuing in the same direction. This family-oriented way of looking at dysfunctional behavior brought family therapy and family systems theory into the treatment of alcohol and substance abuse. Family therapy became both a treatment approach and a theoretical perspective for understanding family behavior in relation to the symptom and the symptomatic family member.

Genetic Studies of the Alcoholic Family

Research on alcoholism presents strong evidence of an active genetic component in the development of certain types of alcoholic disorders. There is equally substantial evidence for the influence of family and environmental factors in alcoholism. A family history of alcoholism is the strongest predictor of future alcoholism (Goodwin and Warnoch 1991; Vaillant and Milofsky 1982). In both sexes, a family history of alcoholism increases the risk in children by a factor of four or five (Goodwin and Warnoch 1991).

A search for the genetic underpinnings of alcoholism can be traced to the 1970s and Goodwin's exploration of the transmission of alcoholism in families (Goodwin et al. 1973). Since the 1970s, genetic inheritance of this disorder has become a significant line of inquiry in family studies of alcoholism (Cadoret et al. 1980, 1986; Goodwin 1985; Goodwin et al. 1973). Evidence for a genetic factor in alcoholism has come from a variety of sources: family studies, twin studies, separation studies involving adoptees or half-sibs, and studies of genetic linkage. Studies of adoptees by Cadoret et al. (1980, 1986) support the existence of a genetic factor in the transmission of alcoholism. The studies established a positive relationship between alcoholism in the biological families and their children who were subsequently adopted (Cadoret et al. 1986) and found that childhood conduct disorder, antisocial personality disorder, and alcoholism in the offspring were related to alcoholic biological backgrounds.

Separation or Adoption Studies

Separation studies of children reared by adoptive parents can separate genetic from environmental factors and measure gene-environment interaction. The adoption model provides the most powerful evidence among these studies (Cadoret et al. 1986). The three major separation studies are the Danish Adoption Study (Goodwin et al. 1973), the Swedish Adoption Studies (Cloninger 1987), and the Iowa Adoption Studies (Iowa Children's and Family Services [ICFA] and Lutheran Social Services [LSS]). These studies demonstrate a significant rate of alcoholism in the target groups adopted at the age of 5 months or later, in contrast to the control groups (Cadoret et al. 1986). For the children with an alcohol-abusing parent, the three studies showed, respectively, alcoholism rates of 18%, 23%, and 64% in comparison to 5%, 14.7%, and 22% for male children with nonalcoholic biological parents.

The Danish Adoptive Studies

In the Danish Adoption Study, Goodwin (1985; Goodwin et al. 1973) studied a sample of 133 Danish men who were all adopted as small children and raised by nonalcoholic parents. The subjects were then separated into groups that had nonalcoholic biological parents and those with at least one alcoholic parent. He then interviewed the men and studied their health records to monitor the development of alcoholism in adulthood. Goodwin's research strongly supports the hypothesis of a genetic factor that contributes to the development of alcoholism in the offspring of alcoholics. Sons of alcoholics had a fourfold greater risk of becoming alcoholics than sons of nonalcoholics. The environmental factor of the presence of an alcoholic parent at home added additional risk for alcoholism. There was a twofold increase in depression in nonadopted daughters of alcoholics when compared with their adopted sisters. Goodwin's study also found a threefold increase in divorce when the adopted-out sons of alcoholics were compared with a matched sample of adopted offspring of nonalcoholic parents. In these cases, the divorce was apparently unrelated to drinking.

The Swedish Adoption Studies

Cloninger (1987) followed children of single women adopted by nonrelatives at an early age. The risk of alcoholism in the children was increased by having a biological parent who abused alcohol, but not by having adoptive parents who abused alcohol. Cloninger (1987) proposed two types of alcoholism. In type I alcoholism, there is a later onset without significant social complications. In type II alcoholism, there is an earlier onset of alcohol abuse and more social complications. These findings point to the complex interaction of genetic and environmental factors.

In the Swedish Adoption Studies, the group of adopted-out sons of alcoholics had a significantly increased number of alcohol abusers compared with the sons of nonalcoholics. The daughters of alcoholic parents showed a nonspecific increase in alcohol abuse when compared with controls, but daughters of alcoholic mothers included a significantly higher number of alcohol abusers than controls did (9.8% vs. 2.8%). The Swedish Adoption Studies also examined the correlation between alcoholism and criminality in biological parents and concluded that a predisposition to alcohol abuse and criminality were independently inherited. Depression did not appear to be more prevalent in biological parents of alcoholics versus the control group.

Twin Studies in Alcoholism

Twin studies in alcoholism are based on the recognition that monozygotic (MZ) twins have all of their genes in common, but dizygotic (DZ) twins have on average only 50% of their genes in common. Meta-analysis of the data from twin studies suggests that genetic factors play a significant role in the ability to regulate alcohol consumption. Twin studies also indicate a significant amount of variability, even in MZ-twin samples. For example, the concordance rate for monozygotic twins (Strachan and Read 1996) was 63%–71.4% versus 26.7%–32.3% for dizygotic twins. In Jonsson and Nilsson (1968), the rate of pairwise concordance for monozygotic twins was 43% versus 35% for dizygotic twins. The extant genetic research has paid very little attention to the role of environment in either enhancing or inhibiting alcoholism. Even less notice has been paid to the complex interaction between genetic and environmental factors.

Psychological Studies of Alcoholic Families

Early Studies of Alcoholic Families

Below, we describe some of the early psychological studies of alcoholic families. The family transmission studies of Steinglass et al. (1987) resulted in the development of two core hypotheses about alcohol-related interactions in families:

1. Alcohol-related interactions among intimates appear to show more patterns, organization, and predictability than sober interactions.
2. Alcohol-related interactions seem to provide adaptive or stabilizing functions for families, helping to reinforce intoxication as an integral part of family life.

Steinglass and colleagues observed dramatic changes in affective expression and relationship rules when alcohol was introduced into the family system. When sober, family members were distant and critical of each other, but while drinking, they expressed warmth and tenderness. The brothers in the study alternated their drinking episodes, with the sober brother providing structure for the intoxicated one. This was in contrast to the chaos observed when they were all sober. Alcohol-related behavior was thus a *stabilizing factor* in the family. During intoxicated states, the interaction between married couples was predictably more exaggerated and more restricted in range. While sober, married partners were more outgoing with staff and each other at a variety of levels of intensity. However, within 30 minutes of becoming intoxicated, the partners would always start to fight in an intense manner. They would attempt to solve problems in a short-term manner while remaining focused on each other and no one else.

Alcoholism Transmission and the Family Ritual Project

Family myths and rituals have been shown to be important processes in the generational transmission of alcoholism. Wolin and his colleagues (Wolin and Bennett 1984; Wolin et al. 1988) identified a number of key mechanisms involved in the transmission of alcoholism across generations, and one of them was the *family ritual process*. Rituals are a symbolic form of communication enacted in a systematic fashion over time (Imber-Black et al. 1988). They contribute to the establishment and preservation of a family's identity and collective sense of itself. These repetitious and symbolic activities transmit culture, religious and familial beliefs, values, and attitudes across generations. Family myths are a series of well-integrated beliefs shared by all family members, concerning each other and their mutual position in the family life—beliefs that go uncontested by everyone involved in spite of the distortions they may conspicuously imply (Ferreira 1971). The family myth and its embodiment in the family ritual symbolically communicate a sense of past history for family members.

Wolin and Bennett (1984) developed the Family Ritual Interview as a structured, individual interview designed to study the relationship between the disruption of family rituals and the transmission of alcoholism. The interview covers the identification of the rituals before heavy drinking occurs and the impact of heavy drinking on those rituals. Questions are asked about each of seven family occasions: dinnertime, holidays, evenings, weekends, vacations, visitors in the home, and discipline.

Characteristics of the drinking periods (Wolin et al. 1979, p. 590) include

1. Presence of the alcoholic parent
2. Intoxication of the alcoholic parent
3. Response of the family to the intoxication
4. Change in level of participation of the alcoholic parent when intoxicated
5. Response of the family to that change
6. Overall change during the period of heaviest drinking

Family celebrations are those holidays and special occasions that are widely practiced throughout the culture and represent the family's connectedness to its religious, cultural, and ethnic community. These include rites of passage such as weddings, funerals, graduations, and annual religious celebrations. These celebrations mark developmental family milestones and assert the family's identity. *Family traditions* are less culture-specific and more individually determined by the family. Family vacations, birthday customs, and family reunions are part of these traditions. Patterned routines include dinner time, bedtime rituals with children, and use of leisure time and weekends.

These traditions provide the family with specific roles and responsibilities and the opportunity to interact and share as a group.

Results of Studies From the Family Ritual Project

Extreme ritual disruption was significantly related to greater intergenerational recurrence of alcoholism, whereas ritual protection was associated with less transmission (Wolin et al. 1980). Three different family types were identified on the basis of the maintenance or discontinuation of rituals under the impact of alcohol consumption: distinctive, subsumptive, and intermediate subsumptive. These family types became markers in the identification and treatment planning needs for the patient and family.

The Alcoholic Family: Definition and Description

The *alcoholic family* is defined as a family in which alcohol has become an inseparable component in the family's daily life. It affects the family's growth and development, imposes itself on the family's way of interacting, and becomes the core of the family's identity.

Four basic principles characterize the alcoholic family (Steinglass et al. 1987):

1. Alcoholic families are behavioral systems whose central organizing principles and structures are determined by alcoholism and alcohol-related behaviors.
2. The presence of alcoholism in the family distorts the family's ability to adjust to changes and crises. The slightest change in the environment pushes the system into an immediate response to maintain stability.
3. Regulatory mechanisms such as rituals, routines, and celebrations are governed by the demands of alcoholism.
4. Any alterations in the family's regulatory behaviors profoundly influence family growth and development.

The family's involvement in alcoholic behaviors is part of daily life and interaction. Similar to the natural life cycle, the alcoholic family passes through phases:

1. Early Phase

The early phase of the family life cycle is a time of intense activity, rapid change, and optimism in the normative family. When one or more members of the family has a history of alcoholism, the decision whether or not to carry over the values of family of origin becomes far more complex. The long-term implications of the generational transmission of alcoholism for the children are obvious in terms of how the child fares psychologically and interpersonally. Generational transmission also affects later relationship choices, mate selection, and the continued identity of the family as alcoholic.

2. The Middle Phase

The middle phase of the family life cycle is when the family becomes committed to a sense of purpose, organization, and regularity in life. Members work toward commitment to a set of stable and consistent rules regarding role behavior and relationships within the family. The alcoholic family faces a most difficult and disruptive time during this phase because rigidity forms in an effort to dull the impact of the alcoholism. During the middle phase the family is faced with *repetitive cycling* between states of intoxication and sobriety. Predictable changes occur in the family's interactional activity rate. These behaviors are actually dependent on what Steinglass et al. (1987, p. 153) refer to as an "alcohol-on" or "alcohol-off" state. The concept is similar to that of state-dependent learning in which a chronic alcoholic can only recover memories of events and places "learned" during a drinking episode by again becoming intoxicated. When sober, he has a total inability or "blackout" of recall for those events. Families report having one life when alcohol is present and another when it is not. During the intoxication cycle families know what to expect and the predictability becomes useful. Alcohol-related behaviors help the family deal with day-to-day problems in a routine fashion and allow for a retreat from problem solving. When a problem arises, the alcoholic drinks rather than interacts, which usually results in a family battle and predictable frustration. This temporarily interrupts the negotiation or problem-solving process, and as a short-term solution to problems this behavior is easily reinforced. The result is a powerful, defensive alternative to conflict resolution.

During the middle phase, the alcoholic usually drinks *at home* and most often in front of all family members at mealtime or while the family is gathered in the evening. Decisions are made about how to handle friends. Should they be allowed in the home or kept away until the drinking stops? Most often the family chooses to adjust to the needs of the alcoholic member. Families tolerate and even subsidize the drinking behavior as if to maintain the role played by alcohol in keeping members at a distance from each other.

3. The Late Phase

In normative families, the late phase of the family life cycle is when the family shifts its focus from the present to the future. The family works to adjust to the losses and gains experienced during the middle phase of family life and incorporates new ideas and philosophies brought in by growing children. The alcoholic family faces a more difficult challenge in this phase than normative families because the alcoholic family does not accommodate to changes. As young members grow and expand their internal and external boundaries, they may need to sever all ties with the family of origin. Alcoholic families are usually not flexible enough to make allowances for the new ways of life. During this phase the family is faced with four options:

1. The stable wet alcoholic family pathway
2. The stable wet or controlled drinking nonalcoholic family pathway
3. The stable dry alcoholic family pathway
4. The stable dry nonalcoholic family pathway

The choice of option one indicates that the family anticipates the continuation of the *stable wet* pathway regardless of the consequences. In effect this is merely a continuation of the behavior evidenced in the middle phase. The pattern continues regardless of the consequences to members such as threats of divorce or heated conflict. During intoxicated periods, family members interrupt family ritual, traditions, and routines; isolate themselves from neighbors, friends, and relatives; and essentially maintain a rigid boundary around the family as if all members were consuming the alcohol. When the *stable wet* pattern is operating, the family can anticipate that its week-to-week schedule of daily routines will have to include periods when the alcoholic member is actively drinking.

Option two, the *stable wet or controlled drinking nonalcoholic* family pathway, is a slight movement away from alcoholism as a central organizer, together with a significant reduction (although not total cessation) of alcohol consumption. Families that once engaged in drinking to the point of intoxication now engage in daily or occasional social drinking. In a large-scale epidemiological study (Steinglass et al. 1987), a substantial percentage of former patients (15%) continued to abstain at the time of follow-up (5–8 years later). Twelve percent of the total sample returned to heavy drinking, and 67% were "continuing alcoholics" as represented by this second option—stable wet or controlled drinking nonalcoholic.

Option three is the *stable dry alcoholic family*. This option describes the situation in which there is an actual cessation of drinking, but the family continues to use alcohol as an organizing principle despite the absence of active drinking. When this option is chosen, families continue their involvement with alcohol through alcoholism-centered self-help groups such as AA (or Al-Anon, Alateen, and Alafam—counterparts to AA groups for spouses, children, and entire families, respectively).

Option four is the *stable dry nonalcoholic family*. It is chosen when families have stopped both active drinking and the preoccupation with alcohol. This choice may be related to the developmental pressure created by a wet-to-dry conversion or an active response to the family's attempts to reorganize itself, possibly as a result of family therapy.

Principles of Family Intervention With Alcoholism

In this section, we discuss the principles of family intervention with alcoholism. The *family systems model* described by Steinglass et al. (1987) views family life as the product of a dynamic interplay between the forces of *morphostasis* and *morphogenesis* (Jackson 1957). Morphostasis or family homeostasis refers to those forces that help with the regulation of family life by providing an organizational structure and determining the rules that govern sequential behavioral processes in the family. In contrast, the forces of morphogenesis refer to growth patterns in the family. These growth patterns are delineated in terms of the family's life cycle and the maturational processes within the life cycle.

Family therapy has been shown to be an effective treatment approach for a wide range of alcohol and substance abuse problems (Corcoran 1989; Kaufman and Kaufman 1979; O'Farrell and Courles 1989; Stanton 1979; Stanton and Todd 1979, 1981; Steinglass et al. 1987; Szapocznik and Kurtines 1980). Research covering different generations of family drinking within different cultures indicates that having the family involved in the treatment of alcoholism has a positive impact in terms of treatment compliance, completion, and outcome. Kaufman (1994) notes that most substance abuse treatment agencies provide some form of family therapy with an effort made to include the entire family. Heath and Stanton (1991) noted that family therapy is recognized as an essential approach in the treatment of a full range of addictive problems in families. Furthermore, accreditation standards of the Joint Commission on the Accreditation of Healthcare Organizations (JCAHO) authorize involvement of family members in the treatment process within a patient's 22-day hospitalization.

Stages of the Progress of Therapy With the Alcoholic Family

Steinglass et al. (1987) describe the four stages of the progress of therapy for the typical alcoholic family.

Stage I: Diagnosing Alcoholism and Labeling It a Family Problem

During stage I, the family and its alcoholic member try to reach a common understanding about problems that they are experiencing. The main focus is whether alcoholism is the primary treatment priority; whether, in fact, family therapy is appropriate; and whether an acceptable treatment contract can be worked out. Evaluation includes identification of patterns of behavior, problem-solving techniques, and family rituals.

Stage II: Removal of Alcohol From the System

Stage II involves a plan to detoxify the family. The task at hand is to stop the alcoholic member's drinking, which necessitates a choice among three options. *Option one* is hospitalization for detoxification because withdrawal symptoms will require medication. Therapists are cautioned not to work with a family that refuses to accept the recommendation of hospitalization for detoxification. *Option two* is to continue working with the family but exclude the alcoholic member from therapy and from patient status. This option is chosen only when the patient is highly resistant to the recommendation of hospitalization, the therapist assesses the addiction to be moderate, or the therapist determines that the family could not manage detoxification on an outpatient basis. *Option three* is outpatient treatment and a trial period of outpatient detoxification of at most 2 or 3 weeks. This option necessitates a clearly understood contract in which cessation of drinking is seen as a remedy that the entire family (including the alcoholic member) must maintain.

The detoxification contract will vary among families; however, rules regarding alcohol in the home will not. Some issues to be covered in the contract include the following:

- What is to be done with alcohol already in the home?
- What is to be done about social entertaining?
- Should the family include alcoholic drinks at parties and offer drinks to friends?
- Should the family impose a rule of abstinence, or is a more flexible policy appropriate?

Vital issues for the success of the contract are clear and simple rules, agreement about criteria in the contract, clearly defined tasks, and, above all, agreement that the home remains alcohol free.

Stage III: The Emotional Desert

"Emotional desert" is the title given to the family experience by Steinglass et al. (1987) following cessation of drinking and the loss of related family mechanisms. Prior to this, all emotional and interactional distance has been regulated by mechanisms tied to the drinking. Once the drinking stops, the intoxicated behavior and interactions associated with it also stop. This creates the sensation of being cut adrift: the family does not know how to respond or react to life. A type of depression and emptiness pervades the system, and there is a wish to return to the old way of life. In view of these phenomena, the therapist must anticipate resistances and regressions and help the family by providing a secure framework within which they can understand why the task is difficult. The therapist should also emphasize the length of time sobriety has been maintained and provide general encouragement. It is also appropriate to seek support from self-help group attendance.

Stage IV: Stability

The family and alcoholic member have learned alternative behaviors, and stability is maintained.

Family Therapy With Adults

Five clinical trials have reported on treatment efficacy with adult drug addiction (Bernal et al., in press; Kang et al. 1991; Stanton and Todd 1979, 1982; Ziegler-Driscoll 1977). The work of Stanton and Todd (1982) has been one of the more promising lines of work and pioneered the exploration of the efficacy of family therapy with adults (Liddle and Dakof 1995a, 1995b).

Stanton's theories and treatment of substance abuse are rooted in systems theory. In his comprehensive literature review, Stanton and Todd (1979) suggested that addicts became locked into a particular family pattern due to the "function" of the symptom in maintaining homeostasis in the family. This clearly indicated the need for family involvement if drug abuse was to be interrupted and siblings prevented from continuing in the same direction. Stanton's way of looking at dysfunctional behavior brought family therapy and family systems theory into the treatment of alcohol and substance abuse. Family therapy became both a treatment approach and a theoretical perspective for understanding family behavior in relation to the symptom and the symptomatic family member.

Many of the early drug abuse studies focused on family dynamics, structural patterns, and interactions. The most systematic work was that of Stanton and Todd (1979), who reported significant symptom reduction through the use of structural-strategic family therapy based on the work of

Minuchin (1974a, 1974d) and Haley (1959, 1963). They reported a doubling of effectiveness in nonfamily treatment (Aponte 1985). Follow-up intervals of 6 and 12 months showed continuation of the effects of treatment. Stanton's work evolved within a clinical research context with young, male heroin addicts (Stanton 1979; Stanton and Todd 1979, 1981, 1982). His approach was an expansion of the use of structural therapy with a variety of problems, including delinquency, psychosomatic illness, and anorexia nervosa, described by Minuchin et al. (1978). Stanton's research with this population of young adult heroin addicts found a consistent pattern in which the family would cling to the addict as he attempted to individuate from the family. Stanton's work was based on the concept of problematic separation between a young person and his or her family described in Haley's (1980b) book *Leaving Home: The Therapy of Disturbed Young People*. In Haley's study, the young person's dysfunctional behavior was viewed as a manifestation of the family's attempt to maintain its sense of organization and balance. The family became unstable and distressed when the young person began to leave home and he or she was triangulated in order to protect the stability or relieve distress. One of the major tasks for the therapist was to free young people from their triangulated position in the family.

Stanton's strategic-structural approach to treatment put parents in charge of solving the young person's problems by setting rules and clearly communicating the consequences for continued substance abuse. Therapy was construed as intense involvement followed by a rapid disengagement, rather than protracted treatment. Reframing and relabeling behaviors that bypassed the family's defenses were typical techniques utilized through this strategic approach. For example, the therapist would reframe the son's drug addiction as an attempt to "protect the family." Developing knowledge of the family's interactional patterns was not as important as changing the family's behavior.

Parents were instructed on how to strengthen their own generational boundaries and work together toward stopping the drug abuse. The function of the therapist was to support the role played by the parents. The parents needed to become more responsible in order to help the patient improve and become more competent in coping with future situations. Stanton found that by emphasizing the positive ways of handling the addicted youth, parents gain a sense of accomplishment. The most lasting and valuable effect of this family work was that the parents would see improvement in the patient as the result of their own efforts. It was the parents and not the therapist who brought about change.

Stanton and Todd's (1979, 1981) approach seems most suited for younger addicts who live with or have regular contact with their parents. It may be less applicable to women, older addicts, or street addicts, particularly those with criminal records (Liddle and Dakof 1995a, 1995b). None of the paid family therapy group dropped out of treatment, in comparison to a 48% dropout rate for the unpaid family therapy groups (which also failed to recruit 39% of families). Paid family therapy groups stayed in treatment much longer than the unpaid groups. However, the unpaid family therapy was nearly as effective as the paid family therapy.

In summary, family therapy trials with adult drug addiction demonstrated that family therapy can engage and retain drug users and their families in treatment, significantly reduce drug use and other related problem behaviors, and enhance biosocial functioning. A small number of studies have shown family therapy to be more effective than nonfamily therapies. A comprehensive intervention package with multiple treatment components, including family therapy, is more effective than standard care (Liddle and Dakof 1995a, 1995b; McLellan et al. 1993). However, a blanket endorsement of family therapy efficacy with adult substance abuse cannot be made at this time. The field has not replicated and expanded on its initial promising work. More importantly, recent promising investigative lines are absent in the treatment of adult addicts, such as exploration of marital and intergenerational interactions as in alcoholism research and multimodal and developmental interventions as in adolescent drug abuse.

Family Therapy With Adolescent Substance Abuse

Family therapy for adolescent drug use is more advanced than that for drug abuse in adult patients. The results of multiple studies have been promising, although a blanket confirmation of family therapy's efficacy for drug abuse cannot be made yet due to the small number of studies and their methodological limitations (Liddle and Dakof 1995a, 1995b). The substantial progress in this area includes the studies by Szapocznik and Kurtines (1980), Friedman (1990), Henggeler et al. (1991), and Liddle and Dakof (1995a, 1995b).

Szapocznik et al. (Szapocznik and Kurtines 1980; Szapocznik et al. 1989b) first reported on the efficacy of family treatment in the treatment of adolescent substance abuse. They reported an abstinence rate of 80% at termination and a high level of improved family functioning in Hispanic families. Their approach included two different time-limited family-based interventions: structural family therapy and on-person family therapy. The positive results were maintained in 6- and 12-month follow-ups for both groups.

Szapocznik et al. (1989a) also reported on the efficacy of structural strategic systems engagement (SSSE) over engagement as usual (EAU). SSSE groups exhibited a 93% engagement of the subjects and 75% treatment completion, in contrast to 42% engagement and 25% completion in EAU groups. SSSE uses structural methods such as *joining* to engage this difficult-to-treat population (see Chapter 2, "Structural Family Therapy," for a description of joining).

Research on Adolescent Substance Abuse

The National Institute on Drug Abuse (1991) showed that adolescents 12–17 years of age are at high risk for addiction, drug-related medical complications, and social and behavioral difficulties. The institute's research indicated that almost 50% of the adolescents entering drug abuse treatment report that family problems are the reason they are seeking help. Despite these figures, research is an area of controversy with few hard data. However, based on the review by Gurman et al. (1986), family therapy—behavioral, psychoeducational, strategic, structural, and functional—was moderately effective in the treatment of substance abuse (see Chapter 36, "The State of Family Therapy Research: A Positive Prognosis," for more information).

Earlier studies found that families of adolescent drug abusers are characteristically different from families in which no drugs or only marijuana has been experimentally used. For example:

- There is a discrepancy between how the parents would like their children ideally to be and how they actually perceive them (Alexander and Dibb 1972).
- Parents are perceived as having less influence than peers, and both parents are perceived to be more approving of drug use (Jessor and Jessor 1977; Liddle and Dakof 1995a).
- Children perceive less love and support from both parents, especially fathers (Streit et al. 1974).
- When the adolescent perceives parental support and positive parent-child relationships exist, low levels of drug use are reported (Bethards 1973; Blum 1972; Streit et al. 1974).
- There is less shared authority and poorer communication (Hunt and Azrin 1973).
- There is less problem solving shown in structured family interaction tasks.

Research has shown that adolescents experiment and use drugs for a variety of reasons including 1) easy availability; 2) the rapid results produced by the drug; 3) peer pressure and the need for social acceptance; 4) alleviation of the problems attached to being an adolescent (e.g., depression, tension and anxiety over success/failure, conflict over sexuality); and 5) coping with the normal stresses of life (Beschner and Friedman 1985). Adolescence has been described as a time in which the major life-cycle task is establishing a separate identity from the family while the family characteristically attempts to keep a close, dependent relationship with the adolescent. Drug abuse becomes a part of the adolescent's struggle within the family.

Therapists are continually challenged to show adolescents that family therapy can help them reach their goals without the use of drugs. However, adolescents frequently see family therapy as antagonistic to their goals, and they prefer group or even individual therapy in place of family therapy. Family therapy alone is unable to make a substantial impact on the multiplicity of problems involved in adolescent substance abuse because adolescents function within a peer group that is even more demanding of its participants than is a family.

Adolescents whose parents had drug, alcohol, or psychiatric problems, or problems with the law were more heavily involved in drug abuse than children of nonabusing parents. There was a significant positive correlation between the number of family problems and the number of different types of drugs being abused (Friedman et al. 1980). In an NIMH-funded study conducted by Szapocznik et al. (1989b), 69 two-parent Hispanic families with boys ages 6–12 were extensively tested at intake, at termination, and at 1-year follow-up. The boys were assigned to one of three treatments: a brief strategic family therapy approach, individual psychodynamic child therapy, or a recreational control group. One year after treatment the brief strategic family therapy approach showed the most dramatic improvements, whereas the child-focused treatment (without family involvement) resulted in deterioration in family functioning. The follow-up assessment was based on parents' reports of children's behavior, children's self-reports, and an independent assessment by a consultant psychologist. The assessment results seem to indicate the need for treatment that combines the use of peer-group or parent-group therapy with family therapy.

Treatment of Adolescent Substance Abuse

Functional Family Therapy

Friedman et al. (1990) selected functional family therapy (FFT) as a method of treatment for adolescent drug abusers because of its effectiveness in a controlled research study of adolescent delinquents. It had already proven to be effective in reducing recidivism rates (Alexander and Parsons 1973) and in reducing adolescent delinquent behavior associated with adolescent substance abuse (Friedman 1990). FFT is a method developed by Alexander and Barton (1976) that integrates systems, behavioral, and cognitive intervention strategies. Friedman used FFT to enhance support and decrease defensiveness within the family (Friedman 1990).

FFT views problems from the perspective of the *function* they serve in the family system. The research underlying FFT found that families with delinquents have higher rates of *defensive communication* in the parent-child and parent-parent communications and exhibit lower rates of *supportive communication*. The goal of treatment is to improve family communication and enhance supportive and reciprocal interactions among family members. The focus is on increasing the drug-abusing adolescent's social competence, problem-solving skills, self-control, and autonomy through positive family relationships (Friedman 1990). The adolescent's individual, family, and social contexts are addressed: peer groups and their influence on the adolescent, family interactions and monitoring of behavior, and the adolescent's individual developmental needs. The approach, therefore, combines individual, group, and family therapy modalities.

Friedman (1990) reported the effectiveness of family therapy and parent groups in the treatment of adolescent drug abuse. His study compared outcomes based on FFT used in combination with procedures such as Parent Effectiveness Training (PET) (Gordon 1970) and the approach of the Parent Communication Project of Canada's Addiction Research Foundation (Shain 1990, 1994). The combined use of programs was found to be more effective in treating the problem than any one program alone.

In the follow-up, Friedman (1990) reported the following findings:

- A reduction in the patient's substance abuse by more than 50% in both the family therapy groups and the parent groups
- A decrease in patient symptomatology
- A decrease in the patient's negative family role
- An improvement in the patient's communication with mother and father

Multisystemic Therapy

Henggeler et al. (1991) applied a new approach, called *multisystemic therapy* (MST), to the treatment of adolescent substance abuse. MST is an intensive family- and community-based treatment. It addresses the multiple determinants of substance abuse and delinquency within the family, individual, peers, school, and neighborhood through a combination of strategic family therapy, parent training, and individual therapy. In comparison to usual community services, MST was more effective (as assessed on self-report measures) in reduction of soft-drug and hard-drug use, reduction of incarceration (46%), and reduction in total days in out-of-home placement (50%). Reduction in repeated arrests (26%) was more modest.

Multidimensional Family Therapy

The use of multidimensional family therapy (MDFT) is being studied in ongoing comprehensive research of adolescent substance abuse by Liddle and colleagues (1991a, 1991b; Liddle and Dakof 1995a, 1995b; Liddle et al. 1991, 2001). MDFT is a multisystemic treatment approach for adolescent substance abuse that focuses on the involvement and engagement of the adolescents in the development of many aspects of their own treatment. The MDFT model looks at the total context of adolescents' lives, as well as multiple problems such as poor social, cognitive, and problem-solving skills, learning and school difficulties, low self-esteem, and family stress. This wide context must be applied in order to understand the complex behavioral problems of adolescents and their families.

Liddle describes adolescent drug abuse in terms of problems with *reconnection versus separation* (Liddle et al. 1995a, 1995b). He sees drug-abusing families as functionally disengaged. The research team helps the family assume responsibility, create an agenda for the treatment, and thereby have some sense of control over their own lives. Work proceeds along several parallel and sometimes intersecting paths. Therapists meet alone with the teenagers to sketch out goals, which differs from the more usual approach of talking to the *parents* in the session. Individual work with the teens usually involves issues such as the peer network, dating, adolescents' feelings about themselves, and, quite commonly, an offer by the therapist to help adolescents get along with their parents. More colloquially stated, the therapist asks, "How can I help get your parents off your back?"

Liddle and Dakof (1995a, 1995b) note that MDFT pays more than usual attention to simultaneously working with parental and adolescent subsystems. Unlike other family approaches, MDFT does not focus on mandating parental control and authority. Placing parents in control is secondary to having adolescents' views heard and having them feel important in their own treatment. One avenue for this is the use of *subsystem therapy*—that is, separate sessions with key subsystems and the use of peer groups. There is an emphasis on initially *motivating* adolescents, as well as *remotivating* them during difficult times.

MDFT is a research-based approach to the treatment of adolescent substance abuse and related problems. It has commonalties with the social learning perspective of Patterson et al. (1982), who view antisocial or delinquent behavior as a precipitant of social failure, which in turn produces a depressed mood. Depressed mood and delinquent behavior occur together and influence each other. Patterson's (1982) research has shown that socially unskilled and aggressive children who are rejected by peers and receive poor parental monitoring of their behavior are most at risk for involvement with "deviant" peers and are most prone to depression. These children are thereby most at risk for drug involvement. MDFT reflects the contemporary view that drug use and delinquency are correlated behaviors.

A randomized clinical trial compared MDFT, multifamily therapy, and peer group therapy over 16 sessions and 4–5 months. Cases were randomly assigned to either MDFT, MFT (two or three families participating in structured activities and discussion), or peer group therapy for adolescents (five to eight adolescents in a standard group psychotherapy format). Results indicated that MDFT was more successful in retaining adolescents and their families in treatment than peer group therapy or MFT.

The attrition rate was 27% with MDFT compared with 40% with MFT and 49% with peer group therapy. Furthermore, MDFT was more effective in reducing substance abuse with adolescents. Peer group treatment was the least effective therapy, although it still produced significant reductions in adolescent drug abuse. Peer group treatment in the absence of considerable family involvement was not the treatment of choice for the adolescents. The research indicated that MDFT interventions were designed to engage both parents and children in treatment, and this was a key factor in outcome success (Liddle and Dakof 1995a, 1995b). Szapocznik et al. (1989a) also suggested that active and focused engagement strategies were a prerequisite for working with adolescents.

The evaluation of substance abusers who may also have additional psychiatric disorders is complex. Diagnosis must clarify if presenting symptoms are part of an underlying disorder, as opposed to manifestations or consequences of drug intoxication or withdrawal. This distinction becomes more difficult in the case of adolescents in whom the history of drug abuse, although shorter in duration than in adults, is mediated by adolescents' developmental problems, withholding of information, or distortion of facts as they are questioned.

Additional Options in Therapeutic Models and Settings

The following therapeutic settings provide the alcoholic or drug-abusing patient with a variety of treatment approaches.

Short-Term and Crisis Intervention

Short-term and crisis intervention involves hospitalization in chemical dependence units. It is designed to treat patients with serious reactions to drugs or overdose reactions for a few days to several weeks.

Hospital-Based Inpatient Programs

Hospital-based inpatient programs are designed to treat more chronic problems or are used when the adolescent's drug abuse cannot be controlled effectively by the family. Family therapy is among the medical and psychiatric options.

Outpatient Programs

Outpatient programs are used to treat 82.5% of adolescent substance abusers (U.S. Executive Office of the President 1989). Services include individual and group therapy, counseling, and family education. There is a growing emphasis on the treatment of chemically dependent women. The Center for Substance Abuse Prevention (CSAP) has funded more than 50 programs nationally to intervene and prevent the many health and social problems attributed to substance abuse among pregnant and postpartum women.

Day Treatment Programs

Day treatment outpatient programs combine group therapy, individual therapy, drug abuse education, and recreation.

Residential Treatment Programs

These residential facilities offer a new environment with self-help peer-group programs in addition to a range of individual and group counseling opportunities and drug education.

Therapeutic Communities

Therapeutic communities are highly structured, nonpermissive, drug-free residential settings based on social learning systems models. Adolescents with strong antisocial or delinquent behavior patterns who need limit-setting and problem-solving skills development benefit most from the therapeutic communities. Other community services include religious treatment programs, alternative activity programs, school-based intervention, and halfway houses.

Alcoholics Anonymous

Alcoholics Anonymous (AA) is one of the earliest and best known of the self-help groups. The "Twelve Step" program has origins in the spiritual exercises of St. Ignatius, the founder of the Jesuit Order of Priests; another source was the teaching of the Oxford Group, a spiritual organization that encouraged the membership of alcoholics. The treatment philosophy is based on the concept of powerlessness over alcohol. The influence of religion can be seen in the approach, which often makes AA appear incompatible with other more psychodynamic approaches. AA and the "Twelve Step" program are widely accepted by the majority of treatment approaches (Galanter et al. 1991).

Al-Anon

Al-Anon is the most common approach to involving the family in treatment; it focuses on self-help rather than involvement with professionals. Al-Anon provides support to the nonalcoholic partner within a group framework (Offord et al. 1975; Rychtarik et al. 1989).

Behavioral Marital Therapy

Behavioral marital therapy has been found to be superior to individual treatment (McCrady et al. 1986; Stout et al. 1987). Involving the spouse has been effective in cessation of drinking and enhancing the motivation for treatment (Sisson and Azrin 1986). Behavioral marital therapy addresses a variety of dysfunctional behaviors of spouses related to their dysfunctional partner, such as nagging about drinking, attempting to control drinking, providing alcohol, or drinking in the presence of the alcoholic partner.

Community Reinforcement Approach

The community reinforcement approach (Azrin et al. 1982) combines treatment with the anti-alcoholism drug disulfiram with job finding, behavioral marital therapy, and encouragement to join an alcohol-free club. Outcome studies showed up to 2 years of improved social adjustment, sobriety, and employment compared with controls.

Conclusion

Substance abuse, including alcoholism, is an enormous and complex public challenge that has resisted community and therapeutic intervention. Investigations with alcoholism have revealed the significance of family interactions and family rituals and their role in the transmission of alcoholism across generations. Family studies with adolescent substance abuse have underlined the significance of developmental factors, as well as multimodal and multisystemic interventions.

Family therapy is an integral part of the broad-based and multimodal approach to treatment-resistant substance abuse. Other helpful therapeutic components include marital therapy, multifamily therapy, peer group therapy, individual therapy, medication, self-help groups based on the AA model, and a range of outpatient and residential services to assist patients and families. Because of high relapse rates and comorbidity, assessments and interventions must reflect knowledge of the family, addiction history in the family, and family dynamics that may maintain the illness. Collaboration among multiple disciplines and social systems can provide a comprehensive approach to the treatment of addictions and comorbid conditions.

A definitive statement about the role of family therapy awaits further investigation. However, more recent studies assign a favorable status to family therapy in the engagement and retention of, and therapeutic impact on, substance-abusing patients and their families. Some family studies have demonstrated more efficacy in comparison to strict therapeutic intervention.

Chapters on Related Topics

The following chapters describe concepts related to alcoholic and substance-abusing families:

- Chapter 2, "Structural Family Therapy"
- Chapter 15, "Functional and Dysfunctional Families"
- Chapter 17, "Family Therapy With Children and Adolescents: An Overview"
- Chapter 35, "Medical Family Therapy"

32

Family Intervention With Incest

G. Pirooz Sholevar, M.D.
Linda D. Schwoeri, Ph.D.

Introduction

Incest is a manifestation of individual personality pathology and a disturbance in the total family unit. This definition reflects the expansion of the individual-based theories of the past to commonly held views today of incest as a disturbance in the familial regulation of sexuality, aggression, and dependency. The behavior of the perpetrator is now understood to inflict a range of psychological harm not only on the victim but also on the family unit. In addition, incest is considered by some health professionals (or theorists) to be a restitutive attempt to maintain family integrity while addressing anxieties and conflicts about abandonment and sexuality. Sholevar (1975) has proposed a comprehensive view that incestuous behavior may develop when coping mechanisms of the family can no longer manage family conflicts without violating the integrity of the system. Thus, in one sense, the incestuous behavior is an expression of the family's effort to solve its problem and create a new equilibrium with a more manageable level of dissonance. But like all primarily defensive behavior, incest does not achieve an enduring pattern balance in the family. The family continues with its defective relationship and erratic communication, further burdened by the consequences of incestuous behavior.

Many investigators erroneously describe the *nature* of an incestuous act as a *sexual one*. More accurately, incest represents the dysfunctions of sexuality, aggression, and dependency needs. In families with incestuous relationships, frequently one spouse believes that attempting to express his or her sexual or dependency needs will be rebuffed by the partner and eventually cause the breakup of the family. Thus, he or she displaces his expectations to the child who most closely *represents* the spouse and "acts out" in a sexual mode toward the child.

There has been strong endorsement for the use of multiple therapeutic interventions in cases of intrafamilial sexual abuse. Individual therapy has been commonly used with the victims, the perpetrators, and other family members. Behavior modification techniques, communication skills training, and problem-solving training have been used with the abusers. Cognitive therapy techniques have also been particularly useful in overcoming multiple cognitive distortions in the perpetrators, including their denial, blaming of others, and tendency to paranoid thinking (Veach 1997). Family therapy can be helpful in the later stages of treatment when the treatment goals are consolidated and the initial resistances modified (Dixen and Jenkins 1981).

The legal involvement in treatment of sexual abuse has resulted in much controversy and confusion in recent years. The controversy is particularly strong in cases of recovered memory—rather than continuous memory, which is consistently present—and therapists have been held liable by the courts for confirming invalidated allegations made against the parents. At the same time, there has been legal action against other therapists for *negligence* in exploring, diagnosing, and treating sexual abuse (Regehr and Glancy 1997). Bowman and Mertz (1996) have called the legal intervention in sexual abuse survivor's therapy a "dangerous direction," an intervention that will ultimately deprive the victims of the opportunity to be heard and validated in a therapeutic situation.

Historical Perspective on Incest

Incest is a familiar theme in mythology, history, and religion. Greek mythology was replete with accounts of incest among close relatives. Zeus, himself born of the union between a brother and sister, raped his mother, Rhea, and married his sister Hera. He produced many children through incestuous relationships, including a child with his daughter Persephone, who was the product of incest between Zeus and his sister. Oedipus' relationship with his mother is the most celebrated case of incest in the psychiatric literature: he killed his father and, unbeknown to him, married his mother, Jocasta. In ancient Egypt, the practice of incest, particularly brother-sister incest, was a common and well-celebrated event among the ruling class. Cleopatra was the product of many generations of incestuous relationships and married one of her siblings. The conservation of wealth and power seemed to be an important motive for incest in Egypt as well as other ancient societies.

Since the early 17th century, parent-child incest has been viewed as an unacceptable sexual intimacy that disrupts childrearing and creates intense intrafamilial bonds that undermine exogamy (Aries and Duby 1989). In the United States, incestuous relationships are illegal.

In the Judeo-Christian (and Moslem) West, incest has long been considered a grave social crime. In recent times, the taboo has been supported by biological, sociological, and psychological theories, some of which claim that the taboo functions to protect the human species. In 1913, Sigmund Freud proposed the theory of the "primal herd," which describes the killing of the tyrannical father by his sons to gain access to the women in the herd (Freud 1913/1946). According to this theory, the incest taboo was a way of regulating rivalry between the sons and fathers for the women. Anthropologist Bronislaw Malinowski (1927) attempted to explain the incest taboo as a method of regulating the balance of power in the family. Margaret Mead (1935) hypothesized that the function of the incest taboo was to minimize the jealousy and rivalry between the children and the parents of the same sex, while maintaining family cohesiveness and integrity.

Definition

The definition of *incest* is at once simple and complex (Sholevar 1975). In defining an act as incest, the following factors must be considered: 1) the nature of the act, 2) the degree of relationship between the parties, and 3) the ages of the parties involved. A narrow definition of *incest* would be *intimate sexual or anal contact or genital intercourse between close relatives*. However, this definition overlooks many forms of inappropriate sexual activity with young children that can be highly arousing (Faller 1988; Meiselman 1978). Therefore, what constitutes a legal definition may be too restrictive clinically (because incestuous behavior can include gestures, looks, and touching of a sexually explicit nature). For example, the fondling of the breasts of a pubescent daughter by a father is an invasive act and can lead to sexual excitation and even orgasm in one or both of the participants. Therefore, *exposure to sexual behavior inappropriate to one's age and the relationship of the parties* should be added to the definition of incest.

Few disagree that the act is incest when close relatives in biologically related families are involved. However, children, adult stepchildren, and foster children are not uniformly or adequately protected by law in all states. This remains a serious clinical problem when unconscious and even conscious sexual attraction between stepchildren and stepparents may have been a major factor in the marital decision from the beginning. It also has tremendous ramifications for the stability of the marriage and the possibility of divorce. The age of the partners involved is also relevant. Sexual contact between younger children (prepubescent) may be considered sex play. Sex play may also occur between an older and younger adolescent as a result of impulsiveness, sexual anxiety, family realignment, or age-related fears about negotiating their position in the adult world. Sex play is not characterized by the use of force and is usually entered into by mutual agreement. The age difference between the parties is less than 4 or 5 years.

Causality

Many theories of causality of incest have been proposed; however, one of the primary factors is the offender's sexual attraction to children. This can be *situational*, or the result of some regressed, vulnerable state in the offender at the time. It can be more *characterological*, as in the case of the pedophile whose behavior is a compulsive pattern of sexual attraction to and victimization of children. The willingness to act on this forbidden sexual attraction depends, in part, on the intensity of the feelings, the character of the offender, and his or her overcoming physical or social constraints on this behavior.

The closeness of the relationship between victim and offender plays a significant role in the initiation, duration, and frequency of the behavior; the nature of the act; the child's reaction to it; the parent's reaction on discovery; and the psychological damage to the child. In the case of father-daughter incest, it is not uncommon for the father to progress from appropriate affectionate behavior to more intrusive sexual behavior, including mutual masturbation, oral or anal sex, and then intercourse. If the biological relationship is close, there is more access to the child, less need for persuasion, and ultimately more harm done because of the abuse of the child's affection and trust.

The mental retardation of the victim or the offender, or both, may also be causative factors. This represents about 2% of cases (Gof and Demetra 1983). Victims who are mentally retarded or physically disabled are 4–10 times more vulnerable and perhaps more prone to victimization than nondisabled children (National Resource Center on Child Sexual Abuse [NRCCSA] 1992). Furthermore, disabled children may be more socially isolated, frustrated, compliant, passive, emotionally unable to claim their rights, or physically unable to protect themselves. These factors increase their vulnerability to abuse.

At-Risk Families

A review of the research by Finkelhor and Browne (1990; Browne and Finkelhor 1986; Finkelhor 1979, 1987) indicated that children are at greater risk for sexual abuse in certain family contexts than in others, specifically, when 1) they live in single-parent homes; 2) they have a poor relationship with their parents or are subject to very punitive disciplinary practices; 3) a stepfather is present in the child's home; 4) the mother is not available because she is working outside the home, is ill, or is disabled; 5) a family member is a sexual abuser with a history of sexual attraction to children that dates back to adolescence; 6) there is a conflicted sexual relationship between the parents; 7) there is problematic drinking in the family; and 8) there is history of sexual and physical abuse in the parent's or parents' family history.

Psychological Impact of Incest

The long-term effect of incest includes disturbances in relating to others, often evidenced by an inability to form trusting adult relationships, withdrawal, depression, and other aberrations in social behavior. Dissociative reaction in stressful situation is common. Abused individuals, perhaps out of feelings of shame and guilt, simply seem to *take it* and do not express indignation when they are exploited. Sexuality becomes disturbed, and the expression of it may run the gamut from lack of interest in sex to excessive or impulsive sexual activity. Greenacre (1969) wrote that traumatized children often "play out" or act out in an attempt to master the event. They may become excessively active and aggressive sexually as a way of gaining temporary relief from the memory of the trauma. Rasmussen et al. (1992) suggest three options for children: 1) they can express and then work through their feelings, 2) they can develop self-destructive behavior such as self-victimization, or 3) they can identify with the aggressor and abuse others (Cosentino et al. 1985).

Posttraumatic stress disorder (PTSD) is a common manifestation with primary features such as intrusive, distressing dreams and flashbacks, increased arousal, avoidant behaviors, and a type of psychological numbing (DSM-IV; American Psychiatric Association 1994). Delayed PTSD symptoms may emerge in later adult life in child abuse victims (Courtois 1988; Goodwin et al. 1981; van der Kolk 1987).

Types of Incest

Types of incest include father-daughter, sibling, mother-son, and incest with extended family members.

Father-Daughter Incest

The literature on father-daughter incest is more abundant than information about other forms of incest, and its occurrence is more often documented. Available figures indicate that 70%–80% of reported incest cases occur between daughters and their stepfathers or natural fathers (Green 1988; Nakashima and Zakus 1977; Swanson and Biaggio 1985). Sgroi et al. (1982) have noted that the abuse moves in a predictable pattern from the engagement phase to sexual interaction to secrecy to disclosure, and then often to suppression. The behaviors progress from less to more sexual forms and are maintained by the powerful reinforcement provided by the inequities in the parent-child relationship. Characteristically, the daughter makes few sexual demands while the paternal figure experiences intense pleasure based on his power and dominance. The secrecy required to protect the relationship, as well as to maintain family cohesion, becomes an equally powerful reinforcer. Summit (1983) has called this an "accommodation" by the victim to the abuse through secrecy, helplessness, and entrapment. It leads finally to the daughter's unconvincing disclosure of the situation and then often to her retractment—a denial that the abuse ever occurred.

Many studies are available about the paternal characteristics of offenders. Finkelhor (1987) concluded in his review of 29 studies of paternal abuse that these fathers do not exhibit one particular psychological profile. Some fathers have *personality disorders* characterized by paranoid thinking, intense involvement, and overcontrolling attitudes toward their daughters. They are also heavily dependent on the family for emotional and social relationships. Others may present with *pedophilic sexual preferences* (Abel et al. 1983; Langevin et al. 1985). This sexual orientation is characterized by disinterest in, disgust with, or conflict over sexual relations with adults (Baker 1985; Marshall et al. 1986). Faller (1988) has disputed the more classical incest pattern in which incest becomes a family defense against disintegration or further disruption. She found paternal preferences for children to be just as potent as the wife's lack of desire or desirability and other, more structural problems in the family. Studies have also found that drug and alcohol abuse is not a major factor in incest (Herman 1981; Lee 1982; Mandel 1986; Parker and Parker 1986).

Parker and Parker (1986) looked at the effect of the father's absence in the early years of a child's life on the development of the early caregiving relationship that provides a bond and a deterrent against possible incestuous abuse. Some fathers who had been in prison when their offspring were young later developed incestuous relationships with their daughters, presumably because this caregiving bond had not been formed. Finkelhor and Baron (1986) and Russell (1984) also note that daughters are at greater risk for sexual abuse at the hands of *stepfathers* than natural fathers due to this weakened bond. Russell (1984) states that a stepdaughter is *seven times* more likely to be abused than a natural daughter because the stepfather's role is unclear, which complicates the relationship between the child and parent.

Other possible factors include social isolation, a limited social network, poor social skills, and a lack of appropriate adult sexual partners (Araji and Finkelhor 1986; Kirkland and Bauer 1982; Langevin et al. 1985; Panton 1979; Parker 1984; Scott and Stone 1986).

Sibling Incest

Although father-daughter incest is the most frequently discussed and reported form of incest, sibling incest is believed to be the *most widespread* (Forward and Buch 1979). Estimates are that it is at least *five times more common* than parent-child incest (Cole 1982; Finkelhor 1979; Smith and Israel 1987). Sibling incest has not been studied or documented as much as other forms of incest, and there are still few theories concerning its occurrence. There is also debate among professionals concerning the traumatic effects of sibling incest. Some mutual sexual exploration among young same-age children is seen as a normal part of a child's psychosexual development and therefore viewed as nonproblematic (Bank and Kahn 1982; Courtois 1988; Forward and Buck 1979; Russell 1986). In some family contexts, sibling incest has been said to provide the mutual nurturance and acceptance that is missing in the relationship with the parents (Bank and Kahn 1982). Incest is common when children live in overcrowded homes, are unsupervised, and are poorly cared for by their parents (Finkelhor 1979; Meiselman 1978; Russell 1986). The playful sexual activities go unrestrained and over time develop into incestuous behavior. Victimization is possible when there are violent, coercive, and power-oriented motives in the incestuous act. Courtois (1988) suggests three variations of this relationship: 1) a pubescent brother who uses a younger, naive sister for sexual experimentation; 2) a misfit or outcast brother who substitutes a sister for female friends and abuses her affection; and 3) a much older brother who forces sexual activity on a sister.

Most often, the incest stops once the brother engages in appropriate peer relationships outside the home. Many times, the brother has modeled his behavior on that witnessed between father and daughter in the home. Incest between siblings is more likely to occur when there is indiscriminate sexuality in the family. The chaos and anxiety related to sexuality in the parents can result in heightened sexuality in the children, who act out by becoming sexually involved with each other as well as sexually preoccupied. Physical proximity, such as shared rooms and beds, helps siblings turn to each other for emotional care. This type of incest is underreported because of parental neglect and lack of recognition.

In the absence of longitudinal studies, it is difficult to predict the long-term effects of sibling incestuous behavior. However, researchers have observed some problems for the sisters in these relationships that are similar to those experienced in father-daughter incest. They are less likely to marry, are more likely to be abused in their marriages if they do marry, and continue to fear sexual assault (Courtois 1988; Russell 1986). In addition to this, they often feel guilty and even suspect themselves of complicity (Courtois 1988), experience low self-esteem (Finkelhor 1980), have difficulties in sexual and intimate relationships and preorgasmic functioning (Cole 1982; Meiselman 1978; Russell 1986), and experience depression and attempt suicide (Cole 1982; Laviola 1989; Loredo 1982). They are often taken advantage of socially and sexually (Cole 1982; DeYoung 1982; Meiselman 1978). Other effects of sibling incest include the following:

- Guilt is greater if this is a first sexual experience.
- The relationship may interfere with the individuals' ability to establish more socially appropriate love relationships because there is a mutual dependency and sense of acceptance granted by the incestuous relationship that hinders development.
- If there is violence or if the relationship is no longer mutually consensual, the victim feels entitled to repair this harm through exploitation in other relationships, holding others responsible for the abuse inflicted in the past.

Williams and Finkelhor (1997) have summarized findings from 29 studies describing the characteristics of *incestuous* fathers. The common findings included a history of childhood abuse, poor relationship with their parents as a child, and multiple family problems. The personality structure of the parents exhibited a strong tendency toward passivity, feelings of inadequacy, and dependence. The feelings of dependence were countered by periodical attempts to be aggressive and dominate others. The personality factors support the recommendation for training in assertiveness, communication skills, and problem solving.

Mother-Son Incest

Mother-son incest is estimated to constitute as much as 10% of all incest. The cases reported in the literature describe repeated separation from the mother (misidentified as maternal psychosis) at significant developmental periods as a possible contributing factor. As a rule, another family member, such as a grandmother, assumes the parental role and the father is absent from the home. The son may see incest as a way of gaining closeness to his mother or as revenge for this separation. This type of incest seldom occurs in intact families because the presence of the father tends to maintain the family structure and establish the appropriate distance between mother and son. However, some female sex offenders have reported abusing children at the insistence of a man.

Incest With Extended Family Members

Incest with extended family members (between children and grandparents, uncles, and aunts) may be discovered by the parents, but they generally do not prosecute the perpetrators or obtain treatment for them. Researchers have concluded that there is less psychological harm attached to incest with relatives who are distant from the nuclear family because of the perpetrator's lack of emotional significance for the abused individual (Landis 1956; Peters 1976). When aunts and uncles become sexually involved with nephews and nieces, victims tend to be younger. Homosexual and heterosexual pairings occur with equal frequency.

Incidence and Prevalence of Incest

Incest is perhaps one of the most emotionally charged words in the literature on child abuse and neglect. Incidence rates (the number of new cases occurring in a time period) rarely reflect the true number of children involved. Furthermore, the total incidence of child sexual abuse known to authorities, whether *validated* or not, is undoubtedly significantly higher than reported in studies. Surveys indicate that within the general population, 16% of women have experienced sexual contact with a relative (Russell 1984).

Abuse by fathers and stepfathers of their daughters constitutes 7%–8% of child abuse cases. The most commonly occurring type of sexual abuse—namely, sibling incest—is significantly underreported.

There is widespread agreement that at least one million children are abused each year, with many cases either never reported or simply dismissed with no further inquiry. In 1991, there were 375,000 reports of children who had been sexually abused. In 85% of these cases, the abuser was a family member or someone close to the family—*an adult in a caregiver position for that child*. Sexual activities included genital exposure, intimate kissing, fondling, masturbation, fellatio, cunnilingus, and digital or penile penetration (NRCCSA 1992). There are many discrepancies in the numbers reported because child abuse itself constitutes several types of maltreatment. Sexual abuse is a part of spectrum of maltreatment grouped with physical abuse, neglect, and emotional maltreatment. The nature of the sexual act in the sexual abuse further complicates the reporting. An interdisciplinary Project on Child Abuse and Neglect that involved some 200 cases in Michigan found that sexual contact represented 41.2% of the cases, followed by oral sex (19.3%), and genital intercourse (15.7%). The victims reported forced sexual contact, but no injury in the largest number of cases. The largest number of offenders were *biological fathers*, followed by stepfathers. Biological fathers represented 35.7% of the cases (number still married [28.1%] plus number longer married [7.6%] to the mother). Stepfathers accounted for 17.3% of the cases, followed by the mother's boyfriends (9.2%).

Prevalence refers to the estimate of the proportion of the population that has been sexually abused. The National Institute of Mental Health funded a data-gathering project to study the incidence and prevalence of intrafamilial and extrafamilial child sexual abuse in women 18 or older. In a sample of 930 women in San Francisco, 16% reported at least one experience of intrafamilial sexual abuse *before* the age of 18. Twelve percent had been sexually abused by a *relative before* age 14. Thirty-one percent reported at least one incident of sexual abuse by a nonrelative before age 18, and 20% reported sexual abuse by a nonrelative before age 14 (NRCCSA 1992).

The first national prevalence study found that 27% of the women and 16% of the men in their sample had experienced some form of child sexual abuse (NRCCSA 1992). The Finkelhor study (Finkelhor 1990) determined the median age at abuse was 9.6 years for girls. Large-scale community surveys indicate that 1 in 4 girls and 1 in 10 boys have been sexually abused before age 18 (Finkelhor 1979, 1984, 1990; Russell 1986). In summary, no figures can accurately reflect the incest problem, and despite numerous studies, the NRCCSA notes that they simply do not know for certain how many children are sexually abused each year (NRCCSA 1992). Children do

Family Intervention With Incest

not readily disclose their victimization because of fear, shame, or lack of understanding of its wrongfulness, among other explanations.

Detection of Incestuous Behavior

Individual Manifestations

Some behaviors should alert the clinician to the possibility of incestuous behavior. These include the child or adolescent who 1) expresses extreme fear for no apparent reason; 2) experiences depression; 3) presents serious runaway behavior; 4) contracts venereal disease, yet denies being sexually active or being a victim of rape; 5) is pregnant and gives vague stories about the father of the child; 6) is unable to trust, as exhibited in poor object relations; 7) is sexually precocious or inhibited; 8) exhibits severe conduct disorders and academic failure following a previous history of good adjustment and success in school; 9) exhibits acute psychotic breaks or sudden self-destructive behavior; 10) has insomnia or excessive sleepiness; 11) has ongoing school truancy as a result of his or her reversed role in the family; 12) acts pseudo-mature at an early age; 13) exhibits depression, guilt, and embarrassment, particularly following sexual behavior; 14) exhibits displaced anger toward others; 15) demonstrates psychosomatic complaints such as headaches or stomachaches; 16) is generally lonely and lacks friends; and 17) tends to be angry with the mother for mistreatment of the father or feels sorry for the father. These children are prone to amnesia from the trauma experience and are prone to dissociation as a defense against the trauma (Spiegel and Wissler 1986).

Detection Through Family Interaction

Incestuous behavior should also be suspected when there is an overly close relationship between a parent and child, particularly when they are of opposite sexes. There may be extreme preferential treatment of one child over other children in the family and extreme jealousy shown by the father as his daughter reaches puberty. Very often the parents have a background of emotional deprivation, neglect, and/or victimization sexually or physically. The clinician should also suspect incest when the parents accuse the child of being a *pathological liar* or the child complains that no one believes him or her.

The denial of incest by the family is a general rule rather than an exception. Even when the child repeatedly has informed the health care professional of incestuous acts, she may retract her statements under parental pressure or because of fear of punishment. Uncovering incest is a difficult task because the denial is a strong defense that serves both interpersonal and intrapsychic purposes. Trepper and Barrett (1989) say that denial takes many forms and appears in multiple stages. In the first stage, there is denial of the *facts*. The family members simply deny that incest ever occurred. As this phenomenon fades away, there is a second stage in which the incest is admitted but blame is projected outward. This is denial of *awareness*. For example, the father may blame his behavior on his drinking or the mother may simply say that she was not at home or was never told about the incidents. The child may say that he or she did not realize that what was happening was sexual. The third stage is a denial of *responsibility*, in which each person involved blames the other. After the truth is revealed, there is a fourth stage in which the family denies the *impact* of the incest by minimizing its traumatic effects. The family holds back and becomes more protective through obfuscation. The clinician must gradually and progressively, as well as cautiously, confront the denial.

Disclosure

If the clinician is in the position of being the first to learn about the incest, it is best to help the individual prepare for the disclosure to her family. Disclosure is not something that should be done without adequate preparation because it can result in retaliation, violence, further denial, or additional scapegoating in the family. Courtois (1988) suggests that the motivation behind the disclosure needs to be explored. Is she doing this to seek relief from guilt? Is she motivated by anger and the need to retaliate? Does she suspect other incest in the family and want to protect someone in the family? Is she attempting to make this a reality rather than deny it any longer? Courtois further recommends a careful assessment of the patient's pretrauma functioning and family history, the traumatic incestuous events, and any other trauma that may have occurred.

Careful documentation of the patient's memories and references to abuse must be made, especially when the patient has a borderline personality. Borderline patients experience high rates of cognitive distortion in addition to dissociation and fragmentation. They experience extreme anxiety about their lost or absent attachment figures. The recovery and integration of traumatic memories and associated affect are necessary for validation of the experience in the patient. This process becomes a primary step toward treatment (Lonie 1993). However, caution is needed because it is possible to pressure patients into the search for confirmation of these ideas, reinforcing false traumatic memories.

Family Configurations and Incest

Structural Considerations

The dysfunctional family structures and patterns that occur commonly in incestuous families (Alexander 1990; Trepper and Barrett 1986, 1989) include the following:

- Weakened generational boundaries that cause poor demarcation of familial roles
- Isolation of family from the social community, dependence on itself for most of its emotional needs, and absence of the appropriate social skills
- Triangulation of children into the emotionally detached parental system
- Disturbances in the marital and sexual relationship
- Distancing maneuvers of provocations, constant strife, and abandonment of parental and marital roles
- Family secrets regarding sexual matters, such as affairs, promiscuity, or abortions
- Disturbances in the sibling subsystem in which the siblings function in a disengaged manner or fuse and lose all identity
- Active denial of feelings, creating an atmosphere of constant doubt and questioning of reality
- Reversal of parental roles and inconsistent, unpredictable, and erratic parenting
- Parentification of the children in childhood and adulthood
- Intimidation of children, leaving them helpless and victimized

Multigenerational Considerations

Incest represents a relational distortion among all family members. The abuse of the children is rooted in the abuse of the parents by their own parents in the past and extends to the siblings and the next generations. The abused child remains vulnerable, distrustful, and confused because of the breach of the parental trust and lack of protective generational boundaries. Parents seem to cast these children in roles that have nothing to do with their own lives—as if the child in some way resembled the father's or mother's own ungiving or absent mother. Or the child may be the helpless victim of the father's rage at being betrayed by his wife and another person. There is an intergenerational reoccurrence rate of 33% in incest.

Interviewing the Victim

Talking to the victims can be especially difficult. The techniques for interviewing should above all place the abused individual at ease while being objective and clear. Walker (1993) has provided a checklist consisting of 21 items, which allows the interviewer to confirm the 1) framing of the event, 2) use of clear language, 3) asking of appropriate questions, 4) listening to the answers and 5) checking of global issues (NRCCA News 1994a).

Identification of Incestuous Behavior

Larson and Maddock (1984) differentiate the following four types of incestuous behavior characterized by particular psychological motivations and functions:

1. *Affection-based* behavior implies positive intention, nonviolence, and little desire for power and control. Probably some anxiety, depression, and strong dependency needs lead to a parent-child *love affair*.
2. *Erotic exchange* behavior also implies positive intention, but with the wish for emotional connection. There may or may not be actual intercourse, only sexual behavior in the form of voyeurism, exhibitionism, or sexual teasing and the family's encouragement to use sex as a way of relating.
3. *Aggression exchange* behavior, a more pathological form, involves the need for power and control on the perpetrator's part. This behavior implies a wish to punish a rejecting wife, using sexual contact with, for example, a daughter.
4. *Rage* behavior, the most pathological form, indicates life-threatening concerns because it is sudden and violent.

Treatment Planning

Treatment planning, suggested by Larson and Maddock (1984), addresses the function of these typologies:

1. With affection-based behavior, the incest is a way of making a connection. Therefore, working on boundary issues, reinforcing attempts to form supportive relationships through networks *outside* the family, and focusing on personal identity and self-esteem issues are paramount. Since there is little need for family separation, therapy can commence quickly and be active.

2. With erotic exchange behavior, there is a need to see family members separately at first and then begin marital and family therapy in the later phase of treatment. Group therapy with incest survivor groups in the early stages is beneficial.
3. With aggression exchange behavior, there needs to be an assessment of the lack of impulse control and the desire for power over others, both of which could lead to greater exploitation. Perpetrators could benefit from residential treatment, and victims should be in a sheltered environment. Family therapy should focus on the power struggles within the generations and the enhancement of problem solving and marital therapy for conflict management. At some point the family needs to address the need to repair ruptured relationships and rebuild trust. Individual therapy is also indicated.
4. With rage behavior, the best option is inpatient treatment for the perpetrator combined with exploratory individual therapy and supportive group therapy. Depending on the degree of parental dysfunction, adequacy of boundaries, support, and nurturing, child protective agencies may need to intervene and authorize separation.

The family's communication patterns are also observed: Do father and mother display a great deal of conflict avoidance, secretiveness, and hostility in their exchanges? Do the children, especially the incest victims, talk to parents and not to each other?

Incestuous behavior is reflected in intergenerational, interpersonal, and intrapsychic disturbances. Some typical characteristics of these disturbances include

- Poor body/self-image based on shame and a negative view of sex and the body
- Disturbed psychosocial interactions among family members
- Exploitation of family members through touch and body contact
- Lack of respect for both physical and emotional privacy evidenced in the adult's intrusive, overly detailed questioning of the adolescents' sexual behavior
- Lack of affective communication, misinformation about sex, and the inability to discuss feelings regarding sex
- Lack of knowledge about sex, often leading to distortions, myths, and stereotypes

In the assessment of the family dynamics, the therapist must especially attend to the patient's presentation of the incest. Incestuous behavior can occur on a continuum, with the most traumatic condition being the act itself. There is a continuum of the wide range of areas in need of clinical investigation. Questions can be raised about sleeping arrangements, bathroom *rules*, attitudes about intercourse, the appropriate age for dating, content of TV and movies, and so forth. The researchers also caution the therapist to not overlook the possibility of false memory and confusion of memory in which the events of childhood can be mislabeled incestuous because of the arousal, fear, or anxiety involved with the whole sexual issue. In addition, information from collateral sources such as other family members and even the children's friends is important. Assessment can include reports from the school authorities, the legal system, and probation offices. Medical consultation should be considered, particularly if infections, pregnancy, anorexia, or bulimia is part of the incest syndrome.

Family Intervention Strategies With Incest

Considering the complexities involved in cases of incest, it is safe to say that no one set of intervention strategies is appropriate for all families. The guidelines should make use of legal, medical, social, and psychological resources.

Step One—Early Intervention

The first step in intervention is to *report* the suspected incestuous relationship to the local child protection service, which in turn will inform state social services. This reporting is mandated by the National Child Abuse Prevention Act of 1974 and by state laws that cover physical and sexual abuse of children, incest, and child neglect. The law requires physicians, mental health professionals, teachers, and others who come in contact with children to report cases of suspected abuse. The incest victim frequently revels in the incestuous relationship after he or she has obtained a promise that the secret will be kept. As a result the mental health professional may consider not reporting the incest. This reenacts the silent pact between the victim and offender, which places the victim at great risk and undermines his or her trust in adult authority.

Protection is a primary concern for the abused individual as well as other siblings and the mother in the home. It may mean that the offender and victim must live apart for a period of time. Removing the offender can actually promote change because it emphasizes an adult's responsibility for the protection of children, holds the offender accountable, reassigns the child's position as a child in the family where parentification existed, and increases motivation for treatment since the offender will want to return to his home. Notifying child protection agencies and establishing a liaison with the necessary personnel informs the family as to the seriousness of the situation, adds to the child's protection under the law, and enlists the protection agency's help to place appropriate conditions on visitation.

Step Two—Crisis Management

Once the report has been made, the second step is *crisis management*. The family may react to the disclosure or suspicion of incest with different forms of acting-out, including suicide attempts by the mother or the victim, new forms of seductive or even promiscuous behavior, violence, threats, or mimicked incestuous behavior between siblings. Once the offender is removed, the mother may become overwhelmed with the responsibilities for family management and neglect or abandon the children. A characteristic pattern is further drinking, emotional withdrawal, and erratic behavior. The therapist will need to set limits on his or her availability, while providing a sense of security for the family during their crisis. This may necessitate the involvement of crisis team members who can respond to different family members as needed.

Step Three—Treatment

The third step is to provide *treatment* for the individual victim, the mother, and the whole family. The mother may need to become involved in group therapy with other mothers or attend parenting-skills classes as part of the total family treatment. The offender will need his own treatment. Family intervention/family therapy will develop as the incest pattern is revealed and the patient feels prepared to speak in front of all of the family members. All decisions regarding the return of the offender to the family home should be made after consideration of how that will affect all members.

Therapists need to remain alert to the family's style of interaction, which includes secrecy, denial, fusion, and enmeshment. A firm boundary between clinician and patient or family is vital. Overly identifying with the victim, feeling sorry for the offender, or simply missing the powerful projections of blame in the family can greatly impede treatment.

Group therapy has been used with the perpetrators, victims, and other family members for the past three decades. Its therapeutic effectiveness has been confirmed and its methodology has been refined. Group therapy provides different family members with support, expanding their cognitive and problem-solving capacities so they can better cope when the level of stress and tension is high (Saxe and Johnson 1999a, 1999b). The group format has also been used preventively to educate and increase the level of children's knowledge about how to recognize the threats to their safety in their environment (MacMillan et al. 1994).

A combination of psychoanalytic and feminist therapies has been used by a number of investigators. They address the victim's strong feelings of shame and negative self-image: "the ugly child within" (Courtois 1988). The impact of sexual abuse on impaired adult interpersonal functioning has also become a central focus of treatment (Davis and Petretic-Jackson 2000). The focus on sexual dysfunction, eating disorders, self-harm, and depression in relation to sexual abuse has remained constant (Kearney-Cooke and Stringel-Moore 1994).

Countertransference issues in the treatment of victims of sexual abuse have received increasing recognition in recent years. The higher than average frequency of sexual abuse of incest victims by their therapist is an alarming finding (Brodew and Agresti 1998). This complex phenomenon underlines the need for extensive training and ongoing supervision and consultation for the therapists (Llewelyn 1997).

Broader Interventions With Incest

Many individual strategies can be applied in treatment that prepare the victim and strengthen his or her attempt to confront the abuser.

Individual Sessions

Individual sessions can include a rehearsal of the confrontation prior to the family session. Solution-based techniques of Bass and Davis (1988), de Shazer (1985, 1988), de Shazer et al. (1986), and Dolan (1991) are helpful, such as imagining the worst that could happen if the offender were confronted and then role-playing this feared confrontational scene with the patient. Psychotherapy for PTSD symptoms includes supporting adaptive coping skills by positive self-talk, relaxation with visualization, normalizing the symptoms, and decreasing avoidance (Witt et al. 1993).

Writing Three-Part Healing Letters

The therapist can encourage writing three-part healing letters in which the details of the incest are described, the feelings and aftermath are outlined, and responses are predicted. This may be possible with pubescent and adolescent victims. These letters, written but never mailed, help prepare the victim for the responses he or she can expect and give him or her a sense of power and some control over the encounter. These techniques aim at offering hope to the abused person while mobilizing his or her own internal resources.

Telling the Truth

Another solution-based strategy described by Dolan (1989) is having the patient write down on a small piece of paper the *truth* that it was not her fault and he or she is not to blame. The patient then carries this with her as a *reminder of truth*.

Making Positive Associations

Associational cues are also part of the repertoire of techniques aimed at providing symbolic sources of comfort and security. As described by Dolan (1991), the patient is helped to identify an experience in which *relative*, but not total, comfort and security was experienced. During this exercise, the patient is directed to 1) "notice and describe all the details of the experience with special attention to sights, sounds, sensations," 2) "take some time to enjoy the experience," 3) "make adjustments, additions, and subtractions of details to further enhance the comfort and security of the experience," and 4) tell the therapist when the experience is "just right." Finally, the therapist invites the patient to "enjoy the experience one more time and, while doing so, to select a little symbol that can serve to remind her of the pleasant experience in the future."

Encouraging the Narrator

Involvement of supportive family members or friends who will listen to the patient's (narrator's) story and help him or her get through discussing the details has also proved to be helpful.

Forgiving

Sessions should be held between mother and daughter in the case of father-daughter incest to help heal wounds through understanding and forgiveness. This reassures the abused individual that she is safe and makes it possible for the mother to assume a parental role in the family. Very often, these mothers are frightened for their physical and financial safety and jeopardize their children's rights rather than risk family integrity.

Conclusion

The phenomenon of incest can be best understood and treated within the context of the family. Incestuous relationships are a sign of disturbances in family relationships in which the family members are unable to negotiate their basic needs for nurturance, trust, affection, sexuality, and aggression. The difficulties with the negotiation of the above functions are the result of the failure of the family and its members to progress in contemporary and historical spheres. Being unable to pursue a developmental course in a normative fashion, the family defensively falls back on the defensive maneuver of regulating aggressive, sexual, and dependency needs, as well as its members' need for affection, in a socially unacceptable manner. The goal of this behavior is generally to prevent family breakup or abandonment by other family members, which is historically a common fear in incestuous families. However, this defensive family maneuver burdens the incestuous family with further social, clinical, and legal consequences.

It has been a major conceptual misperception to treat incestuous behavior solely as a manifestation of the perpetrator's personality deficiencies. In addition to the examination of the perpetrator's role, there is a need to look at the vulnerabilities in the family unit and the victim that promote exploitation of one family member by another.

Chapters on Related Topics

The following chapters describe concepts related to family intervention with incest:

- Chapter 17, "Family Therapy With Children and Adolescents: An Overview"
- Chapter 33, "Family Therapy With Personality Disorders"

33

Family Therapy With Personality Disorders

G. Pirooz Sholevar, M.D.
Linda D. Schwoeri, Ph.D.

Introduction

Early experiences provide the context for the development of a healthy personality as well as a disordered one. Developmental trends established in childhood are further consolidated through continued interactions with parents and other family members. Subsequent social interactions with peers as well as with other individuals in the community are influential in the modification or redirection of personality traits, but they rarely have the decisive impact of early family relationships.

Later life experiences shape the formation of the individual's personality and provide the major tools of social development. In cases of personality constriction or disorders, premarital dating and marital choices are influenced substantially by a replication of former critical experiences with primary objects. A person who chooses a marital partner based on replication may find himself or herself in a harmonious, although constricted, marital interaction with limited capacity for growth. The choice of a marital partner with character traits that are the opposite of early models (primary objects) may hold the promise of personality expansion but can result in significant turmoil and the potential for marital breakup in cases in which the level of difference is significant.

A person with a healthy and resourceful personality establishes a relatively open and unrestricted interaction with a large number of diverse personalities in a broad range of situations, selects an equally healthy marital partner, and produces resourceful children. Such individuals adapt satisfactorily to most circumstances and may only develop transitory symptoms when encountering challenges. Restricted and disordered personalities can become symptomatic in minimally stressful circumstances. They can produce significant symptomatology, depression, or functional breakdown in challenging times. In cases of severe disorders, such as extreme degrees of schizotypal or antisocial personalities, the person may be unable to establish or sustain relationships, which can result in remaining single or divorcing after a short period of marriage or forming a highly pathological family unit.

It is the premise of family and marital therapy that personality and character constrictions are rooted in early developmental failures and lead to marital characteristics that are an extension of personality dysfunction. The interactional and marital disorder creates a relational and social context that perpetuates the intrapsychic conflicts and hinders the forward movement of the couple and their children (Johnson and Lebow 2000; Sholevar 2000).

Borderline Personality Disorder

Borderline personality organization denotes a relatively stable type of personality structure characterized by an unstable image of self and others, poor impulse control, low frustration tolerance, and primitive defenses. Such patients can decompensate emotionally under the stress evoked in close interpersonal relationships. Their developmental history indicates a pervasive fear of abandonment, sense of aloneness, and empty despair. The maturational failure in early life occurs as a consequence of a pathological parent-child relationship before the age of 3 years and undermines the establishment of an autonomous sense of self in the child. Erratic parental practices characterized by intrusiveness, unavailability, and insensitivity to the needs of the young child are the significant elements. For the child, having unstable and inconsistent parents can mean having repeated traumatic situations in early childhood. The deficiency in the resolution of symbiosis, the failure of the separation-individuation process, and the inability to form an autonomous ego have been described by a number of contributors and summarized by Zinner and Shapiro (1972, 1975), Shapiro (1963, 1966), and Lachkar (1992).

Marriage and the family life of patients with borderline personality disorder are marked by impulsivity, violence, suicide attempts, substance abuse, a conflictual and unsatisfactory marriage, and abrupt breakup with the partner at the height of friction (Lachkar 1992). Parents with this disorder tend to parentify their children and excessively bind their children to themselves. Highly pathological parental behaviors result in highly pathological behaviors in children. Children may run away or attempt suicide during adolescence to escape parental control. Parents with borderline personality disorders exert extreme possessiveness and demand absolute, unlimited control while threatening rejection. This rejection is usually rooted in the parents' unresolved grief over their past losses. Painful affects are frequently dormant in the family and emerge disproportionately at the time of frustration and disappointment. The function of such painful affects is to reestablish ties with a frustrating early object (Kissen 1995; Sholevar 1997a)

Families with a borderline member use projection and projective identification in their daily interactions as interpersonal attempts at dealing with loss (Schwoeri and Schwoeri 1982a, 1982b). The unconscious projection of the feared separation or loss culminates in bitter, unexplained arguments and often violent acting out. Very often there is a replay of violent behavior resulting from the shared pathology in the family.

Usually, the *separation-individuation stage* of development has been faulty for several generations in families of borderline patients. Frequently, the separation-individuation process has stagnated at the developmental stage of 18 to 24 months (rapprochement). The child's striving for autonomy is thwarted, and he or she remains highly susceptible to the fear of separation and abandonment. The underlying psychodynamic and structural deficiency is a lack of attainment of *object constancy* that would have allowed the child to maintain an internal image of the parent at the times of separation. The instability of self-image in the growing individual is manifested by vulnerability to depression, anxiety about abandonment, feelings of helplessness, lack of vitality, inability to control impulses, and self-destructive actions. Pain may offer a false sense of aliveness and vitality to counter feelings of despair. Repeated traumatic experience revives the feeling of attachment to early traumatic and disappointing objects (Kissen 1995; Sholevar 1997a). The conflictual and violent marital relationship is a revival of such traumatic ties. The instability of the images of others is manifested by the imagining of people as either ideal or villains, exhibited by oscillating periods of extreme closeness and being *in love* followed by *hatred* when experiencing minor disappointments and threats of separation.

This may be followed by flight into a relationship and marriage to someone of equally diffuse identity or someone interpersonally distant. This person is idealized and viewed as an answer to all the shortcomings and early disappointments in the parents. The selection of a narcissistic partner and establishment of a *narcissistic* borderline marriage facilitates the idealization. This type of marriage prevents the adult phase of development from taking place. It sets the stage for a family in which procreation is expected to directly *compensate* the couple for early disappointments. This idealized stage of marriage breaks down soon. This new phenomenon is reacted to by premature planning for a child to re-create the idealized stage of union. Once the child arrives, the spouses abandon each other for the child, and the triangular stage of family development does not take place. The intense and inappropriate involvement with the child results in the further weakening of the marital relationship. Separation and divorce at this later stage is likely for these individuals. Fearing abandonment, a spouse may flee from the marriage when, as frequently occurs, the other spouse becomes impulsively involved with an inappropriate and emotionally unstable person who lacks self-definition and is willing to become an unwitting partner to the continuation of this psychological drama.

The fight over control and autonomy is resumed between the borderline parent and her child once the child enters school and later in adolescence. It is the intense fighting between the mother and child and the mother's wish to either control or put away her child that frequently bring the borderline family to the clinician's office. As noted by Villeneuve and La Roche (1993) in the case of borderline adolescents, the problem is both an individual one and a family one. Treatment that aims toward the adolescent's separation-individuation involves decisions concerning how and when to involve the family. Family intervention is not a panacea in the treatment of personality disorders in adolescents. However, a flexible family approach based on a psychodynamic understanding of the disorder and its interpersonal manifestations can be very helpful.

Treatment

The ultimate goal of treatment is for family members to learn the value of negotiated agreements. Disappointments are an integral part of human relationships, but they can be resolved through meaningful communication and the application of problem-solving methods. The accomplishment of the above goals requires modification of highly pathological defenses such as projective identification, splitting, idealization, and denial. The psychodynamic family therapists uncover the genetic roots of marital and parent-child disturbances of the family in a multigenerational context. However, the disturbances in the relationship of the borderline family can also be addressed by concentrating on the diffuse boundaries that contribute to repetitive and conflictual communications and on the family's lack of problem-solving skills. The establishment of functional and adequate boundaries between the nuclear and extended families in borderline patients may be an essential task for establishing the integrity of the nuclear family and its members. The resolution of *emotional cut-off* (Bowen 1976b, 1978) is a highly useful concept for reactivating the dormant conflict between the nuclear and the extended families, which is unwittingly played out with the children. Bowen's (1976b, 1978) concept of *differentiation* is highly effective in correcting structural and boundary deficiencies in such families. Equally applicable is the concept of *multigenerational loyalty* (Boszormenyi-Nagy and Spark 1984), which binds the nuclear and extended families along certain lines.

Narcissistic Personality Disorders

Narcissistic personality organization and disorders have received significant attention due to the investigations of Kohut (1971a) and Kernberg (1975). The narcissistically vulnerable individual has a tendency to marry a spouse with narcissistic vulnerability in a collusive manner in order to conceal his or her narcissistic problems and underlying personality issues. The marriages of narcissistically vulnerable people have been described extensively by Lansky (1981, 1986). Narcissistic couples are excessively sensitive to criticism due to their humiliation-prone personalities, which make them very sensitive to shame and criticism. They lack empathy for other people and each other's feelings; instead, they react to each other with blaming or have sympathy but lack genuine empathy. They employ pathological distance regulation and avoid a mutually gratifying relationship due to the fear of experiencing emptiness and personality fragmentation. As children, narcissistic parents experienced neglect and emotional absence from one or both parents. At times, they were parentified and forced to cater to the emotional needs of their parents. A history of sexual or physical abuse, neglect, or exploitation is common.

Narcissistic people frequently choose other narcissistically vulnerable people as partners and enter into a mutually reinforcing and self-perpetuating collusive pattern of painful relationships. Despite the lack of gratification and the rigidity in their marriage, their chronically conflictual marriages tend to endure. Narcissistic couples seek treatment primarily because of a high level of *blaming* but also because of dysfunction, depression, or other symptomatic behaviors in one of the spouses. Impulsive actions such as wrist-slashing, binge drinking, and compulsive gambling are relatively common (Lachkar 1992; Lansky 1981, 1982).

There are several common marital patterns in narcissistic marriages. Most common is *blaming couples*, who show surprising cohesiveness despite their chronic state of marital stress and symptomatology. Impulsive actions and a high level of reactivity are common. Such couples tend to be more treatable than other, more severely disturbed ones, who tend to be treatment-resistant. Demanding and blaming couples tend to alienate their families and be very isolated. Psychotherapy can be difficult with such couples, particularly if there is a high level of manipulativeness and substance abuse.

Preoccupied couples are usually high achievers who are successful vocationally and socially and are active in the community. The external obligation is frequently used as an excuse to avoid intimacy. The treatment can be difficult due to their external successes and rationalization.

The narcissistic interaction in couples generally conceals the underlying developmental arrest marked by the inability to develop a nurturing and intimate relationship. The couples tend to see themselves as cheated, deficient, and in need of attention or recompense. The nurturance provokes feelings of shame and personality fragmentation. The propensity for personality disorganization is countered by pathological distance regulation. A high level of mutual reactivity is a common manifestation. In narcissistic marriages, ordinary disagreements can serve as opportunities to express infantile rage in the form of blame. One aspect of such disorders is to conceal inadequacy and project it onto a spouse or a child. In some narcissistically vulnerable marriages, the conflicts may be covert and difficult to recognize. This occurs particularly when there is a conflict of loyalty between one's job and family.

Treatment

The goals of treatment with narcissistic couples are to reduce reactivity and collusive defenses, to avoid humiliation, and to enhance empathy in order to allow for growth and change. Lansky recommends a *conductor* type of therapeutic style (see Chapter 11, "Techniques of Family Therapy," for the description of this technique) in which the therapist takes command of the treatment situation to prevent overreactivity between the couple.

The therapist may choose the use of the *funneling through the therapist* technique (see Chapter 11 in this volume) in order to undermine the defensive and pathological overactivity and collusion. In this technique, the therapist asks that all transactions go through him or her. The second goal of this technique is the enhancement of empathic listening through which the therapist attempts to understand each spouse and help him or her understand each other.

An important goal of treatment is to address the intergenerational aspects of narcissistic disorders. Intergenerational constructions are particularly helpful and necessary in dealing with humiliation. The use of a genogram in the early phase of treatment is helpful. Narcissistic tendencies and disorders have a high propensity to repeat themselves in the next generation. Therefore, it is necessary to prevent such disorders in the younger generation by reducing blaming and collusion and increasing empathy. A common finding is that the identification of each spouse, as a child, with the same-sex parent was constantly criticized by the parent of the opposite sex, weakening her or his gender identity. Another goal of intergenerational psychotherapy is the reconstruction and resolution of traumatic events in the early life of the spouses such as parental absences, neglect, and abuse.

Mirroring and idealizing transferences (Kohut 1971, 1977) are commonly displaced onto the therapist and the marital partner. The couples tend to develop a special transference reaction to the therapist characterized by overt or covert blaming and provocation of blame. The therapist may find himself or herself competing with the same-sex spouse or may react with blaming or sympathy for the blamed spouse rather than expressing empathy for the feelings of the partners, which is necessary for the enhancement of understanding in the family.

Case Example

The following case example demonstrates the role of intense and unresolved marital transferences in the formation of marital dysfunction that has eluded resolution in the simultaneous psychoanalysis of the marital partners:

> Sally and Paul entered treatment because Sally complained that Paul was nonresponsive to her needs and noncommunicative. Paul admitted to social and sexual inadequacy on the surface but covertly accused Sally of being demanding and critical. The dissatisfaction had prevailed during their marriage of 23 years. Their sexual relationship had ceased in the past few years after a long period of unsatisfactory exchanges. Paul felt inadequate because of "coming too fast" but complained that Sally was hard to arouse. The couple had five children, who had done well educationally: four of them were graduate students in prestigious colleges, and the last one was attending a private high school.
>
> Sally and Paul both had been in psychoanalysis, each for a period of 6 years, prior to seeking marital therapy. The psychoanalytic treatment produced limited results according to the couple. Paul remained aloof and intellectual in his psychoanalytic treatment, and Sally felt that her analyst was cold, detached, and unresponsive to her strong and seemingly immediate needs.
>
> The couple retained a very submissive and childlike position in relation to their fathers, who were both extremely successful businessmen. The image of the mothers of the couple remained in the background because the mothers were not a source of conflict for the couple, as well as a less signif-

icant source of parenting. Paul's father was perceived as dominating Paul (and Sally), and Sally's father was believed to be demeaning and critical of Sally's personality as self-serving.

Sally's major conflict was with her father; she felt he didn't appreciate her and her many good qualities and was cold and subtly sadistic toward her. She had similar transference feelings toward her analyst, which remained unresolved. Paul felt put down and undermined by his father as a child and had become skilled in protecting himself from expected attacks by detaching himself from other people. This aloofness, which has characterized his relationships in general, remained relatively unresolved during his psychoanalysis and limited his success at work and in the marriage. Both spouses were relatively neglected by their mothers and have remained unaware of their unsatisfactory maternal relationships in spite of many years of psychoanalysis.

The marital transference was characterized by the constant attacks by Sally on Paul, who seemed to be blind to what was going on. He remained disengaged from Sally and the therapist, attempting to frustrate them both. The marital transference was further extended and displaced in the marital therapist.

The therapeutic interventions were to:

- Delineate the character traits and structure of both spouses
- Interpret the marital transference, transference to the previous analysts, and transference to the marital therapist on those different occasions when transference was *less heated* and more amenable to interpretation
- Interpret the hidden and unsatisfactory maternal transference that has remained dormant
- Interpret the same transference reactions and phenomena, particularly the maternal ones, when they were displayed toward the siblings and close friends outside of the family

It was the ability to interpret the transference reactions in multiple domains that allowed for a more satisfactory therapeutic outcome than had been achieved in the earlier analyses of the spouses. The marital relationship became more functional and satisfactory by the resolution of marital transference.

Conclusion

Personality is the major tool of social adaptation that is reflected in the selection of and interaction with peers and marital partners. There is a close relationship between both personality and *neurotic* disorders and dysfunctional family relationships. Such families generally represent a midrange level of dysfunction and become symptomatic only when excessive internal and external pressures are placed on them. The nucleus for the development of a personality and its disorders is formed within the families of origin. The continued relationship with the extended family tends to maintain and consolidate the personality disturbances. The personality and neurotic types of interactions are further perpetuated by the choice of a mate who overtly or covertly supports the rigidities in the personality of the spouse. The developmental failures initiated in childhood serve as the basis for the creation of marital disorders, and intensified relational problems further impede developmental progression and intimacy. The interlocking of the neurotic traits in a married couple results in what has been traditionally referred to as the *interlocking neurotic marriage*, in contrast to *marital neurosis*. In a marriage in which the vulnerabilities of a couple do not interlock, the rehabilitative forces in the marriage coupled with the flexibility in the spousal relationship can allow for the gradual resolution of neurotic vulnerabilities.

Chapters on Related Topics

The following chapters describe concepts related to family therapy with personality disorders:

- Chapter 4, "Psychodynamic Family Therapy"
- Chapter 21, "Psychodynamic Couples Therapy"

34

Impact of Culture and Ethnicity on Family Interventions

Linda D. Schwoeri, Ph.D.
G. Pirooz Sholevar, M.D.
Mark P. Combs, Ph.D.

Introduction

The changing racial and ethnic nature of our American society has made cultural diversity a subject relevant to anyone who works in the mental health field. It is irresponsible professional behavior to ignore the cultural sensitivities of patients. Although practitioners are always careful not to overlook the obvious, and may believe that cultural sensitivity is a given, they must still make a special effort to understand psychopathology as expressed in different cultures. This chapter looks at some differences among three cultural groups and asks the reader to reflect on his or her own biases and values when treating these groups. Therapists must consider the possibility that Anglo-American-based rules of behavior and conduct can be against a different culture's ideology.

McIntosh (1988) uses the metaphor of an "invisible knapsack of privilege" for white Americans who do not see, or in many instances acknowledge, their advantaged status. Unfortunately, the vast majority of therapeutic and mental health practices were formulated by white Americans for other white ethnic groups (McGoldrick et al. 1996).

Despite America's history of racism and the enduring state of racial tension in this country, intermarriage abounds. Descriptive statistics indicate that upward of 50% of Americans are forming intimate and marital relationships outside of their family's ethnicity of origin (Hines and Boyd-Franklin 1982).

Diagnosis Is Culture-Bound

Family theory recognizes that the culture, ethnic background, and the sociocultural context in which a family's problem occurs are fundamentally interconnected. The family's culture, values, orientation to the world and everyday issues and conflict, life strategies, and worldview combine to form an approach to life that directs *all* behaviors. The ideology beneath behavior is unquestioned, unconscious, and essentially metaphorical in nature. Ideology is lived out by the individual and family through myths, beliefs, celebrations, and rituals (Schwartzman 1983). Value orientations regarding the character of human nature, the relationship between humanity and nature, the temporal focus of life on earth, and the manner and nature of human activity and human relationships (Kluckhohn 1958; Spiegel 1971) are part of the family culture. These values influence all approaches to problem solving, decision making, and socialization.

Definitions

Understanding the cultural aspects of psychiatric problems requires some basic observations. The first is that psychiatric diagnosis is *culture bound*. *Culture* consists of those patterns of behavior, acquired and transferred over time, which prescribe the norms, customs, roles, and values inherent in the political, economic, religious, and social aspects of family life. Culture provides the set of rules and standards that guide peoples' actions, makes their behavior understandable to one another, and helps to explain individuals' relationship to their sociobiological context.

Ethnicity refers to the sense of belonging and having a rootedness in history that reaches beyond religion, race, or national or geographic origin. Ethnicity is our basic identity—who we are in relation to other minority groups. It frames our manner of dress, style, and communication through language and rituals, as well as how we feel about life, death, and illness (Giordano-Giordano 1977; McGoldrick et al. 1982). The concept is derived from the Greek word *ethnos*, or people of a nation. We are born with an ethnic identity. Throughout life we experience and adopt different cultures, thereby living with expectations and values from both a majority

Impact of Culture and Ethnicity on Family Interventions

culture (i.e., the American culture) and a minority culture—our culture of origin. We carry with us both the values, assumptions, traditions, and worldviews transmitted over generations within our ethnic group and the concurrent—sometimes competing—views of the cultural context in which we live. As noted by McGoldrick et al. (1982) and Herr (1989), ethnic traditions still affect third and fourth generations in subtle ways and are often experienced as cultural conflicts between members of the younger generation.

Cultural context refers to the sociocultural environment in which people live and interact. The combination of ethnic origin and cultural context, together with the pressures imposed by cultural transitions and/or migration, inevitably creates difficulties that family groups must resolve. Landau (1982) discusses the challenge of balancing the demands of living within these two cultures—the culture of origin and the majority culture. She notes that if the stresses and differences are too great, and the family network is too remote or too weak to help, the family must either adapt to the culture or turn inward on itself, becoming isolated and enmeshed as a family group. As a consequence of the ethnocentric defense, very often the family resists accepting help from outsiders unless their problems become too great to handle alone.

Effect of Culture on Help-Seeking

Religion, faith, and healing are often so intertwined that in certain cultures, when a psychiatric condition occurs, diagnosis and remedy may be more related to spiritual than medical interpretation. For example, in Hispanic culture there is a condition called *susto*. This describes a type of terror or fright that occurs through some trauma. The victim of the *susto* or trauma suffers a "soul loss" through fright. As in posttraumatic stress disorder (PTSD), the trauma can manifest clinically as depression, anxiety, or fear (Gobeil 1973). The cure for this condition requires the intervention of a person skilled in healing—a *curander*, or "curer," who allows the patient to release fears and hostilities (Tseng and McDermott 1981). "Treatment" consists of medicine, some ritual or ceremony with friends and relatives, and the support of a network of friends. Ultimately the person is "reassured" through a type of transferential cure—a combined systematic approach that includes a spiritual orientation, the support of friends and family, and faith in the curer.

An example, given by Tseng and McDermott (1981, p. 32), describes a case involving a 60-year-old woman who had lost family members by death and desertion. Being all alone, she began to manifest paranoid symptoms, refused to eat, became sleepless, shouted to herself, and began losing weight.

She feared being poisoned, locked herself in her house, and slept with knives by her bedside. She "regained her reason" through the arrival of a Catholic priest who blessed the house and the help of one of her sisters who brought her food. Although the woman's symptoms could be identified by DSM-IV-TR standards (American Psychiatric Association 2000) as those of a psychiatric depression, her "mental illness" was remedied through nourishing meals and community support.

Moving Beyond Masks to Find the Family

Montalvo and Gutierrez (1983) identified *cultural masks* as an important element in treating families from different cultures. *Cultural mask* refers to the family's use of real elements in their culture to conceal their problematic interactions. For example, the family can use the rationale: "We are Latin, we are expected to have hot tempers." The family thus uses culturally sanctioned behavior in a defensive fashion in order to protect crucial underlying issues. The family presents to the therapist a view of who they are based on what they think is *expected* of them instead of showing how they actually behave when trying to resolve problems or even interact with one another. Montalvo and Gutierrez caution the therapist to search for the *problem-solving approach* of the family and not get caught up in exotic or unusual behavior patterns unique to the family's culture.

Another important treatment issue is making the assessment as culture-free as possible. For example, in conducting a mental status examination, inquiries concerning memory loss, orientation to time and place, or mathematical problems must be relevant to the patient's cultural experience and level of education and/or schooling. What an American may consider common knowledge may not be true in other cultures. It is more culturally sensitive and may be more diagnostic to ask patients to name their own government leaders, the name of their country, and their village of origin rather than apply our standard (American) list of questions (Tseng and McDermott 1981).

Characteristics of Families From Three Cultures

African-American Families

African Americans compose from 12% (Hines and Boyd-Franklin 1982) to 12.8% (U.S. Census Bureau 1999) of the population. A majority of African

Impact of Culture and Ethnicity on Family Interventions

Americans have migrated from the American south to northern and western states (Henderson 1994). Issues of parity and equality with other cultural groups are most evident in the job market, where African Americans made 80% of what whites earned (O'Hare et al. 1991).

A pejorative "deficit view" of African Americans persists in the field of psychology; that is, African Americans are often considered to be hampered by a lack of education, financial stability, good upbringing, and so forth. More recently, there has been a strong upsurge of African Psychology sensibility that seeks to expose African-American culture's richness and strengths for a more balanced perspective (Nobles and Goddard 1984).

There is much diversity in African-American culture. Much of this dates to the history of slavery, which still greatly influences how the African-American family views the world and the values placed on life.

Rich delineations are created within the African-American family by the extended family. Specifically, this arrangement localizes subfamilies within the large family matrix consisting of primary and secondary members (Hill 1977). Other arrangements include households where the children are not related to the head of the household, an arrangement that Billingsley (1968) refers to as "augmented families." Billingsley also identifies the role of non-blood relatives who are integrated into this permeable but very functional boundary of family membership (McAdoo and McAdoo 2002).

Kinship Bonds

Although slavery and its aftermath disrupted the structure and support of the tribal experience for those Africans who were torn from their homeland, the tribal kin "network" remained as a vital part of their heritage (Hines and Boyd-Franklin 1982; Mintz and Price 1992; Nobles 1980; Pinderhughes 1979, 1982). This focus on kin and the kinship network is relived in many parts of African-American life through religion, childcare, and foster family care, and constitutes a significant aspect of African-American life. Kinship bonds are a central residual part of the African culture. In contrast to the widely quoted Cartesian dictum of *cogito ergo sum*, which stresses the individual's lonely perception of his or her own consciousness, the African-American view could be stated as "We are; therefore, I am." This belief in kinship networks extends beyond bloodlines and includes friends, neighbors, and ministers. To ignore the importance of the kinship network operating within African-American culture is to disregard an essential aspect of this culture's identity. This kinship network is often the first place African Americans go when there is a problem.

Mothering and Informal Adoption

Mothering and informal adoption are crucial concepts in African-American culture. Motherhood is a very important role for the African-American woman. It is common within the African culture for women to nurse other women's children as needed. In the United States, informal adoption is quite common and part of a very old slave tradition whereby friends or relatives "took in" children who could not be cared for by their own parents. "Childkeeping," as it is referred to by Stack (1975), is indicative of the strong network operating within this culture. A network of childcare continues today and can often be seen in the appearance of a grandmother who assumes full responsibility for raising her son or daughter's children. The childcare network is also manifest in the foster-parent network, as well as the kinship foster-care network so prevalent in the United States today. The Child Welfare League of America estimates that nearly four million children are raised by relatives nationwide (Woodall 1993). Often, very little funding is available to help support these children; however, kinship care is part of the family's belief in the need to care and protect children.

Upward Mobility

Upward mobility is highly valued in the "American dream" of individualism and ownership of material goods (Boyd-Franklin 1989). However, as described by Pinderhughes (1982), the American dream is always in conflict with the "victim value system." The victim value system is a name given to the struggle to overcome obstacles that threaten self-esteem. Often this struggle leads to the paradoxical erection of barriers to opportunity through inadequate education that limits employment opportunities.

Children and Responsibility

In many African-American families the role of the parent is often delegated to a child who takes on responsibility for other children while the parent(s) works. Boszormenyi-Nagy has named this phenomena *parentification*; it denotes how the child assumes a parental role both emotionally and physically (Boszormenyi-Nagy and Spark 1984). From a young age, children take the task of "mothering" very seriously. The assignment of this role to children must not be dismissed, because it is connected to a cultural value system necessary for survival. Future generations ultimately feel the impact of the loss of childhood through parentification. The family will need to learn how to negotiate tasks and responsibilities as part of their treatment in order to let their children grow up free of guilt and unwarranted feelings of obligation.

Responsibility also extends to aging grandparents and is characterized by respect and recognition for what the grandparents have done for the family as children. Elderly people are respected and cared for within the family network rather than institutions or agencies. It is a family's way of repaying those who helped them and sacrificed for them. An intergenerational view of families is most helpful in working with African-American families because of the issues around loyalty and reciprocity.

Paternity and the African-American Male

Secrets about paternity and informal adoption are difficult issues that may not be discussed by black families. Even within African-American culture, a toxic issue is one of darker and lighter skin color (Boyd-Franklin 1989), reflecting the dominant culture's legacy of racism. Franklin (1998) refers to the plight of African-American males as the "invisibility syndrome," which in essence marginalizes them and treats them as peripheral figures. Subsequently, men are frequently not included in family sessions or even contacted, given the deficit perspectives that prevail in the hegemony of the socially constructed African-American male. These concerns are shared by African-American women, who are careful *not* to reify this perception, yet who struggle to deal with many latent issues in their relationships (see McGoldrick et al. 1989). Nevertheless, issues of sexual prowess and power between spouses in African-American couples reflect an area that African-American men may feel more in control of when juxtaposed against the legacy of external control by racism and the victim status that has prevailed long after emancipation (Boyd-Franklin 1989). A corresponding social myth depicts the black father as peripheral, a myth that has been overemphasized in psychiatric literature and further reifies deficit perspectives (Boyd-Franklin 1989; Gary 1981).

The Role of the Church and Spirituality

The role of the church and spirituality are crucial to this culture and can be traced throughout African history. As Knox (1985, p. 31) wrote, "Spirituality is deeply embedded in the Black psyche." The church is seen as the one institution that remains a refuge against the painful experiences of life, including racism and discrimination. The church and spirituality are part of the complex social, spiritual, educational and family network within African-American culture (DuBois 1903; Frazier 1963). The importance of religion and the role of the church cannot be ignored if the therapist is to gain the family's trust. It is not uncommon to invite the additional services of a minister into treatment, especially if the minister has already been part of the family's approach to problem solving.

Latino-American Families

Latino is the more contemporary term used to refer to a cultural group that shares a language, values, and customs. There are several regional subcultures that are referred to collectively as the "Latino culture." (Note that *Latino* is used to describe the general culture, but *Latina* and *Latino* are used to describe female and male members of the culture, respectively.) Gonzalez (1992) correctly notes that for many in this very diverse population, the word *Hispanic* projects a politically conservative perspective, whereas Latino is considered a much less political demarcation and more in keeping with a sense of vitality and ethnocultural progressiveness. Falicov (1998) ascribes to the Hispanic label as reflecting an inherently Spanish-European superiority versus the conquered and indigenous populations of the Americas associated with Latino. In 1954, Latinos previously associated with whites were reclassified as *Hispanics*, a "colored" or racial designation with roots in desegregation policies (Falicov 1998). Another term frequently misapplied is *Chicano*. Chicano denotes people of American birth but of Mexican descent who do not align themselves with either culture (see Acuna 1996). Puerto Ricans, Mexicans, and Cubans make up the three largest segments of the Latino population. Relatively recent changes to Latino culture include large numbers of immigrants from Central and South American countries, each bringing another nuance to the Latino population (Garcia-Preto 1996).

To recap, Latino culture consists of a diverse mix of Spanish descendants of the European culture, native Indians from Mexico and South and Central America, and the offspring of this union known as *mestizo;* the offspring of black slaves and Spanish descendants; Chicano, the offspring of Mexican and American inhabitants; and the large number of Puerto Rican immigrants.

This diversity requires very careful use of cultural context, since race is no longer a biological concept. For example, when treating an individual who is of Hispanic origin, yet physically looks African American, which cultural lens do we apply?

Beliefs About the Etiology of Illness

Harwood (1981, 1994) observed folk beliefs about the etiology of illness. Some illnesses were seen as "natural," or *males naturales,* and others were associated with the supernatural and witchcraft, *mal puesto.* A nerve attack or *ataque de nervios* is associated with distress and being unable to control oneself. Another common belief in the folk etiology of illness is the evil eye

Impact of Culture and Ethnicity on Family Interventions 733

or *mal de ojo*, which posits that individuals can be influenced by stronger persons. These beliefs are frequently amalgamated with Catholic beliefs into a syncretic worldview of religion and corollary practices. Rituals to remove or cleanse individuals are frequently performed by *espiritistas* and *curanderos* in these rituals, or *limpias*. Some physicians and therapists with traditional Western medical training are unable to blend folk beliefs into their practice (Garcia-Preto 1996).

Family and the Individual

Familismo is a critical component of the Latino fabric of life for construction of a familial self (Falicov 1998). Autonomy and separation from family are not overt movements but rather *personalismo*, which is an inner sense of differentiation maintained in relation to the familial self at all times (Levine and Padilla 1980). Hence, family therapy can be a very powerful ally when presented within this conceptual framework. Therapists who approach these family constellations from a systemic perspective attribute enmeshment to family members. Mothers are honored and imbued with parental status; the mother-son bond is very strong and supported in the culture. Fathers were traditionally the source of authority, with the mother mediating the father's interactions with family members. However, stratification and changes in Latino culture no longer support this monolithic stereotype of the paternal role (Powell 1995).

American ideals of independence and autonomy often clash with the interdependence that is part of Latino culture. Latinos often feel that they are misunderstood and often diagnosed improperly by mental health professionals. As discussed by Sue and Sue (1990), these differences about independence and interdependence present a variety of problems and treatment considerations. For example, the family may identify more with the Anglo culture as noted in their choice of anglicized names, American food, and American music. The family may therefore appear very American and yet may exhibit behavior based on Old World thinking. Such a dichotomy would become evident as stress is placed on the family to think and act like American Anglos. Among the questions therapists should ask themselves are: Would family members feel more comfortable conducting therapy in their native tongue? What has living in the United States done to the family's ethnic heritage? Do they maintain the views of their original culture in relation to family values and worldview? Is questioning a Latina about sexual matters disrespectful? Would it be better to have a female therapist do this? Does a Latina's reluctance to speak about sex mean resistance to getting help?

Spiritism

Spiritism pervades Latino culture and is the belief that the visible world is influenced by powerful good and evil personages who inhabit a larger invisible world. Rituals help maintain this belief. Emotional problems are often attributed to spiritual problems; therefore, the sufferer is more likely to consult a spiritist than a mental health professional. Especially in Puerto Rican culture, spiritism reflects an underlying distrust of organized religion and a belief that God and the supernatural can be contacted without clergy (Garcia-Preto 1982). These beliefs can easily be misunderstood in an evaluation when the patient tells the psychiatrist about his or her conversation with God.

Integrity and Respeto

Personalismo, or individualism, emphasizes inner virtues and enables an individual to respect himself or herself regardless of the level of material success achieved. Respect for authority and self is the basis for dignity in the Puerto Rican culture. It is maintained in the family and community through the enforcement of a system of rules. Respect for men and for elderly people is emphasized. Children learn to respect adults through a system of *compadrazgo*, which is a kinshiplike tradition of copaternity of children by compadres (godparents) and biological parents. In the *compadrazgo* tradition, there are expectations of mutual aid among family members and the practice of the rules of respect (Garcia-Preto 1982).

Kinship Bonds and the Extended Family

Kinship bonds in Latino culture are strong, and the family pledges to support all of its members as long as they remain within the family system (Garcia-Preto 1982). The unity and dignity of the family are highly valued. The extended family, rather than the nuclear family system, is emphasized and includes the godparents (compadres) and adopted children as well as relatives by blood or marriage. During times of crisis, children are often moved from one nuclear family to another within the family system. More so than in the American culture, marriage seems to signify the joining of two families and dependence on each other. It is more common for the mother of the family to turn to other women in her family for help. If other women in the family cannot help the mother, she may ask more of her husband, but she is careful to not make demands of him. It is commonly believed that the mother is, in essence, responsible for taking care of herself emotionally or with the help of her children.

Although Latino women typically work outside the home, the husband is considered the main provider. Conflict may arise if the husband has not been able to support the family through employment. The wife may be unable to complain or to criticize her husband's failure because she must not exhibit disrespect in front of the children or the family. If the couple seeks treatment, it is necessary to bring the conflict between the economic and cultural realities into the open. As noted by McGoldrick et al. (1982), the therapist needs to help the couple see how vital it is for them to work *together* for their family's survival; to criticize or blame produces only further family problems.

The Role of Migration

Migration (e.g., in search of work) can affect family structure and behavior in a variety of ways because it often involves shifts in the male dominance of the marital dyad. The reversal of sex roles (e.g., the wife may earn more money than the husband) may create marital conflict and cultural dissonance. She may become depressed and anxious if she must assume total economic responsibility for the family because of her spouse's poor employment opportunities. Her value system and her family needs are in conflict with the economic and social reality of her immigrant status. This role conflict may not be resolved until a second- or third-generation status in this country is achieved.

The often-used term *machismo*, or the cult of manliness, is well established in the social sciences lore and has iconic symbolism. However, the notion of being a gentleman, or *caballero*, is also essential and more accurate. Corresponding to this is the cult of the Virgin Mary and *Marianismo* or living according to the traits Mary exemplified. Comas-Diaz (1994) observed that at home Latinas are expected to adhere to their "marianista" side and at work they are expected to show their determination, or "hembrismo" side.

When migrating across national borders, difficulties with learning a new language can pose a problem in general for Hispanic parents and their children. Children frequently learn English faster than their parents and must act as interpreters and communicators of the needs of their parents. A reversal of child-parent roles occurs, and the established hierarchical system of children respecting and depending on parents becomes distorted. Furthermore, children of foreign-born parents may adopt American values sooner than their parents and gradually come to reject their parents because they view the new values as superior to traditional values. Under these circumstances, the parents typically respond with even stricter enforcement of traditional values, particularly respect for and obedience to authority.

Immigration itself has had an impact on the structure of Puerto Rican families by precipitating a transformation from an extended to a nuclear family orientation. However, as Latino patients will tell you, not including a family member in treatment is to risk losing family support and understanding.

Children and Childrearing

Children provide a source of closeness for the mother. The Hispanic mother characteristically demonstrates this during the first 3 years of a child's life by doing everything for the child and being very permissive. A dependence on the mother is fostered and maintained, especially for the male child. The male adolescent is given more social freedom than the female, while having his everyday needs met by his mother or sister. The female adolescent more typically is encouraged to begin caring for the younger children. She remains at home with her parents and thinks less about her own independence.

Sacrificing for the Children

Parents are expected to put their needs second to those of their children. This fosters the children's dependence as well as an obligation to the parents and keeps the children close to the family.

Asian-American Families

In Asian cultures, the tenets of Confucianism and Buddhism, symbolism within the language, the cultural view of health and wellness, migration trends, kinship bonds, and sex roles are instrumental in defining behavior. These issues should always be considered while searching for a solution to the family's problems. In addressing the needs of Asian families, it is important to recognize that the value orientations of Asian-American communities in America are very different from the values of mainstream America. Furthermore, the diversity within Asian-American families makes it beneficial to become familiar with the Asian experiences of migration and immigration in order to understand better the part they have played on the family's ability to adjust.

Lee (1982) describes three types of Asian families within the United States: 1) immigrant families who have recently arrived and are in need of basic survival skills; 2) immigrant-American families (usually foreign-born parents with American-born children), who often experience parent-child value conflicts; and 3) immigrant-descended families of American-born parents with children. This third group usually speaks English at home and lives according to Western cultural values, thus experiencing far less value conflict. There are a variety of Asian-American groups to consider when addressing the treatment needs of this culture. There are Chinese, Filipino, Korean, Japanese, Samoan, and Southeast Asian families who have different family values and characteristics. Unfortunately, there is limited intraethnic research. Research presently appears to focus on descriptions of individual traits; however, certain profiles can be useful in becoming familiar with interethnic differences.

The Roles of Confucianism and Buddhism

In Asian culture there is an emphasis, reinforced by religion, on the primacy of the group over the individual. Confucianism and Buddhism assign hierarchical roles for all members and dictate highly formalized rules of behavior and conduct. Autonomy and independence are not encouraged; relationships among and between family members are strictly prescribed. Since forces outside the individual dictate behavior, the feeling of control from within is diminished. Very often the formalization of personal and social behavior contributes to an image of inactivity, dependency, and passivity in the individual.

In the East Asian family the concept of family encompasses many generations. This unlimited familial timeframe is reinforced by such customs as ancestor worship, family record books, and marriage arrangements that are designed to mark the continuation of the family line, not necessarily the start of a new family. It is believed that through marriage, the woman leaves her family of origin and becomes *absorbed* into her husband's family—past and present.

Sex Roles and Family Roles

Within the East Asian family unit, the father assumes the role of leader, decision maker, authority figure, and primary disciplinarian. As such, East Asian fathers can appear stern, distant, and generally less approachable than East Asian mothers (Shon and Ja 1982). The community views the family's successes and failures as the father's responsibility. Mothers, by contrast, are the nurturers of husbands and children and are emotionally devoted caregivers. The children's strongest emotional ties are with the mother. Generally, sons are more highly valued than daughters, since the family name and linkage are passed through the male side. The most important child is the oldest son, since he becomes the head of the family when his father dies. He is also devoted to his mother and is heavily influenced by her. In this way, the mother *indirectly* controls the family upon the death of her husband.

Obligation and Shame

Obligation and shame are strong determinants of interpersonal relationships within the context of East Asian culture. Obligation is incurred through assigned roles or stature and through acts of kindness or helpfulness for which obligation is due (Shon and Ja 1982). A family member's greatest obligation is to his or her parents.

Communication among family members and with the society is shaped by age, sex, education, occupation, social status, and family background. There are many linguistic subtleties in syntax and word endings that reflect the status of the speakers and the nature of their relationship. Unfamiliar or threatening social situations in which little is known about the persons involved are a source of anxiety, because communicators do not know how to respond to each other. There is an ever-present fear that a social error will be committed, resulting in *Tiu Lien* or shame (literally "loss of face"). This can occur through the public exposure of misconduct and can result in the withdrawal of support for an individual from family, community, and society. The loss of support produces tremendous feelings of anxiety and abandonment; therefore, there is a silence and watchfulness for the correct cues to follow in social situations (Shon and Ja 1982).

The Role of Migration and Transition

There are tremendous cultural conflicts imposed on the Asian American in trying to live within two cultures. The experience of migration and the process of transition and acculturation can produce interpersonal and intrapsychic conflict for recently immigrated Asian families. Adaptation to a new culture is a complex process and is determined by several factors: 1) the extent to which the original expectations of migration coincide with reality, 2) the availability of support systems, 3) the degree to which the immigrant family structure is similar to the family structure of the newly adopted culture, and 4) how the cultures fit together within the larger society (Landau 1982). There may be insufficient internal resources to meet the demands of adaptation to the new environment. The act of migration creates a loss of identity, structure, and boundaries. Individual family members' personal goals may conflict with family goals, creating a source of stress. Social relationships are often a problem while the children and adolescents learn the customs of their new cultural context.

View of Psychiatric Symptoms and Psychiatry in Asian Culture

In Asian culture, somatization is the usual manner in which psychological problems and complaints are presented. Rather than using the word *depressed*, the person will talk about his stomach hurting or her head being empty. If a person is angry, he or she may present symptoms related to the gallbladder or liver but *not* present a psychological complaint. Furthermore, the words for psychiatry—*Jing sheng bin shue*—have nothing to do with psychiatry. They mean kidney-heart specialty. Therefore, the person of the psychiatrist is really a kidney-heart doctor who is going to treat the emotions. When Asian Americans come for treatment they are probably expecting some form of physical intervention, not talking therapy, because in China, for instance, there is no psychotherapy (Uzee 1989). The issue of medication is also complex. Telling the patient and family that he or she must take Mellaril and not continue taking ginseng is threatening to existing beliefs. Treatment requires compromises on the part of psychiatrists. They must defer to culture-based treatments, including heat, electroacupuncture, and herbal teas, in an effort to be seen as sensitive to the patient's beliefs and values.

The father in an Asian-American family may resist bringing the children for family therapy because it may be stressful or shameful and the child would be seen as a type of "mental patient." As Uzee (1989) has noted, in Asian culture "there is no concept of being a little bit sick. If you are sick and you go to a psychiatrist or counselor that means you are very, very sick—you are psychotic, suicidal, homicidal, or something is severely wrong. That reflects not only upon you, but your whole family." The customary way to avoid this shame is to hide the person from the community—to save face.

Uzee (1989) notes the reluctance with which many Asian Americans discuss problems as part of Asian culture's bias toward accepting life as it is; complaining is useless since problems are part of life. Many Asian elders believe that too much analytic thinking can cause problems such as depression. Chou (1989) notes that there is an obligation to focus on the future generation and its well-being, *not* the present. This view engenders beliefs about the necessity of *suffering* and *doing without* in order to provide for the future of the family. This could be seen as a stereotypic stoicism in Asian culture, but when put into perspective, it is the family's way of preserving its traditional ideologies while interacting with forces within its sociocultural context. It is not passivity; it is more a loyalty to the culture.

Treatment

There is no single approach to treatment of families from any culture. It is therefore necessary to look into which approach works best and why.

Sue and Sue (1990) described the need for therapists to be aware of their position as authorities, as well as their personal class values, communication style, and use of language. The most important consideration is the level of comfort felt by the family. The issue of racism permeates the therapy from the start. The therapist who feels antagonism toward the family will exhibit it in subtle ways. If the family cannot trust the therapist, or feels it is being patronized, judged, or stereotyped, there will be no treatment. Training in cultural diversity, peer supervision, and consultation requirements is needed to work effectively with different cultural groups.

African-American Families

Given the climate of cultural paranoia that exists based on the legacy of institutional racism (Hines and Boyd-Franklin 1982), therapy can be and frequently is viewed as another oppressive system. Unfortunately, many clinicians fail to acknowledge this salient dimension in therapy, only to find difficulties connecting and engaging African-American families. Differences in ethnic or racial backgrounds between counselor and family should be addressed early in therapy so as to deal with any resulting issues and to allow families the opportunity to seek other options and opinions if desired.

Religiosity has been a steadfast resource for African Americans and continues to be so. Religious communities may be the only source of care used when distress or other issues arise (Larson et al. 1988). One has only to see how Reverend Martin Luther King Jr., Reverend Jesse Jackson, Reverend Al Sharpton, and Reverend Sullivan have been seen as crusaders to understand the relevance of this institution within African-American culture and on everyday lives (Broman 1996).

In terms of treatment approaches, Boyd-Franklin (1989) notes that the structural approach is most effective during the opening phase of treatment. This approach provides a clear focus on the problem and allows for engagement between the therapist and family. It tells the family that the therapist understands the problem. Once focus and understanding have been established, and some progress is made toward solving the initial presenting problem, the family can move into the middle phase of treatment. At this time, a more in-depth exploration of family dynamics can be initiated, which may include the use of a family genogram. Furthermore, white therapists working with African-American families need to explore their own cultural biases and not hide their own concerns about racism and its effects. Boyd-Franklin (1989) advises broaching rather than avoiding the issue of difference in race and exploring the comfort level with the family and/or patient.

In working with African-American families, the therapist should be guided by the values inherent in the family system. In this culture there is much flexibility between systems; however, problems can occur if rules are not clearly established. For example, if the grandmother is very much part of the parental subsystem by functioning as a co-parent for her single daughter's children, the alliance between grandmother and mother must be strengthened, never diminished. This can be accomplished by clarifying roles and tasks. The mother must be made to look competent by encouraging her to parent more effectively through the grandmother's support and definition of her own responsibilities.

The following case illustrates the method of establishing an alliance between a mother and grandmother. The grandmother had custody of her grandchildren by this daughter.

Case Example

The mother had been a drug abuser since adolescence. The children were placed with the maternal grandmother by Child Protective Services, and the mother was initially given limited visitation rights. The children loved the grandmother but were now nearly adolescents and reluctant to follow and totally accept the grandmother's "old-time rules." The mother continued to promise a reunion with the children during the visits. The children could not express any anger toward the mother and displaced it on the grandmother. In sessions with the grandmother and children, loyalty issues concerning the mother were explored. Chores and responsibilities were outlined. The mother and children discussed homework, school activities, problems, and so forth. The proposed changes enlarged significantly the role of the mother, who assumed the responsibility of assisting the children with their studies. The grandmother was willing to support the mother and understood that the children were causing discipline problems as a means of involving their mother and getting attention. Grandmother was seen separately to encourage her to support the mother to deal effectively with the children. She began to accept her daughter as an adult who could be responsible with the children, while the grandmother herself remained the custodial parent. The children learned that no one, especially their grandmother, would try to hurt their mother. The children benefited from relationships with both generations of parental figures. The children's mother began to visit on a more regular basis, which decreased the children's anxiety and disruptive behavior.

Latino-American Families

Therapy with Latino families usually occurs with adolescents who are influenced by both American popular culture and the culture of their parents. This condition of two languages, behaviors, and cultures has been termed *entremundos*, or between two worlds (Zavala-Martinez 1994).

Garcia-Preto (1982) offers some recommendations for addressing cultural issues with Latino families:

- A close working relationship should be established during the initial interview. This may require an extended session in which questions concerning family values, rituals, and beliefs are addressed.
- Respect must be shown for the structure, boundaries, roles, and positions of the family.
- Enlist adults—not children—as interpreters if language is a barrier to communication.
- Latinos seek help for marital problems relatively infrequently. Generally, those who do enter therapy are significantly more acculturated than those who do not. The following principles stress the importance of family involvement: 1) extended family is an important part of therapy; 2) exploration of environmental stressors associated with cultural adaptation will reveal the many family strengths and challenges; 3) a concrete, time-limited, and goal-oriented treatment plan will put needed structure in place and lessen resistance to discussing personal family issues.

Respect for family roles and structure is illustrated in the case example below.

Case Example

A family came for treatment because their preadolescent daughter was disruptive and failing in school, breaking family rules, and associated with friends unacceptable to her parents. These somewhat common problems were exacerbated by the strain placed on the girl to live within the cultural dictates of the family's gender bias: "Boys can date and stay out late," while "girls must be refined, study hard, and remain ladylike and virginal until marriage." As the youngest of three daughters, the patient was expected to stay close to her mother, clean up after her brothers, wait on her father, and love her piano and French lessons. She resented these expectations, yet felt torn because her mother lived by these gender-driven rules.

The parents, a biologist and an attorney, struggled to keep their South American values intact. The mother stayed at home with the family, never sat for her boards, and therefore did not practice law. She was depressed and ambivalent about her career. The father suffered with depression over the loss of his family ties. Life-cycle issues added to the adolescence's struggle for identity in the American sociocultural setting.

This family, although affluent and assimilated into the mainstream, was still struggling with issues of acculturation brought to a head by the youngest child's need to help Mom and Dad become more Americanized. The mother had to face her conflict over fulfilling her professional dreams and accepting her position as a competent woman who was married to a competent man. Family therapy remained focused on commitment to family "unity."

Asian-American Families

As discussed earlier in this chapter, Asian-American families tend to underutilize mental health services, defer to family, or keep quiet about their problems. When working with Asian-American families, therapists should keep in mind that bringing the problem to an outsider creates great shame for the family. This requires a show of respect by not confronting the family's values. Making small talk, overly friendly approaches, and unstructured sessions can hinder treatment. Criticizing the father's role would bring shame to the family; therefore, interventions must be framed in a positive way. Berg and de Shazer (1993) suggest phrasings such as "When your son becomes more respectful of what you are saying, what will he do differently?" The role of the mother must likewise be respected. The concept of distance in relationships needs to be readjusted, since clear boundaries are not upheld in the Asian culture. For example, to see a son's close relationship to his mother as pathological is to disregard the importance placed on that relationship. Sons are expected to be very close to mothers throughout their lives. They also expect to be pampered and have their lives tied into their mother's life; "meddling" by the mother is acceptable and expected (Berg and Jaya 1993). The therapist needs to find out what would contribute to harmony within the family. Consider the questions "What do you think your son would say is the problem between you and him?" and "What do you think he will notice you do differently?" These questions elicit information that is important to the Asian family on the consequences of behavior. An adaptation of the circular questioning technique (Selvini Palazzoli et al. 1980) helps elicit personal impressions of the relation of behaviors to each other and does not challenge or shame the family. Asian-American families often prefer to have the therapist direct the process of the discussion and give information as well as being very clear. A therapist who is less directive and structured will confuse the family.

Training in Cultural Diversity

The complex interrelationship between cultures of origin and the majority sociocultural context warrants special attention by family therapists and all clinicians who expect to be helpful to different individuals. There is an enormous amount of misinformation about different cultures, and when this is combined with ethnic prejudice or mislabeling, the possibilities for treatment errors increase rapidly. There has been a growing appreciation for the need to train clinicians in order to reduce cross-cultural errors. Consciousness raising (Christensen 1989), multicultural skills training (Boyd-Franklin 1989), supervision of family therapy (Liddle et al. 1988), and practice and internships with minorities (Hardy 1989; McGoldrick et al. 1982) have begun to address the need to sensitize clinicians to the impact of their cultural heritage on their work with families from different cultures. Family-of-origin issues revolving around ethnicity and culture are very much a part of how the therapist conducts treatment. Therefore, exercises in multicultural training are intended to make the therapist aware of the broad issues of racial identity, religion, and socioeconomic status. Genograms (McGoldrick and Gerson 1985) are useful in drawing out culturally learned and communicated patterns of behavior and myths about family of origin. Another useful tool has been home videos of family celebrations and holidays.

Falicov (1988) stresses that cultural attunement should include a combination of lectures, readings, and experiential exercises in how to think in cultural terms, as well as how to understand the fit between the family's culture and its sociocultural context. In times of stress, transition, or crisis in the family life cycle, the family's culture will dictate behaviors that may appear poorly adaptive. These behaviors are transferred over generations as appropriate ways of dealing with transitions and changes. For example, as in the case study of the Latino family, the role division along sexual lines became more apparent as the children attempted to become more a part of the American culture. However, through therapy the mother began to resolve her conflict to be part of the professional world yet the center of her family's life.

Conclusion

This chapter describes some principles that can guide therapeutic intervention with families from three different cultures—African-American, Asian-American, and Latino-American. Issues of culture and ethnicity are still alive in the value systems and worldviews of second- or even third-genera-

Impact of Culture and Ethnicity on Family Interventions

tion immigrant families. These views are fundamental to each individual and do not change easily, although the original migration and acculturation process may no longer create adjustment problems. It is becoming increasingly apparent that to understand families we need to differentiate between culture-specific behaviors and a *cultural mask*: that is, the family's real problems and a "mask" of behavior presented to the therapist based on what they think is *expected* of their culture. Training in cultural diversity is necessary if therapists are to be sensitive to and effective with the variety of problems brought to them. No single treatment approach is proposed as the best. Indeed, with some families, it may be best to first work individually with the patient and then consider family therapy. However, if family therapy is the treatment chosen, it appears that taking a more structural approach in the opening phase of therapy and then gently moving into a more intergenerational approach, such as Bowen's, is a productive strategy. Not all families are prepared to explore their feelings. Not all families are ready to see the world through the eyes of the therapist. Conversely, the challenge for family therapists is to understand and see the world through the eyes of the family and to intervene within that framework. Matching different treatment approaches—individual, family, or group—with the family's needs and expectations can lead to the achievement of the desired goals.

Chapters on Related Topics

The following chapter describes concepts related to the impact of culture and ethnicity on family intervention:

- Chapter 9, "Social Network Intervention"

35

Medical Family Therapy

G. Pirooz Sholevar, M.D.
Christoph Sahar, M.D.

Introduction

The term *medical family therapy*, coined by McDaniel et al. (1992), refers to the biopsychosocial treatment of individuals who are affected by medical problems as a member of a family. It emphasizes collaboration between family physicians, other health professionals, and family therapists. The conceptual framework of medical family therapy is intended to provide a practical way of understanding and promoting the relationship among all the parties involved in treatment of a patient with medical or somatoform illness. The concept became particularly influential after the inauguration of the journal *Family Systems Medicine* by Donald Bloch and co-workers. The major foci of medical family therapy are 1) to provide a framework for working with a chronic illness or disability, 2) to recognizing the impact of such disorders on the family unit, 3) to promote collaboration with health care professionals, and 4) to promote *agency* in the patient and the family. The term *agency* (Coyne 1986b) describes active involvement in and commitment to one's own care.

Medical family therapy infuses biological and medical concepts into the field of family therapy, as well as provides a systematic way of including the psychosocial and interpersonal dimensions in the care of medically ill patients.

History

The description of the biopsychosocial model of illness and treatment by George Engel (1980a, 1980b) was the foundational step in the definition of the biopsychosocial perspective on medical illness, in contradistinction to the older, dominant biomedical model. The biopsychosocial model acknowledged the hierarchical, interdependent relationship of biological, psychological, individual, family, and community systems. The broader hierarchical model starts at the bottom with a description of atomic and subatomic particles and ends in the biospheres. The involvement of organ systems, nervous system, the person, two-person relationships, the family system, and the community are important parts of the biopsychosocial paradigm.

The contemporary field of medical family therapy was initiated through the work of many investigators, particularly Minuchin et al. (1978) and Reiss (1981). The roots of this approach are also deeply grounded in the work of many pioneering family therapists who were very aware of the emergence of psychosomatic symptoms in the course of family psychopathology and family therapy, as well as the interpersonal dimension of medical illnesses.

The training of primary care specialists (family physicians) to counter specialization and fragmentation of patient care started to be emphasized in the late 1960s and early 1970s, as reflected in the recognition of family medicine as the twentieth medical specialty in 1968, and provided opportunities for further integration of the biopsychosocial mode. The goal of family medicine was to provide continuing health maintenance and medical care to the entire family.

Medical family therapy drew very heavily from the developments of the 1970s and 1980s. A series of conferences in the early 1980s paved the way for the development of this field. Donald Bloch and colleagues (Bloch 1983) started the publication of the journal *Family Systems Medicine*, which emphasized the collaboration between family physicians, family therapists, and other health care providers. The book *Textbook of Family Therapy and Family Medicine* by Doherty and Baird (1983) was very influential in bringing about this intradisciplinary collaboration. Doherty and Baird emphasized how primary care physicians inevitably become part of a triangle with the family. They recommended the necessary skills for primary care physicians, which included provision of support to the family, systemic assessment, recognition of the appropriate time for referral, planned family intervention, and family therapy in the cases of protracted illness. Chronic illnesses and disabilities were particularly in need of comprehensive family intervention.

Other seminal work was done by Minuchin et al. (1978) on the psychosomatic family model, which described the characteristics of "psychosomatic families." David Reiss and colleagues (1986) contributed pertinent theory, particularly from their work with renal failure. They emphasized *coordination*, or the family's ability to experience themselves as a single unit, especially in times of stress. John Rolland (1987a, 1987b, 1994) described a psychosocial model of illness type: a psychosocial typology of chronic illness with the framework of the family life cycle. His proposed typology used four categories: onset, course, outcome, and degree of incapacitation.

Medical Family Therapy: The Model

Medical family therapy emphasizes the collaborative relationship between family physicians, family therapists, and other health care providers. It requires accessibility on the part of the family therapist and defines the etiquette of collaboration and consultation. In the consultation model, the consultee initiates the consultation and retains the ultimate responsibility for the care (Wynne 1994; Wynne et al. 1986).

The consultation model describes the level of closeness between the physician and the patient (distant, midrange, intense), the initiation of referral (by physician or patient), and the duties the therapist expects to perform (intake, support during the assessment period, frequent feedback and consultation on treatment planning).

The family therapist is expected to recognize and start with the focus on the patient; use the psychoeducational approach to explain the ongoing medical and psychotherapeutic encounters; ask the physician to explain the patient's illness, its prognosis, and its possible course; accept ambiguity and disagreements about diagnosis and treatment course; and accept the possibility of unexplained biological changes. The necessary skills for the family therapist are to solicit the illness history, listen empathetically, respect the patient's defenses, remove blame, accept denial when appropriate, externalize the illness, and normalize negative feelings. Furthermore, the maintenance of communication between family and medical providers, as well as among family members, is an essential therapeutic skill. The therapeutic work is enhanced by the recognition of the developmental issues of the family as well as the impact of the illness on the developmental course of family members.

Related to the concepts of medical family therapy is the concept of family psychiatry (Sholevar 1989b), which describes the relationship of family theory to the understanding of major mental illnesses (Hahlweg et al. 1987), as well as the use of psychotropic medications in treating psychiatric illnesses. An increasing number of psychotropic medications have proved effective intervention agents in a wide range of psychiatric illnesses, such as depression, anxiety, and major mental illnesses. Frequently, the family enters treatment with full understanding of the biological nature of many disorders, such as panic, depression, or mental illnesses and insists on the utilization of the medications. The new "family psychiatry" paradigm recognizes the importance of the use of such agents to enhance individual functioning, reduce the impact of disabling symptoms on the individual and the family, and enhance the family's feelings of optimism and agency. Contrary to early family therapy views, the use of medication can enhance the motivation and optimism of the family rather than increase their resistance to psychological or interpersonal interventions.

When a marital relationship is stable and positive, couples are better able to withstand struggle with serious illness and in some cases report an enhancement in their relationship; conversely, if the relationship is already troubled, it may be destroyed by the addition of illness (Coyne et al. 1994). A study of family relationships 10 years post–coronary incident revealed that less than 20% reported less satisfaction with their marriage, and 25% reported *increased* marital satisfaction, after onset of chronic illness; commitment and relationship were different at the time of evaluation (Sholevar and Perkel 1990).

Locus of Control

Rotter (1966) developed scales for measuring *internal* and *external* loci of control. Patients with an internal locus of control think that the ability to overcome a serious illness is dependent on themselves and their behavior. In the *chance* locus of control, the outcome seems subject to extraneous factors such as luck, fate, or God. People who empower *health care professionals* as an *external* locus of control are less likely to seek second opinions and medical procedures.

The Unique Role of Family Physicians

The unique role and position of the primary care physician in relation to the family has not been adequately researched. In comparison to other professionals offering services to a family, primary care physicians are in a unique position to be maximally helpful at critical times because of their knowledge of and ready access to families. The family physician should capitalize on his long-standing relationship and knowledge of the patient and family and use an educational approach to help prevent emotional, psychosomatic, and physical disorders in patients. Whether the family physician likes it or not, families indeed consider the physician part of the overall family unit and utilize him or her in an adaptive or defensive fashion for their goals.

The family physician's unique relationship with the family has been frequently confused with the role of a family therapist or family psychiatrist. The attempt to use the family physician as a therapist fails to capitalize on the physician's ability to act in a preventive role. Family physicians should make use of their unique role with the family in the following ways:

- Emphasize the natural role of family physicians as a first-line family advisor, and stress the use of their already well-developed evaluative skills and authority.
- Emphasize family physicians' long-standing relationship with the family and their knowledge of family members to establish a diagnosis and motivate change.
- Use their generalized knowledge of the life-cycle events of families—such as pregnancy, departure of an adolescent, or death—to prepare families to deal with such sources of internal stress, thus preventing symptomatic behavior and illness.
- Note information given by different family members about each other.
- Synthesize the psychosocial and physical aspects of the illness.

The major role of a family physician is a *preventive* one. Prevention can take a variety of forms. Physicians can recognize stressful situations that can impair functioning or the developmental progression in family members. Physicians can also perceive the need for new family initiatives in times of change in the family, and recommend special actions to enhance adaptive family interactions at times of need.

A family physician can judiciously use information gained from different family members seen separately to form a diagnosis or propose an intervention strategy. Such information can be used to encourage family communication, multilateral interpersonal observations, and negotiation. For example, the complaints of a wife about the excessive drinking of her husband can sensitize the physician to the symptoms of alcoholism in the husband. Although the family meeting is an important vehicle for assessment and intervention, it should not be the only available tool to the family physician.

Sholevar (1996) reported on a case that summarized 28 years of collaborative treatment of three generations of a family by a primary care physician (PCP) and a family psychiatrist (FP). The mental health assessments by the PCP occurred at times of crisis, medical illness, or routine medical checkups. Referrals to the FP were made when the problems required skills broader than the range practiced by the PCP.

> At the time of the initial referral to the FP, the father and mother were in their 30s; their daughter, Jacqueline, was 16 years old; and their son, David, was 13 years of age.

Intervention 1 (by FP): Referral of the family to the FP by the PCP for Jacqueline's academic problems. Her academic performance improved after a few family sessions.

Intervention 2 (by FP): Marital therapy following Jacqueline's improvement; the parents were undermining each other and had financial expectations in excess of their means. The marriage improved after a few months of marital therapy, but the couple ignored the warnings of the FP about an upcoming serious legal (financial) problem.

Intervention 3 (by FP): Evaluation of David for passivity and social isolation followed by family and individual therapy for several months.

Intervention 4 (by both PCP and FP): The legal problem of the family reached its height, resulting in a severe heart attack in the father. The treatment outcome was very favorable, the marriage improved significantly, and the mother obtained a job and excelled at it.

Intervention 5: Referral of Jacqueline and her husband to a sex therapist for sexual problems.

Intervention 6 (by PCP): The parents' concerns about David's lack of interest in dating revealed he was gay. The parents accepted David's orientation and became closer to him.

Intervention 7 (by PCP): For Jacqueline's marital problems. The husband quickly decided to pursue a divorce, which resulted in a "good divorce" that protected the relationship of the children with both parents.

Intervention 8 (by PCP): David was fearful of AIDS, had been almost asexual, and needed counseling and reassurance.

Intervention 9 (by PCP): Brief interventions during the wife's illness and subsequent death from cancer allowed the husband to grieve effectively.

Intervention 10 (by PCP): Counseling was offered 2½ years following the wife's death to reduce friction between the father and the two children. It allowed the father to move toward a second marriage.

Intervention 11 (by FP): To evaluate and help Jacqueline's son's adjustment and self-esteem on entering college.

This case illustrates the unique relationship of family physicians with patients over many years, helping the families through multiple life-cycle crises, and the advantage of close teamwork between the family, primary care physician, and family therapist. Even in today's managed care environment, families can be treated for many years in the same center, and their records are available to the succession of family physicians who staff such practices.

Family Evaluation

Family evaluation in family practice is best achieved through family meetings including members of the household as well as other significant family members. There are specific indications for holding a family meeting in family practice.

Assessment

Assessment should provide for the inclusion of the family as a unit of observation; they are a crucial dimension for diagnosis and treatment. The assessment should examine role rigidity, clarity of communication, adequacy of problem-solving capacity, clarity of boundaries and power structure, and the existence of recent or chronic family conflicts. (Refer to Chapter 12, "Initial and Diagnostic Family Interviews," and Chapter 13, "Family Assessment," for more detail on assessment.)

The initial family meeting in the primary care physician's office or hospital setting should begin with a gentle conversational style, assessing family strengths, coping styles, and patterns of behavior. The physician should respond sensitively to the family's requests for information about the course of physical illness. The evaluation should include a discussion of family communication, problem solving, and interactional patterns that might heighten or diminish adjustment to the illness, as well as possible systemic interventions aimed at changing dysfunctional family interpersonal patterns. During the first consultation interview, the physician should define the family *as a valuable resource*, and family consultation as a resource for the family. Doherty and Baird (1983) suggest a variety of practical measures to enhance family participation, such as using the hospital setting for family meetings and issuing the invitation for the meetings in a firm but routine manner. To enter a family system, the physician must acknowledge the role of the family's primary health authority and agent and must also identify the chief *overutilizers* and *underutilizers* of medical services in the family. The husbands tend to be the underutilizers of medical care, while one or more of the children may be the overutilizers.

Family assessment instruments can be employed in research-oriented clinical protocols. They include the Family Adaptability Cohesion Evaluation (FACES III) (Olson et al. 1978), The Family Assessment Device (FAD; Epstein et al. 1983), the Family Environment Scale (FES; Moos and Moos 1981), and the Beavers/Timberlawn Family Evaluation Scale (see Chapter 13 for a detailed description).

Indications

Epidemiological research data support the proposition that involvement of the family makes medical treatment more cost-effective. Serious or chronic illness can overload a family's coping mechanisms and produce dysfunctional transactional patterns. Psychosocial factors, especially poor family functioning, are associated with a group of 14 major conditions, in which the factors either contribute to the cause of the disease or initiate a major stressful reaction in the family. These major conditions include pregnancy, failure to thrive, recurrent childhood poisoning, preschool and school behavior problems, adolescent maladjustment, major depression, chronic illness, diabetes, arteriosclerotic heart disease or coronary bypass surgery, poor adherence to medical regimen (noncompliance), "inappropriate" use of health services, terminal illness, and bereavement.

The involvement of the total family in the medical care of patients should not be considered a routine matter. Doherty and Baird (1983) advocate family meetings for the purpose of arriving at a comprehensive assessment of complex disorders, discussion of treatment planning, overcoming the resistance of the medically ill patients and the family, mobilizing the rehabilitative forces within the family, or preparing the family for a family therapy referral. Involvement of the family is essential in treatment planning and treatment of chronic illnesses such as hypertension, serious acute illnesses such as myocardial infarction, psychosocial problems, lifestyle problems such as obesity, and life-cycle crises such as death of a family member. The involvement of the family is also desirable in cases of treatment failure, frequent recurrence of symptoms, and routine preventive, educational care such as prenatal visits. The following are a few useful procedures and tools in family evaluation.

Family APGAR

The family APGAR is a practical family assessment instrument, particularly applicable to family practice, that provides reliable, valid, and clinically useful data. It is a brief (15-item), reliable paper-and-pencil test that is designed to elicit the patient's perceptions of his or her family relationships. APGAR stands for adaptation, partnership, growth, affection, and results. These qualities form the core elements of family functioning. The APGAR can be a helpful tool of prevention when there are indications of abuse, neglect, mental illness, and so forth (Smilkstein 1978).

Family Circle

The family circle method consists of asking the symptomatic family members to draw a circle and place their family members and important related people; the people may be touching or far apart, large or small, near or within the circle. The positions of individuals within the circle, and their size and nearness to or distance from each other, as well as clustering, yield much information about the family dynamics. Family structures are easily elucidated, providing an excellent view of the patient's personal, subjective situation.

Genogram

The family genogram is a well-accepted method for recording family genetic relations and the age, health status, marital status, and relationship status for an entire family across multiple generations. It consists of a drawing that includes squares and circles for males and females, respectively; horizontal lines to indicate marriage; and vertical lines to delineate parentage. A formal system for representing divorce, nonmarital parentage, death, abortion, adoption, and twins exists. Relationship modifiers that add emotional states to the diagram include zigzag lines for conflict, triple lines for overinvolved relationships, arrows to indicate dominance, a circle to enclose the members of one household, and an arrow for the identified patient. Major health issues in the lives of individuals are noted alongside their symbols in abbreviated form (e.g., ALC for alcoholism, CA for cancer). The identified patient's important life events are noted at the bottom of the genogram under "Dynamic Changes" (such as obtaining a full-time job) and "Critical Events" (such as suicide attempts, hospitalizations, divorces). Most of the important information (over 80%) in a complete genogram can be obtained with a high level of accuracy in about 15 minutes. Social and interactional data about multiple generations within a family can be easily recorded and read despite the assessor's never having met the involved persons.

Family Database

The family database should be an essential part of the family-oriented medical record, much as is the traditional history and physical examination for an individual. It includes demographic, psychosocial, and family medical information. In addition to the present history, the family database has special sections for 1) risk factors for family problems, 2) family interviews, 3) conclusions, and 4) plans for family intervention or referral. Risk factors for family problems include stresses, level of family functioning, resources, and family dynamics (Shapiro 1981).

Referral Process

In developing guidelines for referral, the primary care physician should function as an active agent whose relationship with patient and family can influence significantly the outcome of referrals. Physicians should consider the interrelatedness of "the referral triangle," consisting of the referring physician, the patient and family, and the psychiatrist or therapist. Any dysfunction in the referral triangle can result in an eventual failure. The same boundary dysfunctions found in families can apply to the relationship of the primary care physician with the family.

The following guidelines can be used in helping to determine what to refer for and when to refer and can help physicians to differentiate their "comfort zone" in treating certain disorders from their "referral zone." Physicians are cautioned to consider the nature of the problem, their specific knowledge and ability to treat the problem, and their level of outside commitments and resources. Disorders considered appropriate for treatment by family physicians are family life-cycle stresses such as a birth, death of a family member, and acute problems such as depression or behavior problems in a child. Problems that should be referred to a therapist are chronic depression and/or anxiety that has been unresponsive to treatment, severe chemical dependence, chronic family dysfunctions, and serious and acute family symptoms such as child abuse, spouse abuse, and incest.

Chronic Medical Illness

An increasing number of families are coping with chronic illness due to medical advances that have transformed some terminal illnesses into treatable conditions.

The reduction in the mortality rate has increased the number of patients with chronic illness and disability. The National Health Interview Survey (National Center for Health Statistics 1990) reported that 14% of all Americans are limited in their activities by a chronic medical condition. Chronic illness limits the activities of 33.1 million Americans to some degree (National Center for Health Statistics 1993). *Chronic illness* refers to a chronic, progressive, and degenerative disease. The percentage of persons whose activities are limited by their chronic disease increases by 25% between the ages of 35 and 60 and is 45% for people older than 65. Rolland (1987a, 1987b, 1994) described a model for chronic illness by psychosocial type, differentiating illnesses on the basis of incapacitating or non-incapacitating quality and fatal or nonfatal dimensions. An example of a fatal, non-incapacitating illness would be lung cancer with central nervous system metastasis; a non-incapacitating but fatal illness would be acute leukemia; a nonfatal but incapacitating illness would be congenital malformation; and a noncapacitating, nonfatal illness would be a benign arrhythmia. Rolland (1987a, 1987b, 1994) emphasized the developmental phases of illness in terms of a crisis phase, a chronic phase, and a terminal phase. Furthermore, he utilized the transgenerational life-cycle model of the individual and the family in order to understand the developmental course of an illness and its impact on the developmental course of the family and its members.

Wynne et al. (1992) make a distinction between three factors in chronic illness:

1. The *illness experience*, which refers to the distress and suffering of the patient
2. The *illness behavior*, which refers to the impaired functioning due to illness that can be observed by others
3. The *meaning of illness*, which refers to the social and psychological definitions given to the illness and the resultant "scripts" taken on by the family members

The psychological impact of illness on the family includes the isolation of the "sick" family member and the assumption of controlling attitudes by other family members. One impact of illness on the family life cycle is the added *centripetal pull* exerted by progressive disease, which halts normal family disengagement processes such as a child's going to college and freezes a family into a permanent state of fusion (Rolland 1987a, 1987b, 1994).

Strategies for managing chronic illness include respecting defenses, removing blame, accepting unacceptable feelings, maintaining communication, reinforcing family identity, eliciting from the family its history and meaning, provision of psychoeducation and support, increasing the family's sense of agency, and maintaining an empathic presence within the family.

Neurological Disorders

Sholevar and Perkel (1990) reviewed and added to the literature on family therapy with neurological disorders, including work on the treatment of multiple sclerosis and senile dementia. Intervention with Huntington's disease requires special consideration. Kessler and Bloch (1989) examined family factors in Huntington's disease, with particular attention to the then recently developed capacity for presymptomatic genetic testing for this illness. They described three family mechanisms that may come into play with Huntington's disease: patient preselection, denial of disease onset, and induction of suicide.

Patient preselection refers to the singling out in advance of asymptomatic family members who are expected to eventually become "affected" with the disease. The preselected member shares the family consensus in the selection process. This mechanism helps to organize the family's expectation by assigning the respective roles of the "healthy one" and the "sick one" and to contain the overall apprehension about becoming ill. *Denial of disease onset* attempts to protect the family and the patient from the traumatic effects of the illness and may have a short-term adaptive function but a high long-term cost. The period of denial allows the family to prepare for the diagnosis. *Induction of suicide* may partially explain the high rates of suicide and suicide attempts in patients with Huntington's disease—a rate five times higher than that in the general population. In suicide induction both the patient and other family members share the belief that the patient is a burden and that death would bring relief to him or her and to the rest of the family. These beliefs can inhibit the family's attempts to protect the patient.

Chronic Medical Illness in Children

Chronic illness in children is a common feature of childhood. An estimated 10%–15% of all children have a chronic medical disorder, and about 1% of children have a severe disorder. These percentages translate into about 7.5 million children with a chronic illness and about 1 million with a severe chronic illness (Hobbs et al. 1978). Asthma in its moderate to severe form constitutes 10 cases per 1,000 and is the most common disorder in the severe chronic illness category. The special issues for families with a chronically ill child include the management of parental guilt, parental grief over the child's loss of a "normal" childhood and a bright future, fear of "contagion," and developmental issues. Enmeshment, overprotection, family interactional rigidity, poor conflict resolution or conflict avoidance, and triangulation of the children in family conflicts are areas that require special attention and investigation. The initial model described by Minuchin et al. (1978) has been extended by Wood (1995) to give closer attention to "developmental biopsychosocial" issues, particularly in families that are more normative than pathological.

Therapeutic issues with childhood chronic illness include examination of the meaning of the child's health problems in relation to different family members, examination of possible inclusion of child's illness as part of a dysfunctional family triangle, attention to other relationships in the family, the impact of the child's illness on the functioning of siblings, the examination of developmental versus illness-related issues, the parents' relationship with professionals, and promotion of support within the family social network.

Acute Medical Problems

A diagnosis of a life-threatening illness plots a new life trajectory for the patient and the family; for the patient, it is potentially a dying trajectory (Pattison 1977; Wright and Leahey 1987). The trajectory relates to issues of certain or uncertain death at a known or unknown time. The effect of an individual's life-threatening illness on the family differs in intensity depending on the nature of the illness itself, the timing of the illness in the family life cycle, the openness of the family system, and the position of the patient in the family (Hertz 1980). The patient may respond more strongly to his or her family's response to the illness, such as inability to effect a needed change in family roles, than to the condition itself (Wright and Leahey 1987).

Sholevar and Perkel (1990) described the following reactions to the diagnosis of a serious illness. The first phase is one of shock and bewilderment; the second phase is one of disorganized thinking and feelings of loss, grief, and despair; and the third phase is one of denial of circumstances but the acknowledgment of the existence of the health problems. If avoidance and denial are maintained over too long a period of time, they result in the immobilization of the patient. Other family members generally will be forced to take over the decision-making role.

Treatment Adherence and Compliance

Primary adherence refers to adherence to activities that prevent the initial onset of the illness. Secondary and tertiary adherences are generally called compliance and refer to following a prescribed regimen by the physician. Compliance with the regimen results in a feeling of self-confidence and an increased sense of well-being. The simplification of the regimen by health care professionals can enhance compliance. A high level of compliance reduces the likelihood that the patient or family will define the patient as "a diseased" person, and generally results in an increase in new social activities and a new and healthier social life.

Implications for the Family

The fear of illness, abandonment, and death are general feelings that are mobilized by a serious illness. Another important factor in chronic illness is the exhaustion of the caregiver.

The serious illness initially manifests itself in the family as an intruder. Eventually, the illness becomes a functioning member of the family system with its own separate identity, which requires readjustment of schedules, roles, finances, and so forth.

Emotional reactions to chronic illness include blaming other family members, blaming oneself, and eventually blaming caregivers and the health system. Hostility, low self-esteem, and other negative patterns can follow, which results in creation of distance between family members and the shutting down of intrafamilial communications, negotiations, and accommodations. Such a dysfunctional pattern can result in delay of a necessary treatment, depletion of energy, reduction in optimism, and depression. If the chronically ill person experiences depression, it may lead to increased risk for depression in other family members (Coyne 1987).

Understanding how *narrative focus* functions can reveal the crucial role language plays in how people "see" and experience illness and themselves. People revise accounts of life experiences in the face of unexpected or adverse events so as to maintain a sense of coherence, continuity, and meaning (Gergen 1991). Life stories or narratives must recognize events in such a way that they demonstrate a sense of coherence as well as a sense of direction or movement over time (Bruner 1990). The revision of narrative accounts enables each person to act as his or her own historian and interpret past, present, and future experiences in a congruent fashion.

Conventional risk factors in diseases such as coronary heart disease include factors associated with and heightened by certain characteristics in the person and the spouse. This phenomenon has been named "cross-spouse" risk factor (Swan et al. 1986).

Medical family therapists can help families to assume a broader perspective and reduce the tendency to become focused entirely on health problems. Therapists can help the family to remain aware of constraints, seek information, validate and normalize emotional responses, draw forth family support, encourage respite, and reinforce the continuance of family rituals. The pathological disengagements and severe enmeshments can be countered. In severe cases of enmeshment, it is difficult to distinguish between the sick family member and others who are well. Inverted hierarchies are common in chronic illnesses and other family members can take over the decision-making role of the patient for "his/her own good."

Medical personnel and the medical family therapist can become a permanent and important component in the family. They can be triangulated easily, even at times in a dysfunctional way, in order to reduce anxiety and regain stability. The therapist can help the family to make effective rules to govern the family system and prevent the family from becoming centrally or peripherally (depending on the severity of the symptoms) organized around the illness.

The major function of the medical family therapist is to establish beliefs that sustain hope and empower and to help keep at bay the forces that foster blame, shame, or guilt.

Lifestyle Disorders

Lifestyle disorders include smoking and obesity. Management of lifestyle disorders can be facilitated by employment of the FIRO model, which emphasizes *inclusion, control, and intimacy* (Doherty and Colangelo 1984). The inclusion dimension denotes factors such as bonding, organization, structure, connectedness, and shared meaning. The control dimension addresses the importance of power sharing during conflict, as well as the effects of domination, reactivity, and collaboration. The intimacy dimension refers to self-disclosure, personal exchange, and mutuality of feelings and thoughts.

The following factors can strongly enhance therapeutic outcomes when treating smoking: inclusion of multiple family members in treatment, emphasis on the smoker's sense of agency, use of a behavioral contracting strategy, negotiation of ritual alternatives to smoking, reframing of failures and relapses as learning opportunities, avoidance by family members of the urge to be "too persuasive" with the patient, and support for the smoker's decision to try a smoking cessation program.

In treating obesity, it is important to dissociate therapeutic success from the number of pounds lost. The initial focus should be on the patient's decision-making processes about losing weight, and distinguishing the level of weight that contributes to the medical problem from weight that is culturally unacceptable. The physician can also help by promoting family support without overinvolvement and attendance at community weight-loss programs.

In summary, medically compromised patients are a significant challenge to all health care providers. Such patients are frequently overwhelmed by a fear of dying or a fear of living and generally feel uneasy with uncertainty of any kind. These feelings tend to mirror corresponding feelings in the total family unit. The treatment team can enhance therapeutic effectiveness by encouraging the family to remain actively involved with the patient and his or her struggles while facing the issues described above on the familial and individual levels. Close collaboration of health care providers, the family therapist, and the family is necessary to achieve this goal.

Somatoform Disorders

Somatoform disorders are a group of disorders characterized by physical symptoms that cannot be adequately explained by medical findings and are not attributable to conscious malingering. These disorders are associated with emotional factors. The physiological changes involved are those that normally accompany certain emotional states, but in these disorders the changes are more intense and sustained. The individual may not be consciously aware of his or her emotional state (DSM IV-TR; American Psychiatric Association 2000a). Meissner (1977) notes that the patient's emotional involvement in the family system constitutes a major aspect of that ecology which we can no longer afford to ignore. Comprehensive guidelines for treatment of somatoform disorders can be found in Perlmutter's (1996) book *A Family Approach to Psychiatric Disorders.*

The term *somatoform disorder* should be differentiated from the term *psychosomatic medicine*, which refers to a complete approach to the patient and the problem of his or her illness. Psychosomatic medicine includes consideration of the social and psychological factors that may play a role in the predisposition, inception, and maintenance of many diseases. The proponents of the psychosomatic approach are concerned with the adaptation of human beings to stressful personal and interpersonal conditions and the psychological reasons for the failure of this adaptation. They are also more concerned with predisposition to the disease and its inception than with pathophysiology (Weiner 1977).

Interest in the pathology of human illness has more recently expanded into a concern for the ecology of human conditions. Understanding the different aspects of the patient's ecology is deemed necessary for the comprehension of human illness. The family unit constitutes a major part of this ecology.

Family Characteristics of Somatoform Disorders

Important contributions to the understanding of somatoform disorders in families have been made by family theorists with psychodynamic, intergenerational, or structural approaches.

Psychodynamic

The psychodynamic family therapist describes psychosomatic disorders as occurring in *centrifugal* family types. The centrifugal family type is characterized by isolation and early individuation of family members, poor communication of emotions, and early departure of family members from the family unit. The emphasis in such families is on individuation, mobility, and the individual's thrust for success. Youngsters in centrifugal families separate early from their parents in terms of physical closeness, emotional expression, and personal goals. There is only minimal sharing of affect and motivation, which forces the individual to turn to his or her own resources for handling emotions and conflicts. This encourages somatization rather than sharing of painful experiences with other family members. Later in life, these families generally enter a somatically regressive path when they encounter object loss or frustration. Within centrifugal families, two different types have been described: the first places special emphasis on independence; the second emphasizes social success, achievement, and adaptability.

Multigenerational

The multigenerational concepts of Murray Bowen's family systems theory (Bowen 1978) considered "psychosomatic dysfunction" as one of the mechanisms by which people with a low level of differentiation "control the emotion of too much closeness." Bowen is referring to a failure to resolve childhood dependency on parents after adolescence and the resulting functional helplessness, which may find expression in somatic illness. Bowen proposed the notion of physiological reciprocity of overfunctioning and underfunctioning persons in a family system. In families with a seriously ill member, another member must remain healthy while strenuously laboring to maintain the "ill" one in his or her role as the sick member. Bowen also described the function of the mother as "family diagnostician," deciding who is sick and what is to be done and denying the possibility of being mistaken (for further detail, see Chapter 5, "Multigenerational Family Systems Theory of Bowen and Its Application").

Structural

The structural "psychosomatic" model was developed by Minuchin et al. (1978) through the investigation of families with young children who had unstable diabetes, intractable asthma, or anorexia nervosa. The attempts of Minuchin and his colleagues to induce family crisis, rather than shielding patients from stress, were quite successful in controlling these conditions. The "psychosomatic family" was described by Minuchin as an open system (multiple feedback loops) in which illness is seen as serving a function in maintaining dysfunctional patterns within the family. Different illnesses (asthma, anorexia nervosa, and labile diabetes mellitus) can arise in similar family systems, implying that treatment goals for these families will be similar. Regardless of the specific symptom, most families require a similar kind of restructuring. Five characteristics of these families are noted: 1) they are very enmeshed, 2) they tend to be overprotective, 3) they are very rigid and resist change, 4) overt conflict within the family is avoided, and 5) the identified patient is involved in parental conflict (Liebman et al. 1974). These characteristics have been described fully in Chapter 2, "Structural Family Therapy."

Integrative

Sholevar (1980) has proposed an *integrative* view of the three models of family characteristics of somatoform disorders described above. The description of deficiencies and relational patterns in psychosomatic families by individual psychotherapists and psychodynamic and structural family therapists may appear contradictory. However, there are no significant inconsistencies in the observations and conceptualizations of the three systems just described. In fact, recognition of the complementary nature of the systems can assist in arriving at a comprehensive model allowing for scientific research on and effective interventions for these disorders.

One foundational deficiency in somatoform disorder families is the emotional unavailability of the marital partners to each other, usually due to developmental failure on a multigenerational level or overwhelming acute stress in the contemporary scene. As a result of their particular rearing and position in their families of origin, the marital partners have not developed the ability to recognize their needs or satisfy those needs through another person. This deficiency leaves the couple in a state of frustration, tension, isolation, and helplessness, with little vision or hope for satisfaction and fulfillment. They are still aware that they can achieve satisfaction and fulfillment through each other. As a result, the couple drifts away from attending to each other's needs by failing to communicate and by not seeking out and correcting areas of interpersonal conflict. They ultimately attempt other means to reduce marital tension, such as inappropriate overinvolvement (fusion) between a parent and one child or mechanisms such as work compulsion.

The structural and psychodynamic models of family treatment *do not* contradict each other; nor do they preclude individual psychotherapy for family members with somatoform disorder. The best results are accomplished by combining methods according to the needs of specific families and the stage of treatment. Judicious utilization of structural models is helpful and frequently necessary in the initial stage of treatment, particularly with more acute problems. The recognition and delineation of contemporary family patterns often uncovers the dynamic underpinnings of family relationships, and this can be helpful in dealing with the rigid defenses of the more severely and chronically disturbed families. At times the reorganization of the family allows one of the family members to enter family-oriented individual psychotherapy with the hope of further differentiation and individuation.

Psychodynamic approaches, although of great assistance, are slow to help in the acute stage of somatoform disorder, in which quick action and results are needed to protect the lives of some family members as well as to keep the family in treatment. The combination of the psychodynamic family model with structural therapy, and with other treatment modalities such as individual psychotherapy or behavior modification, may prove to be the essential elements of success in treating psychosomatic disorders.

Outcome Research

The major research on outcomes for families whose members have a somatoform disorder is based on the structural model of psychosomatic problems such as anorexia, asthma, and diabetes. Structural therapy claimed the striking therapeutic result of substantial recovery from both the anorexia and its psychosocial components in 86% of cases at follow-up, with the follow-up periods ranging from 1.5 to 7 years (Minuchin et al. 1978; Rosman et al. 1976). Despite the lack of control groups for the psychosomatic research, Gurman and Kniskern (1978) noted that because of the often life-threatening nature of the psychosomatic disorders studied, the objective measures for change (e.g., weight gain, blood sugar levels, respiratory functioning) offered strong evidence of major clinical changes in conditions that have been universally acknowledged as having an extremely poor prognosis when untreated or treated by standard medical procedures.

Managed Care and Family Therapy

The economics of health care has included the rapid expansion in health maintenance organizations (HMOs), preferred provider organizations (PPOs), and other health care organizations. These groups have assumed the contractual responsibility to provide health care for prearranged cost with the expectation that they would reduce unexpected or significant escalation in health care. The negotiations of benefits through such organizations, as well as through traditional indemnity insurance companies, are complex but significant issues. Family therapists may be in a unique position to use the benefits provided by HMOs, PPOs, and employee assistance programs (EAPs) to provide evaluative and therapeutic services to different members of the families. Jodi Aaronson (1996) provides a comprehensive road map through the maze of the health care scene and health care benefits, which would be of interest to all family therapists.

Pressure from managed care organizations has resulted in expanded use of solution-focused therapy. This model allows the therapist to provide the full course of treatment to the family in fewer sessions than in more traditional family therapy approaches. Applications for credentialing used by various managed care companies directly inquire about the practitioner's training and proficiency in this solution-focused therapy.

Solution-focused family therapy encourages and guides the family to move away from "problem talks" to "solution talks" that focus on the patient's resources, strengths, and solutions that are already present but not used by the patient. This allows patients to "construct" a different and more pragmatic view of their problems and situation and "language" their problems differently—"language being the reality" (see Chapter 3, "Constructing Therapy: From Strategic, to Systemic, to Narrative," in this volume). Solution-focused therapy has designed a number of clear-cut techniques to work collaboratively and productively with the client in a future- and solution-oriented way.

Conclusion

The turn of the century has brought about closer collaboration between family therapy and the medical profession. On the theoretical side, evidence for the contributions of biological, interpersonal, and psychological factors to human adaptation and dysfunction is convincing. Evidence for the effectiveness of biological and interpersonal therapies has become increasingly strong. The need for application of biological, psychological, and family therapies in an integrated fashion characterizes the multimodal and multidisciplinary nature of contemporary interventions. The use of combined approaches requires expanded consultation and referral skills for all professionals involved in the care of patients and families. To provide patients with "agency"—that is, the means to actively participate in their own treatment—requires refined communication, education, and psychoeducational skills for physicians. Only then can physicians share accurate information with patients and their families. The new field of medical family therapy has emerged in response to this challenge to provide collaborative biopsychosocial treatment. The challenge stems from the longstanding interest of pioneering family therapists in "psychosomatic" and somatoform disorders.

The contemporary emphasis by managed care organizations to contain cost and possibly enhance the quality of health care has indirectly helped the flourishing of medical family therapy. The partnership between health care professionals and families has the potential to decrease the cost of care and to enhance its quality, a proposition that appeared unrealistic not so long ago.

Chapters on Related Topics

The following chapters describe concepts related to medical family therapy:

- Chapter 2, "Structural Family Therapy"
- Chapter 5, "Multigenerational Family Systems Theory of Bowen and Its Application"

Medical Family Therapy

- Chapter 12, "Initial and Diagnostic Family Interviews"
- Chapter 14, "The Family Life Cycle: A Framework for Understanding Family Development"
- Chapter 16, "Diagnosis of Family Relational Disorders"

VII

Research in Family and Couples Therapy

36

The State of Family Therapy Research

A Positive Prognosis

John F. Clarkin, Ph.D.
Daniel Carpenter, Ph.D.
Eric Fertuck, Ph.D.

Introduction

Advances in the field of family therapy can be measured by the quality and extent of the research investigations. In this chapter, we review family therapy research literature with several goals in mind. First, this chapter updates the previous reviews. Second, while not providing a meta-analysis of family therapy research, we indicate the advances in design sophistication of family outcome research and suggest further improvements. Third, we are interested not only in family therapy outcome studies but also in the research on family systems concepts that can be of assistance in family therapy research. Finally, this review indicates the family disorders and problem areas that call for the application of family intervention in current clinical practice.

The question "Is family therapy effective?" is a poor one because of its imprecision. The questions instead should be "Is the family treatment format, with its specific strategies, techniques, and targeted mediating goals of treatment, effective with particular family problem areas and individual diagnoses?" and "Is family treatment effective compared with no treatment, treatment as usual, or a competing treatment?"

We will never have the resources to empirically compare family therapy with all other competing treatments for every known family condition and individual diagnosis or problem area. Such an all-inclusive approach is neither feasible nor intellectually satisfying. Rather, family therapy researchers must examine those family and individual problem areas that seem by their functional properties most likely to require family therapy as the only part or one part of a treatment package. In the ideal situation, one would have an empirically derived model of the disorder with known family variables before embarking on the development of a family treatment for that condition. Two examples come to mind.

The first example is the research on the family management of schizophrenia, which arose from a conceptualization of the family's role not in the etiology but in the course of the disorder. Studies suggesting that family hostility and overinvolvement with the patient were deleterious to the course of the patient's illness led to family treatments to modify those factors. In the second example, the early work of Patterson (1982) and the more recent investigation by Kazdin et al. (1992; Kazdin 1997) have based a family treatment for children with conduct disorder on an understanding of the role of the family in shaping and reinforcing acting-out behavior.

In preparation for this review, we utilized a computer search of research efforts from 1974 to the present. Searching for "family therapy" articles alone did not adequately cover the literature. Many newer intervention strategies, such as parent training, were not listed under family therapy. One example was the Singer et al. (1989) study, which was described as "Community-Based Support" and did not include family therapy in its descriptors but nonetheless was a true cognitive-behavioral intervention with children and their families. This spoke to widening the net in conducting a review.

Standards for Treatment Development

When creating standards for treatment development, one can conceptualize a number of steps in the process:

1. The treatment is described in written (i.e., manual) form.
2. There are instruments to assess the faithful and skillful execution of the treatment.
3. The treatment is shown to produce clinically significant change in treated subjects.

4. The treatment is shown to be efficacious when compared with treatment as usual in randomized assignment studies.
5. The treatment is efficacious when compared with other competing treatments in a randomized assignment clinical trial.
6. The treatment is effective as delivered in the local community.

In reviewing family therapy outcome studies here, we noted the various areas in which the studies are methodologically sound and sophisticated, and we attempted to arrive at some notion of the current state of family therapy research and its design sophistication.

Manualization of treatment in the individual format was more extensive than that in the family therapy format. Probably the most developed family treatments and their manualization were for schizophrenia (C. M. Anderson et al. 1980, 1986; Falloon et al. 1984) and parent training (Kazdin et al. 1992). Nonetheless, recent authors have clearly made more of an effort to standardize the treatments they were evaluating. For example, Szykula et al. (1987) compared a strategic family therapy with behavioral family therapy for children with various diagnoses. The authors made an effort to check that therapists were adhering to manual form.

Random assignment of patients was necessary in order to equalize the two groups for the influence of known and unknown variables on outcome. While the number of nonrandomized studies of family therapy was large relative to the number of randomized studies, we were able to locate and review a number of family therapy studies that used randomization. Furthermore, the number of randomized studies has been increasing.

Since treatment outcome is multifaceted and sometimes value-laden, it was important to assess outcome from multiple points of view. Individual psychotherapy studies have typically obtained outcome from the patient, therapist, objective observers, family members, and significant others. It seemed all the more important to obtain outcome results from various vantage points when the family is the focus of intervention. This would include not only measures of the identified patient's symptoms and adjustment but also measures of the family interaction patterns that were hypothesized to relate to the individual pathology. Measurement of the mediating goals of treatment must be done in both individual and family therapy outcome research. Examples in individual treatment would be cognitive variables and social relations in the treatment of outpatients with depression. In family treatment, the mediating variables would be changes in family interaction behavior, decrease in family burden, increase in family coping and problem solving, and decrease in family expressed emotion (EE).

Assessments of both clinical significance and statistical significance have received attention recently but are rarely noted in the family therapy studies. A few exceptions are worth noting. Glick et al. (1993) derived criteria based on the Global Assessment Score (GAS) to define clinically significant outcome in seriously disturbed inpatients following family intervention. Kazdin et al. (1992) defined clinical significance as the proportion of children within the range of nonclinic levels of functioning following intervention for conduct disorders.

Assessment of therapist effects in psychotherapy outcome studies has been strongly recommended. Martindale (1978) and Crits-Christoph and Mintz (1991) stressed the importance of determining the extent to which differences between therapists may account for some of the variance in the outcome variables. Specifically, Crits-Christoph and Mintz (1991) recommended that researchers manualize the techniques being evaluated to standardize delivery of the treatment and include the therapist as a random within-subjects variable when different therapists deliver the same treatments. When a preliminary analysis of therapist effects on the outcome variables is undertaken, a P value of 0.2 or greater should be employed.

The Chambless and Hollon (1998) criterion for assessing the *empirical support* of a psychosocial intervention is that an intervention must be demonstrated to be superior to a wait-list control condition in at least two studies conducted by two independent research teams to be labeled as "efficacious." If the intervention is demonstrated to be superior to a placebo, a nonspecific treatment, or rival interventions in two studies conducted by independent research teams, it is labeled as "efficacious and specific." These two labels (efficacious, and efficacious and specific) are qualified by the term "possibly" when all other criteria are met for a designation but when only one study (or two or more by a single research team) has been conducted. Finally, the intervention must be "manualized" to allow researchers to assess whether the clinicians are adhering to the techniques and strategies of the intervention. Thus, manualization is one of the first steps in the stages of treatment development.

Review of Well-Designed Studies

A review of well-designed studies showed that the most informative treatment studies were those using random assignment of patients (and families) to both competing treatments or conditions at the beginning of the study.

Parent-Child Difficulties

Parent-child difficulties (including difficulties between parents and adolescents) make up one problem area that has special appeal for the application of family intervention. These difficulties can take the form of child and adolescent behavioral problems, child abuse and neglect, and difficulties, deficits, or excesses in parenting.

Child and Adolescent Behavior Problems

In one study of the effect of family therapy on child and adolescent behavior problems, filial therapy (i.e., teaching mothers in a "Rogerian" manner to be more empathic and emotionally connected) was compared with a no-treatment control group for mothers and their "emotionally maladjusted" children ages 5 to 10 (Stover and Guerney 1967). Outcome measures were based on audiotaped play sessions with mother and child. Treated mothers show increased reflective behavior, and treated children were less nonverbally aggressive. This was an early study with a behavioral outcome measure. The difficulties of the children were, unfortunately, vaguely defined.

Reiter and Kilmann (1975) randomly assigned 24 families with children ages 8 to 12 with various school adjustment problems to either counseling for mothers or a no-treatment control group. Results indicated improved family relationships, increased positive communications, decreased negative communication, and decreased negative behaviors in the treatment group. Treatment was vaguely defined, and there were no follow-up data.

Families with "problem children" ($N=36$) ages 4 to 12 were randomized (stratified on father involvement, sex, and age of child) to individual family therapy, group family therapy, or a control condition (bibliotherapy) (Christensen et al. 1980). Measures were parent attitude, parent-collected data on defined problem behaviors, and observational data from audio recordings made in the homes of the families. On several measures, all groups improved. The group and individual treatments were about the same, and both were better than the control condition on specific behavioral measures. The authors concluded that group family therapy was more efficient, requiring about half the clinician time.

Hardcastle (1977) randomly assigned 25 families to a mother-child multiple-family group condition or to no treatment. The population was not precisely defined—simply families of children identified by principals and teachers as having behavior and/or attitudinal problems. Fathers were excluded from the treatment, but mothers were encouraged to pass the information and experiences from the group along to their husbands. Results indicated both an improvement in mother and father's family satisfaction and integration and an increase in positive responses. The author noted that fathers dramatically improved their scores on satisfaction and integration without even having been in the groups. This study suffered from poor outcome measures.

In a treatment study of families referred for child behavior problems (Pevsner 1982), subjects were randomly assigned to either parent training plus group behavior therapy or to individual behavioral family therapy. Children in the study evidenced at least three behavior problems (as listed in a modified version of Patterson et al.'s 1975 Behavior Check List) that were not school related. The group condition was more efficient and was more informed by behavioral principles, but otherwise there were no differences. The study groups were small (seven families in the group condition and eight families in the individual family condition), thus reducing power.

Families with children ages 10 to 16 years with nonspecific behavior problems (e.g., parent-child conflict) were randomly assigned to reciprocity training with individual families, group-based family reciprocity training, or a no-treatment control group (Raue and Spence 1985). Treatment involved only four sessions. Treatment subjects showed greater reduction in parent-reported problem behaviors than did controls. The authors concluded that there were no differences between group and individual family reciprocity training. The limitations of this study are clear: the number of subjects was small, the treatment was not described in detail, and the controls were not assessed at follow-up.

Martin (1977) combined enhancement of communication within families with contingency management (behavioral) techniques. Families were randomly assigned to father-not-included family treatment, father-included family treatment, or a no-treatment control group. A fairly low criterion for child-parent behavior problems was used (at least one child-parent problem behavior over each 20-hour period they were together). Outcome measures were based on telephone interviews with parents (usually the mothers), who were asked to report problem behaviors over the past 12 hours and to be specific in their descriptions. They were called every day for a 7-day period. Results indicated a significant reduction in treatment cases relative to the control group for child-prolonged problems, mother-brief problems, and mother-prolonged problems. No differences were found between the two experimental conditions. The authors suggested that some of the variance lay in styles of punishment that each parent employed (i.e., including a father who is extremely punitive might have a different effect than including a father who is a more lax disciplinarian). Unfortunately, the treatment was poorly defined and brief, and outcome measures were weak.

Sayger et al. (1988) compared a 10-week social learning family therapy (including sections on discipline, reinforcement, school consultation and involvement, and encouragement) to a waiting-list control condition for boys in grades two through six who were identified as most aggressive in the classroom by teachers. There was a 9- to 12-month follow-up assessment on the treatment group only. Aggressive behavior decreased significantly more in the treatment group, and gains were maintained at follow-up. These gains included decreased aggressive behavior in the classroom and the home and better family interactions.

A strategic family therapy was compared with behavioral family therapy for children with various diagnoses (Szykula et al. 1987). The only differences found were higher satisfaction scores (rated by families) in favor of behavioral treatment. The authors speculated that the therapists delivered a more seasoned behavioral treatment and that clients had greater expectation of success in the behavioral treatment group. The authors made an effort to check that therapists were adhering to the treatment manuals.

Besalel and Azrin (1981) evaluated the effectiveness of reciprocity training in addressing child behavior problems. They randomly assigned 29 children (25 families) to either a no-treatment control group or a four-session treatment group that promoted mutuality in the parent-child relationship (usually the mother). The treatment was structured and didactic with in-session practicing. The results indicated a reduction in both the number and the severity of problems as rated by parent and child. The authors noted that the only conclusion to come out of the study was that reciprocity training between parents and children is promising.

Child Abuse and Neglect

Research on family therapy and its effect on child abuse and neglect included a comparison of two brief treatments for parents who abuse or neglect their children. The first was a parent training treatment that involved improving parent-child interactions and decreasing aversive child behaviors. The second, called multisystemic therapy (MST), involved addressing the problems as system-determined, with treatment strategies individually developed to address the needs of a given family (Brunk et al. 1987). No control condition was used. Results indicated that people in both treatments showed decreased psychiatric symptoms, reduced stress, and improvement of family problems. MST families manifested improvement in parent-child interaction patterns. Maltreating parents showed greater control over their children. Parents in the parent training condition showed more improvement in social problems, most likely because the treatment was in a group context.

Difficulties in Parenting

The effects of family therapy on various difficulties in parenting were studied by Kazdin et al. (1992), who randomly assigned children (ages 7 to 13) with a variety of conduct disorders and problems to problem-solving skills training (PSST), parent management training (PMT), or a combination of the two. PSST uses cognitive-behavioral strategies to assist the child in negotiating interpersonal situations. The parents were brought in on the sessions to assist the therapist and foster problem-solving steps in the home. In PMT the parent was seen individually in order to improve childrearing practices and to use contingencies to support prosocial behavior by the child. The treatments were manualized, and results were assessed at post-treatment and 1-year follow-up. Both treatments resulted in improved child functioning and increased prosocial competence. However, it was the combination treatment that resulted in more marked changes in child and parent functioning and that placed a larger proportion of children within the range of nonclinic levels of functioning.

Specific Child Problems

The effects of family therapy on specific child problems were examined in several studies. Graziano and Mooney (1980) recruited 33 families of children ages 6 to 12 who had a severe fear of the dark. Families were randomly assigned either to the treatment group or to a no-treatment control group. The treatment consisted of three training meetings that focused on child self-monitored self-control exercises at home while parents supervised, monitored, and rewarded their efforts. Nightly exercises consisted of muscle relaxation, imagining a pleasant scene, and reciting "brave" self-statements. Results indicated a significant reduction in fearful behaviors at night in the treatment group. The effects were magnified at 2-, 6-, and 12-month follow-ups. There was no effect on school and social functioning as rated by parents. The investigators established clinical significance criteria (passing 10 consecutive "fearless" or "perfect" nights). The outcome measures relied exclusively on the parents.

Satin et al. (1989) evaluated a multifamily group intervention either alone (MF) or combined with parent simulation of diabetes (MF+S) as compared with a control group to increase functioning of diabetic adolescents. Adolescents in the MF+S group showed more of a decrease in glycosylated hemoglobin than the control group did; there was some evidence that this decrease also happened in the MF group. Adolescents in the treatment groups also improved in their perceptions of themselves as diabetics. Fathers, by contrast, reported increased negative perceptions of diabetes and of "parents with diabetes" as a result of the treatment. The authors hypothesize that fathers became aware of how little they were doing for their children. No significant changes in reported family environment were found.

Black and Urbanowicz (1987) randomly assigned 45 bereaved families to either brief family therapy focusing on bereavement techniques or a control group. Their rationale was to see whether treatment could affect the impact that a death in the family had on a child. The study reported generally no differences, particularly after a 2-year follow-up. Both the outcome measures and the treatment were vaguely defined.

Singer et al. (1989) randomly assigned parents of school-aged children with severe disabilities to either intensive support groups (standard care offered by local agencies, assistance from community volunteers, and 16 two-hour classes on coping skills, including homework practice) or less intensive support groups (standard care offered by local agencies). Group one was followed 1-year posttreatment. Results indicated that mothers in group one showed a reduction in depression and anxiety that was maintained at follow-up. Results were similar for fathers, although, because of a very small sample size, the results were not statistically significant despite large effect sizes. Efforts were made to be sure the treatment manual was followed, but the authors acknowledge some individualization of treatment plans that precluded strict standardization. Stress management and child behavior management were identified by parents as the most helpful coping skills for them.

Summary

There were a number of studies of child behavior problems (Hardcastle 1977; Pevsner 1982) in which the definition of the child problematic behaviors was either too vague or too broad to allow optimal use of the results. The most impressive results were the reduction of aggressive behavior in the Sayger et al. (1988) study, the statistical and clinically meaningful results that held up at 1-year follow-up in the Kazdin et al. (1992) study, and the reduction of parental anxiety and depression in the Singer et al. (1989) study. These studies suggest that family therapy has promise in reducing specific problematic child behaviors through the use of behavioral techniques, and that the parents have a better personal adjustment after learning parenting skills. The combination of these effects augurs well for the use of family therapy.

Nonspecific Parent-Adolescent Conflicts

Nonspecific parent-adolescent conflicts and the effects of family therapy in these areas were examined in a study of hospitalized adolescents and young adults ages 13 to 22. Patients were randomly assigned to individual therapy or family therapy of 10 sessions in duration (Ro-Trock et al. 1977). Patients who received family treatment showed decreased recidivism and improved school functioning. On follow-up, none of the 14 patients in the family therapy group had been rehospitalized. In comparison, 6 of 14 patients in the individual therapy group had been rehospitalized. This study was conducted before the publication of DSM-III, with an unequal number of patients with schizophrenic reaction, adolescent adjustment reaction, and drug problems.

Foster et al. (1983) randomly assigned 28 families to either a no-treatment control group, a skills-training (ST) group (i.e., seven sessions of problem-solving and communication skills), or a generalization group (i.e., same as skills training with added homework and discussion of homework experiences in sessions). Families were recruited through the newspaper and included in the study if the primary issue was parent-adolescent (ages 10 to 14) conflict. Families were randomly assigned to treatment based on the severity of conflict as measured by information supplied on a questionnaire. The two treatment groups showed a reduction in parent-child conflict. There was also considerable improvement in the no-treatment control group on some measures. Data at follow-up indicates some gains were maintained.

Guldner (1990) randomly assigned families with adolescents to either family treatment with a structural approach or family treatment with a structural approach plus additional action-oriented techniques (e.g., psychodrama). There was some suggestion that action-oriented therapy resulted in better agreement between adolescents and parents about goals that were achieved. The author was a family treatment supervisor who found himself assigned to supervise four therapists of different orientations, so he set up a random assignment of families applying to the clinic. This is a good example of how research can be born of clinical utility.

Szapocznik et al. (1989b) randomly assigned 79 families using a Solomon Four Group Design and employed an intervention/prevention model with Hispanic youths (mostly Cuban) in families deemed at risk for problems. High risk factors included current maladaptive interactions within the family, intergenerational conflict, and intercultural conflict. The treatment lasted 13 weeks. A "minimal contact control" condition with relatively brief contacts on the phone with the family was used. Family Effectiveness Training (FET) as described by the first author did not appear to be related to Parent Effectiveness Training (PET). FET focuses on family interactions and structural concepts. Although the treatment approach was not manualized, there was a description by session of what it entailed. These descriptions included teaching interaction skills that were appropriate to the child's developmental stage. Results indicated that FET was related to increased child self-esteem, decreased parentally reported child behavior problems, and better family functioning with better interaction patterns. There was not so much effect on family climate as rated by parents. The study design (the Solomon Four Group Design) made it possible to measure the effects of the assessment itself by providing a control group for each condition (treatment and control) that did not undergo the pretreatment assessment procedure. Unfortunately, the design involved too many cells (i.e., reduced power), not enough pretreatment data, and complicated data collection. There was no evidence that assessment made any difference. Every subject was eventually given treatment within the design, maximizing the data.

Adolescent Behavior Problems and Delinquency

The effects of family therapy on adolescent behavior problems and delinquency were examined in a study by Parsons and Alexander (1973), who compared a cognitive-behavioral family treatment with bibliotherapy (subjects were given a behavior therapy primer) for predelinquent boys and girls about 15 years of age. Outcome measures were behavior samples from an audiotaped task given to families, as well as some self-report measures that showed no improvement. The treatment led to normalization of family interaction patterns.

Stuart et al. (1976) randomly assigned 60 predelinquent youths to either behavioral family therapy (contracting to modify parent-child and teacher-child interactions) or group therapy. Results indicated improvement on teacher evaluation, counselor evaluation, mother's evaluation of marital adjustment, and mother-adolescent relationship.

Garrigan and Bambrick (1977) compared brief (10 sessions) family therapy using Zuk's go-between method with a no-therapy control group as a treatment for adolescent behavior problems. Children were labeled by the school as emotionally disturbed (children with psychosis, low IQ, poor hearing, or language disorder were excluded). Results indicated a reduction of the child's symptoms in the class and the home, a reduction of anxiety in boys, and an enhanced mutuality and empathic understanding in the marriage of the parents. One of the strengths of the study was an effort to address systemic issues. The authors included a Venn diagram of the family and analyzed the data in terms of each cell in the diagram, which represented where family members interacted. For example, marital issues were addressed in the cell where the mother and father circles overlapped. In a follow-up of this study, Garrigan and Bambrick (1979) provided some separate analysis for single-parent mother-only (SPM) families. Experimental subjects showed greater school attendance or employment, less involvement in the court system, and a significant reduction in trait anxiety. There was a trend toward significant reduction in aggressive behavior, bizarre cognition and thought disorder, and state anxiety. There were no differences on hyperactivity and other scales. The SPM-disturbed boys were not as responsive to therapy as the disturbed boys from intact families. Untreated sons and their mothers in SPM families tended to rate each other as less symptomatic and better adjusted than untreated sons and mothers in intact families. The former may be expected—that boys in intact families showed more improvement in symptoms with treatment (highly significant for unethical behavior, timidity, and anxious self-blame; significant for emotional control and schizoid withdrawal; and trend for bizarre cognition, bizarre action, and paranoid thinking). The latter suggests some kind of shared denial of problems—they see each other as having fewer problems than the other kids. Boys were ages 10 to 17 ($n=14$).

Gant et al. (1981) randomly assigned 20 families who had been referred to them by the court because of their adolescents' behavior to either family treatment (a behaviorally focused, social learning approach) or the usual court-implemented program. Results indicated improved communication (both observed and perceived) for treatment families.

Klein et al. (1977) randomly assigned 86 families of delinquents who had been identified by the courts for "soft" delinquency offenses to one of four groups: 1) a no-treatment control group, 2) a client-centered family group, 3) an eclectic-dynamic approach group, or 4) the primary treatment program, which was described as a behavioral family intervention that focused on improving family interaction patterns. In addition to utilizing a no-treatment control group, the authors used as a contrast the recidivism rate (base rate) for the county where the study took place. This is an interesting alternative to offering no follow-up data on controls and helped put the study in perspective. Results indicated a reduced recidivism rate and reduced rate of sibling court involvement for the fourth group (behavioral treatment) as compared with the other three groups. The eclectic-dynamic condition was by far the worst for recidivism, which occurred at a rate of 73% as compared with 50% in the no-treatment control group, 47% in the client-centered family group, 51% as the base rate, and 26% in the behavioral treatment group. The same was true for rate of sibling court involvement.

Emshoff and Glakely (1983) addressed the problem of adolescent delinquency with a program designed to decrease contact with the courts and police, decrease delinquent behavior, and increase school participation. Adolescents were randomly assigned to either the research project or court processing "as usual." The project defined two types of intervention: contracting and advocacy. The project involved two groups (also randomly assigned). In the first group, intervention applied to "a variety of social domains," including school, family, and work (multifocus). In the second group, intervention focused exclusively on the family (family condition). Nonprofessional volunteers delivered the treatment. Staff for the multifocus group participated in a wider range of interventions (employment, school) than did the staff for the family condition group. Parents were more involved in the treatment of children in the family condition group, and children in the family condition group were involved in more contracting behavior than those in the multifocus group.

Results indicated a reduction in rates of incarceration in the experimental groups and a slowed deterioration in school functioning in the multifocus group. The authors noted a significantly greater decrease in the number of police contacts between the experimental and control groups. However, examination of the data provided indicated that the groups differed on that measure at pretreatment and that at posttreatment the levels of the experimental groups were brought down to that of the controls at pretreatment. It must also be noted that the multifocus condition was able to slow a landslide of school dropouts. That is, in all groups, fewer subjects were enrolled in school at posttreatment than at pretreatment. But in the multifocus group, the increase was significantly less.

Barkley et al. (1992c) randomly assigned 61 adolescents with ADHD (12–18 years of age) to behavior management training (8–10 sessions), structural family therapy, or problem-solving and communication training (PSCT). All three treatments resulted in reduced parent-child conflicts, anger, and intensity of conflicts. Clinically significant change was shown in 5%–30% of the subjects across the three groups, and clinical recovery was seen in 5%–20% of the children. The authors noted,

> These findings are consistent with follow-up studies of hyperactive and aggressive children, which find their disorders quite resistant to most short-term psychologically based single-treatment approaches. Calls for multimodal, long-term, joint-pharmacological-psychological interventions . . . seem well founded given the present results.

PCST families were less cooperative. The major flaw of this investigation was the lack of a control group. As noted by the authors, the only treatment for adolescents with ADHD that has been well-researched has been medication; a natural control group, then, would have been a group receiving medication.

In a well-designed study, Henggeler et al. (1992) compared MST with "treatment as usual" (incarceration and/or probation) for juvenile offenders with records of serious crime. Eighty-four offenders were randomly assigned; pairs of subjects were "yoked" in the two groups. MST had a duration of 3 months and employed intervention strategies similar to family and behavior therapy (i.e., individualized treatment plans sometimes involving home visits in addition to therapy meetings). Results indicated a reduction in incarceration and a decrease in criminal behavior for boys in the treatment condition. MST was manualized (Henggeler et al. 1991), and there was a strong effort to adhere to the manual. The authors discussed clinical significance as different from statistical significance. Authors included follow-up data taken from the subjects' criminal record at an average of 59 weeks posttreatment.

Summary

There are several impressive studies in the area of adolescent behavior problems. Henggeler et al. (1992) showed a reduction in juvenile offenses with the use of multisystemic therapy. The authors provided a strong rationale for family therapy with this problem area, and their family intervention was manualized. Klein et al. (1977) likewise found family therapy effective in reducing adolescent delinquent behavior, but only when behavioral strategies were utilized. These two studies suggest that family therapy that addresses the specific problematic behaviors holds promise for clinically significant change.

Substance Abuse

The effects of family therapy on patients who are involved in substance abuse was addressed in an early work by Stanton (1979, 1982) that is often considered classic in the family field. Stanton randomly assigned males addicted to heroin for at least 2 years to one of four treatment conditions: paid family therapy, unpaid family therapy, paid family movie placebo, and treatment as usual (i.e., unpaid individual counseling and methadone). In general, paid family therapy outperformed unpaid family therapy, and both were better than individual therapy.

Friedman (1989) compared two treatment programs for adolescent drug abusers. The first was functional family therapy (FFT), which is a combination of systems theory and transactional behaviorism and focuses on relabeling of attributions, family communication, self-disclosure, and trust. The second was a parent group that ran 24 weeks and integrated Parent Effectiveness Training, communication, and assertiveness training. Note that the IP was not involved in this. The identified patient was involved to some extent in individual counseling equally in both groups. Results indicated no differences between the two groups despite multiple measures of patient and parent symptoms and functioning. The author concluded that a parents group is just as effective as the family therapy used in the study to treat adolescent drug abusers. Since parents groups are cheaper to run than family treatment, this finding is of practical import. A major strength of the study was that the FFT was manualized (Alexander and Barton 1983) and efforts were made to ensure adherence to the manual.

Kang et al. (1991) examined the efficacy of family therapy as compared within both individual and group therapy for patients with cocaine use disorders. Significant improvements were observed for the cohort of 122 patients who were treated and interviewed 6 and 12 months later. Virtually all of the improvement, however, was shown by the patients (19%) who were abstaining from cocaine at follow-up. The authors concluded that outpatient therapy, of whatever format, is not effective for cocaine use disorder, and that alternative treatments, such as intense outpatient or residential treatment, were needed for this group.

The Community Reinforcement Approach (CRA; Azrin et al. 1976) is a behavioral intervention that involves spouses, family members, and other individuals from drinkers' social networks in the treatment. Azrin et al. have completed four controlled studies evaluating the efficacy of CRA for treatment of male problem drinkers. One study aimed at achieving the engagement of the patient with alcohol abuse in treatment (Sisson and Azrin 1986); two investigated the acute stage of this disorder, focusing on drinking behaviors (Azrin et al. 1982; Hunt and Azrin 1973); and one study included both acute and relapse prevention interventions (Azrin 1976). In all of these studies, CRA evidenced superior outcomes to treatment as usual in terms of treatment engagement, drinking, and subsequent hospitalizations, as well as employment, social, and marital adjustment. CRA met the criteria for a "possibly efficacious and specific treatment" by Chambless and Hollon (1998) as argued in the Baucom et al. (1998) review. The qualifier "possibly" is added because the results have not been replicated by an independent investigator.

Lewis et al. (1990) compared a brief family therapy with a family drug education program and found reduced substance use in the family therapy group only. Structural-strategic family therapy was compared both with adolescent group therapy and with family drug education (Joanning et al. 1992). There were more abstainers in the family therapy condition than in the other two conditions.

In comparing multisystems family therapy with individual therapy, Henggeler et al. (1991) found significantly fewer substance-related arrests in the family approach as compared with the individual approach. Liddle and Dakof (1995a) compared the efficacy of multidimensional family therapy to adolescent group therapy. Family therapy and group therapy both showed reductions in substance use, but greater reductions in substance abuse were found for family therapy as compared with the other two approaches.

Summary

More research is needed with patients and their families in dealing with alcohol and substance abuse, a major problem area in our society. The existing family studies show some promise for the use of family therapy, but it may be most effective with subgroups, possibly those with younger abusers still at home and those whose family assets are substantial. The poor response to any treatment of the cocaine abuse in the Kang et al. (1991) study is particularly disappointing but may suggest that some patients are beyond help with typical verbal therapies regardless of the format (i.e., individual, family, group) of treatment.

Eating Disorders

Eating disorders and how they were affected by family therapy were examined in two randomized studies of family treatment for anorexia/bulimia nervosa. Crisp et al. (1991) randomly assigned 90 patients with DSM-III-R anorexia nervosa to no treatment, behavioral treatment, behavioral treatment coupled with individual therapy, and behavioral treatment coupled with family therapy. All three active treatments were effective as compared with no treatment in regard to weight gain, return of menstruation, and social and sexual adjustment.

Russell et al. (1987) randomly assigned patients (57 with anorexia and 23 with bulimia) to either family therapy or individual supportive treatment following an inpatient treatment intended to bring the patient to normal weight. The results were relevant to differential treatment planning, as those patients whose eating disorder was not chronic and had begun before the age of 19 were more effectively treated with family therapy.

Summary

The paucity of family studies in this area is surprising given the early theoretical and clinical work of Minuchin, one of the leaders of the family movement. It remains for future family therapy research to ascertain in which cases of eating disorders family therapy will be most useful. The findings of Russell et al. (1987) suggest that nonchronic conditions in which the patient is young and still in the parental home might prove amenable to family intervention.

Schizophrenia

In an early, ambitious and impressive series of studies on family therapy and its effects on schizophrenia, Langsley et al. (1968, 1969, 1971) randomly assigned 300 patients seen as needing hospitalization to either outpatient family crisis therapy or standard inpatient care. The authors reported that family crisis therapy succeeded in keeping the patients out of the hospital and, furthermore, made it subsequently less likely as compared with the hospitalized group that the patient would be subsequently hospitalized. Family crisis therapy and hospitalization were equally effective in returning patients to their prior social adjustment. Furthermore, family crisis therapy led to better management of stressful events. The diagnostic information on the patients was less than current standards, and it was difficult to conceptualize the supportive and systemic family treatment. However, this was a large undertaking and a very early attempt to assess serious treatment decisions in a disturbed population. The results suggested the clinical power of working with the family unit under such circumstances.

Family therapy of brief duration for schizophrenic patients and their families has been found to have some beneficial effects. For example, Goldstein et al. (1978) randomly assigned 104 young acutely schizophrenic patients, following brief inpatient care, to one of four aftercare treatments involving two dose levels of fluphenazine enanthate and the presence or absence of crisis-oriented family therapy (during the 6-week treatment period and 6-month follow-up). The relapse rate was the lowest (0%) in the group of patients who received high-dose medication combined with family intervention and highest (48%) in the low-dose no-family-therapy group.

Liberman et al. (1981) randomly assigned 28 males with schizophrenia to social skills training or holistic health therapy (HHT). There were no resulting differences in symptoms, but the HHT patients required more rehospitalizations and had more relapses.

In a randomized study of family intervention during hospitalization, investigators at Cornell Medical Center (Glick et al. 1990, 1993; Haas et al. 1988) found that brief family intervention with schizophrenic patients and their families had some modest effects. A total of 92 schizophrenic patients and their families were randomly assigned to either inpatient treatment with family intervention or inpatient treatment without family intervention. All but two patients were assessed at 18-month follow-up. The authors concluded that those schizophrenic patients with poor prehospital functioning may benefit from inpatient family intervention, but this effect appeared to be limited to female patients and did not appear until 18 months after admission to the hospital. In addition to the benefit to the patient, the families showed benefit from the treatment. This beneficial effect was seen earlier with the family than with the patients and was associated with achieving the goals of family intervention. Although the positive effects in the family treatment group could not be accounted for by improved posthospital medication compliance, they may have been related to the group's greater tendency to obtain further family treatment following discharge. This suggested that if one wishes to introduce family intervention, this could be done effectively during an episode in which the patient is hospitalized.

There are a growing number of studies of family intervention of at least 9 months' duration. For example, Leff et al. (1982, 1985) compared routine care to a package of social interventions with the families. For patients who continued to take medication, the social intervention significantly reduced the relapse rate over 9 months and 2 years. However, when two patients in the experimental group who committed suicide were included, the difference in outcome was not significant at 2 years. In a second study (Leff at al. 1989), schizophrenic patients taking medication who were living in contact with high-EE relatives were randomly assigned to medication only or to medication and social interventions (either family therapy plus education or relatives group plus education). The relapse rate in the family treatment group over 9 months was 8%, compared with a 17% relapse rate in the compliant relatives group. The authors concluded that the reduction in the relapse rate was mediated not by compliance with medication but by reduction in relatives' EE and/or face-to-face contact. Leff's approach is most distinctive in its explicit attempt to lower EE or reduce contact between patient and family members.

The treatment approach articulated by C.M. Anderson et al. (1980, 1986) is broad-based and extensive, including survival-skills workshops for the families, reentry of the patient into the family, enhancing work and social adjustment of the patient, and maintenance of therapeutic gains. Results of their randomized studies (Hogarty et al. 1986, 1991) showed the superiority (in terms of relapse rates and social adjustment of patients) of family therapy or family therapy plus social skills training in comparison to skills training alone or the control condition.

Falloon et al. (1982, 1985) utilized an extensive behavioral approach with the schizophrenic patient and family. Treatment was provided involving the following: assessment of strengths, weaknesses, and goals; education about schizophrenia and its treatment; communication skills training; and problem-solving skills training. The researchers randomly assigned 39 adults with schizophrenia to either individual or family management. Family management included behavioral family therapy conducted in the home. The family management approach showed clear and consistent advantages over a 2-year period.

Tarrier et al. (1988a, 1988b, 1989) also used an approach that was behavioral in orientation, with treatment focused on education, stress management, and training in goal setting and attainment. Families were randomly assigned to family therapy, brief family education, or treatment as usual. Those in family therapy were subsequently differentiated so that half received didactic training only while the other half received didactic training plus actual skills training with rehearsal. Outcome at 1 and 2 years favored the family therapy in terms of reduced relapse rates and improved patient functioning. The two forms of family therapy were equally effective.

Posner et al. (1992) randomly assigned 55 patients with schizophrenia to a psychoeducational support group or to a control group. Subjects in the experimental condition increased their knowledge of schizophrenia and had a more positive view of health care services. However, there was no evidence of improvement in outcome, coping behavior, or psychological well-being. Unfortunately, only 70% of those originally assigned completed the treatment. The authors cautioned that it might not be possible to reproduce positive results of extensive psychoeducational programs in a briefer, psychoeducational support-group format.

Randolph et al. (1994) compared a yearlong behavioral family therapy to usual care for patients and their families in the Veterans Administration system. Whereas only 14% of patients in the family treatment condition experienced a psychotic exacerbation during the year, 53% of patients in usual care had such an exacerbation.

Schooler et al. (1993) compared a group family intervention with an individual family treatment intervention in interaction with three medication treatment conditions. The strength of this National Institute of Mental Health study was the large number of patients ($N=313$) across five hospital sites. Findings supported targeted and early intervention with medication, and there was no differential information from the two family interventions.

Summary

Both the number and the quality of family therapy studies with schizophrenic individuals and their families are impressive. The family treatments have been manualized, and the existing outcome literature suggests that family therapy is a useful and effective part of the overall treatment of these seriously disturbed individuals. Questions remain as to the most important focus of family intervention—for example, lowering EE and increasing family coping. Which families, at what point in the illness of the patient, are most likely to respond positively to family intervention? The family studies to date used predominantly psychoeducational and cognitive-behavioral strategies and techniques.

In the history of family therapy, most impressive is the shift in attitude toward the family of the schizophrenic patient and the rationale for using family therapy. Blaming either the mother (e.g., "schizophrenogenic mother") or the family (e.g., double binds) for the condition of the patient is no longer theoretically nor clinically the rule of the day. The current family treatments assume that the family is coping the best they can with the schizophrenic member, and the treatment is geared to improve those coping strategies.

Long-term family treatment of schizophrenia also meets the criteria for an "empirically supported intervention" (Chambless and Hollon 1998) as reviewed by Baucom et al. (1998). In aggregate, the results of the family therapy of schizophrenia studies indicate that behavioral family interventions are "efficacious and specific" for improving long-term outcomes of schizophrenia. In addition, supportive family treatments are "efficacious and specific" for improving long-term outcomes of schizophrenia. Given that only one study has explored the family systems approach, it is designated as "possibly efficacious and specific." Family interventions are associated with a range of promising outcomes, including reductions in positive and negative symptoms, improved social functioning, and improvements in relatives' distress and knowledge of medication. Taken together, these findings suggest that family intervention techniques can be implemented successfully by trained community clinicians from different disciplines. The many diverse family treatment modalities and manuals that have been developed have prevented any one of them from achieving dominance and becoming the benchmark in the area of schizophrenia treatment research.

Affective Disorders

Most of the studies of family intervention with affective disorder have been done in the marital treatment format (see Chapter 28, "Depression and the Family: Interpersonal Context and Family Functioning"), reflecting the age at onset of affective disorders. However, there are several studies involving families. Anderson et al. (1986) randomly assigned 40 inpatients with a range of affective disorder diagnoses to a traditional process-oriented multifamily group or a more structured psychoeducational multifamily group. The results indicated roughly equivalent treatment effects on the patients' view of themselves and of their families. As the authors noted, the lack of a true control group against which to evaluate the treatments limits conclusions based on these data. In addition, no follow-up information was offered, making it difficult to put the study in a clinical context.

Data from the Cornell Medical Center study of inpatient family intervention with bipolar and unipolar patients (Clarkin et al. 1990) suggested that more extensive inpatient intervention may be fruitful for some subgroups. Twenty-nine unipolar and 21 bipolar patients and their families were randomly assigned to inpatient treatment with or without family intervention. The family intervention was psychoeducational and behavioral in orientation. At both 6- and 18-month follow-up, the bipolar patients with family intervention showed better outcome than those without it. This treatment effect was limited, however, to the female bipolar patients. In contrast, the patients with unipolar depression did better without family intervention.

Summary

The role of family therapy for affective disorders is an area of increasing interest to family therapists and holds real promise. The fact that depressed individuals with and without coexisting personality disorders respond differently to treatment should influence the family (and marital) studies in this area. The application of marital or family treatments to bipolar disorder is an area of current development, with a number of studies in progress.

Family Studies Classified by Strategies and Techniques

The designation "family treatment" indicates a format of treatment in which the family members meet with a therapist to further treatment goals. Within the family treatment format, one can use the whole range of strategies and techniques (e.g., cognitive-behavioral, strategic, systemic, paradoxical, and insight-oriented). We attempted to classify the family treatment studies reviewed here by their strategies and techniques, even though at times this was difficult to do because of lack of specificity in the research report. We arbitrarily defined and classified the techniques into the following three types:

- Cognitive-behavioral (including psychoeducational)
- Dynamic (including psychodynamic, client-centered)
- Structural/strategic/systems (e.g., Zuk's go-between method; combination of systems and behavioral)

Using this system, we found that the vast majority of studies used cognitive-behavioral techniques and that the other techniques were exceptions that can be noted. Exceptions included studies using structural system approaches (Brunk et al. 1987; Crisp et al. 1991; Garrigan and Bambrick 1977; Guldner 1990; Henggeler et al. 1992; Ro-Trock et al. 1977). In three other studies (Barkley et al. 1992c; Stanton et al. 1982; Szykula et al. 1987) structural/systemic was compared with another competing strategy, with little differentiation in outcome due to strategies or techniques.

The randomized family outcome studies examined here have utilized predominantly cognitive-behavioral strategies and techniques. This parallels the preponderance of studies in individual and marital psychotherapy studies. One wonders if the field will see the empirical investigation of family therapy using other than cognitive and behavioral strategies. The difficulties to surmount in such an effort are formidable. First, it is much easier to manualize a highly structured behavioral treatment than a psychodynamic one. Second, most family treatments target specific behaviors in the identified patient (e.g., schizophrenic family member, individual with anorexia/bulimia, acting-out adolescent), and behavioral approaches seem most fitting to address these behaviors.

Meta-Analysis of Family Interventions

The meta-analysis has emerged as a sophisticated way to obtain results on the efficacy of treatments through the statistical aggregation of controlled studies for a particular treatment. This has the effect of improving the power (the likelihood of finding a statistically significant difference when it does exist), and thus validity, of the findings by increasing the number of subjects analyzed. A drawback of the meta-analysis is that there may be bias of the types of studies included, as efficacy studies that do not obtain significant results tend not to get published or included in the meta-analysis. This can lead to a false inflation of the actual efficacy of a particular treatment. Additionally, when there are relatively few studies of a particular modality of treatment for a diagnostic group, different modalities and patients in many diagnostic categories are often grouped together, obscuring possible differential treatment-patient interactions and highlighting more general differences in treatment versus control groups.

Shadish et al. (1993) conducted the most recent, rigorous meta-analysis of family and marital psychotherapy studies. The studies included in their review met the following criteria: subjects were randomly assigned to conditions, subjects were distressed, and the studies examined a marital ($n=62$) or family therapy ($n=101$). The authors developed a manual pertaining to general study characteristics, presenting problem, circumstances of and surrounding treatment, outcome, and effect size, and coded each study accordingly. The main findings were that effect sizes from marital therapies ($n=27$, $d+=0.60$, $SE=0.09$) were nonsignificantly higher than those from family therapies ($n=44$, $d+=0.47$, $SE=0.06$), and these effect sizes are considered moderate to large and are associated with clinically significant improvements for most participants in these treatments compared with control groups. However, family therapies treated a greater range of problems than marital therapies and intervened with more difficult problems such as schizophrenia, juvenile delinquency, and alcohol or substance abuse. In the uncommon instance in which marital and family therapies treated the same problems, they were essentially equivalent. The investigators also calculated effect sizes for theoretical orientation separately for marital and family therapies. All orientations including psychodynamic, behavioral, and systemic (except humanistic) yielded significant effect sizes. The investigators qualified this by stating that if all treatments were equally well designed, implemented, measured, and reported, then differences among orientations may not have been identified.

Conclusion

The methodology in family therapy studies is improving. We were able to find a number of studies with randomized assignment. In terms of the problem area or diagnosis to which family therapy is applied, family therapy has been examined most in randomized designs as applied to schizophrenia, child and adolescent problems, and substance abuse. There is promise of studies in the area of affective disorder. Family outcome studies are needed to further define the usefulness of family therapy in the area of eating disorders, substance abuse, and affective disorders.

With the data in hand, it would appear that family therapy is effective in addressing schizophrenia, parent-child difficulties, and some acting-out disorders involving children and adolescents. There is, however, very little comparison research such as studies in which patients and families are randomly assigned to either family therapy or a competing therapy (e.g., individual or group therapy). When comparison studies are done, it is most usual to compare two forms of family intervention.

Prior reviews of family therapy research have concluded on an optimistic note, suggesting that family therapy is effective. We would add a cautious but optimistic note to the assessment of these prior reviewers. There is growing evidence that family therapy has some positive effects as applied to problem or diagnostic areas such as schizophrenia and child behavioral problems. More impressive than the content of the results, however, is the increasing sophistication of family therapy research designs. Family therapy researchers are beginning to look at clinical significance as opposed to merely statistical significance, so there will be more attention to *how much* family therapy is helpful. Data are needed on the relative effectiveness of family therapy in comparison to other reasonable intervention formats.

Baucom et al. (1998) reviewed the studies evaluating couples and family treatments. In evaluating the efficacy status of couple and family interventions, the investigators used the following categories based on Chambless and Hollon's (1998) criteria:

- If an intervention was demonstrated to be superior to a waiting-list control condition in at least two studies conducted by two independent research teams, it was labeled as *efficacious*.
- If an intervention was demonstrated to be superior to a placebo, nonspecific treatment, or rival interventions in two studies conducted by independent research teams, it was labeled as *efficacious and specific*.

These two labels ("efficacious" and "efficacious and specific") are qualified by the term "possibly" when all other criteria are met for a designation but only one study has been conducted (or two or more by a single research team).

By these criteria, two family interventions were identified as empirically supported, one for substance abuse and one for schizophrenia. The Community Reinforcement Approach (Azrin 1976) is a behavioral intervention that involves spouses, family members, and other individuals from drinkers' social networks in the treatment. Azrin et al. conducted four controlled studies evaluating the efficacy of CRA for treatment of male problem drinkers. One study aimed at achieving the engagement of the alcoholic in treatment (Sisson and Azrin 1986); two investigated the acute phase, targeting drinking behaviors (Azrin et al. 1982; Hunt and Azrin 1973); and one included both acute and relapse prevention interventions (Azrin 1976). In all of these studies, CRA evidenced superior outcomes to treatment as usual in terms of treatment engagement, drinking, and subsequent hospitalizations, as well as employment, social, and marital adjustment. On the basis of the superiority of CRA over treatment as usual, and given that this finding has not yet been replicated by an independent investigator, CRA meets the criteria for a possibly efficacious and specific treatment.

Long-term family treatment of schizophrenia also meets the criteria for an empirically supported intervention. Taken together, the findings of the family therapy of schizophrenia studies indicate that behavioral family interventions should be considered efficacious and specific for improving long-term outcomes of schizophrenia. Similar to the studies involving a behaviorally oriented family intervention, these findings indicate that supportive family interventions are efficacious and specific for improving long-term outcomes of schizophrenia. Given that only one study has explored the family systems approach, however, it is designated as possibly efficacious and specific. Family intervention was associated with a range of positive outcomes, including reductions in positive and negative symptoms, improved social functioning, and improvements in relatives' distress and knowledge of medication. Taken together, these limited findings suggest that family intervention techniques can be implemented successfully by trained community clinicians from different disciplines. It also is possible that the multitude of different family treatment models and manuals available has prevented any one model from achieving prominence and becoming the standard in the field. This may have resulted in less implementation of family intervention than if a single model had been developed and studied more intensively. More work is needed to understand how to implement family intervention programs for the broad range of clinicians working in the field.

Chapters on Related Topics

The following chapters describe concepts related to family therapy research:

- Chapter 7, "Behavioral Family Therapy"
- Chapter 22, "Behavioral Couples Therapy"
- Chapter 27, "Family Variables and Interventions in Schizophrenia"
- Chapter 28, "Depression and the Family: Interpersonal Context and Family Functioning"
- Chapter 29, "Family Intervention and Psychiatric Hospitalization"
- Chapter 37, "Couples Therapy Research: Status and Directions"

37

Couples Therapy Research

Status and Directions

Susan M. Johnson, Ph.D.

Introduction

The goal of this chapter is to summarize, rather than extensively review, what has been learned from couples therapy research and to specify what still needs to be explored. The first broad review of the results of couples therapy (Gurman 1973) was published 30 years ago and identified 15 studies in this area. Since then, studies and reviews have proliferated (Alexander et al. 1994; Baucom and Hoffman 1986; Baucom et al. 1998; Beach and O'Leary 1985; Gurman and Kniskern 1981a; Todd and Stanton 1983). Couples therapy has emerged from the umbrella of family therapy in the last three decades and has grown into a relatively sophisticated treatment modality. It is now used to address not only relationship distress and dysfunction but also individual symptomatology such as depression, agoraphobia, and alcoholism (Baucom et al. 1998; Prince and Jacobson 1995). The growth in clinical techniques and research reflects the demand for this kind of service. Failure to develop a satisfying intimate relationship with one's partner is now the single most frequently presented problem in therapy (Horowitz 1979). Research into family functioning suggests that of the three levels of intervention (individual, couple, and family therapy), the couple level has perhaps the most potential to change not only the couple's relationship but also individual and general family functioning (Lewis et al. 1976; Pinsof and Wynne 1995).

I also discuss in this chapter the question of how far couples therapy has traveled toward becoming a scientific endeavor; that is, an endeavor that addresses the tasks of the accurate description of phenomena and events and the provision of explanations for events. As in other areas of psychological and psychiatric research, progress toward scientific methods has been irregular and inconsistent. The field has not followed the logical path of first describing and empirically examining the phenomena of relationship distress, then creating theories and interventions that lead, in an integrated fashion, to prediction and explanation. Rather, couples therapy started with interventions based on theory taken from individual psychotherapy, and research focused on the efficacy of these interventions. The field is only now turning back toward the accurate description of relationship dysfunction, the tasks of model and theory building, and the explanation of change events in therapy (Johnson 1991; Johnson and Lebow 2000).

The Task of Description: The Nature of Distress/Satisfaction in Relationships

What are the essential differences between a nondistressed and a distressed couple? The work of John Gottman (1991, 1994a, 1994b) is seminal in this area and is supported by the work of others such as Christensen and his colleagues (Heavey et al. 1993, 1995). The findings from Gottman's research underscore the power of negative affect and highly structured interaction patterns, such as criticism and contempt responded to with distancing and stonewalling, to predict the future of a relationship. The typical dance of couple distress involves one partner (usually female) demanding change and being critical of the other spouse, while the other (usually male) partner's facial expression is one of fear; this partner becomes more and more unresponsive. This lack of responsiveness from one partner elicits and maintains the other's frustration and criticism. As this pattern evolves and becomes more encompassing, emotional engagement becomes impossible to sustain (Gottman 1994a, 1994b) and a cycle of polarization and relationship dissolution has begun. Gottman also stresses that, in the most typical cycle, the withdrawing male partner is intensely aroused physiologically and recovers from this arousal at a slower rate than his spouse; withdrawal appears then to be an attempt at affect regulation that, unfortunately, alienates the other partner. The destructiveness of withdrawal becomes apparent here and runs against the conventional wisdom about relationships, which tends to suggest that "keeping the peace" is the best strategy. In fact, the number, content, and resolution or nonresolution of fights do not seem to be that useful in predicting couple distress or happiness and stability.

Besides offering couples therapists a map of the territory of relationship distress, the research discussed above stresses the impact of gender roles and how they operate in marriage. Women are socialized to seek intimacy and affiliation, whereas men tend to be independent and achievement-oriented (Gilligan 1982). Stereotyped gender roles seem to be bad for the health of relationships. It is also interesting to note that when husbands are demanding, their wives tend to react more favorably, perhaps because this signals the male partner's engagement in the relationship.

The power of the patterns described above to predict relationship satisfaction and status is persuasive (Gottman 1994a, 1994b). Gottman's most recent study suggests that the key to stable relationships is not behaviors such as active listening, but factors such as the willingness of the husband to accept influence from his wife and soothe her low-level negative affect (Gottman et al. 1998). A happy and stable relationship, the ultimate goal of couples therapy, seems at last to be tangible, or at least less mysterious. The image of successful couple relationships that emerges depicts partners that can soothe each other when negative emotions arise, rather than becoming absorbed in states of negativity. Partners who calm each other and are open to influence from each other can resist reactive, rigid cycles of blame and create cycles of positive emotional responsiveness in their interaction.

Distressed partners also tend to form distress-maintaining attributions, such as interpreting their partner's behavior in a way that discounts positive events and accentuates negative events. Put another way, distressed partners form attributions consistent with their affect, seeing negative behavior as a reflection of their spouse's character and explaining away positive behavior in terms of situational factors (Holtzworth-Munroe and Jacobson 1985). More specifically, distressed partners are reluctant to grant their spouse credit for positive actions, but tend to view negative actions as intentional and motivated by selfish concerns (Bradbury and Finchan 1990). Distressed partners view their spouses' negative behaviors as global (occurring in all situations) and stable, rather than transient, and their positive behaviors as transient and specific to a few situations. These partners also tend to construct self-enhancing interpretations of relationship events (which may be seen as defensive reactions), whereas happy spouses tend to be self-effacing in their attributional style. The most critical finding is that distressed couples seem to focus selectively on negative events. Holmes and Rempel (1989) suggested that ambivalent or distressed couples are engaged in constant hypothesis testing concerning their partner's caring and responsiveness, and develop a risk-aversive bias to avoid vulnerability. Such a bias then tends to maintain the distress in the relationship.

The research of authors such as Holmes and Rempel represents a marked advance over the time when, lacking good data, discourse about relationships was inevitably reduced to each expert's own value-laden sense of what was important to successful relationships. The couple therapist can now draw on a science of relationships and can more readily assess the status of a relationship. He or she can go to the heart of the matter, to the experiences and actions that constitute distress and the journey of couples therapy.

Turning our attention from the observation of interaction patterns to more abstract variables, we see that the marital therapy literature has begun to be augmented by social psychology research into variables such as love (Sternberg and Barnes 1988), trust (Holmes and Boon 1990; Holmes and Rempel 1989), and intimacy (Descutner and Thelen 1991). This kind of research may eventually be helpful in creating models of marital interaction and other intimate relationships, which can then be used to further elucidate the nature of marital distress and improve therapy interventions.

Couples therapy has evolved without a coherent theory of adult love to inform interventions, similar to the way theories of personality inform interventions in individual therapy. The question of why the phenomena discussed earlier occur in distressed couples may be considered from many theoretical viewpoints. All of the research referred to above may be interpreted in a different light by proponents of different schools of couples therapy, such as those with analytic (J. Scharff 1995), cognitive-behavioral (behavioral marital therapy [BMT; Baucom and Epstein 1990]), systemic (Minuchin and Fishman 1981), experiential (emotionally focused therapy [EFT]; Johnson and Greenberg 1995), narrative (Freedman and Combs 1996), and solution-focused (de Shazer 1991b) approaches. The rigid patterns observed in distressed marriages, for example, may be viewed in terms of patterns of reinforcement, as the projection of distorted perceptions from the past, as an organized system of behaviors in and of themselves, as reflections of the emotional responses and unmet needs of each partner, or as negative stories constrained by culture and the way couples label key events and problems.

Even though it may be interpreted in different ways, the descriptive research on couple distress has directly influenced interventions. Specifically, there is mounting evidence that happy couples do not display a focus on immediate contingencies or short-term reciprocity. The relevance of negotiating quid pro quo contracts, once the cornerstone of behavioral marital therapy, has thus been questioned. As a result, some behavioral approaches have shifted somewhat from an exchange orientation to a focus on general communication skills and even to a new focus on variables such as acceptance (Jacobson and Christensen 1996). If monitoring equality of gains and losses, keeping accounts, and focusing on immediate contingencies is typical of distressed couples, it does not seem logical to reinforce this process in couples therapy (Robinson and Jacobson 1987). As a result of the findings on the key features of marital distress, the field has also generally begun to focus more on phenomena such as interaction patterns and affect, which until recently were eclipsed in empirically validated treatment programs by a focus on cognition and individual behavior.

There is a general consensus that a move to the level of explanation—to a theory of adult love and relatedness—is essential to guide the field of couples therapy (Johnson and Lebow 2000; Roberts 1992). In the last decade, two major contenders for a theory of close relationships have emerged. The first is *exchange theory*, which construes relationships in economic terms, focuses on reward versus cost, and views rational self-interest as the driving force behind close relationships. This theory formed the cornerstone for behavioral approaches and interventions such as behavior contracts and exchange (N. Jacobson 1981). A great deal of data supports the exchange theory model about how people interact at a molecular level. However, exchange theory has been criticized as an inappropriate model for intimate relationships, in which partners depend on responsiveness to each other's needs, rather than acting simply in terms of "profit" for themselves (see S. Johnson 1986; Wood 1995).

The second theory that provides a conceptual framework for close relationships is *attachment theory* (Bartholomew and Horowitz 1991; Bowlby 1969, 1988; Hazan and Shaver 1987). In the 1990s, attachment theory as applied to adult bonds became a powerful force in developmental and social psychology. It has been applied to specific factors in close relationships such as support seeking (Simpson and Rholes 1994) and the ability to take a metaperspective in interactions (Kobak and Cole 1991), as well as to general factors such as the quality of love relationships (Collins and Read 1990) and the regulation of negative affect and stress (Mikulincer et al. 1990). Although attachment theory has only just begun to be widely applied to adult relationships in the last decade, it has already generated a large and rich literature (see Bartholomew and Perlman 1992; Shaver and Hazan 1994 for review). It has also been systematically applied to couples interventions in EFT (S. Johnson 1996), one of the best-validated approaches to couples therapy.

Attachment theory also suggests that there are certain universals wired into human beings, and the need for safe contact with a few responsive people is one of them. This contact is seen as an adaptive survival mechanism that promotes optimal development and mastery of the environment. A secure connection to an accessible and responsive attachment figure fosters a sense of felt security; felt security in turn allows for flexibility and open communication and also encourages autonomy. The building blocks of a secure bond are accessibility and emotional responsiveness. The focus of attachment theory on emotion as an organizer of behavior in relationships (Bowlby 1969, 1988) and on the quality of emotional engagement between intimates also parallels Gottman's (1994b) work on divorce predictors. Attachment theory also converges with the depathologization of dependency needs in feminist literature, and Jordan et al.'s (1991) focus on how the self develops in relation to others.

In the context of attachment theory, distress in close relationships is seen in terms of a threat to attachment security, which triggers powerful emotions that organize responses into predictable sequences. Typically, anger and protest will be the first response to such a threat, followed by some form of clinging and seeking that, if security cannot be reestablished, gives way to depression and despair and finally detachment. Lack of responsiveness in an attachment figure primes automatic fight/flight and freeze responses that limit information processing and constrict interactional behaviors. Attachment theory posits a universal need for a particular kind of relationship, predicts when those needs will be particularly relevant, and describes a set of processes that arise when these needs are not met. The theory appears to offer couple therapists a potential map that encompasses inner experience and interactional patterns, as well as a guide for the process and direction of therapy (Johnson and Whiffen 1999).

Effectiveness of Couples Therapy

Studies of the effectiveness of couples therapy were mostly conducted by proponents of BMT (Baucom et al. 1998). Four outcome studies supporting the efficacy of insight-oriented marital therapy exist in the literature (Boelens et al. 1980; Crowe 1978; Snyder and Wills 1989; Waring et al. 1988). One outcome study of systemic paradox-oriented treatment (Goldman and Greenberg 1992) exists. There is also a set of studies on EFT for couples (Johnson et al. 1999) and another study on the experiential-systemic approach (see Chapter 1, "Family Theory and Therapy: An Overview," and Chapter 3, "Constructing Therapy: From Strategic, to Systemic, to Narrative Models"). The only two interventions accepted by the American Psychological Association as effective are BMT and EFT.

BMT evolved from a focus on behavioral exchange contracts into an approach that combined problem solving and communication skills training with behavioral contracting, for example, to increase the frequency of pleasing interactions. No single behavioral intervention has been isolated as necessary to promote effective treatment, and in fact interventions do not seem to differ from each other in impact (Shadish et al. 1993). The results of BMT have been reviewed in detail in previous reviews (Jacobson and Addis 1993; Lebow and Gurman 1995), as well as in two recent meta-analyses (Dunn and Schwebel 1995; Shadish et al. 1993). Shadish et al. (1993) found that BMT demonstrated an effect size of 0.95. This means that the average person receiving BMT had higher scores on outcome measures than 83% of untreated couples. Dunn and Schwebel (1995) found a lower effect size for BMT of 0.79. However, as Baucom et al. (1998) note, there are questions as to how well these changes are maintained over time. Overall findings suggest that less than half of couples receiving BMT will move into the nondistressed range by the end of treatment, and a proportion of these couples tend to relapse after treatment.

In addition to these behavioral techniques, behavior therapists have added cognitive interventions that may be used alone but are generally used as a supplement to BMT (Baucom et al. 1990; Halford et al. 1993). These interventions teach couples alternative attributions for negative behavior and examine their expectations and standards for a happy relationship. However, research has been unable to demonstrate that these cognitive components add to the effectiveness of BMT. For example, Baucom et al. (1998) found no significant differences between couples who received BMT alone and those receiving BMT plus cognitive interventions. In this research, 42% of couples receiving a combined cognitive and behavioral intervention were no longer distressed at the end of treatment.

The emotionally focused approach, first validated in 1985 (Johnson and Greenberg 1985b), has been identified by Gottman et al. (1998) as consistent with their data on the nature of relationship distress and the importance of emotional engagement and responsiveness in successful relationships. EFT focuses on expanding the constricted emotional responses and interactional cycles that typify relationship distress and developing a secure bond between partners. EFT assumes that attachment insecurities and unmet needs play a major role in relationship distress. It focuses on shaping the accessibility and responsiveness that foster safe emotional engagement. EFT interventions combine experiential humanistic techniques with a systemic structural focus on interactions and the setting of interactional tasks (S. Johnson 1996, 2002; Johnson et al. 1999). The therapist works in a collaborative way to help couples de-escalate the negative cycles that maintain their insecurities, framing these cycles as the enemy that robs both partners of their sense of safety and their ability to be close. The therapist also uses newly formulated emotional responses to expand the positions partners take with each other (for example, hostility expands into desperation and grief), so that new cycles of caring and contact can occur.

EFT has generally proven to be effective with distressed couples (Alexander et al. 1994; Baucom et al. 1998), and in a more recent meta-analysis an effect size of 1.3 was obtained (Johnson et al. 1999). This is a considerable effect size for psychotherapy research and exceeds the average effect size noted for couples therapy, which Dunn and Schwebel (1995) estimated as 0.90. In more recent studies, 70%–73% of couples were found to be recovered from distress at follow-up after 10–12 sessions of EFT. Further studies have found no evidence for deterioration after treatment termination, and a 2-year follow-up on particularly stressed couples with chronically ill children found results to be stable. EFT was also found in one study to be more effective than interventions focusing on behavioral exchange and skill building (Johnson and Greenberg 1985a).

A relatively sophisticated insight approach to couples therapy was rigorously tested by Snyder and Wills (1989) with positive results at termination and at follow-up. This approach is called is insight oriented couple therapy (IOMT; Snyder et al. 1991). It offers the couple interpretations that allow them to understand developmental issues, incongruent expectations and beliefs, and maladaptive relationship rules. In the original study, IOMT was found to be more efficacious than a control condition and as effective as BMT. At 4-year follow-up, 42% of the BMT couples had improved from intake levels of distress (as had 52% of the IOMT couples); however, many more BMT couples (38%) than IOMT couples (3%) had experienced divorce. This approach has been labeled as possibly efficacious (Baucom et al. 1998) by rigorous criteria set out by Chambless and Hollon (1998). There has been some debate about the exact nature of the IOMT interventions. Behavioral commentators have found similarities to BMT (Jacobson 1991b), whereas the originators of IOMT see similarities with EFT, in that couples are asked to explore feelings and thoughts that underlie current interactions and share more vulnerable aspects of themselves. There is very little in the literature specifying the interventions used in IOMT, but this deficiency may be remedied in the future and the research results on this model may be replicated.

Behavioral and nonbehavioral researchers (Jacobson et al. 1984a, 1984b; Johnson and Greenberg 1985b) note the lack of any spontaneous remission in untreated couples. This may reflect the self-reinforcing nature of marital distress. Indeed, longitudinal studies of couple interactions (Markman 1984) suggest that once interaction patterns are established, they are very resistant to change. Behavioral and nonbehavioral reviewers also note the lack of outcome data on other popular approaches to couples therapy, such as narrative and solution-focused therapy. In general, researchers are also stressing the need to assess *clinically* as well as statistically significant change (see Jacobson and Truax 1991; Jacobson et al. 1984a, 1984b).

Couples Therapy as a Treatment for DSM Disorders

Couples therapy has emerged in the last decade as an intervention for individual symptomatology, particularly when the marital relationship may play a role in the etiology, maintenance, or exacerbation of symptoms. Individual diagnoses that may be amenable to couples therapy include alcoholism, agoraphobia (Jacobson et al. 1989a), obsessive-compulsive disorders, and, perhaps most significantly, depression (Baucom et al. 1998; Jacobson et al. 1993).

In the treatment of agoraphobia, the spouse may be involved in therapy as a provider of social support rather than as a participant in reviewing the marital relationship. Spouse involvement, which is not couples therapy per se, does seem to improve treatment outcomes with agoraphobia (Cerney et al. 1988; Craske and Zoellner 1995). At least one study has also shown that communication training with the couple improves the effectiveness of exposure treatments for this disorder (Arnow et al. 1985). There is, however, little evidence that marriages involving an agoraphobic spouse are more troubled than nonpsychiatric control marriages or that husbands reinforce their wives' agoraphobic behavior and general dependency. The role of the marital relationship in the etiology and maintenance of this disorder is unclear, although the inclusion of the spouse in treatment appears to facilitate improvement.

The few findings on the usefulness of couples therapy to address marital distress when one partner is alcoholic are equivocal. For example, one study found that group BMT improved the marital relationship in these couples but did not significantly reduce drinking (O'Farrell et al. 1985). Another study (McCrady et al. 1986) found that while a social learning couples therapy program resulted in improvements in sobriety, effects were not significantly better than an intervention that simply involved the spouse in a passive way in the treatment of the alcoholism. It has been suggested that there may be different subtypes of alcoholic patients, some more positive in their interactions when intoxicated and some more negative (Jacob and Leonard 1988). If this is true, marital therapy may have differential effects for these two groups. In general, involvement of the partner is emerging as a key factor in the treatment of addiction (Lebow and Gurman 1995).

There is now overwhelming evidence concerning the roles relationships play in relation to "individual" disorders. A lack of supportive relationships can potentiate other stressors, elicit the onset of symptoms, and undermine response to individual treatment. Alternatively, symptomatic behavior may elicit relationship distress, which in turn exacerbates such symptomatic behavior. These processes seem particularly clear in relation to depression, the common cold of mental health. The link between depression and marital stress is well documented (Brown and Harris 1978; Paykel et al. 1969). Marital distress often precedes depression, and marital dysfunction is associated with subsequent depression and lack of response to individual treatment. Relapse has been found to be inversely related to the improvement in marital satisfaction that occurs during marital therapy (Rounsaville et al. 1979). Researchers such as Hooley have forged specific links between spouse interactions and relapse (Hooley et al. 1986); they have found that the frequency of criticisms from the nondistressed spouse is as powerful a predictor of relapse as any other variable associated with depression.

Several studies have compared BMT with individual therapies for depression (Jacobson et al. 1991; O'Leary and Beach 1990). The studies show that when marital distress and depression are present, marital therapy is as effective as cognitive individual therapy and that changes in depression are related to changes in relationship quality. These results suggest that BMT, at least, can be a viable treatment for depression. In general, couples therapy has emerged as a useful intervention for depression accompanied by relationship distress, and particularly for depressed women in distressed relationships (Beach and O'Leary 1992; Prince and Jacobson 1995). More specifically, EFT has also been used to address major depression in the context of marital distress, with promising results (L. Johnson et al. 1999).

Apart from marital therapy per se, studies of interpersonal psychotherapy (IPT), which attempts to create insight into personal relationships, found that spouse involvement was as effective as standard individual IPT in alleviating depression and more effective in improving marital quality (Foley et al. 1987). A critical question should be asked at this point: When, if ever, is marital therapy *more* effective than individual therapy for depression? The answer may be related to the prevention of relapse rather than the alleviation of symptoms after treatment. While there is no evidence that treatment of the depressed individual alone will alter marital dissatisfaction, there is accumulating evidence that continuing marital dissatisfaction is related to the return of depression. Another question is, How is it that some couples seem to avoid significant marital stress despite psychological problems? Future research will hopefully define subpopulations in this area that are best treated by marital therapy alone or together with other treatments.

The use of couples therapy to address sexual problems has become standard practice, particularly when relationship problems and sexual problems occur together and impact each other (Baucom et al. 1998). This use of couples therapy is supported by a general recognition of the widespread effects of the quality of our closest relationships on our physical and mental health. For example, marital conflict and separation appears to be associated with suppression of the immune system (Kiecolt-Glaser et al. 1993). For women, deleterious effects on general health have been linked in particular to emotional distancing in relationships; for men, conflictual couple exchanges in particular appear to reduce general health. General findings concerning the power of a positive connection with others to regulate emotion and resilience to stressful events parallel this research (Burman and Margolin 1992; Mikulincer et al. 1993; Walsh 1996).

Who Benefits From Couples Therapy and How

It is important to know who benefits from couples therapy and how the benefit is imparted. Factors that predict success in various forms of couples therapy should be identified, so that it will eventually be possible to match couple characteristics and specific interventions. This kind of research is relatively sparse, and the research we do have is largely on middle-class North Americans. By far the best general predictor of treatment success has been *initial distress level* (Jacobson and Addis 1993). This factor was found to account for 46% of the variance in outcome with BMT, with initially less distressed couples doing better (Whisman and Jacobson 1990). This result is hardly surprising, since it parallels a similar, broadly replicated finding in individual therapy.

The impact of couples therapy on older and more traditional couples has mostly been addressed in studies of BMT (Jacobson et al. 1986). These couples seem to find change more difficult when BMT is used. It is interesting to compare the findings of this study with the results of a more recent study examining predictors of the success in EFT by Johnson and Talitman (1997). They found that EFT seemed to work better for older partners (over 35), that having traditional beliefs and behaviors did not influence outcome, and that initial distress accounted for only 4% of the variance at follow-up. The variables that did predict change in EFT were the female partner's initial level of trust in her partner's caring, and the couple's active engagement with the therapist in the tasks of therapy. This result highlights the general findings that the alliance with the therapist and engagement in therapy are powerful predictors of success in psychotherapy. Emotional disengagement between partners seems to negatively impact success in couples therapy. In general, superficial problem solving or the avoidance of problems and distancing all seem to make relationships and relationship repair more tenuous (Jacobson and Addis 1993). In terms of personality variables, only one was reliably related to outcome. Femininity—that is, a sensitive and emotionally attuned attitude and expressiveness—was found to be related to successful outcome in BMT (Baucom and Aiken 1984).

Explanation: How Does Change Occur in Marital Therapy?

To develop a science of psychotherapy, it is crucial to begin to identify the active ingredients of change and show how such ingredients work (Beach and O'Leary 1985; Greenberg and Pinsof 1986). Without this kind of understanding, it is difficult to specify what kind of interventions lead to what kind of specific changes. There are two approaches to this issue. The first is to focus on therapists' interventions and to track the effectiveness of different interventions, seeking for the active ingredients that create positive outcomes. Behavioral researchers have conducted a number of studies testing the relative effectiveness of different interventions within their school of marital therapy, such as behavior change, communication training, and problem-solving training (Jacobson 1984a). They also examined the effect of adding new components, such as cognitive restructuring and emotional expressiveness training, to BMT (Baucom et al. 1990; Halford et al. 1993). In general, in this research, no one component was found to be more effective than the others, although couples receiving communication and problem-solving training maintained their gains better than couples who received only behavior exchange interventions. Adding new interventions, cognitive restructuring, and emotional expressiveness training to BMT did not increase its effectiveness (Jacobson and Addis 1993). Similarly, adding a communication skills training component to experiential couples therapy (specifically EFT) did not increase efficacy (James 1991). It has been suggested that in the future such studies should match couples to intervention and vary the length of treatment, so that no intervention is given in diluted form (Baucom et al. 1990). Furthermore, studies focusing on the immediate in-therapy effects of specific therapist interventions, rather than correlating a general set of interventions with general therapy outcome, might be more successful in elucidating the process of change in couples therapy.

The second approach to identifying the ingredients of change is to focus on the client process associated with change, rather than the processes of therapist intervention. This kind of research, which is extremely relevant to clinical practice and training and to the construction of theories of change, has only recently been applied to couples therapy. There exist a number of small preliminary studies that examine the in-therapy client processes in EFT associated with positive outcomes and one study identifying key change events in EFT (Greenberg et al. 1993; Johnson and Greenberg 1988). The results of the smaller studies suggest that, as the theory of change in EFT postulates, couples do change their negative interaction cycles in this therapy and become more affiliative, supportive, and self-disclosing. In addition, sessions perceived by clients as productive of change were characterized by a greater depth of experiencing and positive self-focused statements (rather than blaming, other-focused, statements), and that partners tended to respond affiliatively after their spouses disclosed in an intimate manner (this was in contrast to interactions that occurred before the disclosure). This disclosure also was associated with reciprocal self-disclosure by the listener.

One of the smaller studies identified a key change event, which it referred to as *a softening*. The elements that defined this event—higher levels of in-therapy experiencing and the evocation of affiliative behaviors in blaming spouses—were associated with dramatic improvement in EFT. Softening refers to a previously hostile and blaming spouse's asking for an affiliative response from the other in a vulnerable and congruent fashion. The other spouse, previously withdrawn, is then able to be accessible and responsive, thus creating positive emotional engagement (see Johnson and Greenberg 1995 for a transcript of this event). This research supports the basic change principles of EFT, which focus on accessing and reprocessing emotional responses underlying interactional positions in order to facilitate a shift in these positions toward the responsiveness and accessibility that form the basis of a secure bond (Bowlby 1969, 1988).

The softening of hostile emotion, which allows for more emotional engagement, may be the hallmark of all successful couple interventions (Gottman et al. 1998). It is to be hoped that there will be more research on how change occurs across a wider range of models in the next decade. Research that informs us as to how and when change occurs in terms of client processes seems to hold considerable promise for understanding what goes on in therapy and why some couples change so dramatically and others change so little (Friedlander et al. 1994).

Problems in Research on Couples Therapy

What are some of the problems and issues in couples therapy research that have been pinpointed in the last decade? In terms of the general relevance of research to clinicians, commentators single out the omission of relevant clinical variables from research programs. For example, therapist competence is not considered (Jacobson and Addis 1993), and neither is therapist commitment to a specific treatment model. In fact, most comparisons of the outcomes of separate interventions involve similar interventions implemented by the same therapists, rather than by therapists experienced in and committed to the interventions they are using, as is the case in clinical practice. When interventions are truly different, and therapists of varying levels of experience and commitment to their interventions are not compared, differences in effectiveness have been found. These differences are not only in alleviating relationship distress (Johnson and Greenberg 1985a, 1985b) but also in increasing positive factors such as intimacy (Dandeneau and Johnson 1994). Furthermore, in much research, invariant treatments are applied to all couples, whereas sensitive clinicians flexibly tailor treatments to specific clients. This limits the ecological validity of present clinical research. Additionally, clients often present with multiple problems, whereas research couples are screened so they present with only one problem.

In spite of the above difficulties, research gives a field of endeavor accountability and credibility and, more pragmatically, offers the clinician treatment options that are specific and substantiated by more than popular appeal. Pinsof and Wynne (1995) have recommended some specific needs for future research:

- Clearer specifying of the problems, their severity, and their treatments, and careful monitoring of treatment adherence
- A set of core outcome batteries
- More attention to issues such as dropouts (which are often not reported) and relapse
- Outcome studies of longer-term treatments
- Research on the process of change

A different survey of general therapy practitioners also stressed the need for research that focuses on therapist and client behaviors leading up to important moments of change in therapy (Beutler et al. 1993).

Research practices are slowly evolving to address the issues listed above. A significant recent development that increases the ecological validity of clinical research was the elaboration of the concept of clinical significance and how it might be calculated. This development has helped to move research to consider how valuable treatment actually is to clients (Jacobson and Truax 1991). The critical events paradigm (i.e., identifying key moments of change) also appears to offer a promising path for understanding the relationship between therapy process and outcome (Rice and Greenberg 1984). Another useful methodology that has become more sophisticated in recent years is the use of various forms of replicated single-case studies (Goldfried and Wolfe 1996; Jones 1993).

Conclusion and Future Directions

There is no doubt that there has been a quantum leap in the quality and quantity of couples therapy research in the last decade. Methodologically sound research studies from different schools of couples therapy, which include features recommended in first reviews of couples therapy such as random assignment, treatment implemented according to manuals, the use of implementation checks, control groups, follow-up results, and the reporting of rates of deterioration, are now becoming the norm. Outcome criteria are being reviewed and made more rigorous, and our basic understanding of the nature of marital distress is increasing. Nevertheless, this is a young field, and there are still more questions and issues than there are answers. There is a need for more outcome studies of nonbehavioral interventions and for more studies concerning which variables predict outcome success in particular kinds of treatment. There is also a pressing need to understand the process of change, as well as the need to continue to evaluate the use of couples therapy for specific populations.

What, then, are the most significant issues and challenges that this field faces at the present time? First, outcome research and change strategies are proliferating, but it is in the area of theory that perhaps the largest challenge lies. Research without theory is, in the final analysis, a ship without a rudder. Couples therapy needs clear, cogent theories of close adult relationships and of therapeutic change, but it is also necessary to link theory, research, and intervention if couples therapy is to become a systematic and reliable treatment modality. The three extant theoretical perspectives on adult intimacy—the analytic, attachment, and social learning/exchange models, of which only the latter two have been supported by research results (O'Leary and Smith 1991)—imply very different strategies and goals for marital therapy. The question arises as to when each model is appropriate. When is the appropriate goal the teaching of communication skills, and when is it the fostering of secure attachment? To answer such questions we have to know more about the nature of intimate relationships and to understand variables such as trust and intimacy that have only just begun to be clearly defined, researched, and included in the couples therapy literature. Couples therapy has to deal with these questions theoretically and clinically. It has to set out, for example, the interventions and the processes that facilitate intimacy (Dandeneau and Johnson 1994) or repair the effects of betrayals (Johnson et al. 2001) and then place these interventions in the context of a theory of intimate relationships.

The various schools of couples therapy also need to develop their conceptualizations of marriage. It has been suggested that lack of theory development is a major weakness of BMT (Markman et al. 1991). In empirical studies, the central components of BMT, contingency contracting and problem solving, have proved to be less crucial in couples therapy than originally thought, and the role of cognition and affect in marriage has become more and more recognized (Markman 1991). The whole question of whether skill building is an appropriate goal for marital therapy has also been identified. There is some evidence that distressed couples have adequate skills when they are not interacting with their spouse (Birchler et al. 1975) and that skills do not necessarily impact marital happiness (Berely and Jacobson 1984; Harrell and Guerney 1976). Suggestions have been made that managing negative affect (Markman 1991) and promoting the acceptance of problems, rather than always focusing on modifying them (Jacobson 1991b; Jacobson and Christensen 1996), might be useful additions to BMT interventions.

Proponents of systemic perspectives have concerned themselves mostly with family therapy rather than focusing on couples. The basic concepts of systems theory, such as that the behavior of any one person is, to a large extent, constrained and dictated by the behavior of other members of the system (i.e., by how interactions are organized), apply to dyads as well as family groups. However, systemic theory and interventions have been delineated in the context of families, and the issue of individual motivation as it relates to interpersonal behaviors has not been addressed in this model. The analytic orientation to couples therapy has still not addressed the problem of clarifying and operationalizing core theoretical constructs such as enmeshment, collusion, and projective identification (Gurman and Kniskern 1978), and this hampers the building of a technology of change and research efforts. The most developed model of couples therapy from the experiential school, EFT, which is a synthesis of experiential and structural systemic perspectives, is based on attachment theory, which has only recently been applied to adult relationships (Hazan and Shaver 1987). How attachment styles relate to specific interaction patterns in present relationships, and how such patterns might influence and change attachment style, are just beginning to be delineated (Johnson and Whiffen 1999).

A second issue that the field faces is the perspective on emotion and how to address emotion in couples therapy. The importance of emotion is becoming more and more recognized in this modality (Broderick and O'Leary 1986; Greenberg and Paivio 1998). Emotion is also becoming a more differentiated concept (Greenberg and Paivio 1997; Leventhal 1979) and its role in close relationships and couples therapy is being examined, whether from the standpoint of teaching couples how to manage negative affect (Lindahl and Markman 1990), how to express emotion (Baucom et al. 1990), or how to use emotional responses to create new interaction patterns (S. Johnson 1996; Johnson and Greenberg 1994). The issue is not now whether to address emotion at all, but how and when to use/teach/control specific kinds of emotional responses to achieve specific ends. All of the above points can also be applied to the area of attributions, which are also becoming more and more differentiated. Attributions of responsibility, which imply intent and harmful motivation, have been identified as particularly salient in close relationships (Bradbury and Fincham 1990).

Third, it is clear that changing the quality of an intimate relationship can impact individual symptomatology. Indeed, self-definition and relationship definition may be viewed as two sides of the same coin (Guidano and Liotti 1983; Johnson and Greenberg 1995). Findings in social psychology (Swann and Predmore 1985) suggest that the stability of self-concept emanates from forces outside the person, from continuity in the organization of people's social relationships, rather than from intrapsychic forces. It may then be very instructive to assess the intrapsychic change that occurs in successful couples therapy and continue to delineate the link between relationship quality and individual functioning.

Fourth, couple interventions are being applied to more and more diverse client groups, and the needs of such groups, and how the change process should reflect such needs, must be researched. For example, partners from other cultures, partners struggling with posttraumatic stress disorder, and gay and lesbian couples are all seeking couples therapy (Johnson and Lebow 2000).

Fifth, violence in close relationships is now acknowledged as a highly significant issue across diverse cultural groups. The underreporting of couple violence even in therapy is a major finding that emerged in the 1990s. One line of research has differentiated patterns of violent behavior, distinguishing those patterns that are more and less likely to be amenable to treatment (Jacobson and Gottman 1998). Such research may assist the couple therapist in differentiating when and how to intervene. In general, assessment procedures, risk factors, and treatment feasibility issues in violent relationships are now beginning to be addressed (Bograd and Mederos 1999; Holtzworth-Munroe et al. 1995). Experts agree that the overriding principle must be the safety of the victimized partner and that, in general, couple interventions should follow individual or group treatment for the abuser. Couples therapy is recommended only if violence is infrequent and mild, the victim is not fearful of retaliation and willingly enters couples therapy, and the perpetrator admits responsibility and can make a commitment to contain violent impulses.

In brief, couples therapy and couples therapy research have come a long way, but the potential inherent in the task of describing, predicting, and understanding intimate relationships has only just begun to be realized. Researchers are striving toward the goal of specificity in the questions they ask. Questions such as "What are the specific effects of specific interventions, by specified therapists, at specific points in time, with particular types of patients, with particular presenting problems?" (Gurman et al. 1986, p. 601) are still daunting, but at this point not unanswerable. The field of couples therapy is emerging from the shadows of individual and family interventions and coming of age.

Chapters on Related Topics

The following chapters describe concepts related to couples therapy research:

- Chapter 7, "Behavioral Family Therapy"
- Chapter 22, "Behavioral Couples Therapy"
- Chapter 27, "Family Variables and Interventions in Schizophrenia"
- Chapter 28, "Depression and the Family: Interpersonal Context and Family Functioning"
- Chapter 29, "Family Intervention and Psychiatric Hospitalization"
- Chapter 36, "The State of Family Therapy Research: A Positive Prognosis"

38

Conclusion and Future Directions

G. Pirooz Sholevar, M.D.

The fields of family and couples therapy entered the twenty-first century having reached maturity by collaborating with other treatment modalities and participating in the investigation of the biological, psychological, and cultural characteristics of individuals. The family therapy field, which approaches this stage in a reluctant and ambivalent fashion because of its rebellious historical roots, emerged in response to the failure of individual psychotherapy to effectively treat specific groups of disorders such as schizophrenia and entrenched neurotic and other psychopathological disorders of adults. Succeeding where individual therapy has failed, family practitioners soon began to feel omnipotent, claiming they could change complex behavior within the family system by altering the hidden family rules or fantasies. Strong opposition to family therapy from the individual therapists, further, helped force family and marital therapists into an antagonistic position not only toward individual therapy but also toward the individual differences and diagnostic and classification systems that were the tools of mental health professionals working with individuals. In addition, the family therapist was able to ignore the potential use of pharmacotherapy, because in the 1950s and 1960s availability of psychotropic agents was limited. It was also easy to deny the value of hospitalization when it was used primarily as a custodial tool rather than an active therapeutic agent at the time of crisis. The diagnostic classification system could also be ignored readily because of the lack of clear consensus among mental health professionals about different diagnostic criteria. The lack of research in individual psychotherapy, psychodynamic in nature at the time, further diminished the reputation of this approach with some populations and made the failure of this treatment appear inevitable.

The defiant attitude of family therapists, which was necessary in the earliest stages of this discipline, continued for a long time—eventually, family therapists came to ignore one another with the same rigor that they had reserved for nonfamily practitioners. The end result was the evolution along divergent paths of multiple family therapy approaches whose practitioners had no genuine interest in defining their areas of commonality, complementarity, or difference.

This state of affairs changed when the investigations in the field of family therapy began to exhibit a high level of success with some methodologies with certain disorders in some populations, while other populations and families failed to engage in and gain from family therapy methods. In addition, different levels of individual and family dysfunctions became apparent that could explain the relative success or failure of different methods with different populations. Furthermore, the same populations that responded poorly to individual psychotherapy in the past continued to defy the broader approaches of family therapists. These populations particularly included schizophrenia, which had stimulated the bulk of early family investigations.

Horizontal integration of family theories emerged in the 1980s and 1990s. New models of family therapy such as *narrative therapy* incorporated the fundamental elements of divergent family therapy paradigms (e.g., strategic and psychodynamic models—see Chapter 3, "Constructing Therapy: From Strategic, to Systemic, to Narrative Models"). The level of integration is understandably highest in the area of couples therapy because of the greater homogeneity of the clinical population and disorders, leading to higher consensus on treatment effectiveness. Emotionally focused therapy (EFT) and integrative couple therapy (ICT) can be exemplary for the broader field of family therapy, which requires a higher level of refinement in describing the clinical variables, therapeutic interventions, and outcome measures because of extreme levels of diversity in the clinical population (see Chapter 28, "Depression and the Family: Interpersonal Context and Family Functioning"; Chapter 29, "Family Intervention and Psychiatric Hospitalization"; and Chapter 31, "Alcoholic and Substance-Abusing Families"). A *vertical integration* correlating the biological, individual, familial, and sociocultural variable will be made possible based on such a comprehensive family therapy (see Chapter 27, "Family Variables and Interventions in Schizophrenia"; Chapters 28 and 29 mentioned above).

The new advances in the area of psychopharmacotherapy, behavioral therapy, crisis intervention, and short-term hospitalization forced family therapists to abandon their insular position and join the broader range of mental health professionals who brought with them powerful family concepts and intervention techniques. The combined use of family intervention with other therapeutic modalities proved more powerful than family intervention alone (consider, e.g., the use of antipsychotic medication with schizophrenic patients). Such collaborations resulted in the emergence of novel intervention models such as psychoeducational family therapy and interventions to alter expressed emotion and affective style (see Chapter 27, "Family Variables and Interventions in Schizophrenia"). The success of such collaborative interventions, as demonstrated by sophisticated research methodology and its broad acceptance by clinicians, has continued to stimulate further collaboration. The treatment of depression with antidepressant medications, family and interpersonal therapies, cognitive therapy, and at times hospitalization has been another area of successful collaboration (see Chapter 28, "Depression and the Family: Interpersonal Context and Family Functioning").

The combined use of multiple treatment modalities with severely disturbed patients required a common theoretical foundation; the diathesis-stress theory was proposed by Rosenthal (1970) and further refined by Zubin and Spring (1977). The diathesis-stress (or vulnerability-stress) theory facilitated the refinement of the specific impact of different intervention methodologies that would be effective in reducing vulnerability or stress. This model, the application of which has continued to evolve, constitutes a biopsychosocial framework to guide investigations as well as a comprehensive clinical intervention.

The emergence of the National Alliance for the Mentally Ill (NAMI) and the National Depressive and Manic-Depressive Association (now Depression and Bipolar Support Alliance) demonstrated the significance of families in caring for their mentally ill members. These organizations were also effective in forcing third parties to pay for the treatment of mental illness and in convincing legislators of the need to support the investigation of the role played by biological factors in major mental disorders. Also, unfortunate labels used by early family therapists such as *schizophrenogenic mothers* and *double-bind phenomena* were declared to be *impressionistic* and not supported by data. These labels had offended the families of those they were applied to. Furthermore, there was no clear evidence that some of the stressful family interactional patterns such as communication deviance, expressed emotion, and affective style predated or followed the symptomatic behavior in the schizophrenic patients, particularly the ones who were seriously disturbed and refractory to treatment. The above developments resulted in the new understanding of the family of the mentally ill patient as the most important resource for his or her treatment. The family is now regarded as the partner of mental health professionals in the treatment of their mentally ill member. The concept that *the family is the patient* was abandoned as an offensive barrier to communication with families (see Chapter 30, "National Alliance for the Mentally Ill [NAMI] and Family Psychiatry: Working Toward a Collaborative Model").

The refinement of diagnostic and classification systems resulted in the emergence of the DSM process and DSM-IV classification systems (American Psychiatric Association 2000a). The refined diagnostic criteria in turn made it possible to undertake large-scale epidemiological studies to exhibit the level of psychopathology and dysfunction in the general population and differentiate it from the two groups of *healthy* individuals and *vulnerable* ones. Today, the new advances in diagnostic and classification systems and the need for epidemiological studies are challenging the field of family therapy and family theory to provide a classification and diagnostic system acceptable to family and marital therapists as well as other mental health professionals. This should be followed by epidemiological studies to differentiate dysfunctional families with a range of disabilities from the families who are vulnerable or "healthy" (see Chapter 16, "Diagnosis of Family Relational Disorders").

The changes in family configurations and the dramatic shift from a two-parent family to single-parent families, divorcing families, remarried families, and gay/lesbian families necessitated the broadening of the concept of family to include perspectives used in other fields such as sociology. The changes in the family configuration also revealed the limitations of some earlier psychoanalytic and systems theory concepts, which either appeared to be or actually were biased against women and implied that men were in control or were more powerful. The recognition of societal biases related to gender, race, socioeconomic status, and childcare gave rise to gender-sensitive or *feminist* family therapy. The ever-increasing cultural diversity in American families forced therapists to enhance their sensitivity to cultural, ethnic, gender, and economic dimensions of family life. The emergence of new therapeutic systems demonstrates the new flexibility in family therapy approach as well as a movement away from the traditional rigidities of the early theories. Solution-focused family therapy (de Shazer 1988, 1991) has become a favorite of managed care companies. Emotionally focused therapy (Johnson 1999a, 1991b) has bridged the gap between the psychodynamic and empirically oriented behavioral therapies. Narrative therapy (White 1995) has demonstrated the importance of collaboration between patients and therapist in order to reduce resistance and power plays (see Chapter 3, "Constructing Therapy: From Strategic, to Systemic, to Narrative Models," Chapter 20, "Couples Therapy: An Overview," and Chapter 37, "Couples Therapy Research: Status and Directions").

Medical family therapy provides for collaboration between physicians or health care providers and family therapists, in which the exchange of information about biological factors and interpersonal dimension can enhance treatment effectiveness. The advances in investigation of biological factors and family dynamics make the implementation of a true biopsychosocial model feasible (see Chapter 35, "Medical Family Therapy"). This collaborative approach helps the field of family medicine achieve its dream of reducing the cost of medical care and emphasizes the importance of health maintenance.

The changes described above have necessitated a move away from the traditional overemphasis on the role of therapy with families and married couples toward a broader orientation that includes evaluation and prevention; an approach that can be called *family psychiatry* and *family psychology*. This orientation goes beyond interventions, which are primarily oriented to bring about symptomatic *change* in the family. The new orientation requires a true *theory of the family* and intimate relationships and looks at the intricacies of family development, healthy family functioning, vulnerability, and dysfunction. Prevention assumes a significant focus within this framework, particularly as it relates to young children of dysfunctional parents in dysfunctional families.

Future Directions

The future directions of family therapy are in the area of 1) further integration of family theories and techniques; 2) integration of family theories and interventions with other general theories and intervention models; and 3) differentiation between dysfunction, vulnerability, and *healthy* functioning. To achieve the above goals, a true diagnostic system according to a hierarchical developmental model should be developed to differentiate between families according to their level of success in completing their developmental tasks and family formation. This classification system should differentiate between disintegrating families with highly constricted and skewed social networks, families who are highly dependent on their families of origin in one or multiple ways, families made vulnerable by developmental failures in their previous stages, families who are functioning reasonably well in the contemporary sphere but lack sufficient resources to deal with a crisis situation, and resourceful families who can ensure the developmental progression of their children and respond to stressful and challenging situations in optimal or adequate ways. The application of a theoretical mode, such as social network therapy, can enhance the effectiveness of broader interventions such as family preservation and *wraparound* services.

The investigation of transmission of disorders across the generations has been particularly productive in the past three decades with the clinical research of Steinglass, Wolin, and their colleagues. Their methodological and clinically sophisticated approach has made possible the examination of both risk factors and protective factors influencing the intergenerational transmission phenomenon (see Chapter 31, "Alcoholic and Substance-Abusing Families"). The expanded application of their approach to other disorders such as depression and schizophrenia can pave the way for a comprehensive approach to the genetic and psychological pathways to transmission of disorders, which is particularly timely with the completion of the Human Genome Project.

The study of nonshared environment is a timely and well-designed project that provides the psychological and interpersonal counterpart to human genome mapping. It attempts to determine in which ways siblings differ in regard to their exposure to an experience of the environment and which shared or nonshared differences are associated with differential developmental outcomes in individuals. The environment measured here refers to the shared and nonshared environmental components that account for the amount of variance that remains after subtracting the variance accounted for by genetic factors and errors (Reiss et al. 1994, 2000). The book *The Relationship Code*, by Reiss et al. (2000), demonstrates that family investigators have done their job in keeping up with genetic research.

The mapping of the human genome, the new discovery of numerous neurotransmitter systems that are responsive to psychoactive medication, and the recognition of the combined impact of biological and psychological events on the human psyche and behavior have created new tasks. The family theoreticians are challenged to describe the relational correlates of biological and psychological vulnerabilities. The behavioral and interactional correlates of *diseased genes* in an early stage can enhance the implementation of preventive intervention in a timely fashion. Significant contributions in this area will be welcomed heartily as a highly sensitive locus for effective intervention. Family interactions may remain a highly viable area for the emergence of vulnerability and dysfunctions as revealed in investigations on expressed emotion.

References

Aaronson J: Inside Managed Care. New York, Brunner/Mazel, 1996

Abel G, Mittelman M, Becker J, et al: The characteristics of men who molest young children. Paper presented at the World Congress of Behavior Therapy, Washington, DC, December 1983

Achenbach T, Edelbrock C: Manual for the CBCL and Revised Child Behavioral Profile. Burlington, University of Vermont, Department of Psychiatry, 1986

Ackerman NW: The unity of the family. Arch Pediatr 2:51–62, 1938

Ackerman N Character structure in hypersensitive persons in life stress and bodily disease. Research Publications of the Association for Research in Nervous and Mental Disease 29:903–917, 1950

Ackerman N: Interpersonal disturbances in the family: some unresolved problems in psychotherapy. Psychiatry 17:359–368, 1954

Ackerman N: Family psychiatry: some areas of controversy. Compr Psychiatry 7:375, 1955

Ackerman NW: The Psychodynamics of Family Life: Diagnosis and Treatment of Family Relationships. New York, Basic Books, 1958

Ackerman NW: Family psychotherapy and psychoanalysis: the implications of difference. Fam Process 1:30–43, 1962

Ackerman NW: The Good Divorce. New York, HarperCollins, 1966

Ackerman NW, Sobel R: Family diagnosis: an approach to the preschool child. Am J Orthopsychiatry 20:744–753, 1950

Acuna RF: Anything but Mexican: Chicanos in Contemporary Los Angeles. London, Verso, 1996

Ahrons C: The binuclear family: two households one family. Alternative Lifestyles 2:499–515, 1979

Ahrons CR: The Good Divorce. New York, HarperCollins, 1994

Ahrons C, Rodgers R: Divorced Families: A Multidisciplinary Developmental View. New York, WW Norton, 1987

Aichorn A: Wayward Youth. New York, Viking Press, 1935

Ainsworth MDS: Attachment as related to mother-infant interaction, in Advances in the Study of Behavior. Edited by Rosenblatt JB, Hinde RH, Beer C, et al. New York, Academic Press, 1979, pp 1–51

Ainsworth MDS, Bell S: Mother-infant interaction and the development of competence, in The Growth of Competence. Edited by Connelly K, Bruner J. New York, Academic Press, 1974

Ainsworth MD, Bell SM, Stayton DJ: Individual differences in the development of some attachment behaviors. Merrill-Palmer Quarterly 18:123–143, 1972

Ainsworth MDS, Blehar MC, Waters E, et al: Patterns of Attachment: A Psychological Study of the Strange Situation. Hillsdale, NJ, Lawrence Erlbaum, 1978

Alexander JF: Defensive and supportive communications in normal and deviant families. J Consult Clin Psychol 40:223–231, 1973

Alexander J, Barton C: Behavioral systems therapy for families, in Treating Relationships. Edited by Olson D. Lake Mills, IA, Iowa Graphics, 1976

Alexander J, Barton C: Functional Family Therapy Training Manual. Salt Lake City, UT, Western States Family Institute, 1983

Alexander BK, Dibb GS: Interpersonal perception in addict families. Family Process 16:17–28, 1972

Alexander J, Parsons B: Short-term behavioral intervention with delinquent families: impact on family process and recidivism. J Abnorm Psychol 81:219–225, 1973

Alexander JF, Parsons BV: Functional Family Therapy. Monterey, CA, Brooks/Cole, 1982

Alexander J, Barton D, Waldron H: Beyond the technology of family therapy: the anatomy of an intervention model, in Advances in Clinical Behavior Therapy. Edited by Craig K, McMahon R. New York, Brunner/Mazel, 1983, pp 48–73

Alexander JF, Holtzworth-Munroe A, Jameson P: The process and outcome of marital and family therapy: research review and evaluation, in Handbook of Psychotherapy and Behavior Change. Edited by Bergin A, Garfield S. New York, Wiley, 1994, pp 595–607

Alexander JF, Robbins MS, Sexton T: Family-based interventions with older, at-risk youth: from promise to proof to practice. Journal of Primary Prevention 21:185–205, 2000

Alexander PC: The role of the extended family in the evaluation and treatment of incest, in Casebook of Sexual Abuse Treatment. Edited by Freidrick W. New York, WW Norton, 1990, pp 79–87

Allgood S, Craine D: Predicting marital therapy dropouts. J Marital Fam Ther 17:73–79, 1991

Almeida RA, Durkin T: The cultural context model: therapy for couples with domestic violence. J Marital Fam Ther 25:313–324, 1999

Amatea E, Clark J: A dual career workshop for college couples: effects of an intervention program. Journal of College Student Personnel 26:271–272, 1986

Ambelas A: Life events and mania: a special relationship? Br J Psychiatry 150:235–240, 1987

American Psychiatric Association: Diagnostic and Statistical Manual of Mental Disorders, 3rd Edition. Washington, DC, American Psychiatric Association, 1980

American Psychiatric Association: Diagnostic and Statistical Manual of Mental Disorders, 3rd Edition, Revised. Washington, DC, American Psychiatric Association, 1987

American Psychiatric Association, Task Force on DSM-IV: DSM-IV Draft Criteria. Washington, DC, American Psychiatric Association, 1993a

American Psychiatric Association: Practice guideline for major depressive disorder in adults. Am J Psychiatry 150 (suppl):1–26, 1993b

American Psychiatric Association: Diagnostic and Statistical Manual of Mental Disorders, 4th Edition. Washington, DC, American Psychiatric Association, 1994

American Psychiatric Association: Practice guideline for treatment of patients with schizophrenia. Am J Psychiatry 154 (suppl 4), 1997

American Psychiatric Association: Diagnostic and Statistical Manual of Mental Disorders, 4th Edition, Text Revision. Washington, DC, American Psychiatric Association, 2000a

American Psychiatric Association: Practice Guideline for the Treatment of Patients With Major Depressive Disorder, 2nd Edition. Washington, DC, American Psychiatric Association, 2000b

Andersen T: The reflecting team: dialogue and metadialogue in clinical work. Fam Process 26:415–428, 1987

Anderson C: Family intervention with severely disturbed inpatients. Arch Gen Psychiatry 34:697–702, 1976

References

Anderson CM, Hogarty GE, Reiss DJ: Family treatment of adult schizophrenic patients: a psychoeducational approach. Schizophr Bull 6:490–505, 1980
Anderson C, Hogarty G, Bayer T, et al: Expressed emotions and social networks of parents of schizophrenic patients. Br J Psychiatry 144:247–255, 1984
Anderson CM, Reiss DJ, Hogarty GE: Schizophrenia and the Family. New York, Guilford, 1986
Anderson H, Goolishian H, Pulliam G, et al: The Galveston Family Institute: some personal and historical perspectives, in Journeys: Expansion of the Strategic-Systemic Therapies. Edited by Efron DE. New York, Brunner/Mazel, 1986, pp 97–122
Anderson KL: Gender, status, and domestic violence: an integration of feminist and family violence approaches. Journal of Marriage and the Family 59:655–669, 1997
Andreasen NC, Rice J, Endicott J, et al: Familial rates of affective disorder: a report from the National Institute of Mental Health Collaborative Study. Arch Gen Psychiatry 44:461–469, 1987
Andrews G: Talk that works: the rise of cognitive behaviour therapy. BMJ 313:1501–1502, 1996
Antononsky A: Health, Stress and Coping. San Francisco, CA, Jossey-Bass, 1979
Aponte H: The negotiations of values in family therapy. Fam Process 24:323–338, 1985
Araji S, Finkelhor D: Abusers: a review of the research, in A Sourcebook on Child Sexual Abuse. Edited by Finkelhor D and Associates. Newbury Park, CA, Sage, 1986, pp 89–118
Ard BN, Ard CC (eds): Handbook of Marriage Counseling. Palo Alto, CA, Science & Behavior Books, 1969
Arevalo J, Vizcarro C: "Emocion Expresada" y curso de la esquizofrenia en una muestra Espanola. Analisis y Modificacion de Conducta 15:3–23, 1989
Ariel S: Strategic Family Play Therapy. Chichester, West Sussex, England, Wiley, 1992
Aries P, Duby G: A History of Private Life, Vol 3. Cambridge, MA, Belknap Press, 1989
Armsworth M, Holaday M: The effects of psychological trauma on children and adolescents. Journal of Counseling and Development 72:49–56, 1997
Arnow B, Taylor D, Agras W, et al: Enhancing agoraphobia treatment outcome by changing couple communication patterns. Behav Ther 16:452–467, 1985
Asante MK: Kemet, Afrocentricity, and Knowledge. Trenton, NJ, Africa World Press, 1990
Asarnow J, Goldstein M, Ben-Meir S: Parental communication deviance in childhood onset schizophrenia spectrum and depressive disorders. J Child Psychol Psychiatry 29:825–838, 1988
Atkeson B, Forehand R: Parent behavioral training for problem children: an examination of studies using multiple outcome measures. J Abnorm Child Psychol 6:449–460, 1978
Atkinson JM, Coia DA, Gilmour WH, et al: The impact of education groups for people with schizophrenia on social functioning and quality of life. Br J Psychiatry 168:199–204, 1996
Atwood DL, Dershowitz S: Constructing a sex and marital therapy frame: ways to help couples deconstruct sexual problems. J Sex Marital Ther 18:196–218, 1992
Augenbaum B, Tasem M: Differential techniques in family interviewing with both parents and preschool child. Journal of the American Academy of Child Psychiatry 5:721–730, 1966
Ault-Riche M: Women and Family Therapy. Rockville, MD, Aspen, 1986
Avis J: The politics of functional family therapy: a feminist critique. J Marital Fam Ther 11:127–138, 1985
Avis J: "Working together": an enrichment program for dual-career couples. Journal of Psychotherapy and the Family 2:29–46, 1986
Avis J: Power politics in therapy with women, in Feminist Family Therapy: A Casebook. Edited by Goodrich T, Rampage C, Ellman B, et al. New York, WW Norton, 1988
Axline VM: Play Therapy. New York, Ballantine Books, 1969

Azrin NH: Improvements in the community reinforcement approach to alcoholism. Behav Res Ther 14:339–348, 1976

Azrin NH, Naster BJ, Jones R: Reciprocity counseling: a rapid learning-based procedure for marital counseling. Behav Res Ther 11:365–382, 1973

Azrin NH, Schaeffer RM, Wesolowski MD: A rapid method of teaching profoundly retarded persons to dress by a reinforcement-guidance method. Ment Retard 14:29–33, 1976

Azrin NH, Sisson R, Meyers R, et al: Alcoholism treatment by disulfiram and community reinforcement therapy. J Behav Ther Exp Psychiatry 13:105–112, 1982

Baber K, Allen K: Women and Families: Feminist Reconstructions. New York, Guilford, 1992

Bachrach A: Learning theory, in Comprehensive Textbook of Psychiatry/IV, Fourth Edition, Vol 1. Edited by Kaplan HI, Sadock BJ. Baltimore, MD, Williams & Wilkins, 1985, pp 184–197

Bagarozzi DA (ed): Family measurement techniques: the Family Coping Strategies Scale. American Journal of Family Therapy 13(2):69–71, 1985

Bagarozzi DA: Some issues to consider in the assessment of marital/family functioning. American Journal of Family Therapy 14(1):84–86, 1986

Bagarozzi DA: Marital/family developmental theory as a context for understanding and treating sexual desire. Journal of Sex and Marital Theory 13:276–285, 1987

Bagarozzi DA, Giddings CW: Conjugal violence: a critical review of current research and practices. American Journal of Family Therapy 11(1):1–3, 1983

Bahnson C: A historical family systems approach to heart disease and cancer, in A New Image of Man in Medicine. Edited by Shaefer KE. Mount Kisco, NY, Futura Publishing, 1986, pp 101–123

Bahr SJ: SIMFAM as a measure of conjugal power. Paper presented at the National Council on Family Relations, 1969

Bakeman R, Gottman JM: Observing Interaction: An Introduction to Sequential Analysis, 2nd Edition. New York, Cambridge University Press, 1997

Baker D: Father-daughter incest: a study of the father. Unpublished doctoral dissertation, California School of Professional Psychology, San Diego, CA, 1985 [Dissertation Abstracts International 46(03):951B, 1985]

Baker KG, Gippenreiter JB: The effects of Stalin's purge on three generations of Russian families. Family Systems: A Journal of Natural Systems Theory in Psychiatry and the Sciences 3(1):5–35, 1996

Baker LA, Daniels D: Nonshared environmental influences and personality differences in adult twins. J Pers Soc Psychol 58:103–110, 1990

Baker TB, Sobell MB, Sobell LC, et al: Halfway houses for alcoholics: a review, analysis and comparison with other halfway house facilities. Int J Soc Psychiatry 22:130–139, 1976

Baker-Fleming J: Stopping Wife Abuse: A Guide to the Emotional and Psychological Implications. Garden City, NY, Harper, 1979

Bancroft J, Coles L: Three years experience in a sexual problems clinic. BMJ 1:1575–1577, 1976

Bandura A: Principles of Behavior Modification. New York, Holt, Rinehart, & Winston, 1969

Bandura A: Aggression: A Social Learning Analysis. Englewood Cliffs, NJ, Prentice-Hall, 1973

Bandura A: Social Learning Theory. Englewood Cliffs, NJ, Prentice-Hall, 1977

Bandura A: Social Foundations of Thought and Action: A Social Cognitive Theory. Englewood Cliffs, NJ, Prentice-Hall, 1986

Bandura A: Self-Efficacy: The Exercise of Control. New York, WH Freeman, 1997

Bandura A, Walters R: Social Learning and Personality Development. New York, Holt, Rinehart, & Winston, 1963

Bank SP, Kahn M: The Sibling Bond. New York, Basic Books, 1982

Barbaree HE, Marshall WL: Erectile responses amongst heterosexual child molesters, father-daughter incest offenders and matched nonoffenders: five distinct age preference profiles. Can J Behav Sci (in press)

Bardwick J: Psychology of Women: A Study of Bio-Cultural Conflicts. New York, Harper & Row, 1971

Barkley RA: Hyperactive girls and boys: stimulant drug effects on mother-child interactions. J Child Psychol Psychiatry 30:379–390, 1989

Barkley RA: Commentary on the Multimodal Treatment Study of Children With ADHD. J Abnorm Child Psychol 28:595–599, 2000a

Barkley RA: Taking Charge of ADHD: The Complete, Authoritative Guide for Parents, Revised Edition. New York, Guilford, 2000b

Barkley RA, Anastopoulos AD, Guevremont DC, et al: Adolescents with attention deficit hyperactivity disorder: mother-adolescent interactions, family beliefs and conflicts, and maternal psychopathology. J Abnorm Psychol 20:263–288, 1992a

Barkley RA, Anastopoulos AD, Guevremont DC, et al: Frontal lobe functions in attention deficit disorder with and without hyperactivity: a review and research report. J Abnorm Child Psychol 20:163–188, 1992b

Barkley RA, Guevremont DC, Anastopoulos AD, et al: A comparison of three family therapy programs for treating family conflicts in adolescents with attention-deficit hyperactivity disorder. J Consult Clin Psychol 60:450–462, 1992c

Barkley RA, Fischer M, Smallish L, et al: The persistence of attention deficit hyperactivity disorder into young adulthood as a function of reporting source and definition of disorder. J Abnorm Psychol 111:279–289, 2000a

Barkley RA, Shelton TL, Crosswait C, et al: Multi-method psycho-educational intervention for preschool children with disruptive behavior: preliminary results at post-treatment. J Child Psychol Psychiatry 41:319–332, 2000b

Barkley RA, Edwards G, Laneri M, et al: The efficacy of problem-solving communication training alone, behavior management alone, and their combination for parent-adolescent conflict in teenagers with ADHD and ODD. J Consult Clin Psychol 69:926–941, 2001

Barkley RA, Shelton TL, Crosswait C, et al: Preschool children with disruptive behavior: three-year outcome as a function of adaptive disability. Dev Psychopathol 14:45–67, 2002

Barnes J: Social networks, in Urban Situations. Edited by Mitchell JD. Manchester, UK, Manchester University Press, 1969

Barrelet L, Ferrero F, Szigethy L: Expressed emotion and first admission schizophrenia: nine-month follow-up in a French environment. Br J Psychiatry 156:357–362, 1990

Barrowclough C, Tarrier N: Social functioning in schizophrenic patients: the effects of expressed emotion and family intervention. Soc Psychiatry Psychiatr Epidemiol 25:125–130, 1990

Bartholomew K, Horowitz L: Attachment styles among young adults: a test of a four category model. J Pers Soc Psychol 61:226–244, 1991

Bartholomew K, Perlman D: Attachment processes in adulthood, in Advances in Personal Relationships, Vol 5. London, PA, Jessica Kingsley Publications, 1992

Barton C, Alexander J: Functional family therapy, in Handbook of Family Therapy. Edited by Gurman AS, Kniskern DP. New York, Brunner/Mazel, 1981, pp 456–498

Bass E, Davis L: The Courage to Heal. New York, Harper & Row, 1988

Bassi V: The genesis of family therapy: an oral history of the years 1945–1960. Unpublished doctoral dissertation, California School of Professional Psychology, Alameda, CA, 1991

Bassoff E: The memory board: a therapeutic activity for married couples. Journal of Counseling and Development 64:70–71, 1985

Bateson G: Steps to an Ecology of Mind. New York, Ballantine Books, 1972

Bateson G: Mind and Nature: A Necessary Unity. New York, Dutton, 1979

Bateson G, Jackson D, Haley J, et al: Toward a theory of schizophrenia. Behav Sci 1(4):251–264, 1956

Baucom D: The active ingredients of behavioral marital therapy: the effectiveness of problem-solving/communication training, contingency contracting, and their combinations, in Marital Interaction. Edited by Hahlweg K, Jacobson NS. New York, Guilford, 1984, pp 73–87

Baucom D, Aiken P: Sex role identity, marital satisfaction, and response to behavioral marital therapy. J Consult Clin Psychol 52:438–444, 1984

Baucom D, Epstein N: Cognitive Behavioral Marital Therapy. New York, Brunner/Mazel, 1990

Baucom DH, Epstein N: Will the real cognitive behavioral marital therapy please stand up? Journal of Family Therapy 4:394–401, 1991

Baucom D, Hoffman J: The effectiveness of marital therapy: current status and application to the clinical setting, in Clinical Handbook of Marital Therapy. Edited by Jacobson NS, Gurman AS. New York, Guilford, 1986, pp 597–620

Baucom DH, Lester GW: The usefulness of cognitive restructuring as an adjunct to behavioral marital therapy. Behav Ther 17:385–403, 1986

Baucom DH, Epstein NB, Sayers S, et al: The role of cognition in marital relationships: definitional, methodological, and conceptual issues. J Consult Clin Psychol 57:31–38, 1989

Baucom D, Sayers S, Sher T: Supplementing behavioral marital therapy with cognitive restructuring and emotional expressiveness training: an outcome investigation. J Consult Clin Psychol 58:636–645, 1990

Baucom DH, Shoham V, Mueser KT, et al: Empirically supported couple and family interventions for marital distress and adult mental health problems. J Consult Clin Psychol 66:53–88, 1998

Baum CG, Forehand R: Long term assessment of parent training by use of multiple outcome measures. Behavior Therapy 12:643–652, 1981

Bäuml J, Kissling W, Pitschel-Walz G: Psychoedukative Gruppen für schizophrene Patienten: Einfluss auf Wissenstand und Compliance. Nervenheilkunde 15:145–150, 1996

Baumrind D: The development of instrumental competence through socialization, in Minnesota Symposia on Child Psychology, Vol 7. Edited by Pick AD. Minneapolis, University of Minnesota Press, 1973

Beach R, Bauserman S: Enhancing the effectiveness of marital therapy, in The Psychology of Marriage. Edited by Fincham FD, Bradbury TN. New York, Guilford, 1990, pp 349–375

Beach S, O'Leary K: Current status of outcome research in marital therapy, in Handbook of Family and Marital Therapy, Vol 2. Edited by L'Abate L. Homewood, IL, Dorsey Press, 1985, pp 1035–1072

Beach S, O'Leary K: The treatment of depression occurring in the context of marital discord. Behav Ther 17:43–49, 1986

Beach S, O'Leary K: Treating depression in the context of marital discord: outcome and predictors of response for marital therapy vs. cognitive therapy. Behav Ther 23:507–528, 1992

Beach S, Sandeen E, O'Leary K: Treatment for the depressed, maritally discordant client. Paper presented at the Association for Advancement of Behavioral Therapy, Boston, MA, 1987

Beardslee W, Podorefsky D: Resilient adolescents whose parents have serious affective and other psychiatric disorders: importance of self-understanding and relationships. Am J Psychiatry 145:63–69, 1988

Beardslee W, Schwoeri L: Preventive intervention with children of depressed parents, in Depression in Children and Families: Assessments and Interventions. Edited by Sholevar GP, Schwoeri L. New York, Jason Aronson, 1994

Beardslee W, Bemporad J, Keller M, et al: Children of parents with major affective disorder: a review. Am J Psychiatry 140:825–832, 1983

Beardslee W, Keller M, Klerman G: Children of parents with affective disorder. International Journal of Family Psychiatry 6:283–299, 1985

Beardslee W, Klerman G, Keeler M, et al: But are they cases? Validity of DSM-III major depression in children identified in family study. Am J Psychiatry 142:687–691, 1987a

Beardslee W, Schultz L, Selman R: Level of social-cognitive development, adaptive functioning, and DSM-III diagnoses in adolescent offspring of parents with affective disorders: implications of the development of the capacity for mutuality. Dev Psychol 23:807–815, 1987b

Beardslee W, Keller M, Lavori P, et al: Psychiatric disorder in adolescent offspring parents with affective disorder in a non-referred sample. J Affect Disord 15:313–322, 1988

Beardslee WR, Wright EJ, Salt P, et al: Examination of children's responses to two preventive intervention strategies over time. J Am Acad Child Adolesc Psychiatry 36:196–204, 1996a

Beardslee WR, Wright E, Rothberg PC, et al: Response to families to two preventive intervention strategies: long-term differences in behavior and attitude change. J Am Acad Child Adolesc Psychiatry 35:774–782, 1996b

Beardslee WR, Salt P, Versage EM, et al: Sustained change in parents receiving preventive interventions for families with depression. Am J Psychiatry 154:510–515, 1997

Beardslee WR, Swatling S, Hoke L, et al: From cognitive information to shared meaning: healing principles in prevention intervention. Psychiatry 61:112–129, 1998a

Beardslee WR, Versage EM, Gladstone TRG: Children of affectively ill parents: a review of the past 10 years. J Am Acad Child Adolesc Psychiatry 37:1134–1141, 1998b

Beattie M: Codependent No More. Baltimore, MD, Harper/Hazeldon, 1987

Beavers JS, Hampson RB, Hulgus YF, et al: Coping in families with a retarded child. Fam Process 25:365–378, 1986

Beavers WR: Psychotherapy and Growth: A Family Systems Perspective. New York, Brunner/Mazel, 1977

Beavers WR: Healthy, midrange, and severely dysfunctional families, in Normal Family Processes. Edited by Walsh F. New York, Guilford, 1982

Beavers WR: Successful Marriage: A Family Systems Approach to Marital Therapy. New York, WW Norton, 1985

Beavers WR: A clinically useful model of family assessment, in Family Systems in Medicine. Edited by Ramsay C. New York, Guilford, 1988

Beavers WR, Hampson RB: Successful Families. New York, WW Norton, 1990

Beavers WR, Hampton RB: The Beavers System Model of Family Functioning. Journal of Family Therapy 22:128–143, 2000

Beavers WR, Hampton RB: Measuring daily competence, in Normal Fam Processes, 3rd Edition. Edited by Walsh F. New York, Guilford (in press)

Beavers WR, Kaslow FW: The anatomy of hope. J Marital Fam Ther 7:119–126, 1981

Beavers WR, Voeller MN: Family models: comparing the Olson Circumplex Model with the Beavers System Model. Fam Process 22:85–98, 1983

Beavers WR, Lewis JM, Phillips VA, et al: Developing a family evaluation scale: a preliminary report. Paper presented at Southwestern Regional Meeting, American Orthopsychiatric Association, Galveston, TX, 1972

Bebbington P: Marital status and depression: a study of English national admission statistics. Acta Psychiatr Scand 75:640–650, 1987a

Bebbington P: Misery and beyond: the pursuit of disease theories of depression. Int J Soc Psychiatry 33:13–20, 1987b

Beck A: Love Is Never Enough: How Couples Can Overcome Misunderstandings, Resolve Conflicts and Solve Relationship Problems Through Cognitive Therapy. New York, Harper & Row, 1988

Beck A, Ward C, Mendelson M, et al: An inventory for measuring depression. Arch Gen Psychiatry 4:561–571, 1961

Beck A, Rush A, Shaw B, et al: Cognitive Therapy of Depression. New York, Guilford, 1979

Beels C: Family and social management of schizophrenia. Schizophr Bull 13:97–118, 1975

Beels C, Ferber A: What family therapists do, in The Book of Family Therapy. Edited by Ferber A, Mendelsohn M, Napier A. Boston, MA, Houghlin Mifflin, 1972

Beels C, McFarlane W: Family treatments of schizophrenia: background and state of the art. Hospital and Community Psychiatry 33:541–550, 1982

Behar D, Stewart M: Aggressive conduct disorder of children. Acta Psychiatr Scand 65: 210–220, 1982

Bell JE: Family Therapy. New York, Jason Aronson, 1975

Bellack AS, Mueser KT: Psychological treatment. Schizophr Bull (in press)

Bem D: Self-perception: an alternative interpretation of cognitive dissonance phenomenon. Affective Psychological Review 74:183–200, 1967

Bemporad J, Sholevar G, Schwoeri L: Psychodynamic psychotherapy with depressed children and adolescents, in The Transmission of Depression in Families and Children. Edited by Sholevar GP, Schwoeri L. New York, Jason Aronson, 1994

Bennett L, Wolin S: Family culture and alcoholism transmission, in Alcohol and the Family. Edited by Collins RL, Leonard KE, Searles JS. New York, Guilford, 1987

Bennett LA, Wolin SJ, McAvity K: Family identity, ritual, and myth: a cultural perspective on life cycle transitions, in Family Transitions. Edited by Falicov CJ. New York, Plenum, 1988, pp 221–234

Bennett SR: Cognitive style of incestuous fathers. Unpublished doctoral dissertation, Texas Tech University. [Dissertation Abstracts International 42(2):778B, 1985]

Bennun I, Rust J, Golombok S: The effects of marital therapy on sexual satisfaction. Scandinavian Journal of Behavior Therapy 14:65–72, 1985

Benson M, Schindler-Zimmerman T, Martin D: Accessing children's perceptions of their family: circular questioning revisited. J Marital Fam Ther 17:363–372, 1991

Bentsen H, Notland TH, Munkvold OG, et al: Guilt-proneness and expressed emotion in relatives with schizophrenia and related psychoses. Br J Med Psychol 71:125–138, 1998

Berely R, Jacobson N: Causal attributions in intimate relationships, in Advances in Cognitive Behavioral Research and Therapy, Vol 3. Edited by Kendall PC. New York, Academic Press, 1984

Berg IK, de Shazer S: Making numbers talk: language in therapy, in The New Language of Change: Constructive Collaboration in Psychotherapy. Edited by Friedman S. New York, Guilford, 1993, pp 5–24

Berg IK, Jaya A: Different and same: family therapy with Asian-American families. J Marital Fam Ther 19:31–38, 1993

Berglund N: How early intervention in psychiatric long-term illness patients and their families influences relapse, medication and family burden. Unpublished manuscript, 1996

Berkowitz D: An overview of the psychodynamics of couples—bridging concepts, in Marriage and Divorce, A Contemporary Perspective. Edited by Nadelson C, Polonsky D. New York, Guilford, 1984

Berkowitz R, Eberlein-Fries R, Kuipers L: Educating relatives about schizophrenia. Schizophr Bull 10:418–429, 1984

Berman CM: An animal model for the intergenerational transmission of maternal style? Family Systems 3:125–140, 1996

Berman E, Lief H: Marital therapy from a psychoanalytic perspective: an overview. Am J Psychiatry 132:583–592, 1975

Berman E, Lief H, Williams A: A model of marital interactions, in Handbook of Marriage and Marital Therapy. Edited by Sholevar GP. New York, SP Medical & Scientific Books, 1981, p 3

Berman J, Luna AM: Suicide diaries and the therapeutics of anonymous self-disclosure. Journal of Psychoanalysis of Culture & Society 1(1):63–76, 1996

Bernal G, Alvarez A: Culture and class in the study of families, in Cultural Perspectives in Family Therapy. Edited by Hansen FC, Falicov C. San Francisco, University of California/Aspen Systems, 1983

Bernal G, Flores-Ortiz Y, Sorenson JL, et al: Intergenerational family therapy with methadone maintenance patients and family members: findings of a critical outcome study (in press)

Bernal ME, Williams DE, Miller WH, et al: The use of videotape feedback and operant learning principles in training parents in management of deviant children, in Advances in Behavior Therapy. Edited by Rubin RD, Festerheim H, Henderson JD, et al. New York, Academic Press, 1972

Berne E: Games People Play. New York, Grove Press, 1964

Bernheim D, Lehman A: Working With Families of the Mentally Ill. New York, WW Norton, 1985

Bernheim KF: The Caring Family: Living With Chronic Mental Illness. New York, Random House, 1982

Berns SB, Jacobson NS, Gottman JM: Demand/withdraw interaction patterns between different types of batterers and their spouses. Journal of Marriage and Family Therapy 25:337–348, 1999

Bertalanffy L von: General System Theory. New York, George Braziller, 1968

Bertrando P, Bressi C, Clerici M, et al: Terapia familare sistemica ed emotivita espressa nella schizofrenia cronica. Uno studio preliminare. Attraverso lo Specchio 25:511–562, 1989

Bertrando P, Beltz J, Bressi C, et al: Expressed emotion and schizophrenia in Italy, a study of an urban population. Br J Psychiatry 161:223–229, 1992

Besalel VA, Azrin NH: The reduction of parent-youth problems by reciprocity counseling. Behav Res Ther 19:297–301, 1981

Beschner GM, Friedman AS: Treatment of adolescent drug abusers. International Journal of the Addictions 20:971–993, 1985

Besharov DJ: Recognizing Child Abuse: A Guide for the Concerned. New York, Free Press, 1990

Bethards JM: Parental support and the use of drugs. Humboldt Journal of Social Relations 28:234–238, 1973

Beutler L, Williams R, Wakefield P: Obstacles to disseminating applied psychological science. Applied and Preventative Psychology 2:53–58, 1993

Biglan A, Hops H, Sherman L: Problem solving interactions of depressed women and their husbands. Behavior Therapy 16:431–451, 1988

Billings A: Conflict resolution in distressed and nondistressed married couples. J Consult Clin Psychol 47:368–376, 1979

Billings AG, Moos RH: The role of coping responses and social resources in attenuating the stress of life events. J Behav Med 4:139–157, 1981

Billings A, Cronkite RC, Moos RH: Social-environmental factors in unipolar depression: comparisons of depressed patients and nondepressed controls. J Abnorm Psychol 92:119–123, 1983

Billingsley A: Black Families in White America. Englewood Cliffs, NJ, Prentice-Hall, 1968

Bion WR: Learning From Experience. London, Tavistock, 1962

Birchler GR: Behavioral-systems marital therapy. Advances in Family Intervention, Assessment and Theory 3:1–40, 1983

Birchler GR: Handling resistance to change, in Handbook of Behavioral Family Therapy. Edited by Falloon IRH. New York, Guilford, 1988

Birchler GR, Weiss RL, Vincent JP: Multimethod analysis of social reinforcement exchange between distressed and non-distressed spouse and stranger dyads. J Pers Soc Psychol 31:349–360, 1975

Birtchnell J: Depression and family relationships: a study of young, married women in a London housing estate. Br J Psychiatry 153:758–769, 1988

Birtchnell J, Kennard J: Does marital maladjustment lead to mental illness? Soc Psychiatry 18:79–88, 1983

Black D, Urbanowicz MA: Family intervention with bereaved children. J Child Psychol Psychiatry 28:467–476, 1987

Black E: Women's relationships with larger systems, in Women in Families. Edited by Black E. New York, WW Norton, 1989, pp 335–353

Blackburn IM, Bishop S, Glenn MI, et al: The efficacy of cognitive therapy in depression: a treatment trial using cognitive therapy and pharmacotherapy, each alone and in combination. Br J Psychiatry 139:181–189, 1981

Blaney NT, Goodkin K, Feaster D, et al: A psychosocial model of distress over time in early HIV-1 infection: the role of life stressors, social support and coping. Psychology and Health 12:633–653, 1997

Blashfield RK: The Classification of Psychopathology: Neo-Kraepelinian and Quantitative Approaches. New York, Plenum, 1984

Bleiberg A: Psychodynamic psychotherapy, in Conduct Disorders in Children and Adolescents. Edited by Sholevar GP. Washington, DC, American Psychiatric Press, 1995, pp 147–172

Bloch DA: Including the children in family therapy, in Family Therapy. Edited by Guerin P. New York, Gardner Press, 1976, pp 168–181

Bloch D: Family systems medicine: the field and the journal. Family Systems Medicine 1:3–12, 1983

Bloom BL, Kindle KR: Demographic factors in the continuing relationship between spouses. Family Relations: Journal of Applied Family and Child Studies 34:375–381, 1985

Bloomquist ML, Harris WG: Measuring family functioning with the MMPI: a reliability and concurrent validity study of three MMPI scales. J Clin Psychol 40:1209–1303, 1984

Blum RH: Horatio Alger's Children. San Francisco, CA, Jossey-Bass, 1972

Blume S: Women, alcohol and drugs. Paper presented at the annual meeting of the American Psychiatric Association, Philadelphia, PA, May 21–26, 1994

Boake C, Salmon PG: Demographic correlates and factor structure of the Family Environment Scales. J Clin Psychol 39:95–100, 1983

Bodin AM: Conjoint family assessment, in Advances in Psychological Assessment, Vol 1. Edited by McReynolds P. Palo Alto, CA, Science & Behavior Books, 1968

Bodin A, Ferber A: How to go beyond the use of language, in The Book of Family Therapy. Edited by Ferber A, Mendolsohn M, Napier A. Boston, MA, Houghlin Mifflin, 1971

Boelens W, Emmelkamp P, MacGillavry D, et al: A clinical evaluation of marital treatment: reciprocity counselling versus system-theoretic counseling. Behavioral Analysis and Modification 4:85–96, 1980

Bograd M: Strengthening domestic violence theories: intersections of race, class, sexual orientation, and gender. Journal of Marriage and Family Therapy 25:275–289, 1999

Bograd M, Mederos F: Battering and couples therapy: universal screening and selection of treatment modality. J Marital Fam Ther 25:291–312, 1999

Boscolo L, Cecchin G, Hoffman L, et al: Milan Systemic Family Therapy. New York, Basic Books, 1987

Boss PA: Clarification of the concept of psychological-father presence in families experiencing ambiguity of boundary. Journal of Marriage and the Family 37:141–151, 1977

Boszormenyi-Nagy I: Hospital Organization and Family Oriented Psychotherapy of Schizophrenia. 1961

Boszormenyi-Nagy I: Loyalty implications of the transference model in psychotherapy. Arch Gen Psychiatry 27:374–380, 1972

Boszormenyi-Nagy I: A theory of relationships: experience and transactions (1965), in Intensive Family Psychotherapy. Edited by Boszormenyi-Nagy I, Framo J. New York, Harper & Row, 1985, pp 33–86

Boszormenyi-Nagy I: Between Give and Take: Clinical Guide to Contextual Therapy. New York, Brunner/Mazel, 1986

Boszormenyi-Nagy I: Contextual therapy and the unity of therapies (1966), in Foundations of Contextual Therapy. Edited by Boszormenyi-Nagy I. New York, Brunner/Mazel, 1987a, pp 319–332
Boszormenyi-Nagy I: Correlations between mental illness and intracellular metabolism (1958), in Foundations of Contextual Therapy. Edited by Boszormenyi-Nagy I. New York, Brunner/Mazel, 1987b, pp 3–7
Boszormenyi-Nagy I: Foundation of contextual therapy (1958), in Foundations of Contextual Therapy. Edited by Boszormenyi-Nagy I. New York, Brunner/Mazel, 1987c, pp 8–19
Boszormenyi-Nagy I: Transgenerational solidarity: the expanding context of therapy and prevention (1986), in Foundations of Contextual Therapy. Edited by Boszormenyi-Nagy I. New York, Brunner/Mazel, 1987d, pp 292–318
Boszormenyi-Nagy I, Spark GM: Invisible Loyalties: Reciprocity in Intergenerational Family Therapy, Second Edition. New York, Brunner/Mazel, 1984
Bott E: Family and Social Network. London, Tavistock, 1957
Boughner SR, Hayes SF, Bubenzer DL, et al: Use of standardized assessment instruments by marital and family therapists: a survey. J Marital Fam Ther 20:69–75, 1994
Boutselis M, Zarit SH: Burden and distress of dementia caregivers: effects of gender and relationship. Paper presented at the meeting of the Gerontological Society of America, San Antonio, TX, November 1984
Bowen GL: Navigating the Marital Journey, MAP: A Corporate Support Program for Couples. New York, Praeger, 1991
Bowen M: Family psychotherapy. Am J Orthopsychiatry 31:40–60, 1961
Bowen M: The use of family theory in clinical practice. Compr Psychiatry 7:345–374, 1966
Bowen M: Family reaction to death, in Family Therapy: Theory and Practice. Edited by Guerin P. New York, Gardner Press, 1976a, pp 335–350
Bowen M: Theory in the practice of psychotherapy, in Family Therapy: Theory and Practice. Edited by Guerin P. New York, Gardner Press, 1976b
Bowen M: Family Therapy in Clinical Practice. New York, Jason Aronson, 1978
Bowen M, Kerr K, Nowakowski L, et al: Aging: A Symposium. Georgetown Medical Bulletin 30:6–29, 1977
Bowlby J: The study and reduction of group tensions in the family. Hum Relat 2:123–128, 1949
Bowlby J: Attachment and Loss, Vol 1: Attachment. New York, Basic Books, 1969
Bowlby J: The making and breaking of affectional bonds, II: some principles of psychotherapy. Br J Psychiatry 130:421–431, 1977
Bowlby J: A Secure Base: Parent-Child Attachment and Healthy Human Development. New York, Basic Books, 1988
Bowman CG, Mertz E: A dangerous direction: legal intervention in sexual abuse. Harvard Law Review 109:549–639, 1996
Bowman ES: Delayed memories of child abuse, Part II: an overview of research findings related to understanding their reliability and suggestibility. Dissociation: Progress in Dissociative Disorders 9:232–243, 1996
Boyd-Franklin N: The contribution of family therapy models to the treatment of black families. Psychotherapy 24:621–629, 1987
Boyd-Franklin N: Black Families in Therapy: A Multisystems Approach. New York, Guilford, 1989
Boyle M, Offord D: Primary prevention of conduct disorder: issues and prospects. J Am Acad Child Adolesc Psychiatry 29:227–233, 1990
Bradbury TN: The Developmental Course of Marital Dysfunction. New York, Cambridge University Press, 1998
Bradbury TN, Fincham FD: Affect and cognition in close relationships: towards an integrative model. Cognition and Emotion 1:59–87, 1987a

Bradbury TN, Fincham FD: Assessment of affect in marriage, in Assessment of Marital Discord: An Integration for Research and Clinical Practice. Edited by O'Leary KD. Hillsdale, NJ, Lawrence Erlbaum, 1987b, pp 59–108
Bradbury T, Fincham F: Attributions in marriage: review of critique. Psychol Bull 107:3–33, 1990
Bradbury TN, Fincham FD: A contextual model for advancing the study of marital interaction, in Cognition in Close Relationships. Edited by Fletcher GJO, Fincham FD. Hillsdale, NJ, Lawrence Erlbaum, 1991, pp 127–147
Brandon C: Sex role identification in incest: an empirical analysis of the feminist theories. Unpublished doctoral dissertation, California School of Professional Psychology, Fresno, CA [Dissertation Abstracts International 47(7):3099B, 1985]
Brant RST, Tisza VB: Sexually misused child. Am J Orthopsychiatry 47:80–90, 1977
Bray J: Children's development during early remarriage, in Impact of Divorce, Single Parenting, and Stepparenting on Children. Edited by Hetherington EM, Arasteh J. Hillsdale, NJ, Lawrence Erlbaum, 1988, pp 279–298
Bray JH, Kelly J: Stepfamilies: Love, Marriage, and Parenting in the First Decade. New York, Broadway Books, 1998
Brent D: The aftercare of adolescents with deliberate self-harm. J Child Psychol Psychiatry 38:277–286, 1997
Brent DA, Roth CM, Holder D, et al: Psychosocial interventions for treating adolescent suicidal depression: a comparison of three psychosocial interventions, in Euthymia: Psychosocial Treatments for Child and Adolescent Disorders. Edited by Hibbs JP. Washington, DC, American Psychological Association, 1996, pp 187–206
Brent D, Holder D, Kolko D, et al: A clinical psychotherapy trial for adolescent depression comparing cognitive, family, and supportive psychotherapy. Arch Gen Psychiatry 54:877–885, 1997
Brewin CR: Changes in attribution and expressed emotion among the relatives of patients with schizophrenia. Psychol Med 24:905–911, 1994
Briere J: Child Abuse Trauma: Theory and Treatment of the Lasting Effects. Newbury Park, CA, Sage, 1992
Briggs-Myers I, McCauley M: Manual: A Guide to the Development and Use of the Myers-Briggs Type Indicator. Palo Alto, CA, Consulting Psychologists Press, 1985
Brock GW: Beavers-Timberlawn Family Evaluation Scale. American Journal of Family Therapy 14:271–273, 1986
Brock G, Joanning H: A comparison of the Relationship Enhancement Program and the Minnesota Couple Communication Program. J Marital Fam Ther 9:413–421, 1983
Broddy G, Pillegrini A, Sigel I: Marital quality and mother-child and father-child interactions with school-aged children. Dev Psychol 22:291–296, 1986
Broderick CB, Schrader SS: The history of professional marriage and family therapy, in Handbook of Family Therapy. Edited by Gurman AS, Kniskern DP. New York, Brunner/Mazel, 1981
Broderick J, O'Leary K: Contributions of affect, attitudes and behavior to marital satisfaction. J Consult Clin Psychol 54:514–517, 1986
Brodew MJ, Agresti AA: Responding to therapists' sexual abuse of incest survivors. Psychotherapy 35:96–104, 1998
Brodsky A, Hare-Mustin RT (eds): Women and Psychotherapy. New York, Guilford, 1980
Brody EM: The family at risk, in Alzheimer's Disease, Treatment and Family Stress: Directions for Research. Edited by Light E, Lebowitz B. Rockville, MD, U.S. Department of Health and Human Services, 1989, pp 2–49
Brody EM, Schoonover CB: Patterns of parent-care when adult daughters work and when they do not. Gerontologist 26:372–381, 1986
Brody EM, Spark G: Institutionalization of the aged: a family crisis. Fam Process 5:76–90, 1966
Brody S: Simultaneous psychotherapy of married couples in current psychiatric therapy, in Current Psychiatric Therapy. Edited by Masserman J. New York, Grune & Stratton, 1980

Broman CL: Coping with personal problems, in Mental Health in Black America. Edited by Neighbors HW, Jackson JS. Thousand Oaks, CA, Sage, 1996, pp 117–129

Bronfenbrenner U: Toward an experimental ecology of human development. Am Psychol 32:513–531, 1977

Brooker C, Tarrier N, Barrowclough C, et al: Training community psychiatric nurses for psychosocial intervention: report of a pilot study. Br J Psychiatry 160:836–844, 1992

Brooker C, Falloon I, Butterworth A, et al: The outcome of training community psychiatric nurses to deliver psychosocial intervention. Br J Psychiatry 165:222–230, 1994

Brown G, Birley J: Crises and life change and the onset of schizophrenia. J Health Soc Behav 9:203–214, 1968

Brown G, Harris T: Social Origins of Depression. New York, Free Press, 1978

Brown GW, Rutter M: The measurement of family activities and relationships. Human Relations 19:241–263, 1966

Brown G, Monck E, Carstairs G: Influence of family life on the course of schizophrenic illness. Br J Prev Soc Med 16:55–68, 1962

Brown G, Birley J, Wing J: Influence of family life on the course of schizophrenic disorders: a replication. Br J Psychiatry 121:241–258, 1972

Brown GW, Harris T, Copeland JR: Depression and loss. Br J Psychiatry 130:1–18, 1977

Brown JH, Christensen DN: Family Therapy: Theory and Practice, 2nd Edition. Pacific Grove, CA, Brooks/Cole Publishing, 1999

Browne A: Violence against women by male partners: prevalence, outcomes, and policy implications. Am Psychol 48:1077–1087, 1993

Browne A, Finkelhor D: Impact of child sexual abuse: a review of the research. Psychol Bull 99:66–77, 1986

Browne KD, Foreman L, Middleton D: Predicting treatment drop-out in sex offenders. Child Abuse Review 7:402–419, 1998

Bruner J: Acts of Meaning. Cambridge, MA, Harvard University Press, 1968

Bruner J: Culture and human development: a new look. Human Development 33:344–355, 1990

Brunk M, Henggeler SW, Whelan JP: Comparison of multisystemic therapy and parent training in the brief treatment of child abuse and neglect. J Consult Clin Psychol 55:171–178, 1987

Buber M: Guilt and guilt feelings. Psychiatry 20:114–129, 1957

Buchkremer G, Schultze-Monking H, Holle R, et al: The impact of therapeutic relative's groups on the course of illness of schizophrenic patients. Eur Psychiatry 10:17–27, 1995

Burg JE, Sprenkle DH: Sex therapy, in Family Therapy Sourcebook. Edited by Piercy F, Sprenkle DH, Wetchler JL. New York, Guilford, 1996, pp 153–180

Burgess EW: The family as a unity of interacting personalities. Family 7:3–9, 1926 (Reprinted in Family Therapy: An Introduction to Theory and Technique. Edited by Erikson GD, Hogan TP. New York, Jason Aronson, 1976)

Burgess RL, Conger RD: Family interaction in abusive, neglectful, and normal families. Child Dev 49:1163–1173, 1978

Burman B, Margolin G: Analysis of the association between marital relationships and health problems: an interactional perspective. Psychol Bull 112:39–63, 1992

Burns DD, Sayers SL: Development and validation of a brief relationship satisfaction scale. Unpublished manuscript, 1992

Burns RC, Kaufman SH: Actions, Styles and Symbols in Kinetic Family Drawings (K-F-D). New York, Brunner/Mazel, 1972

Burvill PW: An appraisal of the NIMH Epidemiologic Catchment Area Program. Aust N Z J Psychiatry 21:175–184, 1987

Butzlaff RL, Hooley JM: Expressed emotion and psychiatric relapse. Arch Gen Psychiatry 55:547–552, 1998

Cadoret RJ: Genetics of alcoholism, in Alcohol and the Family. Edited by Collins RL, Leonard KE, Searles JS. New York, Guilford, 1987

Cadoret R, Caine CA, Grove WM: Development of alcoholism in adoptees raised apart from alcoholic biologic relatives. Arch Gen Psychiatry 37:561–563, 1980

Cadoret R, Troughton E, O'Gorman TW, et al: An adaptation study of genetic and environmental factors in drug abuse. Arch Gen Psychiatry 43:1131–1136, 1986

Calhoun JB: Population density and social pathology. Sci Am 206:139–148, 1962

Calof D: Treating adult survivors of sexual abuse. Workshop presentation at the Family Therapy Network Symposium, Washington, DC, 1987

Calvo G: Marriage Encounter. St Paul, MN, Marriage Encounter, 1975

Campbell D, Draper R, Crutchley E: The Milan systemic approach to family therapy, in Handbook of Family Therapy, Vol 2. Edited by Gurman AS, Kniskern DP. New York, Brunner/Mazel, 1991, pp 325–362

Camper PM, Jacobson NS, Holtsworth-Munroe A, et al: Causal attribution and interactional behaviors in married couples. Cognitive Therapy and Research 12:195–209, 1988

Candib L, Glenn M: Family medicine and family therapy: comparative development methods, and roles. J Fam Pract 16:772–779, 1983

Cantos A, Neidg P, O'Leary D: Injuries of women and men in a treatment program for domestic violence. Journal of Family Violence 9:113–124, 1994

Caplan PJ, Hall-McCorquodale I: Mother-blaming in major clinical journals. Am J Orthopsychiatry 55:345–353, 1985a

Caplan PJ, Hall-McCorquodale I: The scapegoating of others: a call for change. Am J Orthopsychiatry 55:610–613, 1985b

Carey TC, Kempton TL, Gemmill WD: The significance of emotions in the affective presentation of sexually abused girls. Child Psychiatry Hum Dev 27:115–124, 1996

Cargo M: Psychopathology in married couples. Psychol Bull 77:114–138, 1972

Carter EA, McGoldrick M (eds): The Family Life Cycle. New York, Gardner Press, 1980a

Carter EA, McGoldrick M: The family life cycle and family therapy: an overview, in The Family Life Cycle. Edited by Carter EA, McGoldrick M. New York, Gardner Press, 1980b, pp 3–21

Cartwright C, Harary F: Structural balance: a generalization of Heider's theory. Psychol Rev 63:277–293, 1956

Cascardi M, Langhinrichsen J, Vivain D: Marital aggression: impact, injury, and health correlates for husbands and wives. Arch Intern Med 152:1178–1184, 1992

Cecchin G: Hypothesizing, circularity, neutrality revisited: an invitation to curiosity. Fam Process 26:405–413, 1987

Cerney J, Barlow D, Craske M, et al: Couples treatment of agoraphobia: at two year follow-up. Behavior Therapy 18:401–416, 1988

Chambless DL, Hollon SD: Defining empirically supported therapies. J Consult Clin Psychol 66:7–18, 1998

Chasin R: Involving latency and preschool children in family therapy, in Questions and Answers in the Practice of Family Therapy. Edited by Gurman A. New York, Brunner/Mazel, 1981, pp 32–35

Chasin R: Interviewing families with children: guidelines and suggestions, in Children in Family Therapy: Treatment and Training. Edited by Zilbach J. New York, Haworth, 1989, pp 15–30 Also in Journal of Psychotherapy and the Family 5(3/4):15–30, 1989

Chasin R, Roth S: Past perfect, future perfect: a positive approach to opening couple therapy, in One Couple, Four Realities: Multiple Perspectives on Couple Therapy. Edited by Chasin R, Grunebaum H, Herzig M. New York, Guilford, 1990, pp 129–144

Chasin R, White TB: The child in family therapy: guidelines for active engagement across the age span, in Children in Family Contexts. Edited by Combrinck-Graham L. New York, Guilford, 1988, pp 5–25

Chasin R, Roth S, Bograd M: Action methods in systemic therapy: dramatizing ideal futures and reformed pasts with couples. Fam Process 28:121–136, 1989

Chodorow N: The Reproduction of Mothering: Psychoanalysis and the Sociology of Gender. Berkeley, University of California Press, 1978

Chollak H: Stepfamily Adaptability and Cohesion: A Normative Study. Ann Arbor, MI, University Microfilms, 1985
Chou J: Videotaped discussion of working with Asian-American families. Working With Minority Families. Symposium conducted at the 142nd annual meeting of the American Psychiatric Association, San Francisco, CA, May 6–11, 1989
Christensen A: Assessment of behavior, in Assessment of Marital Discord. Edited by O'Leary KD. Hillsdale, NJ, Lawrence Erlbaum, 1987, pp 130–157
Christensen A: Dysfunctional interaction patterns in couples, in Perspectives on Marital Interaction. Edited by Noller P, Fitzpatrick MA. Philadelphia, PA, Multilingual Matters, 1988, pp 31–52
Christensen A: Cross-cultural awareness development: a conceptual model. Counselor Education and Supervision 28:270–287, 1989
Christensen A, Johnson SM, Phillips S, et al: Cost effectiveness in behavioral family therapy. Behavior Therapy 11:208–226, 1980
Christian J, O'Leary K, Vivian D: Depressive symptomatology in maritally discordant women and men: the role of individual relationship variables. J Fam Psychol 1994
Chubb H, Nauts PL, Evans EL: The practice of change: a working MRI/brief therapy clinic. Australian Journal of Family Therapy 5:181–184, 1984
Clarke MS, Mills J: Interpersonal attraction in exchange and communal relationships. J Pers Soc Psychol 37:12–24, 1979
Clarkin JF, Glick ID: Instruments for the assessment of family malfunction, in Measuring Mental Illness: Psychometric Assessment for Clinicians. Edited by Wetzler S. Washington, DC, American Psychiatric Press, 1989, pp 213–227
Clarkin JF, Miklowitz DJ: Marital and family communication difficulties, in DSM-IV Sourcebook, Vol 3. Edited by Widiger TA, Frances AJ, Pincus HA, et al. Washington, DC, American Psychiatric Association, 1997, pp 631–672
Clarkin JF, Glick ID, Haas GL, et al: A randomized clinical trial of inpatient family intervention: results for affective disorders. J Affect Disord 18:17–28, 1990
Cloninger C: Neurogenetic adaptive mechanisms in alcoholism. Science 236:410–416, 1987
Coatsworth JD, Szapocznik J, Kurtines W, et al: Culturally competent psychosocial interventions with antisocial problem behavior in Hispanic youth, in Handbook of Antisocial Behavior. Edited by Stoff DM, Breiling J. New York, Wiley, 1997, pp 395–404
Cobb LA, Rose RM: Hypertension, peptic ulcer and diabetes in air traffic controllers. JAMA 224:489–492, 1973
Coché J: Group therapy with couples, in Clinical Handbook of Couple Therapy. Edited by Jacobson NS, Gurman AS. New York, Guilford, 1995, pp 197–211
Cohan CL, Bradbury TN: Negative life events, marital interaction, and the longitudinal course of newlywed marriage. J Pers Soc Psychol 73:114–128, 1997
Colapinto J: The relative value of empirical evidence. Fam Process 18:427–441, 1979
Cole E: Sibling incest: the myth of benign sibling incest. Women and Therapy 5:79–89, 1982
Coleman M, Ganong L: The cultural stereotyping of stepfamilies, in Remarriage and Stepparenting: Current Research and Theory. Edited by Pasley K, Ihinger-Tallman M. New York, Guilford, 1987, pp 19–41
Coleman M, Ganong L: Remarriage and stepfamily research in the 1980s: increased interest in an old family form. Journal of Marriage and the Family 50:925–940, 1990a
Coleman M, Ganong L: The uses of juvenile fiction and self-help books with stepfamilies. Journal of Counseling and Development 68:327–331, 1990b
Coleman D, Straus M: Marital power, conflict and violence in a nationally representative sample of American couples. Violence Vict 1(2), 1986
Coleman S: Milan in Bucks County. Family Therapy Networker 11:42–47, 1987
Coleman SB, Stanton MD: An index for measuring agency involvement in family therapy. Fam Process 17:479–483, 1978

Colletta ND: Divorced mothers at two income levels: stress, support and child-rearing practices. Dissertation Abstracts 38(12-B), 1978
Colletta ND: The impact of divorce: father absence or poverty? Journal of Divorce 3:27–35, 1979
Collins N, Read S: Adult attachment, working models and relationship quality in dating couples. J Pers Soc Psychol 58:644–663, 1990
Collins RL, Leonard KE, Searles JS: Alcohol and the Family: Research and Clinical Perspectives. New York, Guilford, 1990
Comas-Diaz L: Lati Negra. Journal of Feminist Family Therapy 5(3/4):35–74, 1994
Combrinck-Graham L: A developmental model for family systems. Fam Process 24:131–151, 1985
Comella PA: Natural selection, technology, and anxiety. Family Systems 2:138–152, 1995
Comella PA: Naturally constrained social systems. Family Systems 4:19–33, 1997
Cook J, Tyson R, White J, et al: The mathematics of marital conflict: qualitative dynamic mathematical modeling of the marital interaction. Journal of Family Psychology 9:110–130, 1995
Cookerly J: Does marital therapy do any lasting good? J Marital Fam Ther 6:393–397, 1980
Coombe PD: Monitoring family therapy in clinical practice: a note on the use of the Beavers-Timber Family Evaluation Scale. Australian and New Zealand Journal of Family Therapy 8:23–28, 1987
Cooper CL, Cooper R, Faragher B: Stress and life events methodology: parent-child attachment and healthy human development. Stress Medicine 1:287–289, 1985
Copans S: The invisible family member: children in families with alcohol abuse, in Children in Family Contexts: Perspectives on Treatment. Edited by Combrinck-Graham L. New York, Guilford, 1989, pp 227–298
Coppersmith EI: "We've got a secret!": a nonmarital marital therapy, in Casebook of Marital Therapy. Edited by Gurman AS. New York, Guilford, 1985, pp 369–386
Corcoran M: Association of stated reason for treatment, family involvement, and stress to self concept changes in alcoholics. Dissertation Abstracts 50(1):341B–343B, 1989
Cordova JV: In-session couple interaction in integrative versus traditional behavioral couple therapy, in Proceedings of the 30th Annual Convention of the Association for the Advancement of Behavior Therapy. New York, Association for the Advancement of Behavior Therapy, 1996, p 138
Cosentino C, Heino F, Meyer-Bahlburg D: Sexual behavior problems and psychopathology symptoms in sexually abused girls. J Am Acad Child Adolesc Psychiatry 34:1033–1039, 1985
Couper-Smartt J, Rodham R: A technique for surveying side-effects of tricyclic drugs with reference to reported sexual effects. J Int Med Res 1:473–476, 1973
Courtois C: Healing the Incest Wound: Adult Survivors in Therapy. New York, WW Norton, 1988
Coverdale JH, Falloon IRH: Home or hospital-based emergency care for chronic psychiatric patients? N Z Med J 106:218–219, 1993
Cox M, Cox R: The aftermath of divorce, in Mother-Child, Father-Child Relations. Edited by Stevens JH Jr, Matthews M. Washington, DC, National Association for the Education of Young Children, 1978, pp 149–176
Coyne J: Depression and the response of others. J Abnorm Psychol 85:186–193, 1976
Coyne J: Strategic therapy with depressed married persons: initial agenda, themes and interventions. J Marital Fam Ther 10:153–162, 1984
Coyne J: The significance of the interview in strategic marital therapy. Journal of Strategic and Systemic Therapies 5(1–2):63–70, 1986a
Coyne J: Studying the role of cognition in depression: well-trodden paths and cul-de-sacs. Cognitive Therapy and Research 10:695–705, 1986b
Coyne J: Evoked emotion in marital therapy: necessary or even useful. J Marital Fam Ther 12:11–13, 1986c

Coyne J: Depression, biology, marriage, and marital therapy. J Marital Fam Ther 13:393–407, 1987
Coyne J: Concepts for understanding marriage and developing techniques of marital therapy: cognition ueber alles? Journal of Family Psychology 4:185–194, 1990
Coyne J, DeLongis A: Going beyond social support: the role of social relationships in adaptation. J Consult Clin Psychol 54:454–460, 1986
Coyne J, Kahn J, Gotlib I: Depression, in Family Interaction and Psychotherapy. Edited by Jacob T. New York, Plenum, 1986, pp 509–533
Coyne J, Kessler R, Tal M, et al: Living with a depressed person. J Consult Clin Psychol 55:347–352, 1987
Coyne J, Schwoeri L, Sholevar GP: The treatment of depression within a family context, in Transmission of Depression in Families and Children. Edited by Sholevar GP, Schwoeri L. New York, Jason Aronson, 1994
Cozolino LJ, Goldstein MJ: Family education as a component of extended family-orientated treatment programmes for schizophrenia, in Treatment of Schizophrenia: Family Assessment and Intervention. Edited by Goldstein MJ, Hand I, Hahlweg K. Berlin, Springer-Verlag, 1986, pp 38–67
Craske M, Zoellner ZA: Anxiety disorders: the role of marital therapy, in Clinical Handbook of Couple Therapy. Edited by Jacobson NS, Gurman AS. New York, Guilford, 1995, pp 394–410
Crews D: Biology and relationships: adaptation in nature. Family Systems 4:99–106, 1998
Crews FC (ed): Unauthorized Freud: Doubters Confront a Legend. New York, Viking, 1998
Crisp AH, Norton K, Gowers S, et al: A controlled study of the effect of therapies aimed at adolescent and family psychopathology in anorexia nervosa. Br J Psychiatry 159:325–333, 1991
Crits-Christoph P, Mintz J: Implications of therapist effects for the design and analysis of comparative studies of psychotherapies. J Consult Clin Psychol 59:20–26, 1991
Cromwell RE, Olson DH, Fournier DG: Tools and techniques for diagnosis and evaluation in marital and family therapy. Fam Process 15:1–49, 1976
Cronbach LJ: Essentials of Psychological Testing. New York, Harper & Row, 1960
Crosbie-Burnett M: The centrality of the step relationship: a challenge to family theory and practice. Family Relations 33:459–464, 1984
Crowe M: Conjoint marital therapy: a controlled outcome study. Psychol Med 8:623–636, 1978
Crowley SL: A psychometric investigation of the FACES III: confirmatory factory analysis with replication. Early Education and Development 9:161–178, 1998
Crowne DP, Marlowe D: The Approval Motive. New York, Wiley, 1967
Crowther J: The relationship between depression and marital maladjustment: a descriptive study. J Nerv Ment Dis 173:227–231, 1985
Cuber JF, Harroff PB: Sex and the Significant Americans. Baltimore, MD, Penguin, 1966
Cuber JF, Harroff PB: Five types of marriage, in Family in Transition: Rethinking Marriage, Sexuality, Childrearing. New York, HarperCollins, 1992
Culp LN, Beach SRH: Marriage and depressive symtoms: the role and bases of self-esteem differ by gender. Psychology of Women Quarterly 22:647–663, 1998
Curran J: Social skills training and behavioral family therapy for schizophrenia: a field trial. Paper presented at World Congress of Behaviour Therapy, Edinburgh, Scotland, September 1988
Dandeneau M, Johnson S: Facilitating intimacy: interventions and effects. J Marital Fam Ther 20:17–33, 1994
Dare C: Psychoanalytic marital therapy, in Clinical Handbook of Marital Therapy. Edited by Jacobson N, Gurman AS. New York, Guilford, 1986
Dausch BM, Miklowitz DJ, Richards JA: Global Assessment of Relational Functioning Scale (GARD), II: reliability and validity in a sample of families of bipolar patients. Fam Process 35:175–189, 1996

Davis JL, Petretic-Jackson PA: The impact of child sexual abuse on interpersonal functioning. Journal of Aggressive and Violent Behavior 5:291–328, 2000
DeFrancis V: Protecting the Child Sex Victim. Denver, CO, American Humane Association, 1965
Degler CN: Remaking American history. Journal of American History 67:7–25, 1980
DeLongis A, Coyne JC, Dakof G, et al: Relationship of daily hassles, uplifts and major life events to health status. Health Psychol 1:119–136, 1982
Derogatis L, Melisaratos N: The Brief Symptom Inventory: an introductory report. Psychol Med 13:595–605, 1983
Descutner C, Thelen M: Development and validation of a fear of intimacy scale. J Consult Clin Psychol 3:218–225, 1991
de Shazer S: Patterns of Brief Family Therapy. New York, Guilford, 1982
de Shazer S: Creative misunderstanding: there is no escape from language, in Therapeutic Conversations. Edited by Gilligan SG, Price R. New York, WW Norton, 1983, pp 81–94
de Shazer S: Keys to Solution in Brief Therapy. New York, WW Norton, 1985
de Shazer S: Clues: Investigating Solutions in Brief Therapy. New York, WW Norton, 1988
de Shazer S: Muddles, bewilderment, and practice theory. Fam Process 30:453–458, 1991a
de Shazer S: Putting Differences to Work. New York, WW Norton, 1991b
de Shazer S, Berg I, Lipchick E, et al: Brief therapy: focused solution development. Fam Process 25:207–222, 1986
Dessaulles A, Johnson S: The treatment of clinical depression in the context of marital distress. Unpublished doctoral dissertation, University of Ottawa, Ottawa, Ontario, Canada, 1991
Detre, Sayer, Norton, Lewis: An experimental approach to the treatment of the acutely ill psychiatric patient. Conn Med 25:613–619, 1961
Devila J, Bradbury TN, Cohan CL, et al: Marital functioning and depressive symptoms: evidence for a stress generation model. J Pers Soc Psychol 73:849–861, 1977
de Wall F, Embree M: The triadic nature of primate social relationships. Family Systems 4:5–18, 1997
De Young M: Self-injurious behavior in incest victims: a research note. Child Welfare 62:577–584, 1982
Diamond G, Liddle HA: Resolving a therapeutic impasse between parents and adolescents in multidimensional family therapy. J Consult Clin Psychol 64:481–488, 1996
Dicks H: Concepts of marital diagnosis of therapy as developed at the Tavistock Family Psychiatric Clinic, London, England, in Marriage Counseling in Medical Practice. Edited by Nas E, Jessner L, Abse D. Chapel Hill, University of North Carolina Press, 1964
Dicks H: Marital Tensions: Clinical Studies Towards a Psychological Theory of Interaction. New York, Basic Books, 1967
Dilley JW, Ochitill HN, Perl M, et al: Findings in psychiatric consultations with patients with acquired immune deficiency syndrome. Am J Psychiatry 142:82–86, 1985
Dilworth-Anderson P, Burton LM: Rethinking family development. Journal of Social and Personal Relationships 13:325–354, 1996
Dinnerstein D: The Mermaid and the Minotaur: Sexual Arrangements and Human Malaise. New York, Harper & Row, 1976
Diop CA: The Cultural Unity of Black Africa: The Domains of Patriarchy and of Matriarchy in Classical Antiquity. Chicago, IL, Third World Press, 1990
Dixen J, Jenkins JO: Incestuous child sexual abuse: a review of treatment strategies. Clin Psychol Rev 1:211–222, 1981
Dixon LB, Lehman AF: Family interventions for schizophrenia. Schizophr Bull 21:631–643, 1995
Dixon L, Goldman H, Hirad A: State policy and funding services to families of adults with serious and persistent mental illness. Psychiatr Serv 50:551–553, 1999
Dixon LB, Lyles A, Smith C, et al: Use and costs of ambulatory care services among Medicare enrollees with schizophrenia. Psychiatr Serv 52:786–792, 2001

Doane JA: Family interaction and communication deviance in disturbed and normal families: a review of research. Fam Process 17:357–376, 1978
Doane J, West K, Goldstein M: Parental communication deviance and affective style: predictors of subsequent schizophrenia-spectrum disorders in vulnerable adolescents. Arch Gen Psychiatry 38:679–685, 1981
Doane J, Falloon I, Goldstein M: Parental affective style and treatment of schizophrenia: predicting course of illness and social functioning. Arch Gen Psychiatry 42:34–42, 1985
Doane J, Goldstein M, Miklowitz D: The impact of individual and family treatment on the affective climate of families of schizophrenics. Br J Psychiatry 148:279–287, 1986
Dobash RP, Dobash RE, Wilson M, et al: The myth of sexual symmetry in marital violence. Social Problems 39:71–91, 1992
Dobson KS, Jacobson NS, Victor J: Integration of cognitive therapy and behavioral marital therapy, in Affective Disorders and the Family: Assessment and Treatment. Edited by Clarkin JF, Haas GL, Glick ID. New York, Guilford, 1988, pp 53–88
Dobson DJG, McDougall G, Busheikin J, et al: Effects of social skills training and social milieu treatment on symptoms of schizophrenia. Psychiatr Serv 46:376–380, 1995
Doherty DW, Colangelo N: The family FIRO model: a modest proposal for organizing family treatment. J Marital Fam Ther 10:19–29, 1984
Doherty W, Baird M: Family Therapy and Family Medicine: Toward the Primary Care of Families. New York, Guilford, 1983
Doherty WJ, Hovander D: Why don't family measures of cohesion and control behave like they're supposed to? American Journal of Family Therapy 18:5–18, 1990
Doherty WJ, McCabe P, Ryder RG: Marriage Encounter: a critical appraisal. J Marital Fam Ther 4:99–107, 1978
Dolan Y: A Path With a Heart: Ericksonian Utilization With Resistant and Chronic Clients. New York, Brunner/Mazel, 1985
Dolan Y: Resolving Sexual Abuse. New York, WW Norton, 1991
Doty P: Family care of the elderly: the role of public policy. Milbank Q 64:34–75, 1986
Doty P: Family caregiving and access to publicly funded home care: implicit and explicit influences on decision making, in Family Caregiving in an Aging Society. Edited by Kane RA, Penrod JD. Baltimore, MD, Williams & Wilkins, 1995, pp 92–122
Dowling E, Jones H: Small children seen and heard in family therapy. Journal of Child Psychotherapy 4:87–96, 1978
Downey G, Coyne J: Children of depressed parents: an integrative review. Psychol Bull 108:50–76, 1990
Dreikurs R, Soltz V: Children, the Challenge. New York, Dutton, 1964
DuBois W: The Souls of Black Folk. Chicago, IL, McClurg, 1903
Ducommun-Nagy C, Schwoeri L: Contextual therapy into the 1990s, in Evaluation of Family System and Genogram. Edited by Guerin GP. New York, Gardner Press, 1990
Duhl F, Kantor D, Duhl B: Learning and action in family therapy: a primer of sculpture, in Techniques of Family Psychotherapy. Edited by Block D. New York, Grune & Stratton, 1973
Dulz B, Hand I: Short-term relapse in young schizophrenics: can it be predicted and affected by family (CFI), patient, and treatment variables? An experimental study, in Treatment of Schizophrenia: Family Assessment and Intervention. Edited by Goldstein MJ, Hahlweg K. Berlin, Springer-Verlag, 1986, pp 59–77
Dunn R, Schwebel A: Meta-analytic review of marital therapy outcome research. Journal of Family Psychology 9:58–68, 1995
Dunn J, Stocker C, Plomin R: Nonshared experiences within the family: correlates of behavioral problems in middle childhood. Dev Psychopathol 2:113–126, 1990
Duvall EM: Family Development. Chicago, IL, JB Lippincott, 1962
Duvall E: Marriage and Family Development, 5th Edition. Philadelphia, PA, JB Lippincott, 1977

Dwyer TF: Assessing distress in couples with cancer: a life cycle view. Dissertation Abstracts 56(9-A):3756, 1996
Dyer KF: Changing patterns of marriage and mating within Australia. Australian Journal of Sex, Marriage and Family 9:107–119, 1988
D'Zurilla TJ, Goldfried MR: Problem solving and behavior modification. J Abnorm Psychol 78:107–126, 1976
Eaton WW, Neufeld K, Chen L, et al: A comparision of self-report and clinical diagnostic interviews for depression: Diagnostic Interview Schedule and Schedules for Clinical Assessment in Neuropsychiatry in the Baltimore Epidemiologic Catchment Area Follow-Up. Arch Gen Psychiatry 57:217–222, 2000
Eaton WW, Mutaner C, Bovasso G, et al: Socioeconomic status and depressive syndrome: the role of inter- and intra-generational mobility, government assistance, and work environment. J Health Soc Behav 42:277–295, 2001
Eaton WW, Anthony JC, Gallo J, et al: Natural history of Diagnostic Interview Schedule/DSM-IV major depression: the Baltimore Epidemiologic Catchment Area Follow-Up. Arch Gen Psychiatry 54:993–999, 1997
Eddy JM, Heyman RE, Weiss RL: An empirical evaluation of the Dyadic Adjustment Scale: exploring the differences between marital "satisfaction" and "adjustment." Behavioral Assessment 13:199–220, 1991
Edmonds VH: Marital conventionalization: definition and measurement. Journal of Marriage and the Family 29:681–688, 1967
Edwards JR, Cooper CL: Research in stress, coping, and health: theoretical and methodological issues. Psychol Med 1:15–20, 1988
Education and gender: does the educational system shortchange females? Congressional Quarterly 4(21):481–504, 1994
Ehlert U: Psychologische Intervention bei den Angelhorigen schizophrener Patienten. Franfurt am Main, Peter Lang Verlag, 1989
Ehrensaft MK, Vivian D: Spouses' reasons for not reporting existing marital aggression as a marital problem. Journal of Family Psychology 10:443–453, 1996
Eichel E: Assessment with a family focus. Journal of Psychiatric Nursing and Mental Health Services 16:11–15, 1978
Eidelson RJ, Epstein N: Cognition and relationship maladjustment: development of a measure of dysfunctional relationship beliefs. J Consult Clin Psychol 50:715–720, 1982
Eissler K (ed): Searchlights on Delinquency. New York, International Universities Press, 1949
Eiswirth-Neems N, Handel F: Spouse's attitudes toward maternal occupational status and effect on family climate. Journal of Community Psychology 6:168–172, 1978
Elion D: Therapy with remarriage families with children: positive interventions from the client perspective. Unpublished thesis, Menomonie, University of Wisconsin–Stout, 1990
Ellis A: Reason and Emotion in Psychotherapy. New York, Lyle Stuart, 1962
Ellis A: Rational-emotive therapy applied to relationship therapy. Journal of Rational-Emotive Therapy 4:4–21, 1986
Ellis H: Studies in the Psychology of Sex. New York, Random House, 1906
Embree BG, De Wit ML: Family background characteristics and relationship satisfaction in Native community of Canada. Social Biol 44:42–54, 1997
Emde R, Harmon R (eds): Continuities and Discontinuities in Development. New York, Plenum, 1984
Emery RE, Laumann-Billings L: An overview of the nature, causes, and consequences of abusive family relationships: toward differentiating maltreatment and violence. Am Psychol 53:121–135, 1998
Emery RE, Weintraub S, Neale JM: The Family Evaluation Form: construction and normative data. Presented at the annual meeting of the American Psychological Association, Montreal, Quebec, Canada, 1980

Emmelkamp PMG, Van Linden van den Heuvel C, Ruphan M, et al: Cognitive and behavioral interventions: a comparative evaluation with clinically distressed couples. Journal of Family Psychology 4:365–377, 1988

Emshoff JG, Glakely CH: The diversion of delinquent youth: family focused intervention. Children and Youth Services Review 8:343–356, 1983

Endicott J, Spitzer RL, Fleiss JL, et al: The Global Assessment Scale: a procedure for measuring overall severity of psychiatric disturbance. Arch Gen Psychiatry 33:766–771, 1976

Engel GL: The clinical application of the biopsychosocial approach. Am J Psychiatry 137:535–544, 1980a

Engel GL: A group dynamic approach to teaching and learning about grief. Journal of Death and Dying 11:45–49, 1980b

Epstein N: Cognitive therapy with couples. American Journal of Family Therapy 10:5–16, 1982

Epstein NB, Bishop D: Problem-centered systems therapy of the family, in Handbook of Family Therapy. Edited by Gurman AS, Kniskern DP. New York, Brunner/Mazel, 1981, pp 444–482

Epstein N, Williams AM: Behavioral approaches to treatment of marital discord, in Handbook of Marriage and Marital Therapy. Edited by Sholevar GP. Jamaica, NY, SP Medical & Scientific Books, 1981, pp 219–287

Epstein NB, Baldwin LM, Bishop DS: The McMaster Family Assessment Device, Version 3 (Copyright Registration Number 82-315). 1981

Epstein NB, Baldwin LM, Bishop DS: The McMaster Family Assessment Device. J Marital Fam Ther 9:171–180, 1983

Epstein N, Keitner G, Bishop D, et al: Combined use of pharmacology and family therapy, in Affective Disorders and the Family: Assessment and Treatment. Edited by Clarkin J, Haas G, Glick I. New York, Guilford, 1988

Epston D: Collected Papers. Adelaide, South Australia, Dulwich Center Publications, 1989

Erickson G: Against the grain: decentering family therapy. J Marital Fam Ther 14:255–236, 1988

Erickson MJ: Re-visioning the family life cycle theory and paradigm in marriage and family therapy. Am J Family Therapy 26:341–355, 1998

Erikson EH: Childhood and Society. New York, WW Norton, 1950

Eron J, Lund T: Narrative Solution in Brief Therapy. New York, Guilford, 1996

Everstine DS, Everstine L: Sexual Trauma in Children and Adolescents: Dynamics and Treatment. New York, Brunner/Mazel, 1989

Eyberg SM, Johnson SM: Multiple assessment behavior modification with families: effects of contingency contracting and order of treated problems. J Consult Clin Psychol 42:594–606, 1974

Eyberg S, Edwards D, Boggs S, et al: Maintaining the treatment effects of parental training: the role of booster sessions and other maintenance strategies. Clinical Psychology: Science and Practice 5:544–554, 1998

Fadden G: Research update: psychoeducational family interventions. Journal of Family Therapy 20:293–309, 1998

Fadden G, Bebbington P, Kuipers L: The burden of care: the impact of functional psychiatric illness on the patient's family. Br J Psychiatry 150:285–292, 1987a

Fadden G, Bebbington P, Kuipers L: Caring and its burdens: a study of the spouses of depressed patients. Br J Psychiatry 151:660–667, 1987b

Fairbairn WRD: Psychoanalytic Studies of the Personality. London, Tavistock, 1952

Falicov C: Learning to think culturally, in Handbook of Family Therapy Supervision. Edited by Liddle H, Breunlin R, Schwartz R. New York, Guilford, 1988, pp 335–357

Falicov CJ: Latino Families in Therapy: A Guide to Multicultural Practice. New York, Guilford, 1998

Falicov C, Karrer B: Cultural variations in the family life cycle, in The Family Life Cycle: A Framework for Family Therapy. Edited by Carter E, McGoldrick M. New York, Gardner Press, 1980

Faller KC: Child Sexual Abuse: An Interdisciplinary Manual for Diagnosis, Case Management, and Treatment. New York, Columbia University Press, 1988

Falloon IRH: Communication and problem solving skills training with relapsing schizophrenics and their families, in Family Therapy and Major Psychopathology. Edited by Lansky MR. New York, Grune & Stratton, 1981, pp 35–56

Falloon IRH: Family Management of Schizophrenia: A Study of Clinical, Social, Family and Economic Benefits. Baltimore, MD, Johns Hopkins University Press, 1985

Falloon IRH: Expressed emotion: current status. Psychol Med 18:269–274, 1988

Falloon IRH, Coverdale JH: Cognitive-behavioral family interventions for major mental disorders. Behavior Change 11:213–222, 1994

Falloon IRH, Fadden G: Integrated Mental Health Care. Cambridge, UK, Cambridge University Press, 1993

Falloon IR, Graham-Hole UG: Family care as an alternative to the mental hospital, in The Closure of Mental Hospitals. Edited by Hall P, Brockington I. London, Gaskill, 1990

Falloon IRH, Liberman RP: Behavioral family interventions in the management of chronic schizophrenia, in Family Therapy in Schizophrenia. Edited by McFarlane WR, Beels CC. New York, Guilford, 1984

Falloon IRH, McGill CW: Family stress and the course of schizophrenia: a review, in Family Management of Schizophrenia. Edited by Falloon IRH. Baltimore, MD, Johns Hopkins University Press, 1985

Falloon IRH, the Optimal Treatment Project Collaborators: Optimal treatment for psychosis in an international multisite demonstration project. Psychiatr Serv 50:615–618, 1999

Falloon IR, Pederson J: Family management in the prevention of morbidity of schizophrenia: the adjustment of the family unit. Br J Psychiatry 147:156–163, 1985

Falloon I, Watt DC, Shepherd M: A comparative controlled trial of pimozide and fluphenazine decanoate in the continuation therapy of schizophrenia. Psychol Med 8:59–70, 1978

Falloon IRH, Boyd JL, McGill CW, et al: Family management in the prevention of exacerbations of schizophrenia. N Engl J Med 306:1437–1440, 1982

Falloon IRJ, Boyd JL, McGill CW: Family Care of Schizophrenia: A Problem-Solving Approach to the Treatment of Mental Illness. New York, Guilford, 1984

Falloon I, Boyd J, McGill C, et al: Family management in the prevention of morbidity of schizophrenia: clinical outcome of a two-year longitudinal study. Arch Gen Psychiatry 42:887–896, 1985

Falloon I, McGill C, Boyd J, et al: Family management in the prevention of morbidity of schizophrenia: social outcome of a two-year longitudinal study. Psychol Med 17:59–66, 1987

Falloon IRH, Brooker C, Graham-Hole V: Psychosocial interventions for schizophrenia. Behaviour Change 9:238–245, 1993

Falloon IRH, McGill CW, Matthews SM, et al: Family treatment for schizophrenia: the design and research application of therapist training models. J Psychother Pract Res 5:45–56, 1996

Falloon IRH, Falloon NCH, Lussetti M, et al: Integrated Mental Health Care: A Guidebook for Consumers. Perugia, Italy, ARIETE Publications, 1998

Falloon IRH, Held T, Coverdale JH, et al: Family interventions of schizophrenia: a review of long-term benefits of international studies. Psychiatric Rehabilitation Skills 3:268–290, 1999

Faludi S: Backlash: The Undeclared War Against American Women. New York, Crown, 1992

Farber RS: An integrated perspective on women's career development within the family. American Journal of Family Therapy 24:329–342, 1996

Farrington D: The family background of aggressive youths, in Aggressive and Antisocial Behavior in Childhood and Adolescence. Edited by Hersov L, Berger M, Shaffer D. Oxford, England, Pergamon, 1978, pp 73–93

Farrington D, Gundry G, West D: The familial transmission of criminality. Med Sci Law 15: 177–186, 1975

Feldman JB: The work of Milton Erickson: a multisystem model of eclectic therapy. Psychotherapy 22:154–162, 1985

Fendrich M, Warner V, Weissman M: Family risk factors. parental depression, and psychopathology in offspring. Dev Psychol 26:40–50, 1990

Ferreira AJ: Family myths and homeostasis, in Theory and Practice of Family Psychiatry. Edited by Howells JG. New York, Brunner/Mazel, 1971

Filsinger EE, Thoma SJ: Behavioral antecedents of relationship stability and adjustment: a five-year longitudinal study. Journal of Marriage and the Family 50:785–795, 1988

Fincham FD, Bradbury TN: The assessment of marital quality: a reevaluation. Journal of Marriage and the Family 49:797–809, 1987

Fincham FD, Bradbury TN: Marital conflict: towards a more complete integration of research and treatment, in Advances in Family Intervention, Assessment and Theory. Edited by Vincent JP. London, Jessica Kingsley Publishers, 1991, pp 1–23

Fincham FD, Bradbury TN: Assessing attributions in marriage: the Relationship Attribution Measure. J Pers Soc Psychol 62:457–468, 1992

Fincham FD, Bradbury TN, Beach SRH: To arrive where we began: a reappraisal of cognition in marriage and in marital therapy. Journal of Family Psychology 4:167–184, 1990

Finkelhor D: Sexually Victimized Children. New York, Free Press, 1979

Finkelhor D: Sex among siblings: a survey report on its prevalence, variety, and effects. Arch Sex Behav 9:171–194, 1980

Finkelhor D: Child Sexual Abuse: New Theory and Research. Beverly Hills, CA, Sage, 1984

Finkelhor D: The sexual abuse of children: current research reviewed. Psychiatric Annals 17:233–241, 1987

Finkelhor D: Early and long term effects of clinical sexual abuse. Professional Psychology 5: 325–330, 1990

Finkelhor D: A comparison of the responses of preadolescents and adolescents in a national victimization survey. Journal of Interpersonal Violence 13:362–382, 1998

Finkelhor D, Baron L: High-risk children, in A Sourcebook on Child Sexual Abuse. Edited by Finkelhor D and Associates. Newbury Park, CA, Sage, 1986, pp 60–88

Finkelhor D, Berliner L: Research on the treatment of sexually abused children: a review and recommendations. J Am Acad Child Adolesc Psychiatry 34:1408–1423, 1995

Finkelhor D, Moore D, Hamby SL, et al: Sexually abused children in a national survey of parents: methodological issues. Child Abuse Negl 21:1–9, 1996

Finney J, Moos R, Mewborn R: Posttreatment experiences and treatment outcome of alcoholic patients six months and two years after hospitalization. J Consult Clin Psychol 48:17–29, 1980

Fisch R, Weakland J, Segal L: The Tactics of Change: Doing Therapy Briefly. San Francisco, CA, Jossey-Bass, 1982

Fischer J, Corcoran K: Measures for Clinical Practice: A Sourcebook, Vol 1: Couples, Families and Children. New York, Free Press, 1994

Fischmann-Havstad L, Marston A: Weight loss maintenance as an aspect of family emotion and process. Br J Clin Psychol 23:265–271, 1984

Fish LS, Piercy FP: The theory and practice of structural and strategic family therapies: a Delphi study. J Marital Fam Ther 13:113–125, 1987

Fisher H: The Anatomy of Love. New York, WW Norton, 1992

Fisher L: Dimensions of family assessment: a critical review. Journal of Marriage and Family Counseling 2:367–382, 1976

Fisher L: On the classification of families. Arch Gen Psychiatry 34:424–433, 1977

Fisher R, Ury W: Getting to Yes: Negotiating Agreement Without Giving in. New York, Penguin, 1981

Fishman HC: Intensive Structural Therapy: Treating Families in Their Social Context. New York, Basic Books, 1993

Fishman HC, Andes F, Knowlton R: Enhancing family therapy: the addition of a community resource specialist. J Marital Fam Ther 27:111–116, 2001

Fishman KD: Therapy for children. Atlantic Monthly, June 1991, pp 47–81

Fleck S: Family functioning and family pathology. Psychiatric Annals 10:17–35, 1980

Fleming J: Stopping Wife Abuse: A Guide to the Emotional, Psychological and Legal Implications for the Abused Woman and Those Helping Her. New York, Anchor Press, 1979

Flugel JC: Psycho-Analytic Study of the Family. London, Hogarth Press, 1921

Foley S, Rounsaville B, Weissman M, et al: Individual vs conjoint interpersonal psychotherapy for depressed patients with marital disputes. Paper presented at the 140th annual meeting of the American Psychiatric Association, Chicago, IL, May 1987

Fordyce WE: Behavioral Methods for Chronic Pain and Illness. St Louis, MO, CV Mosby, 1976

Forehand R: Child non-compliance to parental requests: behavioral analysis and treatment, in Progress in Behavior Modification, Vol 5. Edited by Hersen M, Eisler RM, Miller PM. New York, Academic Press, 1977, pp 111–143

Forehand R, McMahon R: Helping the Noncompliant Child: A Clinician's Guide to Parent Training. New York, Guilford, 1981a

Forehand R, McMahon RJ: Teaching parents to modify child behavior problems: an examination of some follow-up data. J Pediatr Psychol 6:313–322, 1981b

Forehand R, King HE, Reed S, et al: Mother-child interactions: comparison of a noncompliant clinic group and a nonclinic group. Behav Res Ther 13:79–85, 1975

Forehand R, Weeks K, Guest D: An examination of the social validity of a parent training program. Behavior Therapy 11:488–502, 1980

Forehand R, Breiner J, McMahon RJ, et al: Predictors of cross setting behavior change in treatment of child problems. Journal of Behavior Therapy and Experimental Psychiatry 12:311–313, 1981

Forgatch M, Patterson G: Parents and Adolescents Living Together, Part 2: Family Problem Solving. Eugene, OR, Castalia Publishing, 1989

Forman B: Assessing perceived patterns of behavior exchange in relationships. J Clin Psychol 44:992–981, 1988

Forman B, Hagan B: Measure for evaluating total family functioning. Family Therapy 11:34–69, 1984

Forman SG, Forman BD: Family environment and its relation to adolescent personality factors. J Pers Assess 45:163–167, 1983

Forward S, Buch S: Betrayal of Innocence: Incest and Its Devastation. New York, Tarcher, 1979

Fosson A: Family therapy in family practice: a solution to psychosocial problems. J Fam Pract 15:461–465, 1982

Foster SL, Prinz RJ, O'Leary KD: Impact of problem-solving communication training and generalization procedures on family conflict. Child and Behavior Therapy 5:1–23, 1983

Foucault M: The Birth of the Clinic: An Archeology of Medical Perception. London, Tavistock, 1973

Foucault M: Power/Knowledge: Selected Interviews and Other Writings, 1972–1977. New York, Pantheon Books, 1980

Fowler PC: Maximum likelihood factor structure of the Family Environment Scale. J Clin Psychol 37:160–164, 1981

Fowler PC: Factor structure of the Family Environment Scale: effects of social desirability. J Clin Psychol 38:285–292, 1982

Fox JE: Outpatient alcoholism coverage to be tried. US Medicine 19:24–25, 1983

Framo J: Explorations in Marital and Family Therapy. New York, Springer, 1982

Frances RJ, Galanter M, Miller SI: Psychosocial approaches to treatment and rehabilitation (Part III: Alcoholism, Meyer RE, ed), in American Psychiatric Press Review of Psychiatry, Vol 8. Edited by Tasman A, Hales RE, Frances AJ. Washington, DC, American Psychiatric Press, 1989, pp 341–358

Frank E, Anderson C, Kupfer D: Profiles of couples seeking sex therapy and marital therapy. Am J Psychiatry 133:559–562, 1976

Frank E, Anderson C, Rubinstein D: Frequency of sexual dysfunction in "normal" couples. N Engl J Med 299:111–115, 1978

Franklin AJ: The invisibility syndrome. Family Therapy Networker, 1983, pp 33–39

Fraser JS: Integrating system-based therapies: similarities, differences and some critical questions, in Journeys: Expansion of the Strategic-Systemic Therapies. Edited by Efron DE. New York, Brunner/Mazel, 1986, pp 125–149

Frazier E: The Negro Church in America. New York, Schocken, 1963

Frederick C, Pynoos R, Nader K: Child Post-Traumatic Stress Disorder Reaction Index (Available from R. Pynoos, Adult Psychiatry, 300 UCLA Medical Plaza, Los Angeles, CA 90024-6968), 1992

Freedman J, Combs G: Narrative Therapy: The Social Construction of Preferred Realities. New York, WW Norton, 1996

Frese FJ: Advocacy, recovery, and the challenges of consumerism for schizophrenia. Psychiatr Clin North Am 21:233–249, 1998

Freud A: The ego and the mechanisms of defense (1936), in The Writings of Anna Freud, Vol 2. New York, International Universities Press, 1966

Freud S: Three essays on the theory of sexuality (1905), in The Standard Edition of the Complete Psychological Works of Sigmund Freud, Vol 7. Translated and edited by Strachey J. London, Hogarth Press, 1953, pp 135–243

Freud S: The dynamics of transference (1912), in The Standard Edition of the Complete Psychological Works of Sigmund Freud, Vol 12. Translated and edited by Strachey J. London, Hogarth Press, 1958, pp 97–108

Freud S: Tolem and Taboo (1913). Translated by Brill AA. New York, Vintage, 1946

Friedlander ML, Wildman J, Heatherington L, et al: What we do and don't know about the process of family therapy. Journal of Family Psychology 8:390–416, 1994

Friedman A: Interaction of drug therapy with marital therapy in depressive patients. Arch Gen Psychiatry 32:619–637, 1975

Friedman AS: Family therapy vs parent groups: effects on adolescent drug abusers. American Journal of Family Therapy 17:335–347, 1989

Friedman A: The Adolescent and the Family in Family Therapy for Adolescent Drug Abuse. Lexington, MA, Lexington Books, 1990

Friedman A, Sonne J, Speck K: Therapy With Families of Sexually Acting-Out Girls. New York, Springer, 1971

Friedman AS, Pomerance E, Sanders R, et al: The structure and problems of the families of adolescent drug abusers. Contemporary Drug Problems 9:327–356, 1980

Friedman M: Intervening with families of school-aged children with cancer, in Families and Life-Threatening Illness. Springhouse, PA, Springhouse, 1987

Friedman M, Rosenman RH: Association of overt behavior pattern with blood and cardiovascular findings. JAMA 169:1286–1296, 1959

Friedman SL, Amateo J: The child-care environment: conceptualizations, assessments, issues, in Measuring Environment Across the Life Span: Emerging Methods and Concepts. Edited by Friedman SL, Wachs TD. Washington, DC, American Psychological Association, 1999, pp 127–165

Friedrich WN: Sexual victimization and sexual behavior in children: a review of recent literature. Child Abuse Negl 17:59–66, 1993

Friedrich WN, Beilke RL, Urquiza AJ: Behavioral comparisons of children from sexually abusive and distressed families. Journal of Interpersonal Violence 2:39–42, 1988

Fromm E: Escape From Freedom. New York, Rinehart, 1941
Fromm-Reichmann F: Notes on the development of treatment of schizophrenics by psychoanalytic therapy. Journal for the Study of Interpersonal Processes 11:263–273, 1948
Fruzzetti A, Jacobson N: Toward a behavioral conceptualization of adult intimacy, in Emotion and the Family: For Better or Worse. Edited by Blechman E. Hillsdale, NJ, Lawrence Erlbaum, 1990, pp 117–136
Fruzzetti AE, Levensky ER: Dialectical behavior therapy for domestic violence: rationale and procedures. Cognitive and Behavioral Practice 7:435–447, 2000
Furstenberg FF Jr, Nord CW: Parenting apart. Journal of Marriage and the Family 47:893–904, 1985
Furstenberg FF Jr, Morgan SP, Allison PD: Paternal participation and children's well-being after marital dissolution. American Sociological Review 52:695–701, 1987
Gagnon J, Pomeroy WC, Christenson C, et al: Sex Offenders: An Analysis of Types. New York, Harper & Row, 1965
Galanter M, Castaneda R, Franco H: Group therapist and self-help groups, in Clinical Textbook of Adult Disorders. Edited by Frances R, Miller S. New York, Guilford, 1991
Gant BL, Barnard JD, Kuehn FE, et al: A behaviorally based approach for improving intrafamilial communication patterns. J Clin Child Psychol 10:102–106, 1981
Garcia-Preto N: Puerto Rican families, in Ethnicity and Family Therapy. Edited by McGoldrick M, Pearce JK, Giordano J. New York, Guilford, 1982, pp 164–186
Garcia-Preto N: Latino families: an overview, in Ethnicity and Family Therapy, 2nd Edition. Edited by McGoldrick M, Giordano J, Pearce JK. New York, Guilford, 1996, pp 141–154
Gardner RA: Children of divorce: some legal and psychological considerations. J Clin Child Psychol 6(2):3–6, 1977
Garmezy N: Stressors of childhood, in Stress, Coping, and Development in Children. Edited by Garmezy N, Rutter M. New York, McGraw-Hill, 1983, pp 43–84
Garnica O: Some prosodic and paralinguistic features of speech of young children, in Talking to Children: Language Input and Acquisition. Edited by Snow C, Ferguson C. Cambridge, England, Cambridge University Press, 1977, pp 63–88
Garrigan JJ, Bambrick AF: Family therapy for disturbed children: some experimental results in special education. Journal of Marriage and Family Counseling 3:83–93, 1977
Garrigan JJ, Bambrick AF: New findings in research on go-between process. International Journal of Family Therapy 1:76–85, 1979
Gary L (ed): Black Men. Beverly Hills, CA, Sage, 1981
Geerstma RH: Family functioning, in Encyclopedia of Clinical Assessment. Edited by Woody RH. San Francisco, CA, Jossey-Bass, 1980
Geismar LL, Ayers B: A method of evaluating the social functioning of families under treatment. Soc Work 4:102–108, 1959
Gelinas L: The persisting negative effects of incest. Psychiatry 46:312–332, 1983
Gelles R: The Violent Home: A Study of Physical Aggression Between Husbands and Wives. Newbury Park, CA, Sage, 1972
Gelles RJ: Methodological issues in the study of family violence, in Depression and Aggression in Family Interaction. Edited by Patterson GR. Hillsdale, NJ, Lawrence Erlbaum, 1990, pp 49–74
Gelles RJ: Through a sociological lens: social structure and family violence, in Current Controversies on Family Violence. Edited by Gelles RJ, Loseeke DR. Newbury Park, CA, Sage, 1993, pp 31–46
Gelles RJ, Straus MA: Intimate Violence: The Causes and Consequences of Abuse in the American Family. New York, Touchstone/Simon & Schuster, 1988
Gelles R, Straus M: Physical Violence in American Families: Risk Factors and Adaptations to Violence in 8,145 Families. New Brunswick, NJ, Transaction Publishers, 1990
Gergen K: The saturated family. Networker, September/October 1991, pp 26–35

Gerson R: The family life cycle: phases, stages, and crises, in Integrating Family Therapy: Handbook of Family Psychology and Systems Theory. Edited by Mikesell RH, Lusterman DD. Washington, DC, American Psychological Association, 1995, pp 91–111

Giblin, et al: Enrichment outcome research: a meta-analysis of premarital, marital and family interventions. J Marital Fam Ther 11:257–271, 1985

Gigy L, Kelly JB: Reasons for divorce: perspectives of divorcing men and women. Journal of Divorce and Remarriage 18:169–187, 1992

Gil E: Etiologic theories in sexualized children: assessment and treatment of sexualized children and children who molest. Child Abuse Negl 12:163–170, 1993

Gil E: Play in Family Therapy. New York, Guilford, 1994

Gilligan C: In a Different Voice: Psychological Theory and Women's Development. Cambridge, MA, Harvard University Press, 1982

Gingerick WJ, de Shazer S: The Briefer Project: using expert systems as theory construction tools. Fam Process 30:241–250, 1991

Giordano-Giordano GP: The Ethno-Cultural Factor in M.H.: A Literature Review and Bibliography. New York, Institute on Pluralism and Group Identity, 1977

Glaser R: Family, spouse, and individual Rorschach responses of families with and without young adult schizophrenic offspring. Unpublished doctoral dissertation, University of California, Berkeley, 1976

Gleidman L, Rosenthal D, Frank S, et al: Group therapy of alcoholics with concurrent group meetings with their wives. Quarterly Journal of Studies on Alcohol 17:655–670, 1956

Glick I, Kessler D: Marital and Family Therapy, 2nd Edition. New York, Grune & Stratton, 1980

Glick ID, Clarkin JF, Spencer J, et al: A controlled evaluation of inpatient family intervention, I: preliminary results of a 6-month follow-up. Arch Gen Psychiatry 42:882–886, 1985a

Glick I, Clarkin J, Spencer J: Recent developments in family therapy: a review. Hospital and Community Psychiatry 33:550–556, 1985b

Glick ID, Clarkin JF, Kessler DR: Family intervention and the psychiatric hospital system, in Marital and Family Therapy, 3rd Edition. New York, Grune & Stratton, 1987, pp 370–391

Glick ID, Spencer J, Clarkin JF, et al: A randomized clinical trial of inpatient family intervention, IV: follow-up results for subjects with schizophrenia. Schizophr Res 3:187–200, 1990

Glick ID, Clarkin JF, Haas G, et al: A randomized clinical trial of inpatient family intervention, VI: mediating variables and outcome. Fam Process 30:85–99, 1991

Glick ID, Clarkin JF, Haas GL, et al: Clinical significance of inpatient family intervention: conclusions from a clinical trial. Hosp Community Psychiatry 44:869–873, 1993

Glick P: Children of divorced parents in demographic perspective. Journal of Social Issues 35:170–184, 1980

Glick P: Marriage, divorce, and living arrangements: prospective changes. Journal of Family Issues 5:7–26, 1984

Glick P: Remarried families, stepfamilies, and stepchildren: a brief demographic analysis. Family Relations 38:24–27, 1989

Glick P: American families: as they are and were, in Family in Transition. Edited by Skolnick JH. New York, HarperCollins, 1992, pp 93–105

Glueck S, Glueck E: Unravelling Juvenile Delinquency. Cambridge, MA, Harvard University Press, 1950

Glueck S, Glueck E: Delinquents and Nondelinquents in Perspective. Cambridge, MA, Harvard University Press, 1968

Gobeil O: El susto: a descriptive analysis. Int J Soc Psychiatry 9:38–43, 1973

Gof G, Demetra D: Personal communication to KC Faller, in Child Sexual Abuse. Edited by Faller KC. New York, Columbia University Press, 1983

Goldenberg I, Goldenberg H: Family Therapy: An Overview, 5th Edition. Belmont, CA, Wadsworth, 2000
Goldfried M, Norcross JC (eds): Handbook of Psychotherapy Integration. New York, Basic Books, 1992
Goldfried M, Wolfe B: Psychotherapy practice and research: repairing a strained alliance. Am Psychol 51:1007–1016, 1996
Goldman A, Greenberg LS: Comparison of interactional systemic and emotionally focused approaches to couples therapy. J Consult Clin Psychol 60:962–969, 1992
Goldman CR, Quinn FL: Effects of a patient education program in the treatment of schizophrenia. Hosp Community Psychiatry 39:282–286, 1988
Goldman HH: Mental illness and family burden: a public health perspective. Hosp Community Psychiatry 33:557–559, 1982
Goldman S, Beardslee WR: Suicide in children and adolescents, in The Harvard Medical School Guide to Suicide Assessment and Intervention. Edited by Jacobs D. San Francisco, CA, Jossey-Bass, 1999, pp 141–156
Goldner V: Feminism and family therapy. Fam Process 24:37–47, 1985a
Goldner V: Warning: family therapy may be dangerous to your health. Family Therapy Networker 9:19–23, 1985b
Goldstein H: Parental composition, supervision and conduct problems in youths 12 to 17 years old. Journal of the American Academy of Child Psychiatry 23:679–684, 1983
Goldstein M: New Developments in Interventions With Families of Schizophrenics. San Francisco, CA, Jossey-Bass, 1980
Goldstein MJ: Family interaction patterns that antedate the onset of schizophrenia and related disorders: a further analysis of data from a longitudinal prospective study, in Understanding Major Mental Disorder: The Contribution of Family Interaction Research. Edited by Hahlweg K, Goldstein MJ. New York, Family Process Press, 1987, pp 11–32
Goldstein M, Miklowitz D: The effectiveness of psychoeducational family therapy in the treatment of schizophrenic disorders. J Marital Fam Ther 21:361–376, 1995
Goldstein MJ, Strachan AM: The family and schizophrenia, in Family Interaction and Psychopathology: Theories, Methods, and Findings. Edited by Jacob T. New York, Plenum, 1987, pp 481–508
Goldstein M, Rodnick E, Evans J, et al: A method for studying social influences and coping patterns within families of disturbed adolescents. J Nerv Ment Dis 147:233–251, 1968
Goldstein M, Rodnick E, Evans J, et al: Drug and family therapy in the aftercare of acute schizophrenics. Arch Gen Psychiatry 35:1169–1177, 1978
Goldstein M, Talovic S, Nuechterlein K, et al: Family interaction vs. individual psychopathology: do they indicate the same processes in the families of schizophrenics? Br J Psychiatry 161 (suppl 18):97–102, 1992
Goldstein MJ, Strachan AM, Wynne LC: Relational problem related to a mental disorder or general medical condition, in DSM-IV Sourcebook, Vol 3. Edited by Widiger TA, Frances AJ, Pincus HA, et al. Washington, DC, American Psychiatric Association, 1997, pp 531–567
Gonzalez D: What is the problem with Hispanic? Just ask a Latino. New York Times 1992
Gonzalez S, Steinglass P, Reiss D: Putting the illness in its place: discussion groups for families with chronic medical illnesses. Fam Process 14:69–87, 1989
Goodall J: The Chimpanzees of Gombe. Cambridge, MA, Belknap Press of Harvard University, 1986
Goodman S, Brogan D, Lynch M, et al: Social and emotional competence in children of depressed mothers. Child Dev 64:516–531, 1993
Goodrich T: Women, power, and family therapy: what's wrong with this picture? in Women and Power: Perspectives for Family Therapy. Edited by Goodrich T. New York, WW Norton, 1991, pp 3–12
Goodwin D: Alcoholism and genetics: the sins of the father. Arch Gen Psychiatry 42:171–174, 1985

Goodwin D, Warnoch J: Alcoholism: a family disease, in Clinical Textbook of Addictive Disorders. Edited by Frances RJ, Miller SI. New York, Guilford, 1991, pp 485–500

Goodwin D, Schulsinger F, Hermansenk L, et al: Alcohol problems in adoptees raised apart from alcoholic biological parents. Arch Gen Psychiatry 28:238–242, 1973

Goodwin J, McCarthy, DiVasto P: Physical and sexual abuse of the children of adult incest victims, in Sexual Abuse. Edited by Goodwin J. Boston, MA, John Wright PSG, 1981

Goolishian H, Anderson H: J Marital Fam Ther 18, 1992

Gordon L: Identifying hidden expectations in marital therapy, in Questions and Answers in the Practice of Family Therapy. Edited by Gurman A. New York, Brunner/Mazel, 1981

Gordon L: Heroes of Their Own Lives: The Politics and History of Family Violence. New York, Viking, 1988

Gordon SB, Davidson N: Behavioral parent training, in Handbook of Family Therapy. Edited by Gurman AS, Kniskern DP. New York, Brunner/Mazel, 1981, pp 517–555

Gordon T: Parent Effectiveness Training (PET). New York, New American Library, 1970

Gotlib IH, Whiffen VE: Depression and marital functioning: an examination of specificity and gender differences. J Abnorm Psychol 98:23–30, 1989

Gottman J: Marital Interaction: Experimental Investigations. New York, Academic Press, 1979

Gottman J: Predicting the longitudinal course of marriages. J Marital Fam Ther 17:3–7, 1991

Gottman J: The roles of conflict engagement: escalation and avoidance in marital interaction: a longitudinal view of five types of couples. J Consult Clin Psychol 61:6–16, 1993

Gottman J: An agenda for couples therapy, in The Heart of the Matter: Perspectives on Emotion in Marital Therapy. Edited by Johnson S, Greenberg L. New York, Brunner/Mazel, 1994a

Gottman J: What Predicts Divorce? Hillsdale, NJ, Lawrence Erlbaum, 1994b

Gottman JM: The Marriage Clinic: A Scientifically Based Marital Therapy. New York, WW Norton, 1999

Gottman J: An agenda for marital therapy, in Emotion in Marriage and Marital Therapy. Edited by Johnson SM, Greenberg LS. New York, Brunner/Mazel (in press)

Gottman J, Krokoff L: Marital interaction and satisfaction: a longitudinal view. J Consult Clin Psychol 57:47–52, 1989

Gottman J, Levenson RW: Assessing the role of emotion in marriage. Behavioral Assessment 8:31–48, 1986

Gottman JM, Levenson RW: Marital processes predictive of later dissolution: behavior, physiology, and health. J Pers Soc Psychol 63:221–233, 1992

Gottman J, Notarius C, Gonso J, et al: A Couple's Guide to Communication. Champaign, IL, Research Press, 1976a

Gottman J, Notarius C, Markman H, et al: Behavior exchange theory and marital decision making. J Pers Soc Psychol 34:14–23, 1976b

Gottman J, Markman H, Notarius C: The topography of marital conflict: a sequential analysis of verbal and nonverbal behavior. Journal of Marriage and the Family 39:461–477, 1977

Gottman JM, Jacobson NS, Rushe RH, et al: The relationship between heart rate reactivity, emotionally aggressive behavior, and general violence in batterers. Journal of Family Psychology 9:227–248, 1995

Gottman J, Coan J, Carrere S, et al: Predicting marital happiness and stability from newlywed interactions. Journal of Marriage and the Family 60:5–22, 1998

Gould E, Glick ID: The effects of family presence and family therapy on outcome of hospitalized schizophrenic patients. Fam Process 16:503–510, 1979

Grad J, Sainsbury P: Mental illness and the family. Lancet :544–547, 1963

Gray J: Men Are From Mars, Women Are From Venus. New York, HarperCollins, 1989

Graziano AM, Mooney KC: Family self-control instruction for children's nighttime fear reduction. J Consult Clin Psychol 48:206–213, 1980

Green AH: Overview of the literature on child sexual abuse, in Handbook for Health Care and Legal Professionals. Edited by Schetky DH, Green H. New York, Brunner/Mazel, 1988, pp 30–54

Green K, Beck S, Forehand R, et al: Validity of teacher nomination of child behavior problems. J Abnorm Child Psychol 8:397–404, 1980

Green RJ: An overview of major contributions to family therapy, in Family Therapy: Major Contributors. Edited by Green RJ, Framo JL. Madison, WI, International Universities Press, 1981

Green RJ: Correspondence in reply to Grunebaum. Fam Process 31:189–191, 1992

Green RJ, Herget M: Outcomes of systemic/strategic team consultation, I: overview and one-month results. Fam Process 28:37–58, 1989a

Green RJ, Herget M: Outcomes of systemic/strategic team consultation, II: three-year follow-up and a theory of "emergent design." Fam Process 28:419–437, 1989b

Green RJ, Herget M: Outcomes of systemic/strategic team consultation, III: the importance of therapist warmth and active structuring. Fam Process 30:321–336, 1991

Greenacre P: The prepuberty trauma in girls, in Trauma, Growth and Personality (1950). Edited by Greenacre P. New York, International Universities Press, 1969, pp 204–223

Greenberg L, Johnson S: Affect in marital therapy. J Marital Fam Ther 12:1–10, 1986a

Greenberg LS, Johnson SM: When to evoke emotion and why: process diagnosis in couples therapy. J Marital Fam Ther 12:19–23, 1986b

Greenberg LS, Johnson SM: in Clinical Handbook of Marital Therapy. Edited by Jacobson NS, Gurman AS. New York, Guilford, 1986c, pp 253–279

Greenberg L, Johnson S: Emotional change processes in couples therapy, in Emotions and the Family. Edited by Blechman E. Hillsdale, NJ, Lawrence Erlbaum, 1990, pp 137–154

Greenberg LS, Paivio SC: Working With Emotions in Psychotherapy. New York, Guilford, 1997

Greenberg L, Pinsof W (eds): The Psychotherapeutic Process: A Research Handbook. New York, Guilford, 1986

Greenberg L, Safran J: Emotionally Focused Therapy for Couples. New York, Guilford, 1988

Greenberg L, Fine SB, Cohen C, et al: An interdisciplinary psychoeducation program for schizophrenic patients and their families in an acute care setting. Hosp Community Psychiatry 39:277–281, 1988

Greenberg LS, Ford C, Alden L, et al: Change processes in emotionally focused therapy. J Consult Clin Psychol 61:78–84, 1993

Greene B, Broadhurts B, Lustig N: Treatment of marital disharmony, in Psychotherapy of Marital Disharmony. Edited by Greene B. New York, Free Press, 1982

Greenson RR: Empathy and its vicissitudes. International Journal of Psychoanalysis 44:418–424, 1960

Greenson RR: The problem of working through, in Drives, Affects, and Behavior. Edited by Schus M. New York, International Universities Press, 1965, pp 217–314

Greenspan SI, Nover RA, Scheuer AQ: A developmental diagnostic approach for infants, young children, and their families. Clinical Infant Reports 3:431–498, 1987

Griest DL, Wells KC: Behavioral family therapy with conduct disorders in children. Behavior Therapy 14:37–53, 1983

Group for the Advancement of Psychiatry: The Family, the Patient, and the Psychiatric Hospital: Toward a New Model. New York, Brunner/Mazel, 1985, pp 27–29

Group for the Advancement of Psychiatry, Committee on the Family: The classification of families. Unpublished monograph, 1991

Group for the Advancement of Psychiatry, Committee on the Family: A model for the classification and diagnosis of relational disorders. Psychiatr Serv 46:926–931, 1995

Grunebaum H: Family psychiatry, in Psychiatry, Vol 3, Section 1. Michael R, editor-in-chief. Philadelphia, PA, JB Lippincott, 1991, pp 1–16

Grunebaum H, Belfer ML: What family therapists might learn from child psychiatry. Journal of Marriage and Family Therapy 12:415–423, 1986
Gubernick DJ: A natural family system. Family Systems 3(23):109–124, 1996
Guerney BG: Relationship Enhancement. San Francisco, CA, Jossey-Bass, 1977
Guerney BG Jr, Maxson P: Marital and family enrichment research: a decade review and look ahead. Journal of Marriage and the Family 52:1127–1134, 1990
Guidano V, Liotti G: Cognitive Processes and Emotional Disorders. New York, Guilford, 1983
Guldner CA: Family therapy with adolescents. Journal of Group Psychotherapy, Psychodrama, and Sociometry 43:142–150, 1990
Gunderson J, Singer M: Defining borderline patients: an overview. Am J Psychiatry 132:1–10, 1975
Gunderson JG, Berkowitz C, Ruiz-Sancho A: Families of borderline patients: a psychoeducational approach. Bull Menninger Clin 61:446–457, 1997
Guntrip H: Schizoid Phenomena, Object Relations and the Self. New York, International Universities Press, 1969
Gurman A: The effects and effectiveness of marital therapy: a review of outcome research. Fam Process 12:145–170, 1973
Gurman AS: Contemporary marital therapies, a critique and comparative analysis of psychoanalytic, behavioral and systems theory approaches, in Marriage and Marital Therapy. Edited by Paolino TJ, McCrady BS. New York, Brunner/Mazel, 1978
Gurman AS: Family therapy research and the "new epistemology." J Marital Fam Ther 9:227–234, 1983
Gurman AS: Back to the future, ahead to the past: is marital therapy going in circles? Journal of Family Psychology 4:402–406, 1991
Gurman A, Kniskern D: Research on marital and family therapy: progress, perspective and prospect, in Handbook of Psychotherapy and Behavior Change, 2nd Edition. Edited by Garfield SL, Bergin A. New York, Wiley, 1978
Gurman AS, Kniskern DP: Family therapy outcome research, in Handbook of Family Therapy. Edited by Gurman AS, Kniskern DP. New York, Brunner/Mazel, 1981a, pp 742–775
Gurman AS, Kniskern DP (eds): Handbook of Family Therapy. New York, Brunner/Mazel, 1981b
Gurman A, Kniskern D, Pinsof W: Research on the process and outcome of marital and family therapy, in Handbook of Psychotherapy and Behavior Change. Edited by Garfield SL, Bergin A. New York, Wiley, 1986, pp 565–624
Guttmann HA, Spector RM, Sigal JJ, et al: Reliability of coding affective communication in family therapy sessions. J Consult Clin Psychol 37:397–402, 1971
Haas G, Clarkin J, Glick I: Marital and family treatment of depression, in Handbook of Depression. Edited by Beckham E, Leber W. Homewood, IL, Dorsey Press, 1985, pp 151–182
Haas G, Glick I, Clarkin J: Inpatient family intervention: a randomized clinical trial, II: results at hospital discharge. Arch Gen Psychiatry 45:217–224, 1988
Hahlweg K, Markman HJ: Effectiveness of behavioral marital therapy: empirical status of behavioral techniques. J Consult Clin Psychol 56:440–447, 1988
Hahlweg K, Revensdorf D, Schindler L: Effects of behavioral marital therapy on couples' communication and problem solving skills. J Consult Clin Psychol 52:553–566, 1984a
Hahlweg K, Schindler L, Revenstorf D, et al: The Munich Marital Therapy Study, in Marital Interaction: Analysis and Modification. Edited by Hahlweg K, Jacobson N. New York, Guilford, 1984b
Hahlweg K, Nuechterlein KH, Goldstein MJ, et al: Parental expressed emotion attitudes and intrafamilial communication behavior, in Understanding Major Mental Disorder: The Contribution of Family Interaction Research. Edited by Hahlweg K, Goldstein MJ. New York, Family Process Press, 1987, pp 45–79

Hahlweg K, Goldstein MJ, Nuechterlein KH, et al: Expressed emotion and patient-relative interaction in families of recent onset schizophrenics. J Consult Clin Psychol 57:11–18, 1989
Hahlweg K, Durr H, Müller U: Familienbetreuung Schizophrener Patienten. Weinheim, Germany, Psychologie Verlags Union, 1995
Hahlweg K, Markman HJ, Thurmaier F, et al: Prevention of marital distress: results of a German prospective longitudinal study. J Fam Psychol 12:543–556, 1998
Haig RA: The Anatomy of Humor: Biopsychosocial and Therapeutic Perspectives. Springfield, IL, Charles C Thomas, 1988
Haley J: The family of the schizophrenic: a model system. J Nerv Ment Dis 129:257–374, 1959
Haley J: Whither family therapy. Fam Process 1:69–100, 1962
Haley J: Strategies of Psychotherapy. New York, Grune & Stratton, 1963
Haley J: Research on family patterns: an instrument measurement. Fam Process 3:41–62, 1964
Haley J (ed): Advanced Techniques of Hypnosis and Therapy: Selected Papers of Milton H Erickson. New York, Grune & Stratton, 1967
Haley J: Uncommon Therapy. Toronto, ON, Canada, WW Norton, 1973
Haley J: Problem Solving Therapy: New Strategies for Effective Family Therapy. San Francisco, CA, Jossey-Bass, 1976
Haley J (ed): Advanced Techniques of Hypnosis and Therapy: The Selected Papers of Milton H Erickson. New York, Grune & Stratton, 1980a
Haley J: Leaving Home: The Therapy of Disturbed Young People. New York, McGraw-Hill, 1980b
Haley J: Reflections on Therapy. Chevy Chase, MD, The Family Therapy Institute of Washington, DC, 1981
Haley J: Ordeal Therapy. San Francisco, CA, Jossey-Bass, 1984
Haley J, Hoffman L: Techniques of Family Therapy. New York, Basic Books, 1981
Halford WK: The ongoing evolution of behavioral couples therapy: retrospect and prospect. Clin Psychol Rev 18:613–633, 1998
Halford WK, Sanders MR: Assessment of cognitive self-statements during marital problem solving: a comparison of two methods. Cognitive Therapy and Research 12:515–530, 1988
Halford W, Sanders M, Behrens B: A comparison of the generalization of behavioral marital therapy and enhanced behavioral marital therapy. J Consult Clin Psychol 61:51–60, 1993
Halford WK, Sanders MR, Behrens BC: Self-regulation in behavioral couples therapy. Behavior Therapy 25:431–452, 1994
Halford WK, Harrison C, Kalyansundaram M, et al: Preliminary results from a psychoeducational program to rehabilitate chronic patients. Psychiatr Serv 46:1189–1191, 1995
Hall AM, Neuharth-Prichett S, Berlfiore PJ: Reduction of aggressive behaviors with changes in activity: linking descriptive and experimental analyses. Education and Training in Mental Retardation and Developmental Disabilities 32:331–339, 1997
Hallam RS, Hinchcliffe R: Emotional stability: its relationships to confidence in maintaining balance. J Psychosom Res 35:421–434, 1991
Halvorsen JG: The Family Stress and Support Inventory (FSSI). Family Practice Research Journal 11:255–277, 1991
Hamilton B: Ethnicity and the family life cycle: the Chinese-American family. Family Therapy 23:199–212, 1996
Hamilton M: A rating scale for depression. J Neurol Neurosurg Psychiatry 23:56–62, 1960
Hamilton M: Development of rating scale for primary depressive illness. British Journal of Social and Clinical Psychology 6:278–296, 1968
Hammen C, Gordon D, Burge D: Maternal affective disorders, illness, and stress: risk for children's psychopathology. Am J Psychiatry 144:736–741, 1987

Hammen C, Burge D, Stansbury K: Relationship of mother and child variables to child outcomes in a high risk sample: a causal modeling analysis. Dev Psychol 26:24–30, 1990

Hampson RB, Beavers WR: Comparing males' and females' perspectives through family self-report. Psychiatry 50:24–30, 1988

Hampson RB, Beavers WR, Hulgus YF: Insiders' and outsiders' views of family: the assessment of family competence and style. Journal of Family Psychology 3:118–136, 1989

Hampson RB, Beavers WR, Hulgus YF: Cross ethnic family differences: interactional assessment of white, black, and Mexican-American families. J Marital Fam Ther 12:187–199, 1990

Hardcastle DR: A mother-child, multiple-family, counseling program: procedures and results. Fam Process 16:67–74, 1977

Hardesty JP, Falloon IRH, Shirin K: The impact of life events, stress, and coping on the morbidity of schizophrenia, in Family Management of Schizophrenia: A Study of Clinical, Social, Family and Economic Benefits. Edited by Falloon IRH. Baltimore, MD, Johns Hopkins University Press, 1985

Hardy KV: The theoretical myth of sameness: a critical issue in family therapy treatment and training, in Minorities and Family Therapy. Edited by Saba GW, Karrer BM, Hardy KV. Binghamton, NY, Haworth, 1989, pp 79–90

Hare-Mustin RT: A feminist approach to family therapy. Fam Process 17:181–194, 1978

Hare-Mustin R: Family therapy may be dangerous to your health. Professional Psychology 2:935–938, 1988

Harrell J, Guerney B: Training marital couples in conflict negotiation skills, in Treating Relationships. Edited by Olson DH. Lake Mills, LA, Graphic Publisher, 1976

Harrington R, Fudge H, Rutter M, et al: Adult outcomes of childhood and adolescent depression: psychiatric status. Arch Gen Psychiatry 47:465–473, 1986

Harris SL: Families of the Developmentally Disabled: A Guide to Behavioral Intervention. New York, Pergamon, 1983

Hartmann H: Essays on Ego Psychology: Selected Problems in Psychoanalytic Theory. New York, International Universities Press, 1964

Harwood A: Ethnicity and Medical Care. Cambridge, MA, Harvard University Press, 1981

Harwood A: Acculturation in the postmodern world: implications for mental health research, in Theoretical and Conceptual Issues in Hispanic Mental Health. Edited by Malgady RG, Rodriquez O. Malabar, FL, Krieger, 1994

Hatfield A: Help-seeking behavior in families of schizophrenics. Am J Community Psychol 7:563–569, 1979

Hatfield AB: Coping effectiveness in families of the mentally ill: an exploratory study. Journal of Psychiatric Treatment and Evaluation 3:11–19, 1981

Hatfield A: What families want of a family therapist, in Family Therapy of Schizophrenia. Edited by McFarlane WR. New York, Guilford, 1983

Hatfield A: The family as partner in the treatment of mental illness. Hosp Community Psychiatry 30:338–340, 1986a

Hatfield A: Semantic barriers to family and professional collaboration. Schizophr Bull 12:325–333, 1986b

Hatfield A: The National Alliance for the Mentally Ill: the meaning of a movement. Journal of Mental Health 15(4):79–93, 1987

Hatfield A: Coping With Mental Illness in the Family: A Family Guide. Arlington, VA, National Alliance for the Mentally Ill, 1991

Hatfield A: Coping With Aggressive Behavior. Arlington, VA, National Alliance for the Mentally Ill, 1992a

Hatfield A: Family Education in Mental Illness: Stress, Coping and Adaptation. New York, Guilford, 1992b

Hatfield AB: Working collaboratively with families. Soc Work Health Care 25(3):77–85, 1997

Hatfield AB, Lefley H (eds): Families of the Mentally Ill: Coping and Adaptation. New York, Guilford, 1987

Hatfield A, Feinstein R, Johnson D: Meeting the needs of families of the psychiatrically disabled. Psychosocial Rehabilitation Journal 4(1):27–40, 1982

Hawton K: The behavioral treatment of sexual dysfunction. Br J Psychiatry 140:94–101, 1982

Hayes SC, Nelson RO, Jarrett RB: Evaluating the quality of behavioral assessment, in Conceptual Foundations of Behavioral Assessment. Edited by Nelson RO, Hayes SC. New York, Guilford, 1986

Hazan C, Shaver P: Romantic love conceptualized as an attachment process. J Pers Soc Psychol 52:511–524, 1987

Hazelrigg MD, Cooper HM, Borduin CM: Evaluating the effectiveness of family therapies: an integrative review and analysis. Psychol Bull 101:428–442, 1987

Heath A, Ayers T: MRI brief therapy with adolescent substance abusers, in Family Therapy Approaches With Adolescent Substance Abusers. Edited by Todd T, Seleckman M. Boston, MA, Allyn & Bacon, 1991, pp 49–69

Heath A, Stanton D: Family therapy, in Clinical Textbook of Addictive Disorders. Edited by Frances R, Miller S. New York, Guilford, 1991, pp 406–430

Heavey C, Layne C, Christensen A: Gender and conflict structure in marital interaction: a replication and extension. J Consult Clin Psychol 61:16–26, 1993

Heavey C, Christensen A, Malamuth N: The longitudinal impact of demand and withdraw during marital conflict. J Consult Clin Psychol 63:797–801, 1995

Heilbrun CG: Writing a Woman's Life. New York, WW Norton, 1988

Heiman J, Lo Piccolo J: The treatment of sexual dysfunction, in Handbook of Family Therapy. Edited by Gurman AS, Kniskern DP. New York, Brunner/Mazel, 1981

Held BS: The relationship between individual psychologies and strategic/systemic therapies reconsidered, in Journeys: Expansion of the Strategic-Systemic Therapies. Edited by Efron DE. New York, Brunner/Mazel, 1986, pp 222–260

Held BS: The problem of strategy in strategic therapy. J Marital Fam Ther 18:24–34, 1992

Held T: Schizophreniebehandlung in der Familie. Frankfurt am Main, Peter Lang, 1995

Helzer JE, Pryzbeck TR: The co-occurrence of alcoholism with other psychiatric disorders in the general population and its impact on treatment. J Stud Alcohol 49:219–224, 1988

Henderson P: Counseling children of parents with severe mental illness. School Counselor 42:147–154, 1994

Henggeler SW: The development of effective drug abuse services for youth, in Treating Drug Abusers Effectively. Edited by Egeston JA, Fox DM, Leshner AI. New York, Blackwell, 1997, pp 253–279

Henggeler SW, Santos AB (eds): Innovative Approaches for "Difficult-to-Treat" Populations. Washington, DC, American Psychiatric Press, 1997

Henggeler SW, Schoenwald SK: The MST Supervisory Manual: Promoting Quality Assurance at the Clinical Level. Charleston, SC, MST Institute, 1998

Henggeler SW, Borduin CM, Melton GB, et al: Effects of multisystemic therapy on drug use and abuse in serious juvenile offenders: a progress report from two outcome studies. Family Dynamics of Addiction Quarterly 1:40–51, 1991

Henggeler SW, Melton GB, Smith LA: Family preservation using multisystemic therapy: an effective alternative to incarcerating serious juvenile offenders. J Consult Clin Psychol 60:953–961, 1992

Henggeler SW, Pickrel SG, Brondino MJ, et al: Eliminating treatment dropouts of substance abusing or dependent delinquents through home-based multisystemic therapy. Am J Psychiatry 153:427–428, 1996

Henggeler SW, Mihalic SF, Rone L, et al: Blueprint for Violence Prevention Multi-Systemic Therapy (DSD; Eliot S, series ed). Boulder, University of Colorado, Center for Study and Prevention of Violence, 1998a

Henggeler SW, Schoenwald SK, Borduin CM, et al: Multisystemic Treatment of Antisocial Behavior in Children and Adolescents. New York, Guilford, 1998b

Henggeler SW, Rowland MD, Randall J, et al: Home-based multi-systemic therapy as an alternative to the hospitalization of youth in psychiatric crises: clinical outcomes. J Am Acad Child Adolesc Psychiatry 38:1331–1339, 1999

Henserson L: African Americans in the urban milieu: conditions, trends, and development needs, in The State of Black America. Edited by Tidwell B. New York, Urban League, 1994, pp 11–26

Herman JL: Father-Daughter Incest. Cambridge, MA, Harvard University Press, 1981

Herr E: Cultural diversity from an international perspective. Journal of Multicultural Counseling and Development 15:99–109, 1989

Hertz F: The impact of death and serious illness on the family life cycle, in The Family Life Cycle: A Framework for Family Therapy. Edited by Carter ES, McGoldrick M. New York, Gardner Press, 1980

Hesselbrock M, Meyer R, Keener J: Psychopathology in hospitalized alcoholics. Arch Gen Psychiatry 42:1050–1055, 1985

Hetherington EM: Family relations six years after divorce, in Remarriage and Stepparenting Today: Current Research and Theory. Edited by Pasley K, Ihinger-Tollman M. New York, Guilford, 1987, pp 185–205

Hetherington EM: Parents, children and siblings six years after divorce, in Relationships Within Families. Edited by Hinde R, Stevenson-Hinde J. Cambridge, UK, Cambridge University Press, 1988

Hetherington EM: Coping with family transitions: winners, loser, survivors. Child Dev 60:1–14, 1989

Hetherington EM, Anderson ER: The effects of divorce and remarriage on early adolescents and their families, in Early Adolescent Transitions. Edited by Levine MD, McArney ER. Lexington, MA, DC Heath, 1987, pp 49–67

Hetherington EM, Clingempeel WG: Coping with remarriage: the first two years. Symposium presented at the Southeastern Conference on Human Development, Charleston, SC, 1988

Hetherington EM, Clingempeel WG: Coping with marital transition. Monogr Soc Res Child Dev 57(227):1–242, 1992

Hetherington E, Martin B: Family interaction, in Psychopathological Disorders of Childhood, 2nd Edition. Edited by Quay H, Werry J. New York, Wiley, 1979, pp 247–302

Hetherington EM, Cox M, Cox R: The aftermath of divorce, in Contemporary Readings in Child Psychology. Edited by Hetherington EM, Parke RD. New York, McGraw-Hill, 1981

Hetherington EM, Cox M, Cox R: Effects of divorce on parents and children, in Nontraditional Families. Edited by Lamb M. Hillsdale, NJ, Lawrence Erlbaum, 1982, pp 233–288

Hetherington EM, Cox M, Cox R: Long-term effects of divorce and remarriage on the adjustment of children. Journal of the American Academy of Child Psychiatry 24:518–530, 1986

Hetherington E, Stanley-Hagan M, Anderson E: Marital transitions: a child's perspective. Am Psychol 44:303–312, 1989

Heyman RE: Cognitive and behavioral differences between abusive and non-abusive early married couples. Unpublished doctoral dissertation, University of Oregon, Eugene, 1992

Heyman RE: Observation of couple conflicts: clinical assessment applications, stubborn truths, and shaky foundations. Psychol Assess 13:5–35, 2001

Heyman RE, Weiss RL: Video-Recall Cognitive Coding System. Unpublished coding manual, Oregon Marital Studies Program, University of Oregon, Eugene, 1991

Heyman RE, Sayers SL, Bellack AS: Global marital satisfaction vs marital adjustment: an empirical comparison of three measures. Journal of Family Psychology 8:432–446, 1994

Hill D, Black D: The effect of an education program for the families of chronically mentally ill on stress and anxiety. Psychosocial Rehabilitation Journal 10:25–40, 1987

Hill R: Families Under Stress. New York, Harper Press, 1949
Hill R: Informal Adoption Among Black Families. Washington, DC, National Urban League, 1977
Hill R, Rodgers RH: The developmental approach, in Handbook of Marriage and the Family. Edited by Christensen HT. Chicago, IL, Rand McNally, 1964
Hillard R: Validity of two psychological screening measures in family practice: Personal Inventory and Family APGAR. J Fam Pract 23:345–349, 1986
Hinchliffe M, Hooper D, Roberts F: A study of the interaction between depressed patients and their spouses. Br J Psychiatry 126:164–172, 1975
Hinchliffe M, Vaughan P, Hooper D: The melancholy marriage: an inquiry into the interaction of depression, II: expressiveness. Br J Med Psychol 50:125–142, 1977
Hinchliffe M, Hooper D, Roberts F: The Melancholy Marriage: Depression in Marriage and Psychosocial Approaches to Therapy. New York, Wiley, 1978a
Hinchliffe M, Hooper D, Roberts F: The melancholy marriage: an inquiry into the interaction of depression, III: responsiveness. Br J Med Psychol 51:1–13, 1978b
Hines P, Boyd-Franklin N: Black families, in Ethnicity and Family Therapy. Edited by McGoldrick M, Giordano J. New York, Guilford, 1982, pp 84–107
Hinshaw SP, Owens EB, Wells KC, et al: Family processes and treatment outcome in the MTA: negative/ineffective parenting practices in relation to multimodal treatment. J Abnorm Psychol 28:555–568, 2000
Ho T, Chow V, Fung C, et al: Parent management training in a Chinese population: application and outcome. J Am Acad Child Adolesc Psychiatry 38:1165–1172, 1999
Hobbs N, Perrin JM, Ireys HT: Chronically Ill Children and Their Families: Problems, Prospects, and Proposals From the Vanderbilt Study. San Francisco, CA, Jossey-Bass, 1978
Hodas G: Psychosomatic families, in Continuing Education in Family and Marital Therapy. Edited by Sholevar GP. New York, Medical Examination Publishing (in press)
Hodes M, Le Grange D: Expressed emotion in the investigation of eating disorders: a review. Int J Eat Disord 13:279–288, 1993
Hodges B, Regehr G, Hanson M, et al: An objective structured clinical examination for evaluating psychiatric clinical clerks. Acad Med 78:715–721, 1997
Hoenig J, Hamilton MW: Elderly psychiatric patients and the burden on the household. Psychiatric Neurology (Basel) 154:281–293, 1966
Hof L, Berman E: The sexual genogram. J Marital Fam Ther 12:39–47, 1986
Hoffman L: Foundations of Family Therapy: A Conceptual Framework for Systems Change. New York, Basic Books, 1981
Hoffman L: Beyond power and control: toward a second-order family systems therapy. Family Systems Medicine 3:381–396, 1985
Hoffman L: A reflective stance for family therapists. Journal of Strategic and Systemic Therapies 10:4–17, 1991
Hogarty GE, Anderson CM, Reiss DJ, et al: Family psychoeducation, social skills training, and maintenance chemotherapy in the aftercare treatment of schizophrenia, I: one-year effects of a controlled study on relapse and expressed emotion. Arch Gen Psychiatry 43:633–642, 1986
Hogarty GE, McEvoy J, Munetz M: Dose of fluphenazine, familial expressed emotion, and outcome in schizophrenia: results of 2-year controlled study. Arch Gen Psychiatry 45:797–805, 1988
Hogarty GE, Anderson CM, Reiss D, et al: Family psychoeducation, social skills training, and maintenance chemotherapy in the aftercare treatment of schizophrenia, II: two-year effects of a controlled study on relapse and adjustment. Arch Gen Psychiatry 48:340–347, 1991
Hogarty GE, Kornblith SJ, Greenwald D, et al: Personal therapy: a disorder-relevant psychotherapy for schizophrenia. Paper presented to XIth International Symposium for the Psychotherapy of Schizophrenia, Washington, DC, June 12–15, 1994

Hogue A, Liddle HA, Rowe C, et al: Treatment adherence and differentiation in individual versus family therapy for adolescent substance abuse. J Couns Psychol 45:104–114, 1998

Holden DF, Lewine RRJ: How families evaluate mental health professionals, resources, and effects of illness. Schizophr Bull 8:626–633, 1982

Holder D, Anderson C: Psychoeducational family intervention for depressed patients and their families, in Depression and Families: Impact and Treatment. Edited by Keitner GI. Washington, DC, American Psychiatric Press, 1990, pp 159–184

Holmes J, Boon S: Developments in the field of close relationships. Personality and Social Psychology Bulletin 16:23–41, 1990

Holmes J, Rempel J: Trust in close relationships. Review of Personality and Social Psychology 19:187–220, 1989

Holmes TH, Masuda M: Life change and illness susceptibility, in Separation and Depression. Edited by Scott JP, Senay EC. Washington, DC, American Association for the Advancement of Science, 1973

Holtz H, Dobro J, Palinkas R, et al: Psychosocial impact of acquired immune deficiency syndrome (letter). JAMA 250:167, 1983

Holtzworth-Munroe A, Jacobson N: Causal attributions of married couples. J Pers Soc Psychol 48:1398–1412, 1985

Holtzworth-Munroe A, Jacobson NS: Toward a methodology for coding spontaneous causal attributions: preliminary results with married couples. Journal of Social and Clinical Psychology 7:101–112, 1987

Holtzworth-Munroe A, Jacobson NS, DeKlyen M, et al: Relationship between behavioral marital therapy outcome and process variables. J Consult Clin Psychol 57:658–662, 1989

Holtzworth-Munroe A, Beatty SB, Anglin K: The assessment and treatment of marital violence, in Clinical Handbook of Couple Therapy, 2nd Edition. Edited by Jacobson NS, Gurman AS. New York, Guilford, 1995

Holzman P: Recent studies of psychophysiology in schizophrenia. Schizophr Bull 13:49–75, 1987

Homans G: Social Behavior: Its Elementary Forms. New York, Harcourt, Brace & World, 1961

Hooley J: Expressed emotion: a review of the critical literature. Clin Psychol Rev 5:119–139, 1985

Hooley J: The nature of expressed emotion, in Understanding Major Mental Disorder: The Contribution of Family Interaction Research. Edited by Hahlweg K, Goldstein MJ. New York, Family Process Press, 1987, pp 176–194

Hooley J: Stability of expressed emotion. Paper presented at the annual meeting of the Society for Research in Psychopathology, Coral Gables, FL, 1989

Hooley J: Attributions about illness in the high- and low-EE spouses of depressed patients. Paper presented at the annual meeting of the Association for the Advancement of Behavior Therapy, New York, November 1991

Hooley J: Expressed emotion and locus of control. J Nerv Ment Dis 186:374–378, 1998

Hooley JM, Hahlweg K: Marital satisfaction and marital communication in German and English couples. Behavioral Assessment 11:119–133, 1989

Hooley J, Richters J: Expressed emotion: a developmental perspective, in Emotion, Cognition and Representations. 1985, pp 133–166

Hooley J, Teasdale J: Predictors of relapse in unipolar depressives: expressed emotion, marital distress, and perceived criticism. J Abnorm Psychol 98:229–235, 1989

Hooley J, Orley J, Teasdale J: Levels of expressed emotion and relapse in depressed patients. Br J Psychiatry 148:642–647, 1986

Hooley JM, Richters JE, Weintraub S, et al: Psychopathology and marital distress: the positive side of positive symptoms. J Abnorm Psychol 96:27–33, 1987

Hooper D, Roberts F, Hinchliffe M, et al: The melancholy marriage: an inquiry into the interaction of depression, I: introduction. Br J Med Psychol 50:113–124, 1977

Hoopes M, Fisher B, Barlow S: Structured Family Facilitation Programs: Enrichment, Education and Treatment. Rockville, MD, Aspen Systems, 1984

Hoover C, Fitzgerald R: Dominance in the marriage of affective patients. J Nerv Ment Dis 169:624–628, 1981

Hopps J, Wills T, Patterson GR, et al: Marital Interaction Coding System. Eugene, University of Oregon and Oregon Research Institute, 1972

Hops H, Biglan A, Sherman L, et al: Home observations of family interactions of depressed women. J Consult Clin Psychol 55:341–346, 1987

Horney K: New Ways in Psychoanalysis. New York, WW Norton, 1939

Hornung WP, Holle R, Schulze-Mönking H, et al: Psychoedukativ-psychotherapeutische Behandlung von schizophrenen Patienten und ihren Bezugspersonen. Ergebnisse einer 1-jahres-Katamnese. Nervenartz 66:828–834, 1995

Horowitz L: On the cognitive structure of interpersonal problems treated in psychotherapy. J Consult Clin Psychol 47:5–15, 1979

House RM, Pinyuchon M: Counseling Thai Americans: an emerging need. Journal of Multicultural Counseling and Development 26:194–203, 1998

Houts AC, Follette WC: Mini-series on philosophical and theoretical issues in behavior therapy. Behavior Therapy 23:145–262, 1992

Howells J: Family Psychiatry. Edinburgh, Scotland, Oliver & Boyd, 1963

Hubbard W: C Is for Curious: An ABC of Feelings. San Francisco, CA, Chronicle Books, 1990

Huber CH, Milstein B: Cognitive restructuring and collaborative set in couples' work. American Journal of Family Therapy 13:17–27, 1985

Hudgens A: The social worker's role in a behavioral management approach to chronic pain. Soc Work Health Care 3:77–85, 1977

Hudgens A: Family oriented treatment of chronic pain. J Marital Fam Ther 5(4):67–68, 1979

Hunt GM, Azrin NH: A community reinforcement approach to alcoholism. Behav Res Ther 11:91–104, 1973

Hunt RA, Hof L, DeMaria R: Marriage Enrichment: Preparation, Mentoring and Outreach. New York, Brunner/Mazel, 1998

Hurley JR, Palonen DJ: Marital satisfaction and child density among university parents. Journal of Marriage and the Family 29:483–484, 1967

Hyde A: The management of violence in mentally ill people who live at home. Psychiatric Times, October 2, 1994, pp 44–47

Imber-Black E: Families and Larger Systems: A Therapist's Guide Through the Labyrinth. New York, Guilford, 1988

Imber-Black E, Roberts J, Whiting RA: Rituals in Families and Family Therapy. New York, WW Norton, 1988

Imber-Mintz L, Liberman R, Miklowitz D, et al: Expressed emotion: a call for partnership among relatives, patients, and professionals. Schizophr Bull 13:227–235, 1987

Ito J, Oshima I: Distribution of EE and its relationship to relapse in Japan. International Journal of Mental Health 24:23–37, 1995

Iversen A, Baucom DH: Behavioral marital therapy outcomes: alternative interpretations of the data. Behavior Therapy 21:129–138, 1990

Jackson D: The question of family homeostasis. Psychiatr Q Suppl 31 (part 1):79–90, 1957

Jackson DD (ed): The Etiology of Schizophrenia. New York, Basic Books, 1960

Jackson D: Family illness and the principles of homeostasis. Unpublished manuscript, 1964

Jackson D: The study of the family. Fam Process 4:1–20, 1965

Jackson DN: Personality Research Form Manual. New York, Research Psychologists Press, 1974

Jackson DN, Messick S: Differential Personality Inventory. London, Ontario, Jackson DN, Messick S, 1971

Jackson D, Weakland J: Conjoint family therapy: some consideration on theory, technique, and results. Psychiatry 24 (2 suppl):30–35, 1961

References

Jackson D, Yalom I: Family research on the problem of ulcerative colitis. Arch Gen Psychiatry 15:410–415, 1966

Jacob T: Alcoholism and family interaction: clarification resulting from subgroup analyses and multi-method assessments, in Understanding Major Mental Disorder: The Contribution of Family Interaction Research. Edited by Hahlweg K, Goldstein MJ. New York, Family Process Press, 1987, pp 212–227

Jacob T, Leonard K: Alcohol-spouse interaction as a function of drinking style and drinking setting. J Abnorm Psychol 97:231–237, 1988

Jacob T, Tennenbaum D: Family Assessment: Rationale, Methods, and Future Directions. New York, Plenum, 1988

Jacobs J, Wolin S: Alcoholism and family factors: a critical review, in Recent Developments in Alcoholism, Vol 7. Edited by Galanter M. New York, Plenum, 1989, pp 147–164

Jacobson J, Dobson K, Fruzzetti A, et al: Marital therapy as a treatment for depression. J Consult Clin Psychol 59:547–557, 1991

Jacobson N: A review of the research on the effectiveness of marital therapy, in Marriage and Marital Therapy. Edited by Paolino T, McCrady B. New York, Brunner/Mazel, 1978, pp 395–444

Jacobson N: Increasing positive behavior in severely distressed adult relationships. Behavior Therapy 10:311–326, 1979

Jacobson N: Behavioral marital therapy, in Handbook of Family Therapy. Edited by Gurman AS, Kniskern DP. New York, Brunner/Mazel, 1981, pp 556–591

Jacobson N: A component analysis of behavioral marital therapy: the relative effectiveness of behavior exchange and communication/problem/solving training. J Consult Clin Psychol 52:295–305, 1984a

Jacobson NS: The modification of cognitive processes in behavioral marital therapy: integrating cognitive and behavioral intervention strategies, in Marital Interaction: Analysis and Modification. Edited by Hahlweg K, Jacobson N. New York, Guilford, 1984b, pp 285–308

Jacobson N: Behavioral versus insight-oriented marital therapy: labels can be misleading. J Consult Clin Psychol 59:142–145, 1991a

Jacobson NS: To be or not to be behavioral when working with couples: what does it mean? Journal of Family Psychology 4:436–445, 1991b

Jacobson N: Towards enhancing the efficacy of marital therapy and marital therapy research. American Journal of Family Psychology 4:373–393, 1991c

Jacobson N, Addis M: Research on couples and couple therapy: what do we know? Where are we going? J Consult Clin Psychol 61:85–93, 1993

Jacobson N, Christensen A: Integrative Couples Therapy. New York, WW Norton, 1996

Jacobson NS, Gottman JM: When Men Batter Women: New Insights Into Ending Abusive Relationships. New York, Simon & Schuster, 1998

Jacobson N, Gurman AS: Clinical Handbook of Marital Therapy. New York, Guilford, 1986

Jacobson NS, Margolin G: Marital Therapy: Strategies Based on Social Learning and Behavior Exchange Principles. New York, Brunner/Mazel, 1979

Jacobson N, Truax P: Clinical significance: a statistical approach to defining meaningful change in psychotherapy research. J Consult Clin Psychol 59:12–19, 1991

Jacobson N, Waldron H, Moore D: Toward a behavioral profile of marital distress. J Consult Clin Psychol 48:696–703, 1980

Jacobson N, Follette W, MacDonald D: Reactivity to positive and negative behavior in distressed and nondistressed married couples. J Consult Clin Psychol 50:706–714, 1982

Jacobson N, Follette W, Revenstorf D: Psychotherapy outcome research: methods for reporting variability and evaluating clinical significance. Behavior Therapy 15:336–352, 1984a

Jacobson NS, Follette WC, Revenstorf D, et al: Variability in outcome and clinical significance of behavioral marital therapy: a reanalysis of outcome data. J Consult Clin Psychol 52:497–504, 1984b

Jacobson N, Follette W, Pagel M: Predicting who will benefit from behavioral marital therapy. J Consult Clin Psychol 54:518–522, 1986

Jacobson N, Schmaling K, Holtzworth-Munroe A: Component analysis of behavioral marital therapy: two year follow-up and prediction of relapse. J Marital Fam Ther 13:187–195, 1987

Jacobson N, Holtzworth-Munroe A, Schmaling K: Marital therapy and spouse involvement in the treatment of depression, agoraphobia and alcoholism. J Consult Clin Psychol 57:5–10, 1989a

Jacobson NS, Schmaling KB, Holtzworth-Munroe A, et al: Research—structured versus clinically flexible versions of social learning–based marital therapy. Behav Res Ther 2:173–180, 1989b

Jacobson NS, Fruzzetti AE, Dobson K, et al: Couple therapy as a treatment for depression, II: the effects of relationship quality and therapy on depressive relapse. J Consult Clin Psychol 61:516–519, 1993

Jacobson NS, Cordova JV, Prince SE, et al: The impact of acceptance-based interventions on traditional behavioral couple therapy, in Proceedings of the 30th Annual Convention of the Association for Advancement of Behavior Therapy. New York, Association for the Advancement of Behavior Therapy, 1996, p 136

Jacobson NS, Christensen A, Prince SE, et al: Integrative behavioral couple therapy: an acceptance-based, promising new treatment for couple discord. J Consult Clin Psychol 68:351–355, 2000

James P: Effects of a communication training component added to an emotionally focused couples therapy. J Marital Fam Ther 17:263–276, 1991

Janes C, Hesselbrock V: Perceived family environment and school adjustment of children of schizophrenics. Paper presented at the American Psychological Association Annual Convention, Washington, DC, 1976

Jensen SB: Diabetic sexual dysfunction: a comparative study of 160 insulin-treated diabetic men and women and an age-matched control group. Arch Sex Behav 10:493–504, 1981

Jensen SB: Sexual dysfunction in insulin-treated diabetics: a six-year follow-up study of 101 patients. Arch Sex Behav 15:271–284, 1986

Jessor R, Jessor SL: The social-psychological framework, in Problem Behavior and Psychosocial Development: A Longitudinal Study of Youth. Edited by Jessor R, Jessor SL. New York, Academic Press, 1977, pp 17–42

Joanning H, Thomas F, Quinn W, et al: Treating adolescent drug abuse: a comparison of family systems therapy, group therapy, and family drug education. J Marital Fam Ther 18:345–356, 1992

Johnson A, Szurek SA: The genesis of antisocial acting out in children and adults. Psychoanal Q 21:313–343, 1952

Johnson D: The family's experience of living with mental illness. Paper presented at the National Alliance for the Mentally Ill/National Institute of Mental Health Colloquium, Rockville, MD, 1986

Johnson L, Thomas V: Influences on the inclusion of children in family therapy. J Marital Fam Ther 21:260–266, 1999

Johnson L, Bruhn R, Winek J, et al: The use of child centered and filial therapy with Head Start families: a brief report. J Marital Fam Ther 25:169–176, 1999

Johnson PL, O'Leary KD: Behavioral components of marital satisfaction: an individualized assessment approach. J Consult Clin Psychol 64:417–423, 1996

Johnson S: Bonds and bargains' relationship paradigms and their significance for marital therapy. J Marital Fam Ther 12:259–267, 1986

Johnson S: Marital therapy: issues and challenges. J Psychiatry Neurosci 16:176–181, 1991

Johnson S: The Practice of Emotionally Focused Marital Therapy: Creating Connection. New York, Brunner/Mazel, 1996

Johnson S: Emotionally Focused Couple Therapy for Trauma Survivors: Strengthening Attachment Bonds. New York, Guilford, 2002

Johnson S, Greenberg L: Differential effects of experiential and problem solving interventions in resolving marital conflict. J Consult Clin Psychol 53:175–184, 1985a

Johnson S, Greenberg L: Emotionally focused couples therapy: an outcome study. J Marital Fam Ther 11:313–317, 1985b

Johnson S, Greenberg L: Emotionally focused marital therapy: an overview. Psychotherapy 24:552–560, 1987

Johnson S, Greenberg L: Relating process to outcome in marital therapy. J Marital Fam Ther 14:175–183, 1988

Johnson S, Greenberg L: There are more things in heaven and earth than are dreamed of in BMT: a reply to Jacobson. American Journal of Family Psychology 4:407–415, 1991

Johnson SM, Greenberg LS: The Heart of the Matter: Perspectives on Emotion in Marital Therapy. New York, Brunner/Mazel, 1994

Johnson SM, Greenberg LS: The emotionally focused approach to problems in adult attachment, in The Clinical Handbook of Marital Therapy, 2nd Edition. Edited by Jacobson NS, Gurman AS. New York, Guilford, 1995, pp 121–141

Johnson S, Lebow J: The "coming of age" of couple therapy: a decade review. J Marital Fam Ther 26:23–38, 2000

Johnson SM, Talitman E: Predictors of success in emotionally focused marital therapy. J Marital Fam Ther 23:135–152, 1997

Johnson S, Whiffen V: Made to measure: adapting emotionally focused couples therapy to couples attachment styles. Clinical Psychology: Science and Practice 6:366–381, 1999

Johnson S, Hunsley J, Greenberg L, et al: Emotionally focused couples therapy: status and challenges. Clin Psychol 6:67–79, 1999

Johnson S, Makinen J, Millikin J: Attachment injuries in couple relationships: a new perspective on impasses in couples therapy. J Marital Fam Ther 27:145–155, 2001

Johnston M, Holzman P: Assessing Schizophrenic Thinking. San Francisco, CA, Jossey-Bass, 1979

Johnston T: Retirement: what happens to the marriage. Issues in Mental Health Nursing 11:347–359, 1990

Joint Commission on Accreditation for Healthcare Organizations: Accreditation Manual for Hospitals. Chicago, IL, Joint Commission on Accreditation for Healthcare Organizations, 1989

Jones EE: Introduction to special section: single case research in psychotherapy. J Consult Clin Psychol 61:371–372, 1993

Jones J: Patterns of transactional style deviance in the TATs of parents of schizophrenics. Fam Process 16:327–337, 1977

Jones JM: Affect as Process. Hillsdale, NJ, Analytic Press, 1995

Jonsson E, Nilsson T: Alkolkonsumtion hos monozgota och dizgota tvillingpar (Alcohol consumption in monozygotic and dizygotic pairs of twins). Nord Hyg Tidskr 49:21–25, 1968

Jonsson G: Delinquent Boys, Their Parents and Grandparents. Copenhagen, Denmark, Munkgaard, 1967

Jordan J, Kaplan A, Miller J, et al: Women's Growth in Connection: Writings From the Stone Centre. New York, Guilford, 1991

Jouriles EN, O'Leary KD: Interspousal reliability of reports of marital violence. J Consult Clin Psychol 53:419–421, 1985

Jouriles EN, Norwood WD, McDonald R, et al: Physical violence and other forms of marital aggression: links with children's behavior problems. J Fam Psychol 10:223–234, 1996

Justice B: The Broken Taboo. New York, Human Sciences Press, 1979

Kadushin P: Toward a family diagnostic system. Family Coordinator 20:279–289, 1971

Kagan J: Behavioral inhibition to the unfamiliar. Child Dev 55:2212–2225, 1984

Kahler CW, Epstein EE, McCrady BS: Loss of control and the inability to abstain: the measurement of and the relationship between two constructs in male alcoholics. Addiction 90:1025–1036, 1995

Kang S, Kleinman P, Woody G, et al: Outcomes for cocaine abusers after once-a-week psychosocial therapy. Am J Psychiatry 148:642–647, 1991

Kantor J: Interbehavioral Psychology. Granville, OH, Principia Press, 1959

Kaplan HS: The New Sex Therapy. New York, Brunner/Mazel, 1974

Kaplan H: Disorders of Sexual Desire. New York, Brunner/Mazel, 1979

Kaplan H: The Evaluation of Sexual Disorder: Psychological and Medical Aspects. New York, Brunner/Mazel, 1983

Kaplan H: The Sexual Desire Disorders: Dysfunctional Regulation of Sexual Motivation. New York, Brunner/Mazel, 1995

Kaplan H, Sadock B: Comprehensive Group Psychotherapy. Baltimore, MD, Williams & Wilkins, 1971, pp 460–500

Karasu B: Developmentalist metatheory of depression and psychotherapy. Am J Psychother 46:37–57, 1992

Karno M, Jenkins J, De la Selva A: Expressed emotion and schizophrenic outcome among Mexican-American families. J Nerv Ment Dis 175:143–151, 1985

Karoly P: Mechanisms of self-regulation: a systems view. Annu Rev Psychol 44:23–52, 1993

Kaufman E (ed): Power to Change: Family Case Studies in the Treatment of Alcoholism. New York, Gardner Press, 1984

Kaufman E: Substance Abuse and Family Therapy. Orlando, FL, Grune & Stratton, 1985

Kaufman E: Psychotherapy of Addicted Persons. New York, Guilford, 1994

Kaufman E, Kaufman P (eds): Family Therapy of Drug and Alcohol Abuse. New York, Gardner Press, 1979

Kavanagh DJ, Piatkowska O, Clark D, et al: Application of a cognitive-behavioural family intervention for schizophrenia in multi-disciplinary teams: what can the matter be? Australian Psychologist 28:181–188, 1993

Kazdin A: Conduct disorders, in International Handbook of Behavior Modification and Therapy. Edited by Bellack A, Hersov A, Kazdin A. New York, Plenum, 1983, pp 669–706

Kazdin A: Problem solving and parent management in treating aggressive and antisocial behavior, in Psychosocial Treatments for Child and Adolescent Disorders: Empirically Based Strategies for Clinical Practice. Edited by Hibbs E, Jensen P. Washington, DC, American Psychological Association, 1996, pp 377–408

Kazdin AE: Parent management training: evidence, outcomes, and issues. J Am Acad Child Adolesc Psychiatry 36:1349–1356, 1997

Kazdin AE, Siegel TC, Bass D: Cognitive problem-solving skills training and parent management training in the treatment of antisocial behavior in children. J Consult Clin Psychol 60:733–747, 1992

Kazdin AE, Holland L, Crowley M: Family experience of barriers to treatment and premature termination from child therapy. J Consult Clin Psychol 68:553–463, 1997

Kearney-Cooke A, Striegel-Moore RH: Treatment of childhood sexual abuse in anorexia nervosa and bulimia nervosa: a feminist psychodynamic approach. Int J Eat Disord 15:305–319, 1994

Keith DV: Are children necessary in family therapy?, in Treating Young Children in Family Therapy. Edited by Combrinck-Graham L. Rockville, MD, Aspen, 1986, pp 1–10

Keitner G, Miller I: Family functioning and major depression. Am J Psychiatry 147:1128–1137, 1990

Keitner G, Miller I, Epstein N, et al: The functioning of families in patients with major depression. International Journal of Family Psychiatry 7:11–15, 1986

Keitner G, Miller I, Epstein N, et al: Family functioning and the course of major depression. Compr Psychiatry 28:54–64, 1987a

Keitner G, Miller I, Fruzzetti A, et al: Family functioning and suicidal behavior in psychiatric inpatients with major depression. Psychiatry 50:242–255, 1987b

Kellam SG, Adams RG, Brown CH, et al: The long-term evolution of the family structure of teenage and older mothers. Journal of Marriage and the Family 4:539–554, 1982

Keller M: Trends in the treatment of alcoholism, in Second Special Report to the U.S. Congress on Alcohol and Health (DHEW Publ No ADM 75-212). Edited by Keller M. Washington, DC, U.S. Government Printing Office, 1974, pp 111–127

Keller M: Undertreatment of major depression. Psychopharmacol Bull 24:75–80, 1988

Keller MB, Klerman GL, Lavori PW, et al: Long-term outcome of episodes of major depression: clinical and public health significance. JAMA 252:788–792, 1984

Keller MB, Beardslee WR, Dorer DJ, et al: Impact of severity and chronicity of parental affective illness on adaptive functioning and psychopathology in children. Arch Gen Psychiatry 43:930–937, 1986

Keller M, Beardslee W, Lavori P, et al: Course of major depression in non-referred adolescents. J Affect Disord 15:235–243, 1988

Keller M, Lavori P, Mueller T, et al: Time to recovery, chronicity, and levels of psychopathology in major depression: a 5-year prospective follow-up of 431 subjects. Arch Gen Psychiatry 49:809–816, 1992

Kelly GR, Scott JE: Medication compliance and health education among outpatients with chronic mental disorders. Med Care 28:1181–1197, 1990

Kelly J: Longer-term adjustment in children of divorce: converging findings and implications for practice. Journal of Family Psychology 2:119–140, 1988

Kelly J, Wallerstein J: The effects of parental divorce: experiences of the child in early latency. Am J Orthopsychiatry 46:20–32, 1976

Kelsey-Smith M, Beavers WR: Family assessment: centripetal and centrifugal family systems. American Journal of Family Therapy 9:3–21, 1981

Kennett KF: The Family Behavior Profile: an initial report. Ment Retard 15:36–40, 1977

Kernberg OF: Borderline Conditions and Pathological Narcissism. New York, Jason Aronson, 1975

Kernberg P: Conduct Disorders in Children and Adolescents. New York, Basic Books, 1991

Kerr ME: Aspects of biofeedback physiology and its relationship to family systems theory. Am J Psychoanal 37:23–35, 1977a

Kerr M: The use of videotape in psychotherapy, in Georgetown Family Symposia: A Collection of Selected Papers, Vol II. Edited by Lorio P, McClenathan L. Washington, DC, Georgetown University, 1977b

Kerr M: Cancer and the family emotional system, in Psychotherapeutic Treatment of Cancer Patients. Edited by Goldberg J. New York, Free Press, 1981

Kerr M: Physical illness and the family emotional system: psoriasis as a model. Behav Med 41:113–142, 1992

Kerr ME: Bowen theory and evolutionary theory. Family Systems 4:119–179, 1998

Kerr ME, Bowen M: Family Evaluation: An Approach Based on Bowen Theory. New York, WW Norton, 1988

Kessler S, Bloch M: Social system responses to Huntington disease. Fam Process 14:59–67, 1989

Kety SS: Interactions between stress and genetic processes, in Stress in Health and Disease. Edited by Zales MR. New York, Brunner/Mazel, 1984

Khantzian E: A contemporary psychodynamic approach to drug abuse treatment. Am J Drug Alcohol Abuse 12:213–222, 1986

Khantzian E, Mach S: Self preservation and the care of the self-ego: instinct reconsidered. Psychoanal Study Child 38:209–232, 1983

Khantzian E, Mach S: Alcoholics Anonymous and contemporary psychodynamic theory, in Recent Developments in Alcoholism, Vol 7. Edited by Galanter M. New York, Plenum, 1989, pp 67–89

Khantzian EJ, Treece A: Psychodynamics of drug dependence: an overview, in Psychodynamics of Drug Dependence (NIDA Res Monogr 12). Edited by Blaine JD, Julius DA. Rockville, MD, National Institute on Drug Abuse, 1977, pp 11–25

Khantzian EJ, Treece C: DSM-III psychiatric diagnosis of narcotic addicts: recent findings. Arch Gen Psychiatry 42:1067–1071, 1985

Kiecolt-Glaser J, Malarkey W, Chee M, et al: Negative behavior during marital conflict is associated with immunological down-regulation. Psychosom Med 55:395–409, 1993

Kiev A: Curanderismo: Mexican-American Folk Psychiatry. New York, Free Press, 1968

Kinney J, Leaton G: Loosening the Grip. St Louis, MO, CV Mosby, 1987

Kirkland K, Bauer C: MMPI traits of incestuous fathers. Journal of Criminal Psychology 38:645–649, 1982

Kissen M: Affect, Object, and Character Structure. Madison, CT, International Universities Press, 1995

Kleckner T, Frank L, Bland C, et al: The myth of the unfeeling strategic therapist. J Marital Fam Ther 18:41–51, 1992

Klein NC, Alexander JF, Parsons BV: Impact of family systems intervention on recidivism and sibling delinquency: a model of primary prevention and program evaluation. J Consult Clin Psychol 45:469–474, 1977

Klerman G, Weissman M: Interpersonal psychotherapy (IPT) and drugs in the treatment of depression. Pharmacopsychiatry 20:3–7, 1987

Klerman G, Weissman M: The course, morbidity, and cost of depression. Arch Gen Psychiatry 49:831–834, 1992

Klerman G, Weissman M, Rounsaville B, et al: Interpersonal Psychotherapy of Depression. New York, Basic Books, 1984

Kluckhohn F: Variations in the basic values of family systems. Social Casework 39:63–72, 1958

Kluft R: Childhood Antecedents of Multiple Personality. Washington, DC, American Psychiatric Press, 1985

Knight R: The psychodynamics of chronic alcoholism: read at Central Neurological Association, Topeka, Kansas, October 1935. J Nerv Ment Dis 86:538–548, 1937

Knowles M: The Adult Learner: A Neglected Species. Houston, TX, Gulf Publishing, 1978

Knox D: Spirituality: a tool in the assessment and treatment of black alcoholics and their families. Alcoholism Treatment Quarterly 2(3/4):31–44, 1985

Kobak R, Cole H: Attachment and meta-monitoring: implications for autonomy and psychopathology, in Disorder and Dysfunctions of the Self. Edited by Cicchetti D, Toth S. Rochester, NY, University of Rochester Press, 1991, pp 267–297

Koenig J, Sachs-Ericsson N, Miklowitz D: Do psychiatric patients experience family interactions in the same way as observers?

Koenigsberg H, Handley R: Expressed emotion: from predictive index to clinical construct. Am J Psychiatry 143:1361–1373, 1986

Kohut H: The Analysis of the Self. New York, International Universities Press, 1971a

Kohut H: Peace prize 1969. Laudation. J Am Psychoanal Assoc 19:806–818, 1971b

Kohut H: Reflections on narcissism and narcissistic anger. Psyche: Zeitschrift für Psychoanalyse und ihre Anwendungen 27:513–554, 1973

Kohut H: The Restoration of the Self. New York, International Universities Press, 1977

Kolko DJ, Brent DA, Baugher M, et al: Cognitive and family therapies for adolescent depression: treatment specificity, mediation, and moderation. J Consult Clin Psychol 68:603–614, 2000

Kolodny RC: Textbook of Sexual Medicine. Boston, MA, Little, Brown, 1979

Koocher GP: Pediatric oncology: medical crisis intervention, in Health Psychology Through the Life Span: Practice and Research Opportunities. Edited by Resnick RJ, Rozensky H. Washington, DC, American Psychological Association, 1997, pp 213–225

Koocher GP, Goodman GS, White CS, et al: Psychological science and the use of anatomically detailed dolls in child sexual-abuse assessments. Annual Progress in Child Psychiatry and Child Development, 1996, pp 367–425

Koss MP, Goodman LA, Browne A, et al: No Safe Haven: Male Violence Against Women at Home, at Work, and in the Community. Washington, DC, American Psychological Association, 1994

Kottgen C, Sonnichsen I, Mollenhauer K: The family relations of young schizophrenic patients: results of the Hamburg Camberwell Family Interview Study 1. International Journal of Family Psychiatry 5:61–94, 1984

Kovacs M, Goldston D: Cognitive and social cognitive development of depressed children and adolescents. J Am Acad Child Adolesc Psychiatry 30:388–392, 1991

Krauss MW, Seltzer MM: Life course perspectives in mental retardation research: the case of family caregiving, in Handbook of Mental Retardation and Development. Edited by Burack JA, Hodapp RM. New York, Cambridge University Press, 1998, pp 504–520

Kreisman D, Joy V: Family response to the mental illness of a relative: a review of the literature. Schizophr Bull 10:35–57, 1975

Kreitman N, Sainsbury P, Pearce K, et al: Hypochondriasis and depression in outpatients at a general hospital. Br J Psychiatry 3:607–615, 1965

Kubler-Ross E: On Death and Dying. New York, Macmillan, 1969

Kuder GF, Richardson MW: The theory of estimation of test reliability. Psychometrika 2:151–160, 1937

Kuhn JS, Singleton GL, Meyer P, et al: Divorce: a symposium. Georgetown Medical Bulletin 32:5–34, 1979

Kuhn TS: The structure of scientific revolutions, in International Encyclopedia of Unified Science, Vol 2. Chicago, IL, University of Chicago, 1970

Kuipers L, Bebbington P: Expressed emotion research in schizophrenia: theoretical and clinical implications. Psychol Med 18:893–909, 1988

Kurtines WM, Szapocznik J: Family interaction patterns: Structural Family Therapy in contexts of cultural diversity, in Psychosocial Treatments for Child and Adolescent Disorders: Empirically Based Strategies for Clinical Practice. Edited by Hibbs ED, Jensen PS. Washington, DC, American Psychological Association, 1996, pp 671–697

L'Abate L: Screening couples for marriage enrichment programs, in Questions and Answers in the Practice of Family Therapy. Edited by Gurman A. New York, Brunner/Mazel, 1981

L'Abate L: Programmed Writing: A Self-Administered Approach to Interventions With Individuals, Couples and Families. Pacific Grove, CA, Brooks/Cole Publishing, 1992

L'Abate L, McHenry S: Handbook of Marital Interventions. New York, Grune & Stratton, 1983

L'Abate L, Weinstein S: Structured Enrichment Programs for Couples and Families. New York, Brunner/Mazel, 1987

Lachkar J: The Narcissistic/Borderline Couple. New York, Brunner/Mazel, 1992

Lahey B, Green K, Forehand R: On the independence of ratings of hyperactivity, conduct problems, and attention deficits in children: a multiple regression analysis. J Consult Clin Psychol 48:566–574, 1980

Lahey B, Piacentini J, McBurrett K, et al: Psychopathology in the parents of children with conduct disorder and hyperactivity. J Am Acad Child Adolesc Psychiatry 27:163–170, 1988

Lahey B, Russo M, Walker J, et al: Personality characteristics of the mothers of children with disruptive behavior disorders. J Consult Clin Psychol 57:512–515, 1989

Lam DH: Psychosocial family intervention in schizophrenia: a review of empirical studies. Psychol Med 21:423–441, 1992

Lamb HR, Goertzel V: Discharged mental patients—are they really in the community? Arch Gen Psychiatry 24:29–34, 1971

Lambert MJ: Psychotherapy outcome research: implications for integrative and eclectic therapists, in Handbook of Psychotherapy Integration. Edited by Norcross JC, Goldfried MR. New York, Basic Books, 1992

Landau J: Therapy with families in cultural transition, in Ethnicity and Family Therapy. Edited by McGoldrick M, Pearce JK, Giordano J. New York, Grune & Stratton, 1982, pp 552–571

Landis JT: Experiences of 500 children with adult sexual deviation. Psychiatr Q Suppl 30: 91–109, 1985

Langes R: Classics in Psychoanalytic Technique. New York, Jason Aronson, 1981

Langevin R, Handy L, Horah H, et al: Are fathers pedophilic and aggressive?, in Erotic Male Gender Identity and Aggression. Edited by Langevin R. New York, Lawrence Erlbaum, 1983

Langevin R, Handy L, Day P, et al: Are incestuous fathers pedophilic, aggressive, and alcoholic?, in Erotic Preference, Gender Identity, and Aggression. Edited by Langevin R. Hillsdale, NJ, Lawrence Erlbaum, 1985

Langhinrichsen-Rohling J, Neidig P, Thorn G: Violent marriages: gender differences in levels of current violence and past abuse. Journal of Family Violence 10:159–176, 1995

Langsley D, Kaplan R: The Treatment of Families in Crisis. New York, Grune & Stratton, 1968

Langsley DG, Pittman FS III, Machotka P, et al: Family crisis therapy—results and implications. Fam Process 7:145–158, 1968

Langsley DG, Flomenhaft K, Machotka P: Followup evaluation of family crisis therapy. Am J Orthopsychiatry 39:753–759, 1969

Langsley DG, Machotka P, Flomenhaft K: Avoiding mental hospital admission: a follow-up study. Am J Psychiatry 127:127–130, 1971

Lansky MR (ed): Family Therapy and Major Psychopathology. New York, Grune & Stratton, 1981

Lansky M: The role of the family in the evaluation of suicidality. International Journal of Family Psychiatry 3, 1982

Lansky MR: Marital therapy for narcissistic disorders, in Clinical Handbook of Marital Therapy. Edited by Jacobson N, Gurman A. New York, Guilford, 1986

Lansky MR: Family therapy, in Comprehensive Textbook of Psychiatry/IV, 4th Edition. Edited by Kaplan HI, Sadock BJ. Baltimore, MD, Williams & Wilkins, 1989, pp 1535–1541

Laporta M, Falloon IRH, Shanahan W, et al: The NIMH Behavior Family Therapy Skill Assessment: reliability and validity. Paper presented at the World Congress of Psychiatry, Athens, Greece, 1989

Laqueur H: Mechanisms of change in multiple family therapy, in Progress in Group and Family Therapy. New York, Brunner/Mazel, 1972

Laqueur H, Laburt H, Morong E: Multiple family therapy: further developments. Int J Soc Psychiatry 10:69–80, 1964

Larner G: Narrative child therapy. Fam Process 35:423–440, 1996

Larson DB, Hohmann A, Kessler LG, et al: The couch and the cloth: the need for linkage. Hosp Community Psychiatry 45:1015–1020, 1988

Larson N, Maddock J: Incest management and treatment. Paper presented at the annual meeting of the Association for Marriage and Family Therapy, San Francisco, CA, October 1984

Lasegue C, Falret J: La folie à deux à folie communiquee. Am Med Psychol 17:321–329, 1877

Lau S, Kwok IK: Relationship of family environment to adolescent depression and self concept. Social Behavior and Personality 28:41–50, 2000

Laumann EO, Gagnon JH, Michaels R, et al: Social Organization of Sexuality: Sexual Practices in the United States. Chicago, IL, University of Chicago Press, 1994

Laviola M: Effects of older brother–younger sister incest: a review of cases. Journal of Family Violence 4:259–274, 1989

Law DD, Crane DR: The influence of marital and family therapy on health care utilization in a health-maintenance organization. J Marital Fam Ther 26:281–291, 2000

Lawrence E, Eldridge K, Christensen A, et al: Short-Term Couple Therapy. New York, Guilford, 1999

Lawton MP: The Philadelphia Geriatric Center Morale Scale: a revision. J Gerontol 30:85–89, 1975

Lazarus A: The treatment of a sexually inadequate man, in Case Studies in Behavior Modification. Edited by Ullmann LP, Krasner L. New York, Holt, Rinehart & Winston, 1965
Lazarus A: The Practice of Multimodal Therapy: Systematic, Comprehensive and Effective Psychotherapy. New York, McGraw-Hill, 1981
Lazarus A: Marital Myths. San Luis Obispo, CA, Impact Publishers, 1985
Lazarus A: The multimodal approach to treatment of minor depression. Am J Psychother 46:50–57, 1992
Lebow J: Training family therapists as feminists, in Women and Family Therapy. Edited by Ault-Riche M. New York, Aspen, 1986
Lebow J, Gurman A: Research assessing couple and family therapy, in Annual Review of Psychology. Palo Alto, CA, Annual Reviews, 1995, pp 27–57
Lebrun LJ, Leladhar-Singh M, Luke A: Schizophrenia outpatient education. Can Nurse 87: 25–27, 1991
Lederer W, Jackson D: The eight myths of marriage, in The Mirages of Marriage. Edited by Lederer W, Jackson DD. New York, WW Norton, 1968a
Lederer W, Jackson DD (eds): The Mirages of Marriage. New York, WW Norton, 1968b
Lee E: A social systems approach to assessment and treatment for Chinese-American families, in Ethnicity and Family Therapy. Edited by McGoldrick M, Pearce JK, Giordano J. New York, Grune & Stratton, 1982, pp 552–571
Lee R: The family therapy trainer as coaching double. Journal of Group Psychotherapy, Psychodrama and Sociometry 39:52–57, 1986
Leff JP, Vaughn CE: Expressed Emotion in Families. New York, Guilford, 1985
Leff J, Kuipers L, Berkowitz R, et al: A controlled trial of social intervention in the families of schizophrenic patients. Br J Psychiatry 141:121–134, 1982
Leff J, Kuipers L, Berkowitz R, et al: A controlled trial of social intervention in the families of schizophrenic patients: two year follow up. Br J Psychiatry 146:594–600, 1985
Leff JP, Wig N, Ghosh A: II. Influence of relatives' expressed emotion on the course of schizophrenia in Chandigarh. Br J Psychiatry 151:166–173, 1987
Leff J, Berkowitz R, Shavit N, et al: A trial of family therapy versus a relatives' group for schizophrenia. Br J Psychiatry 154:58–66, 1989
Leff J, Berkowitz R, Shavit N, et al: A trial of family therapy versus a relatives' group for schizophrenia: two-year follow-up. Br J Psychiatry 157:571–577, 1990
Lefley H: Etiological and prevention views of clinicians with mentally ill relatives. Am J Orthopsychiatry 55:363–370, 1985
Lefley H (ed): Families Coping With Mental Illness: The Cultural Context. San Francisco, CA, Jossey-Bass/Pfeiffer, 1998a
Lefley H: Families, culture, and mental illness: constructing new realities. Psychiatry: Interpersonal and Biological Processes 61:335–355, 1998b
Lefley H, Sandoval MC, Charles C: Traditional healing systems in a multicultural setting, in Clinical Methods in Transcultural Psychiatry. Edited by Okpaku SO. Washington, DC, American Psychiatric Press, 1998, pp 88–110
Lehman AF, Carpenter WT, Goldman HH, et al: Treatment outcomes in schizophrenia: implications for practice, policy and research. Schizophr Bull 21:669–675, 1995
Leiblum S: The sexual difficulties of women. J Med Assoc Ga 81:221–225, 1992
Leiblum SR, Rosen RC (eds): Principles and Practices of Sex Therapy, 2nd Edition: Update for the 1990s. New York, Guilford, 1989
Leigh G, Loewen IR, Lester M: Caveat emptor: values and ethics in family life education and enrichment. Family Relations 35:573–580, 1986
Leighton AH: An Introduction to Social Psychiatry. Springfield, IL, Charles C Thomas, 1960
Lerner H: The Dance of Anger. New York, Harper & Row, 1986
Lester GW, Beckham E, Baucom DH: Implementation of behavioral marital therapy. J Marital Fam Ther 6:189–199, 1980

Letich L: A clinician's researcher: the work of Jose Szapocznik may transform your everyday practice. Family Therapy Networker 17(5):77–82, 1993

Leung GM, Rastogi SC, Woods J: Relative support group of long-stay psychiatric patients. Psychiatric Bulletin 13:417–419, 1989

Levenson E: The Fallacy of Understanding. New York, Basic Books, 1972

Levenson RW, Gottman JM: Physiological and affective predictors of change in relationship satisfaction. J Pers Soc Psychol 49:85–94, 1985

Leventhal H: A perceptual motor processing model of emotion, in Advances in the Study of Communication and Affect, Vol 5: Perception of Emotions in Self and Others. Edited by Pliner P, Blankstein K, Spigal I. New York, Plenum, 1979, pp 1–46

Levin EC: Therapeutic multiple family groups. Int J Group Psychother 16:203–208, 1966

Levine ES, Padilla AM: Crossing Cultures in Therapy: Pluralistic Counseling for the Hispanic. Belmont, CA, Wadsworth, 1980

Levinger G: A social psychological perspective on divorce. Journal of Social Issues 32:21–47, 1976

Levy D: Maternal Overprotection. New York, Columbia University Press, 1943

Lewis D, Shanok S, Pincus J: Violent juvenile delinquents: psychiatric, neurological, psychological, and abuse factors. Journal of the American Academy of Child Psychiatry 18:307–319, 1979

Lewis JM, Beavers WR, Gossett JT, et al: No Single Thread: Psychological Health in Family Systems. New York, Brunner/Mazel, 1976

Lewis RA, Piercy F, Sprenkle D, et al: Family based interventions and community networking for helping drug abusing adolescents: the impact of near and far environments. Journal of Adolescent Research 5:82–95, 1990

Li F, Wang M: A behavioural training programme for chronic schizophrenic patients: a three-month randomised controlled trial in Beijing. Br J Psychiatry 165 (suppl 24):32–37, 1994

Liberman RP: Behavioral approaches to family and couple therapy. Am J Orthopsychiatry 40: 106–118, 1970

Liberman RP: Managing resistance to behavioral family therapy, in Questions and Answers in the Practice of Family Therapy. Edited by Gurman AS. New York, Brunner/Mazel, 1981

Liberman RP, Wallace CJ, Falloon IRH, et al: Interpersonal problem-solving therapy for schizophrenics and their families. Compr Psychiatry 22:627–630, 1981

Liberman R, Mueser K, Wallace C, et al: Training skills in the psychiatrically disabled: learning coping and competence. Schizophr Bull 12:631–646, 1986

Lickona T (ed): Moral Development and Behavior. New York, Holt, Rinehart & Winston, 2000, pp 31–52

Liddle HA: The Adolescents and Families Project: multidimensional family therapy in action, in ADAMHA Monograph From the First National Conference on the Treatment of Adolescent Drug, Alcohol and Mental Health Problems. Washington, DC, U.S. Government Printing Office, 1991a

Liddle HA: Engaging the adolescent in family systems therapy, in Interventions in Family Therapy. Edited by Nelson T. New York, Haworth, 1991b

Liddle HA, Dakof GA: Efficacy of family therapy for drug abuse: promising but not definite. J Marital Fam Ther 21:511–543, 1995a

Liddle HA, Dakof GA: Family-based treatment for adolescent drug use: state of the science, in Adolescent Drug Abuse: Assessment and Treatment (NIDA Res Monogr 156). Edited by Rahdert E, Czechowicz D. Rockville, MD, National Institute on Drug Abuse, 1995b, pp 218–254

Liddle H, Brenlin D, Schwartz R: Handbook of Family Therapy Training and Supervision. New York, Guilford, 1988

Liddle HA, Dakof G, Parker K, et al: Anatomy of a clinical research project. Paper presented at the American Psychological Association Meeting, San Francisco, CA, August 1991

Liddle HA, Dakof GA, Parker KB, et al: Multidimensional family therapy for adolescent drug abuse: results of a randomized clinical trial. Am J Drug Alcohol Abuse 27:651–688, 2001

Lidz T: The Family and Human Adaptation. New York, International Universities Press, 1963

Lidz T: The Person: His Development Throughout the Life Cycle. New York, Basic Books, 1968

Lidz T, Rubinstein R: Psychology of gastrointestinal disorders, in American Handbook of Psychiatry, Vol 1. Edited by Arieti S. New York, Basic Books, 1959, pp 678–689

Lidz T, Parker B, Cornelison AR: The role of the father in the family environment of the schizophrenic patient. Am J Psychiatry 113:126–132, 1956

Lidz T, Cornelison A, Fleck S, et al: The intrafamilial environment of schizophrenic patients, II: marital schism and marital skew. Am J Psychiatry 114:241–258, 1957

Liebman RS, Minuchin, Baker L: The role of the family in the treatment of anorexia nervosa. Journal of the American Academy of Child Psychiatry 13:264–274, 1974

Liebman R, Minuchin S, Baker L: The use of structural family therapy in the treatment of intractable asthma. Am J Psychosom Med 19:531–537, 1978

Lindahl K, Markman H: Communication and negative affect regulation in the family, in Emotions and the Family. Edited by Blechman E. Hillsdale, NJ, Lawrence Erlbaum, 1990, pp 99–116

Lindolm BW, Touliatos J: Measurement trends in family research. Psychol Rep 72(3):1265–1266, 1993

Linszen D, Dingemans P, Van Der Does JW, et al: Treatment, expressed emotion and relapse in recent onset schizophrenic disorders. Psychol Med 26:333–342, 1996

Linszen D, Dingemans P, Nutger MA, et al: Patient attributes and expressed emotion as risk factors for psychotic relapse. Schizophr Bull 23:119–130, 1997

Lipchik E, de Shazer S: The purposeful interview. Journal of Strategic and Systemic Therapies 5:88–89, 1986

Lipnack J, Stamps J: Networking. New York, Doubleday, 1982

Lippman S, Manshadi M, Christie S, et al: Depression in alcoholics by the NIMH Diagnostic Interview Schedule and Zung Self-Rating Depression Scale. Int J Addict 22:273–281, 1987

Lipsitt DR, Lipsitt MD: The family in consultation-liaison psychiatry. Gen Hosp Psychiatry 3:231–236, 1981

Litwak E: The use of extended family in the achievement of social goals: some social implications. Social Problems 7:177–187, 1959

Llewelyn SP: Sexual abuse treatment: training and supervisory needs. J Consult Clin Psychol 5:32–41, 1997

Locke HJ: Predicting Adjustment in Marriage. New York, Henry Holt, 1951

Locke HJ, Wallace KM: Short marital adjustment and prediction tests: reliability and validity. Marriage and Family Living 21:251–255, 1959

Loeber R, Dishion T: Early predictors of male delinquency: a review. Psychol Bull 94:68–99, 1983

Logan SL: Strenthening family ties: working with Black female single-parent families, in The Black Family: Strengths, Self-Help, and Positive Change. Edited by Logan SL. Boulder, CO, Westview Press, 1996, pp 164–180

Lonie I: Borderline disorder and PTSD: an equivalence? Aust N Z J Psychiatry 27:233–245, 1993

Lopez SR, Nelson K, Snyder K, et al: Attributions and affective reactions of family members and course of schizophrenia. J Abnorm Psychol 108:307–314, 1999

LoPiccolo J: From psychotherapy to sex therapy. Society 14(5):60–68, 1977

LoPiccolo J, Friedman JM: Broad-spectrum treatment of low sexual desire: integration of cognitive, behavioral, and systemic theory, in Sexual Desire Disorders. Edited by Leiblum SR, Rosen RC. New York, Guilford, 1988, pp 107–144

LoPiccolo J, Lobitz WC: The role of masturbation in the treatment of orgasmic dysfunction. Arch Sex Behav 2:163–171, 1972

LoPiccolo J, Steger JC: The Sexual Interaction Inventory: a new instrument for assessment of sexual dysfunctions. Arch Sex Behav 3:585–595, 1974

Loredo C: Sibling incest, in Handbook of Clinical Intervention of Child Sexual Abuse. Edited by Sgroi S. Lexington, MA, DC Heath, 1982, pp 181–188

Lorenz K: The Foundations of Ethology. New York, Simon & Schuster, 1981

Louv R: Childhood's Future. Boston, MA, Houghton Mifflin, 1990

Lupri E, Grandin E, Brinkerhoff MB: Socioeconomic status and male violence in the Canadian home: a reexamination. Canadian Journal of Sociology 19:47–73, 1994

MacCarthy B, Kuipers L, Hurry J, et al: Counselling relatives of the long-term adult mentally ill, I: evaluation of the impact on relatives and patients. Br J Psychiatry 154:768–775, 1989

Mace D: Training and certification of enrichment leaders. Family Coordinator 25:117–125, 1976

Mace D: Marriage and family enrichment—a new field? Family Coordinator 28:409–419, 1979

Mace D: Training families to deal creatively with conflict, in Prevention in Family Services: Approaches to Family Wellness. Edited by Mace D. Beverly Hills, CA, Sage, 1983

Mace D: Three ways of helping married couples. J Marital Fam Ther 13:179–185, 1987

MacGregor R: Multiple impact psychotherapy with families. Fam Process 1:15–29, 1962

MacGregor R: Progress in multiple impact therapy, in Expanding Theory and Practice in Family Therapy. Edited by Ackerman N, Beatman F, Sherman S. New York, Family Service Association of America, 1967

MacGregor R, Ritchie A, Serrano A, et al: Multiple Impact Therapy With Families. New York, McGraw-Hill, 1964

Machal M, Feldman R, Sigal J: The unraveling of a treatment program: a follow-up study of the Milan approach to family therapy. Fam Process 28:457–470, 1989

MacKinnon L: Contrasting strategic and Milan therapies. Fam Process 22:425–441, 1983

MacLean PD: The Triune Brain in Evolution: Role in Paleocerebral Functions. New York, Plenum, 1989

MacMillan J, Crow T, Johnson A: Expressed emotion and relapse in first episodes of schizophrenia. Br J Psychiatry 151:320–323, 1987

MacMillan HL, MacMillan JH, Offord DR, et al: Primary prevention of child sexual abuse: a critical review. J Child Psychol Psychiatry 35:835–876, 1994

MacVicar MG, Archbold P: A framework for family assessment in chronic illness. Nursing Forum 15:180–194, 1976

Madanes C: The prevention of rehospitalization of adolescents and young adults. Fam Process 19:179–191, 1980

Madanes C: Strategic Family Therapy. San Francisco, CA, Jossey-Bass, 1981

Madanes C: Behind the One-Way Mirror: Advances in the Practice of Strategic Therapy. San Francisco, CA, Jossey-Bass, 1984a

Madanes C: Strategic Family Therapy. San Francisco, CA, Jossey-Bass, 1984b

Madanes C: Sex, Love and Violence. New York, WW Norton, 1990

Madanes C: Strategic family therapy, in Handbook of Family Therapy, Vol 2. Edited by Gurman AS, Kniskern DP. New York, Brunner/Mazel, 1991, pp 396–416

Magana A, Goldstein M, Karno M: A brief method for assessing expressed emotion in relatives of psychiatric patients. Psychiatry Res 17:203–212, 1986

Mahler MS: On the current status of the infantile neurosis. J Am Psychoanal Assoc 23:327–333, 1975

Main T: Mutual projection in a marriage. Compr Psychiatry 7:432–439, 1966

Malinowski B: Sex and Repression in Savage Society. London, Routledge & Kegan, 1927

Malone CA: Observations on the role of family therapy in child psychiatric training. Journal of the American Academy of Child Psychiatry 13:437–458, 1974

Malone CA: Child psychiatry and family therapy: an overview. Journal of the American Academy of Child Psychiatry 18:4–21, 1979

Malone CA: Family therapy and childhood disorder (Part III: Family Psychiatry, Grunebaum H, ed), in Psychiatry Update: The American Psychiatric Association Annual Review, Vol 2. Edited by Grinspoon L. Washington, DC, American Psychiatric Association, 1983, pp 228–241

Mandel M: An object relation study of sexually abusive fathers. Unpublished doctoral dissertation, California School of Professional Psychology, San Diego, CA, 1986 [Dissertation Abstracts International 47 (suppl 5):2173B, 1986]

Maney A, Wells SJ (eds): Professional responsibilities in protecting children: a public health approach to child sexual abuse. Sexual Medicine 9:125–137, 1988

Maracek J, Hare-Mustin RT: A short history of the future: feminism and clinical psychology. Psychology of Women Quarterly 15:521–536, 1991

Margolin G: Behavioral exchange in happy and unhappy marriages: a family cycle perspective. Behavior Therapy 12:329–343, 1981

Margolin G: Behavioral marital therapy: is there a place for passion, play, and other non-negotiable dimensions. Behavior Therapist 6:65–68, 1983

Margolin G: Marital therapy: a cognitive-behavioral-affective approach, in Psychotherapists in Clinical Practice. Edited by Margolin G. New York, Guilford, 1987, pp 232–285

Margolin G, Wampold BE: Sequential analysis of conflict and accord in distressed and nondistressed marital partners. J Consult Clin Psychol 49:554–567, 1981

Margolin G, Weiss RL: Comparative evaluation of therapeutic components associated with behavioral marital treatments. J Consult Clin Psychol 46:1476–1486, 1978

Margolin G, John RS, Gleberman L: Affective responses to conflictual discussion in violent and nonviolent couples. J Consult Clin Psychol 56:24–33, 1998

Marjoribanks K, Walberg HJ: Ordinal position, family environment and mental abilities. J Soc Psychol 95:77–84, 1975

Markman HJ: The prediction of marital distress: a five year follow-up. J Consult Clin Psychol 49:760–762, 1981

Markman HJ, Renick MJ, Floyd FJ, et al: Preventing marital distress through communication and conflict management training: a four- and five-year follow-up. J Consult Clin Psychol 61:70–77, 1993

Markman H: The longitudinal study of couples interactions, in Marital Interaction. Edited by Hahlweg K, Jacobson N. New York, Guilford, 1984, pp 253–281

Markman H: Backwards into the future of couples therapy and couples therapy research. Journal of Family Psychotherapy 4:416–425, 1991

Markman HT: Marital and family psychology: burning issues. J Fam Psychol 5:264–275, 1992

Markman H, Floyd F: Possibilities for the prevention of marital discord: a behavioral perspective. American Journal of Family Therapy 8:29–48, 1980

Markman H, Stanley S, Storaasli R: Restrictive conflict predicts divorce: results of a six-year follow-up. Unpublished manuscript, 1991

Markman H, Stanley S, Blumberg SL: Fighting for Your Marriage: Positive Steps for Preventing Divorce and Preserving a Lasting Love. New York, Jossey-Bass, 1994

Marsh DT: Families of children and adolescents with serious emotional disturbance: innovations in theory, research, and practice, in Families and the Mental Health System for Children and Adolescents: Policy, Services, and Research. Edited by Hefliger CA, Nixon CT. Thousand Oaks, CA, Sage, 1996, pp 75–95

Marshak LE, Seligman M, Prezant F: Disability and the Family Life Cycle: Recognizing and Treating Developmental Changes. New York, Basic Books, 1999

Marshall W, Barbarel H, Christopher D: Sexual offenders against female children: sexual preferences for age of victims and type of behavior. Canadian Journal of Behavioral Science 18:424–428, 1986

Martin B: Brief family intervention: effectiveness and the importance of including the father. J Consult Clin Psychol 45:1002–1010, 1977

Martin D: Battered Wives. San Francisco, CA, New Glide Publication, 1976

Martin P, Bird H: An approach to the psychotherapy of marriage partners—the stereoscopic technique. Psychiatry 16:123–127, 1953

Martindale C: The therapist-as-fixed-effect fallacy in psychotherapy research. J Consult Clin Psychol 46:1526–1530, 1978

Mashal M, Feldman RB, Sigal JJ: The unraveling of a treatment paradigm: a followup study of the Milan approach to family therapy. Fam Process 28:457–470, 1989

Mason M: Family therapy as the emerging context for sex therapy, in Handbook of Family Therapy, Vol 2. Edited by Gurman AS, Kniskern DP. New York, Brunner/Mazel, 1991, pp 567–612

Masters W, Johnson V: Human Sexual Inadequacy. Boston, MA, Little, Brown, 1970

Masters W, Johnson V, Kolodny R: On Sex and Human Loving. Boston, MA, Little, Brown, 1986

McAdams CR, Foster VA: The safety session: a prerequisite to progress in counseling families with physically aggressive children and adolescents. Family Journal of Counseling and Therapy for Couples and Families 10:49–56, 2002

McAdoo HP, McAdoo JI (eds): Black Children: Social, Educational and Parental Environments. Beverly Hills, CA, Sage, 2002

McCarthy BW: Cognitive-behavioral strategies and techniques in the treatment of early ejaculation, in Principles and Practices of Sex Therapy, 2nd Edition: Update for the 1990s. Edited by Leiblum SR, Rosen RC. New York, Guilford, 1989, pp 141–167

McClory R: The history of NAMI. Ways, 1986, pp 16–19

McCord W, McCord J, Zola I: Origins of Crime. New York, Columbia University Press, 1959

McCord W, McCord J, Howard A: Familial correlates of aggression in nondelinquent male children. J Abnorm Soc Psychol 62:79–93, 1961

McCrady BS: The Marital Relationship and Alcoholism Treatment: Research and Clinical Perspectives. New York, Guilford, 1990

McCrady BS, Hay W: Coping with problem drinking in the family, in Coping With Disorder in the Family. Edited by Offord J. Croom Helm, 1987

McCrady B, Noel N, Abrams D, et al: Comparative effectiveness of three types of spouse involvement in outpatient behavioral alcoholism treatment. J Stud Alcohol 47:459–467, 1986

McCreadie RG, Phillips K, Harvey JA, et al: The Nithsdale Schizophrenia Surveys VIII: do relatives want family intervention—and does it help? Br J Psychiatry 158:110–113, 1991

McCreary ML, Maffuid J, Stepter TA: Bridges to effective treatment: family therapy and family psychoeducational interventions with maltreating and substance-abusing families, in Substance Abuse, Family Violence and Child Welfare: Bridging Perspectives. Edited by Hampton RL, Senatore V. Thousand Oaks, CA, Sage, 1998, pp 220–248

McCubbin HI, Joy CB, Cauble AE, et al: Family stress and coping: a decade review. Journal of Marriage and the Family 42:855–871, 1980

McDaniel SH, Speice J: What family psychology has to offer women's health: the examples of conversion, somatization, infertility treatment, and genetic testing. Prof Psychol 32:44–51, 2001

McDaniel SH, Hepworth D, William J: Medical Family Therapy: A Biopsychological Approach to Families With Health Problems. New York, Basic Books, 1992

McDermott JF Jr: Family therapy and child psychiatry: introduction. Journal of the American Academy of Child Psychiatry 18:1–3, 1979

McDermott JF Jr, Char WF: The undeclared war between child and family therapy. Journal of the American Academy of Child Psychiatry 13:422–436, 1974

McElroy E: A comparison of families and nurses perceptions of the educational needs of the families of the seriously mentally ill. Paper presented at the 6th Annual Psychiatric Nursing Professional Day at the Brattleboro Retreat, Brattleboro, VT, 1985

McFarlane W: Family psycho-educational treatment, in Handbook of Family Therapy, Vol 2. Edited by Gurman AS, Kniskern DP. New York, Brunner/Mazel, 1991
McFarlane WR: Fact: integrating family psychoeducation and assertive community treatment. Administration Policy of Mental Health 25:191–198, 1997
McFarlane W, Link B, Dushay R, et al: Psychoeducational multiple family groups: four year relapse outcome in schizophrenia. Fam Process 34:127–144, 1995a
McFarlane WR, Lukens E, Link B, et al: Multiple-family groups and psychoeducation in the treatment of schizophrenia. Arch Gen Psychiatry 52:679–687, 1995b
McFarlane WR, Dushay RA, Stastny P, et al: A comparison of two levels of family-aided assertive community treatment. Psychiatr Serv 47:744–750, 1996
McGee R, Feehan M, William S, et al: DSM-III disorders in a large sample of adolescents. J Am Acad Child Adolesc Psychiatry 29:611–619, 1990
McGill D: Cultural concepts for family therapy, in Cultural Perspectives in Family Therapy. Edited by Hansen J, Falicov C. Rockville, MD, Aspen Systems, 1983, pp 108–121
McGoldrick M, Gerson R: Genograms in Family Assessment. New York, WW Norton, 1985
McGoldrick M, Pearce J, Giordano J (eds): Ethnicity and Family Therapy. New York, Guilford, 1982
McGoldrick M, Anderson C, Walsh F (eds): Women in Families. New York, WW Norton, 1989
McGoldrick M, Garcia-Preto NC, Hines PM, et al: Ethnicity and family therapy, in Handbook of Family Therapy, Vol 2. Edited by Gurman AS, Kniskern DP. New York, Brunner/Mazel, 1991, pp 546–582
McGorry PD, Edwards J, Mihalopoulos C, et al: EPPIC: an evolving system of early detection and optimal management. Schizophr Bull 22:305–326, 1996
McIntosh P: White privilege and male privilege: a personal account of coming to understand correspondes through work in women's studies (Work in Progress No 189). Wellesley, MA, Stone Center, Wellesley College, 1988
McKnew D, Dytryn L, Epion A: Offspring of patients with affective disorders. Br J Psychiatry 134:148–152, 1979
McLaughlin M: Graduate school and families: issues for academic departments and university mental health professionals. Journal of College Student Personnel 26:488–491, 1985
McLellan AT, Arndt I, Metzger D, et al: The effects of psychosocial services in substance abuse treatment. JAMA 269:1953–1959, 1993
McPhee D: The use of marital therapy for low sexual desire. Doctoral thesis proposal, University of Ottawa, Ottawa, Ontario, Canada, 1992
McWhinney I: An Introduction to Family Medicine. Oxford, UK, Oxford University Press, 1981, pp 3–9
Mead M: Sex and Temperament in Three Primitive Societies. New York, Mentor Books, 1935
Mederos F: Differences and similarities between violent and nonviolent men: an exploratory study. Unpublished doctoral thesis, Harvard University, Boston, MA, 1995
Meiselman KC: Incest: A Psychological Study of Causes and Effects With Treatment Recommendations. San Francisco, CA, Jossey-Bass, 1978
Meissner WW: Psychobiology and Human Disease. New York, Elsevier North Holland, 1977
Meissner W: The conceptualization of marriage and family dynamics from a psychoanalytic perspective, in Marriage and Marital Therapy. Edited by Paolino T, McCrady B. New York, Brunner/Mazel, 1978, p 35
Melman A, Tiefer L: Surgery for Erectile Disorders: Operation Procedures and Psychological Issues. 1992
Merikangas K, Ranelli C, Kupfer D: Marital interaction in hospitalized depressed patients. J Nerv Ment Dis 167:689–695, 1979

Merikangas K, Bromet E, Spiker D: Assortative mating, social adjustment, and course of illness in primary affective disorder. Arch Gen Psychiatry 40:795–800, 1983

Merikangas K, Prusoff BA, Weissman MM: Parental concordance of affective disorders: psychopathy in the offspring. J Affective Disord 15:279–290, 1988

Meyer J: Impotence: assessment in the private practice office. Postgrad Med 84:87–91, 1988

Meyerstein L: The family behavioral snapshot: a tool for teaching family assessment. American Journal of Family Therapy 7:48–56, 1979

Midelfort CF: The Family in Psychotherapy. New York, McGraw-Hill, 1957

Miklowitz DJ: Psychotherapy in combination with drug treatment for bipolar disorder. J Clin Psychopharmacol 16 (2, suppl 1):56S–66S, 1996

Miklowitz DJ, Alloy LB: Psychosocial factors in the course and treatment of bipolar disorder: introduction to the special section. J Abnorm Psychol 108:555–557, 1999

Miklowitz DJ, Goldstein M: Behavioral family treatment for patients with bipolar affective disorder. Behav Modif 14:457–489, 1990

Miklowitz D, Goldstein M: Mapping the intrafamilial environment of the schizophrenic patient, in Schizophrenia: Origins, Processes, Treatment, and Outcome. Edited by Cromwell R. London, Oxford University Press, 1993, pp 313–332

Miklowitz DJ, Goldstein MJ: Bipolar Disorder: A Family Focused Treatment Approach. New York, Guilford, 1997

Miklowitz DJ, Hooley JM: Developing family psychoeducational treatments for patients with bipolar and other severe psychiatric disorders: a pathway from basic research to clinical trials. J Marital Fam Ther 24:419–435, 1998

Miklowitz D, Stackman D: Communication deviance in families of schizophrenic and other psychiatric patients: current state of the construct, in Progress in Experimental Personality and Psychopathology Research, Vol 15. Edited by Walker EF, Dworkin RH, Cornblatt BA. New York, Springer, 1992, pp 1–46

Miklowitz D, Goldstein M, Falloon I: Premorbid and symptomatic characteristics of schizophrenics from families with high and low levels of expressed emotion. J Abnorm Psychol 92:359–367, 1983

Miklowitz D, Goldstein M, Falloon I: Interactional correlates of expressed emotion in the families of schizophrenics. Br J Psychiatry 144:482–487, 1984

Miklowitz DJ, Goldstein MJ, Nuechterlein KH, et al: Family factors and the course of bipolar affective disorder. Arch Gen Psychiatry 45:225–231, 1988

Miklowitz D, Goldstein M, Doane J: Is expressed emotion an index of a transactional process?, I: parents' affective style. Fam Process 28:153–167, 1989

Miklowitz DJ, Velligan DI, Goldstein MJ, et al: Communication deviance in families of schizophrenic and manic patients. J Abnorm Psychol 100:163–173, 1991

Miklowitz DJ, Simoneau TL, George EA, et al: Family-focused treatment of bipolar disorder: one-year effects of a psychoeducational program in conjunction with pharmacotherapy. Biol Psychiatry 48:582–592, 2000

Mikulincer M, Florian V, Tolmacz R: Attachment styles and the fear of death: a case of affect regulation. J Pers Soc Psychol 58:273–280, 1990

Mikulincer M, Florian V, Weller A: Attachment styles, coping and post-traumatic psychological distress: the impact of the Gulf War in Israel. J Pers Soc Psychol 64:817–826, 1993

Miller G, Prinz R: Enhancement of social learning family interventions for childhood conduct disorder. Psychol Bull 108:291–307, 1990

Miller I, Kabacoff R, Keitner G: Family functioning in the families of psychiatric patients. Compr Psychiatry 27:302–312, 1986

Miller IV, Ryan CE, Keitner GI, et al: Why fix what is not broken? A rejoinder to Ridenour, Daley, and Reich. Fam Process 39:381–384, 2000

Miller N, Chappel J: History of the disease concept. Psychiatric Annals 21:196–205, 1991

Miller SM: Case studies: profiles of women recovering from drug addiction. J Drug Educ 25:139–148, 1995

Miller S: Marriage and Families: Enrichment Through Communication. Beverly Hills, CA, Sage, 2000

Mino Y, Inoue S, Tanaka S, et al: Expressed emotion among families and course of schizophrenia in Japan: a 2-year cohort study. Schizophr Res 24:333–339, 1997

Mintz L, Liberman R, Miklowitz D: Expressed emotion: a call for partnership among relatives, patients, and professionals. Schizophr Bull 13:227–235, 1987

Mintz S, Price R: The Birth of African-American Culture: An Anthropological Perspective. Boston, MA, Beacon Press, 1992

Minuchin S: Families and Family Therapy. Cambridge, MA, Harvard University Press, 1974a

Minuchin S: Forming the therapeutic system, in Families and Family Therapy. Cambridge, MA, Harvard University Press, 1974b, pp 123–137

Minuchin S: The initial interview, in Families and Family Therapy. Edited by Minuchin S. Cambridge, MA, Harvard University Press, 1974c

Minuchin S: Structural family therapy, in American Handbook of Psychiatry, Vol 2. Edited by Arieti S. New York, Basic Books, 1974d

Minuchin S, Fishman HC: The psychosomatic family in child psychiatry. Journal of the American Academy of Child Psychiatry 18:76–90, 1979

Minuchin S, Fishman HC: Family Therapy Techniques. Cambridge, MA, Harvard University Press, 1981

Minuchin S, Nichols MP: Structural family therapy, in Case Studies in Couple and Family Therapy: Systemic and Cognitive Perspectives. Edited by Dattilio FM. New York, Guilford, 1998, pp 108–131

Minuchin S, Montalvo B, Guerney B: Families of the Slums: An Exploration of Their Structure and Treatment. New York, Basic Books, 1967

Minuchin SL, Baker BL, Rosman R, et al: A conceptual model of psychosomatic illness in children. Arch Gen Psychiatry 32:1031–1038, 1975

Minuchin S, Rosman BL, Baker L: Psychosomatic Families: Anorexia Nervosa in Context. Cambridge, MA, Harvard University Press, 1978

Mishler E: Families and schizophrenia. Harvard Mental Health Letter 7(11) May 3–6, 1991

Mishler E, Waxler N: Interaction in Families. New York, Wiley, 1968

Mitchell J (ed): Social Networks in the Urban Situations. Manchester, UK, Manchester University Press, 1969

Mitchell JE, Popkin MK: Antidepressant drug therapy and sexual dysfunction in men: a review. J Clin Psychopharmacol 3:76–79, 1983

Mitchell SA: Relational Concepts in Psychoanalysis: An Integration. Cambridge, MA, Harvard University Press, 1988

Mittleman B: Complementary neurotic reactions in intimate relationships. Psychoanalytic Quarterly 13:479, 1944

Mittleman B: The concurrent analysis of married couples. Psychoanal Q 17:182–197, 1948

Mohamed SN, Weisz GM, Waring EM: The relationship of chronic pain to depression, marital adjustment, and family dynamics. Pain 5:285–292, 1978

Moline RA, Singh S, Morris A, et al: Family expressed emotion and relapse in schizophrenia in 24 urban American patients. Am J Psychiatry 142:1078–1081, 1985

Montalvo B, Gutierrez M: A perspective for the use of the cultural dimension in family therapy, in Cultural Perspectives in Family Therapy. Edited by Hansen IJ, Falicov CJ. Rockville, MD, Aspen Systems, 1983, pp 15–31

Montalvo B, Haley J: In defense of child therapy. Fam Process 12:227–244, 1973

Montero IP, Asencio A: Home-based psychoeducation versus relatives groups: a long-term controlled trial. Presentation at Optimal Treatment Project conference, Athens, Greece, December 12, 1996

Montero I, Gomez-Beneyto M, Ruiz I, et al: The influence of family expressed emotion on the course of schizophrenia in a sample of Spanish patients, a two-year follow-up study. Br J Psychiatry 161:217–222, 1992

Moore BE, Fine BD: Psychoanalytic Terms and Concepts. New Haven, CT, American Psychoanalytic Association and Yale University Press, 1990

Moore J, Chaney E: Outpatient group treatment of chronic pain: effects of spouse involvement. J Consult Clin Psychol 53:326–334, 1985

Moos R: The Social Climate Scales: An Overview. Palo Alto, CA, Consulting Psychologists Press, 1974

Moos RH, Moos BS: Family Environment Scales Manual. Palo Alto, CA, Consulting Psychologists Press, 1981

Moos RH, Solomon GF: Psychologic comparison between women with rheumatoid arthritis and their non-arthritic sisters, II: content analysis of interviews. Psychosom Med 27:150–164, 1965

Moos RH, Insel PM, Humphrey B: Combined Preliminary Manual for Family, Work, and Group Environment Scales. Palo Alto, CA, Consulting Psychologists Press, 1974

Moos R, Bromet E, Tsu V, et al: Family characteristics and the outcome of treatment for alcoholism. J Stud Alcohol 40:78–88, 1979a

Moos RH, Clayton J, Max W: The Social Climate Scales: An Annotated Bibliography, 2nd Edition. Palo Alto, CA, Consulting Psychologists Press, 1979b

Morgan L: Ancient Society. Chicago, IL, Kerr, 1977

Morgan SA, Macey MJ: Three assessment tools for family therapy. Journal of Psychiatric Nursing 16(3):39–42, 1978

Morgan SP, Allison PD: Paternal participation and children's well-being after marital dissolution. American Sociological Review 52:695–701, 1987

Morisky DE: Five year blood pressure control and mortality following health education for hypertensive patients. Am J Public Health 73:153–162, 1983

Moser J: Prevention of Alcohol-Related Problems. Toronto, ON, Canada, Alcoholism and Drug Addiction Research Foundation, 1980

Most R, Guerney B Jr: An empirical evaluation of the training of lay volunteer leaders for premarital relationship enhancement. Family Relations: Journal of Applied Family and Child Studies 32:239–251, 1983

Moustakas CE: Psychotherapy With Children. New York, Harper & Row, 1959

Mozny P, Votypkova P: Expressed emotion, relapse rate and utilization of psychiatric inpatient care in schizophrenia, a study from Czechoslovakia. Soc Psychiatry Psychiatr Epidemiol 27:174–179, 1992

Muhammad MH: Wife abuse and its psychological consequences as revealed by the first Palestinian National Survey on Violence Against Women. J Fam Psychol 13:642–662, 1999

Munir KM, Beardslee WR: Developmental psychiatry: is there any other kind? Harv Rev Psychiatry 6:250–262, 1999

Murstein B, Cerreto M, MacDonald M: A theory and investigation of the effect of exchange-orientation on marriage and friendship. Journal of Marriage and the Family 39:543–548, 1977

Myers JK, Weissman MW, Tischler GL, et al: Six-month prevalence of psychiatric disorders in three communities. Arch Gen Psychiatry 41:959–967, 1984

Nadelson CC: Marital therapy from a psychoanalytic perspective, in Marriage and Marital Therapy. Edited by Paolino TJ, McCrady BS. New York, Brunner/Mazel, 1978

Nadelson C, Polonsky D, Mathews M: Marriage as a developmental process, in Marriage and Divorce—A Contemporary Perspective. Edited by Nadelson C, Polonsky D. New York, Guilford, 1984

Nakashima I, Zakus G: Incest: review and clinical experience. Pediatrics 60:696–701, 1977

Nameche GF, Waring M, Ricks DF: Early indicators of outcome in schizophrenia. J Nerv Ment Dis 139:232–240, 1964

Napier A: The rejection-intrusion pattern: a central family dynamic. Journal of Marriage and Family Counseling 14:5–12, 1978

References 877

National Center for Health Statistics: Questionnaires From the National Health Interview Survey, 1980–84 (PHS 90-1302). Chyba MM, Washington LR. Hyattsville, MD, National Center for Health Statistics, March 1990 (Report #24; PB90-245028 PC A10 MF A02)

National Center for Health Statistics: Questionnaires From the National Health Interview Survey, 1985–89 (PHS 93-1307). Chyba MM, Washington LR. Hyattsville, MD, National Center for Health Statistics, August 1993 (Report #31, PB94-104486 PC A22 MF AO5)

National Institute on Drug Abuse: National Household Survey on Drug Abuse: Main Findings 1985 (DHHS Publ No ADM-88-1586). Rockville, MD, U.S. Department of Health and Human Services, 1988

National Institute on Drug Abuse: National Household Survey on Drug Abuse: NIDA 1990 Findings (DHHS Publ No ADM-91-1732). Washington, DC, U.S. Government Printing Office, 1991

National Institute of Mental Health: Mental Health in the United States. Edited by Manderscheid RW, Sonnenschein M. Washington, DC, U.S. Department of Health and Human Services, 1990

National Marriage Project: The State of Our Unions, 1999. The Social Health of Marriage in America. New Brunswick, The National Marriage Project/Rutgers, The State University of New Jersey, 1999

National Resource Center on Child Sexual Abuse: Personal communication: The Incidence and Prevalence of Child Sexual Abuse; No Easy Answer, 1992

National Resource Center on Child Sexual Abuse News 1 (suppl 4), November/December 1992

National Resource Center on Child Sexual Abuse News 3 (suppl 2), July/August 1994a

National Resource Center on Child Sexual Abuse News 3 (suppl 3), September/October 1994b

Navarre SE: Salavador Minuchin's structural family therapy and its application to multicultural family systems. Issues Ment Health Nurs 19:567–570, 1998

Needle RH, Su S, Doherty WJ: Divorce, remarriage, and adolescent substance abuse: a prospective longitudinal study. Journal of Marriage and the Family 52:157–169, 1990

Neill JR, Kniskern DP (eds): From Psyche to System: The Evolving Therapy of Carl Whitaker. New York, Guilford, 1982

Nelson GM, Beach SRH: Sequential interaction in depression: effects of depressive behavior on spousal aggression. Behavior Therapy 21:167–182, 1991

Nelson KE, Landsman MJ: Alternative Models of Family Preservation: Family-Based Services in Context. Springfield, IL, Charles C Thomas, 1992

Nichols MP: The Self in the Systems: Expanding the Limits of Family Therapy. New York, Brunner/Mazel, 1987

Nichols MP, Schwartz RC: Family Therapy: Concepts and Methods, 4th Edition. Needham Heights, MA, Allyn & Bacon, 1998

Nichols SE: Psychiatric aspects of AIDS. Psychosomatics 24:1083–1089, 1983

Niedermeier T, Watzl H, Cohen R: Prediction of relapse of schizophrenic patients: Camberwell Family Interview versus content analysis of verbal behavior. Psychiatry Res 41: 275–282, 1992

Nobles W: African philosophy: foundations for black psychology, in Black Psychology, 2nd Edition. Edited by Jones RL. New York, Harper & Row, 1980

Nobles W, Goddard IL: Understanding the Black Family: A Guide to Scholarship and Research. Oakland, CA, Black Family Institute Publishers, 1984

Noone RJ: Symbiosis, the Family, and Natural Systems. Fam Process 27:285–292, 1988

Noone RJ: The family unit and the transmission of indivdual variation in adaptiveness. Family Systems 2:116–137, 1995

Norfleet MA, Payne B: Chronic pain and the family: a review. Pain 26:1–22, 1986

Norfleet MA, et al: Helping families cope with chronic pain: an integral part of an interdisciplinary and multimodal treatment program, in Group and Family Therapy. Edited by Wolberg L, Aronson M. New York, Brunner/Mazel, 1982, pp 302–321

North CS, Pollio DE, Sachar B, et al: The family as caregiver: a group psychoeducation model for schizophrenia. Am J Orthopsychiatry 68:39–46, 1998

Norton R: Measuring marital quality: a critical look at the dependent variable. Journal of Marriage and the Family 45:141–151, 1983

Notarius C, Pellegrini D: Differences between husbands and wives: implications for understanding marital discord. Fam Process 14:231–249, 1987

Notarius CI, Vanzetti NA: The Marital Agendas Protocol, in Marriage and Family Assessment: A Sourcebook for Family Therapy. Edited by Filsinger EE. Beverly Hills, CA, Sage, 1983, pp 191–208

Notman MT, Nadelson CC: Reproductive choices and development: psychodynamic and psychoanalytic perspectives, in Psychological Aspects of Women's Health Care: The Interface Between Psychiatry and Obstetrics and Gynecology. Edited by Stewart DE, Stotland NL. Washington, DC, American Psychiatric Press, 1993, pp 331–349

Nuechterlein K, Dawson J: A heuristic vulnerability/stress model of schizophrenic episodes. Schizophr Bull 10:300–312, 1984

Nuechterlein K, Snyder K, Dawson M: Expressed emotion, fixed dose fluphenazine decanoate maintenance, and relapse in recent-onset schizophrenia. Psychopharmacol Bull 22:633–639, 1986

Nuechterlein K, Goldstein M, Ventura J: Patient-environment relationships in schizophrenia. Br J Psychiatry 155 (suppl 5):84–89, 1989

Nuechterlein KH, Snyder KS, Mintz J: Paths to relapse: possible transactional processes connecting patient illness onset, expressed emotion, and psychotic relapse. Br J Psychiatry 161:88–96, 1992

Nugter MA, Dingemans P, Linszen D, et al: Parental communication deviance: its stability and the effect of family treatment in recent-onset schizophrenia. Acta Psychiatr Scand 95:199–204, 1997

Nugter A, Dingemans P, Van der Does JW, et al: Family treatment, expressed emotion and relapse in recent onset schizophrenia. Psychiatry Res 72:23–31, 1997

Nunnally E, de Shazer S, Lipchik E, et al: The study of change: therapeutic theory in process, in Journeys: Expansion of the Strategic-Systemic Therapies. Edited by Efron DE. New York, Brunner/Mazel, 1986, pp 77–92

Nurnberg HG, Prudic J, Fiori M, et al: Psychopathology complicating acquired immune deficiency syndrome (AIDS). Am J Psychiatry 141:95–96, 1984

Nye F: Families and Family Therapy, Cambridge, MA, Harvard University Press, 1958

Oberndorf CP: Psychoanalysis of married couples. Psychoanal Rev 25:453–475, 1938

O'Farrell T, Courles K: Marital and family therapy, in Handbook of Alcoholism Treatment Approaches. Edited by Hester R, Miller W. Elmsford, NY, Pergamon, 1989, pp 183–205

O'Farrell T, Cutter H, Floyd F: Evaluating behavioral marital therapy for male alcoholics. Behavior Therapy 16:147–167, 1985

O'Farrell TJ, Hooley J, Fals-Stewart W, et al: Expressed emotion and relapse in alcoholic patients. J Consult Clin Psychol 66:744–752, 1998

Offord J, Guthrie S, Nicholls P, et al: Self-reported coping behavior of wives of alcoholics and its association with drinking outcome. J Stud Alcohol 36:1254–1267, 1975

O'Hare W, Pollard K, Mann T, et al: African Americans in the 1990s. Popul Bull 46:8–10, 1991

O'Leary KD: Assessment of Marital Discord. Hillsdale, NJ, Lawrence Erlbaum, 1987

O'Leary K, Arias I: The influence of marital therapy on sexual satisfaction. J Sex Marital Ther 9:171–182, 1983

O'Leary K, Beach R: Marital therapy: a viable treatment for depression and marital discord. Am J Psychiatry 147:183–186, 1990

O'Leary KD, Jacobson NS: Partner relational problems with physical abuse, in DSM-IV Sourcebook, Vol 3. Edited by Widiger TA, Frances AJ, Pincus HA, et al. Washington, DC, American Psychiatric Association, 1997, pp 673–692

O'Leary KD, Murphy CM: Clinical issues in the assessment of spouse abuse, in Assessment of Family Violence: A Clinical and Legal Sourcebook. Edited by Ammerman RT, Hersen M. New York, Wiley, 1992, pp 26–46

O'Leary K, Smith D: Marital interactions. Annu Rev Psychol 42:191–212, 1991

O'Leary KD, Fincham FD, Turkewitz H: Assessment of positive feelings toward spouse. J Consult Clin Psychol 51:949–951, 1983

O'Leary KD, Vivian D, Malone J: Assessment of physical aggression against women in marriage: the need for multimodal assessment. Behavioral Assessment 14:5–14, 1992

O'Leary KD, Heyman RE, Jongsma A: The Couples Psychotherapy Treatment Planner. New York, Wiley, 1998

Oliver JE: Intergenerational transmission of child abuse: rates, research, clinical implications. Am J Psychiatry 150:1315–1324, 1993

Olivieri M, Reiss D: Family concepts and their measurement are seldom what they seem. Fam Process 23:33–48, 1984

Ollendick DG, LaBerteaux PJ, Howe AM: Relationships among maternal attitudes, perceived family environments, and preschoolers' behavior. Percept Mot Skills 46:1092–1094, 1978

Olson D: Marital and family therapy: integrative review and critique. Journal of Marriage and the Family 32:501–538, 1970

Olson DH: Prepare-Enrich: Counselor's Manual. Minneapolis, MN, Prepare-Enrich, 1982a

Olson D: Training Lay Couples to Work With Premarital and Newlywed Couples. Minneapolis, MN, Prepare-Enrich, 1982b

Olson DH, Bell R, Porter J: FACES: Family Adaptability and Cohesion Evaluation Scales (manual). St Paul, University of Minnesota, 1978

Olson DH, Sprenkle DH, Russell CS: Circumplex Model of Marital and Family Systems, I: cohesion and adaptability dimensions, family types and clinical applications. Fam Process 18:3–28, 1979

Olson DH, Russell CS, Sprenkle DH: Marital and family therapy: a decade review. Journal of Marriage and the Family 42:923–993, 1980

Olson DH, McCubbin HL, Barnes H, et al: Faces II: Family Adaptability and Cohesion Evaluation Scales. St Paul, University of Minnesota, Family Social Science, 1982a

Olson D, Portner J, Bell R: Faces II: Family Adaptability and Cohesion Evaluation Scales. St Paul, MN, Family Social Services, 1982b

Olson DH, McCubbin HL, Barnes H, et al: Family Inventories. St Paul, University of Minnesota, Family Social Science, 1985

Onnis L, DiGennaro A, Crspa G, et al: Sculpting present and future: a systemic intervention model applied to psychosomatic families. Fam Process 33:341–355, 1994

Orvaschel H: Early onset psychiatric disorder in high risk children and increased familial morbidity. J Am Acad Child Adolesc Psychiatry 29:184–188, 1990

Orvaschel H, Walsh-Allis G, Ye W: Psychopathology in children of parents with recurrent depression. J Abnorm Child Psychiatry 16:235–230, 1988

Oxford Dictionary. Oxford, England, Clarendon Press, 1991

Painter JR, Seres JL, Newman RI: Assessing benefits of the pain center: why some patients regress. Pain 8:101–113, 1980

Palazzoli MS: A Systemic Course of Family Therapy. Northvale, NJ, Jason Aronson, 1988a

Panton J: MMPI profile configurations associated with incestuous and non-incestuous child molesting. Psychol Rep 45:335–338, 1979

Paolino TJ, McCrady B: Marriage and Marital Therapy. New York, Brunner/Mazel, 1978

Papernow P: Becoming a Stepfamily: Patterns of Development in Remarried Families. San Francisco, CA, Jossey-Bass, 1993

Papero DV: Bowen Family Systems Theory. Boston, MA, Allyn & Bacon, 1990

Papero DV: Stress and instability. Family Systems 3:64–68, 1996
Papp P: Paradoxes, in Family Therapy Techniques. Edited by Minuchin S, Fishman HC. Cambridge, MA, Harvard University Press, 1981, pp 244–261
Parens H: Aggression in Our Children. Northvale, NJ, Jason Aronson, 1987
Parker G: Parental Overprotection: A Risk Factor in Psychosocial Development. New York, Grune & Stratton, 1983
Parker G, Hadzi-Pavlovic D: Expressed emotion as a predictor of schizophrenia relapse: an analysis of aggregated data. Psychol Med 20:961–965, 1990
Parker G, Johnston P, Hayward L: Parental "expressed emotion" as a predictor of schizophrenic relapse. Arch Gen Psychiatry 45:806–813, 1988
Parker H: Intrafamilial sexual abuse: a study of the abusive father. Unpublished doctoral dissertation, Salt Lake City, UT, University of Utah, 1984 [Dissertation Abstracts International 45(12):3751, 1984]
Parker H, Parker S: Father-daughter abuse: an emerging perspective. Am J Orthopsychiatry 56:531–549, 1986
Parsons BV, Alexander JF: Short-term family intervention: a therapy outcome study. J Consult Clin Psychol 41:195–201, 1973
Parsons T, Bales R: Family Socialization and Interaction Process. Glencoe, IL, Free Press, 1965
Paitich D, Langeven R, Freeman R, et al: The Clark Sexual History Questionnaire: a clinical sex history questionnaire for males. Arch Sex Behav 6:421–435, 1977
Pasch LA, Bradbury TN: Social support, conflict, and the development of marital dysfunction. J Consult Clin Psychol 66:219–230, 1998
Pasch LA, Bradbury TN, Davila J: Gender, negative affectivity, and observed social support behavior in marital interaction. Personal Relationships 4:361–378, 1997
Pasley K: Family boundary ambiguity: perceptions of adult remarried family members, in Remarriage and Stepparenting: Current Research and Theory. Edited by Pasley K, Ihinger-Tallman M. New York, Guilford, 1987, pp 206–224
Pasley K, Rhoden L, Visher EB, et al: Successful stepfamily therapy: clients' perspectives. J Marital Fam Ther 22:343–357, 1996
Paterson R, Moran G: Attachment theory; personality development and psychotherapy. Clin Psychol Rev 8:611–636, 1992
Patterson GR: Coercive Family Process: A Social Learning Approach to Family Intervention, Vol 3. Eugene, OR, Castalia Publishing, 1982
Patterson GR: Performance models for antisocial boys. Am Psychol 41:432–444, 1986
Patterson GR: Foreword, in Handbook of Behavioral Family Therapy. Edited by Falloon IRH. New York, Guilford, 1988
Patterson GR (ed): Depression and Aggression in Family Interaction (Advances in Family Research). Hillsdale, NJ, Lawrence Erlbaum, 1990a
Patterson GR: Some comments about cognitions as causal variables. Am Psychol 45(8):984–985, 1990b
Patterson GR, Chamberlain P: A functional analysis of resistance during parent training therapy. Clinical Psychology: Science and Practice I:53–70, 1994
Patterson G, Forgatch M: Parents and Adolescents Living Together, Part I: The Basics. Eugene, OR, Castalia Publishing, 1987
Patterson GR, Ray RS, Shaw DD, et al: Manual for Coding Family Interactions. Eugene, Oregon Research Institute, 1969
Patterson GR, Reid JB, Jones RR, et al: A Social Learning Approach to Family Interaction, Vol 1: Families With Aggressive Children. Eugene, OR, Castalia Publishing, 1975
Patterson G, Reid J, Chamberlain D: A comparative evaluation of a parent-training program. Behavior Therapy 13:638–650, 1982
Patterson G, Reid J, Dishion T: Antisocial Boys. Eugene, OR, Castalia Publishing, 1992
Pattison EM: The Experience of Dying. Englewood Cliffs, NJ, Prentice-Hall, 1977
Pattison EM, Kaufman E: The Encyclopedic Handbook of Alcoholism. New York, Gardner Press, 1982

Pattison M, DeFrancisco D, Wood P, et al: A psychosocial kinship model for family therapy. Am J Psychiatry 132:1246–1251, 1975

Paul N, Grosser G: Operational mourning and its role in conjoint family therapy. Community Ment Health J 1:339–345, 1965

Paul NL, Paul BB: Normal Family Processes. New York, Guilford, 1968

Paykel E, Myers J, Dienelt M, et al: Life events and depression: a controlled study. Arch Gen Psychiatry 21:753–760, 1969

Payne BA: A transpersonal family treatment program for chronic pain patients. Unpublished doctoral dissertation, California Institute of Transpersonal Psychology, Menlo Park, 1982

Pearlin LI, Schooler C: The structure of coping. J Health Soc Behav 19:2–21, 1978

Pelto VL: Male incest offenders and non-offenders: a comparison of early sexual history. Dissertation Abstracts International 42 (suppl 3B):1154, 1981

Penk W, Robinowitz R, Kidd R, et al: Perceived family environment among ethnic groups of compulsive heroin users. Addict Behav 4:297–309, 1979

Penn DL, Mueser KT: Research update on the psychosocial treatment of schizophrenia. Am J Psychiatry 153:607–617, 1996

Penn P: Feed-forward: future questions, future maps. Fam Process 24:299–310, 1985

Perlmutter RA: A Family Approach to Psychiatric Disorders. Washington, DC, American Psychiatric Press, 1996

Perosa L: The development of a questionnaire to measure Minuchin's structural family concepts and the application of his psychosomatic family model to learning disabled families. Unpublished doctoral dissertation, State University of New York at Buffalo, 1980

Perosa L, Perosa S: Structural interaction patterns in families with a learning disabled child. Family Therapy 9:175–187, 1982

Perosa L, Hansen J, Perosa S: Development of the Structural Family Interaction Scale. Family Therapy 8:77–90, 1981

Perry SW, Tross S: Psychiatric problems of AIDS inpatients at the New York Hospital: preliminary report. Public Health Rep 99:200–205, 1984

Peters J: Children who are victims of sexual assault and the psychology of offenders. Am J Psychother 30:398–421, 1976

Peters L, Esses L: Family environment as perceived by children with a chronically ill parent. Journal of Chronic Disability 38:301–308, 1985

Pettle S: Thinking about the future when death is inevitable: consultations in terminal care. Clinical Child Psychology and Psychiatry 3:131–139, 1998

Pevsner R: Group parent training versus individual family therapy: an outcome study. J Behav Ther Exp Psychiatry 13:119–122, 1982

Pharoah FM, Mari JJ, Streiner D: Family intervention for schizophrenia, in The Cochrane Library, Issue 2. Oxford, UK, Update Software, 2000

Phillips M, Xiong W: Expressed emotion in mainland China: Chinese families with schizophrenic patients. International Journal of Mental Health 24:54–75, 1995

Piercy R, Sprenkle D: Family Therapy Sourcebook. New York, Guilford, 1986, pp 213–242

Piercy F, Sprenkle D, Avis J, et al: Divorce therapy, in Family Therapy Sourcebook. New York, Guilford, 1986

Piercy F, Sprenkle DH, Wetchler JL: Family Therapy Sourcebook, 2nd Edition. New York, Guilford, 1996

Pilsecker C: Hospital classes educate schizophrenics about their illness. Hosp Community Psychiatry 32:60–61, 1981

Pinderhughes E: Afro-American and economic dependency. Urban and Social Change Review 12:24–27, 1979

Pinderhughes E: Afro-American families and the victim system, in Ethnicity and Family Therapy. Edited by McGoldrick M, Pearce J, Giordano J. New York, Guilford, 1982, pp 108–122

Pinsof W: What is wrong with family therapy? Paper presented at AAMKT Annual Conference, Washington, DC, 1990
Pinsof W, Wynne L: The efficacy of marital and family therapy: an empirical overview, conclusions and recommendations. J Marital Fam Ther 21:585–613, 1995
Pinsof W, Wynne LC, Hambright AB: The outcomes of couple and family therapy: findings, conclusions, and recommendations. Psychotherapy: Theory, Research, Practice, and Training 33:321–331, 1966
Piotrowski C: Use of tests and measures in family and marital research. Psychol Rep 84 (3, part 2):1251–1252, 1999
Pittman F: Introduction to Keynote Address by Salvador Minuchin. Presentation at the Family Therapy Network Symposium "Metamorphosis," Washington, DC, March 1993
Pless IB, Satterwhite BB: A measure of family functioning and its application. Soc Sci Med 7:613–621, 1973
Pollio DE, North CS, Foster DA: Content and curriculum in psychoeducation groups for families of persons with severe mental illness. Psychiatr Serv 49:816–822, 1998
Polonsky DC, Nadelson CD: An integrative approach to couples therapy, in New Clinical Concepts in Marital Therapy. Edited by Bjorksten OJW. Washington, DC, American Psychiatric Press, 1985, pp 151–165
Posner CM, Wilson KG, Kral MJ, et al: Family psychoeducational support groups in schizophrenia. Am J Orthopsychiatry 62:206–218, 1992
Powell DR: Including Latino fathers in parent education and support programs: development of a program model, in Understanding Latino Families. Edited by Zambrana RE. Thousand Oaks, CA, Sage, 1995
Powell K, Wampler K: Marriage enrichment participants: levels of marital satisfaction. Family Relations 31:389–393, 1982
Preli R, Bernard J: Making multiculturalism relevant for majority culture graduate students. J Marital Fam Ther 19:5–16, 1993
Prest L, Carruthers W: The case of the sneaky sleep thief: White's externalizing technique within a broad strategic frame. Journal of Strategic and Systemic Therapies 10:66–75, 1991
Pretzer JL, Epstein N, Fleming B: The Marital Attitude Survey: a measure of dysfunctional attributions and expectancies. Journal of Cognitive Psychotherapy 14(3):123–136, 1992
Price G: Multiple sclerosis: the challenge to the family. Am J Nurs 80:283–285, 1980
Prince SE, Jacobson NS: A review and evaluation of marital and family therapies for affective disorders. J Marital Fam Ther 21:377–401, 1995
Prozan CK: Response, in Construction and Reconstruction of Memory: Dilemmas of Childhood Sexual Abuse. Edited by Prozan CK. Northvale, NJ, Jason Aronson, 1997, pp 223–228
Psychiatric News 29(10, May):6–7, 1994
Puig-Antich J, Chambers W: Schedule for Affective Disorders and Schizophrenia for School-Aged Children, Epidemiological Version (K-SADS-E, 3rd Version). Washington, DC, National Institute of Mental Health, 1978
Puig-Antich J, Lukens E, Davies M, et al: Psychosocial functioning in prepubertal depressive disorders, I: interpersonal relationships during the depressive episode. Arch Gen Psychiatry 42:500–507, 1985a
Puig-Antich J, Lukens E, Davies M, et al: Psychosocial functioning in prepubertal depressive disorders, II: interpersonal relationships after sustained recovery from affective episode. Arch Gen Psychiatry 42:511–517, 1985b
Puig-Antich J, Kaufman J, Ryan N: The psychosocial functioning and family environment of depressed adolescents. J Am Acad Child Adolesc Psychiatry 32:244–253, 1993
Racker H: The meaning and uses of countertransference: essential papers on countertransference, in Classics in Psychoanalytic Technique. Edited by Wolstein B. New York, New York University Press, 1981, pp 158–201

Radke-Yarrow M, Nottelmann E, Martinez P, et al: Young children of affectively ill parents: a longitudinal study of psychosocial development. J Am Acad Child Adolesc Psychiatry 31:66–77, 1992

Randall J, Henggeler SW, Cunningham PB, et al: Adapting multisystemic therapy to treat adolescent substance abuse more effectively. Cognitive and Behavioral Practice 8:359–366. 2001

Randolph ET, Eth S, Glynn SM, et al: Behavioural family management in schizophrenia: outcome of a clinic-based intervention. Br J Psychiatry 164:501–506, 1994

Rapoport JL: American abortion applicants in Sweden. Arch Gen Psychiatry 13:24–32, 1965

Rapoport R, Rapoport R, Strelitz Z: Fathers, Mothers and Society. New York, Basic Books, 1977

Raschke HJ: Divorce and marital separation. Unpublished manuscript, Department of Psychology and Sociology, Austin College, Sherman, TX, 1983

Rasmussen LA, Burton JE, Christopherson BJ: Precursors to offending and the trauma outcome process in sexually reactive children. Journal of Sexual Abuse 1:33–48, 1992

Raue J, Spence SH: Group versus individual applications of reciprocity training for parent-youth conflict. Behav Res Ther 23:177–186, 1985

Rauseo L: Relationships as primary regulators of physiology. Family Systems 2:101–115, 1995

Rausch HL, et al: Adaptation to the first years of marriage. Psychiatry 26:368–380, 1963

Rausch HL, Barry W, Hertel R, et al: Communication Conflict and Marriage. San Francisco, CA, Jossey-Bass, 1974

Ravenscroft K: Family therapy, in Child and Adolescent Psychiatry. Edited by Lewis M. Baltimore, MD, Williams & Wilkins, 1991, pp 850–868

Ravich R: Predictable Pairing. New York, Peter H Wyden, 1974

Redl F, Wineman D: Children Who Hate. New York, Free Press, 1951

Regehr C, Antle B: Coercive influences: informed consent in court-mandated social work practice. Social Work 42:300–306, 1997

Regehr C, Glancy G: Survivors of sexual abuse allege therapist negligence. J Am Acad Psychiatry Law 25:49–58, 1997

Reid J, Hendricks A: Preliminary analysis of the effectiveness of direct home intervention for the treatment of predelinquent boys who steal, in Behavior Change: Methodology, Concepts and Practice. Edited by Hamerlynck L, Handy L, Mash E. Champaign, IL, Research Press, 1973, pp 20–21

Reiss AJ, Roth JA (eds): Understanding and Preventing Violence, Vol 3: Social Influences. National Research Council Commission on Behavioral and Social Sciences and Education Committee on Law and Justice, Panel on the Understanding and Control of Violent Behavior. Washington, DC, National Academy Press, 1994a

Reiss AJ, Roth JA (eds): Understanding and Preventing Violence, Vol 4: Consequences and Control. National Research Council Commission on Behavioral and Social Sciences and Education Committee on Law and Justice, Panel on the Understanding and Control of Violent Behavior. Washington, DC, National Academy Press, 1994b

Reiss AJ, Miczek KA, Roth JA (eds): Understanding and Preventing Violence, Vol 2: Biobehavioral Influences. National Research Council Commission on Behavioral and Social Sciences and Education Committee on Law and Justice, Panel on the Understanding and Control of Violent Behavior. Washington, DC, National Academy Press, 1994

Reiss D: Models of consensual experience, III: contrasts between families of normals, delinquents, and schizophrenics. J Nerv Ment Dis 152:73–90, 1971

Reiss D: The Family's Construction of Reality. Cambridge, MA, Harvard University Press, 1981

Reiss D: The working family. Am J Psychiatry 139:1412–1420, 1982

Reiss D: The represented and practicing family: contrasting visions of family continuity, in Early Relationship Disorders. Edited by Sameroff AJ, Emde RM. New York, Basic Books, 1988

Reiss D, Klein D: Paradigm and pathogenesis: a family centered approach to problems of etiology and treatment of psychiatric disorders, in Family Interaction and Psychopathology: Theories, Methods, Findings. Edited by Jacob T. New York, Plenum, 1987

Reiss D, Olivieri M: Sensory experience and family process. Fam Process 22:289–308, 1983

Reiss D, Gonzalez S, Kramer N: Family process, chronic illness, and death. Arch Gen Psychiatry 43:795–804, 1986

Reiss D, Plomin R, Hetherington EM: Genetics and psychiatry: an unheralded window on the environment. Am J Psychiatry 148:283–291, 1991

Reiss D, Plomin R, Hetherington EM, et al: The separate social worlds of teenage siblings, in Separate Social Worlds of Siblings: Impact of the Nonshared Environment on Development. Edited by Hetherington EM, Reiss D, Plomin R. Hillsdale, NJ, Lawrence Erlbaum, 1994, pp 63–109

Reiss D, Neiderhiser JM, Hetherington EM, et al: The Relationship Code: Deciphering Genetic and Social Influences on Adolescent Development. Cambridge, MA, Harvard University Press, 2000

Reiter GF, Kilmann PR: Mothers as family change agents. Journal of Counseling Psychology 22:61–65, 1975

Renshaw D: Profile of 2376 patients treated at Loyola Sex Clinic between 1972 and 1987. Sexual and Marital Therapy 3:111–117, 1988

Revenstorf D, Hahlweg K, Schindler K, et al: Interactional analysis of marital conflict, in Marital Interaction: Analysis and Modification. Edited by Hahlweg K, Jacobson NS. New York, Guilford, 1984

Rice L, Greenberg L: Patterns of Change: Intensive Analysis of Psychotherapy Process. New York, Guilford, 1984

Ridenour T, Daley JG, Reich W: Further evidence that the Family Assessment Device should be reorganized: response to Miller and colleagues. Fam Process 39:375–380, 2000

Ridenour T, Daley JG, Reich W: Factor analysis of the Family Assessment Device. Fam Process 38:497–510, 1999

Rioch J: The transference phenomenon in psychoanalytic therapy. Journal for the Study of Interpersonal Processes 6:147–156, 1943

Riskin JM, Flaunce EE: An evaluative review of family interaction research. Fam Process 11:365–455, 1972

Rist K: Incest: theoretical and clinical views. Am J Orthopsychiatry 49:680–691, 1979

Ritvo R, Al-mateen C, Ascherman L, et al: Report of the Psychotherapy Task Force of the American Academy of Child and Adolescent Psychiatry. J Psychother Pract Res 8:93–102, 1999

Roberts J: An evolving model: links between the Milan approach and strategic models of family therapy, in Journeys: Expansion of the Strategic-Systemic Therapies. Edited by Efron DE. New York, Brunner/Mazel, 1986, pp 150–173

Roberts T: Sexual attraction and romantic love: forgotten variables in marital therapy. J Marital Fam Ther 18:357–364, 1992

Robertson DU, Hyde JS: The factorial validity of the Family Environment Scale. Educational and Psychological Measurement 42:1233–1241, 1982

Robins LN: Deviant Children Grown Up: A Sociological and Psychiatric Study of Sociopathic Personality. Baltimore, MD, Williams & Wilkins, 1966 (Reprint: Huntington, NY, Krieger Publishing, 1974)

Robins LN, Reiger DA (eds): Psychiatric Disorders in America. New York, Free Press, 1990

Robinson CA, Thorne S: Strengthening family "interference." J Adv Nurs 9:597–602, 1984

Robinson E, Jacobson N: Social learning theory and family psychopathology, in Family Interaction and Psychopathology. Edited by Jacob T. New York, Plenum, 1987, pp 117–140

Rolland JS: Chronic illness and the family: an overview, in Families and Chronic Illness. Springhouse, PA, Springhouse, 1987a

Rolland JS: Family systems and chronic illness: a typological model. Journal of Psychotherapy and the Family 3:143–168, 1987b
Rolland J: Family intervention with chronic physical, psychiatric disorders. Psychiatric Times, October 1994, pp 43–45
Roncone R, Rossi L, Muiere E, et al: The Italian version of the Family Assessment Device. Soc Psychiatry Psychiatr Epidemiol 33:451–461, 1998
Rose D (ed): Assessing families of school-aged children with cancer, in Families and Life-Threatening Illness. Springhouse, PA, Springhouse, 1987
Rosen RC, Leiblum SR (eds): Case Studies in Sex Therapy. New York, Guilford, 1995
Rosenberg ML, Fenely MA (eds): Violence in America: A Public Health Approach. New York, Oxford University Press, 1991
Rosenblatt PC: Metaphors of Family Systems Theory. New York, Guilford, 1994
Rosenfarb I, Goldstein M, Mintz J, et al: Expressed emotion and subclinical psychopathology observable within the transactions between schizophrenic patients and their family members. J Abnorm Psychol 104:259–267, 1995
Rosenthal D: Genetic Theory and Abnormal Behavior. New York, Brunner/Mazel, 1970
Rosman B, Minuchin S, Liebman R, et al: Input and outcome of family therapy in anorexia nervosa, in Successful Psychotherapy. Edited by Claghorn JL. New York, Brunner/Mazel, 1976
Rostworowska M, Barbaro B, Cechnicki A: The influence of expressed emotion on the course of schizophrenia: a Polish replication. Poster presented at the 17th Congress of the European Association for Behavior Therapy, Amsterdam, August 1987
Rothman D: The Discovery of the Asylum: Social Order and Disorder in the New Republic. Boston, MA, Little, Brown, 1971
Ro-Trock GK, Wellisch DK, Schoolar JC: A family therapy outcome study in an inpatient setting. Am J Orthopsychiatry 47:514–522, 1977
Rotter J: A new scale for the measurement of interpersonal trust. J Pers 35:651–665, 1967
Rounsaville B, Weissman M, Prescott B, et al: Marital disputes and treatment outcome in depressed women. Compr Psychiatry 20:483–490, 1979
Rounsaville B, Prusoff B, Weissman M: The course of marital disputes in depressed women: a 48-month follow-up study. Compr Psychiatry 21:111–118, 1980
Roy M: Battered Women: A Psychological Study of Domestic Violence. New York, Van Nostrand Reinhold, 1977
Rubenstein JS, Watson FG, Fletcher G, et al: Young adolescents' sexual interests. Adolescence 11:487–496, 1976
Rueveni R: Networking Families in Crisis. New York, Human Sciences Press, 1979
Ruiz R: Cultural and historical perspectives in counseling Hispanics, in The Culturally Different. Edited by Sue D. New York, Wiley, 1981
Rund BR, Moe L, Sollien T, et al: The Psychosis Project: outcome and cost-effectiveness of a psychoeducational programme for schizophrenic adolescents. Acta Psychiatr Scand 89:211–218, 1994
Rund BR, Oie M, Borchgrevink TS, et al: Expressed emotion, communication deviance and schizophrenia. Psychopathology 28:220–228, 1995
Rush HL, Barry WA, Hertel RK, et al: Communication, Conflict and Marriage. San Francisco, CA, Jossey-Bass, 1974
Russell CS: Circumplex Model of Marital and Family Systems, III: empirical evaluation of families. Fam Process 18:29–45, 1979
Russell C, Bagarozzi DA, Atilano RB, et al: A comparison of two approaches to marital enrichment and conjugal skills training: Minnesota couples communication program and structured behavioral exchange contracting. Am J Family Therapy 12:13–25, 1984
Russell DEH: The prevalence and seriousness of incestuous abusive stepfathers vs biological fathers. Child Abuse Neglect 8:15–22, 1984
Russell DEH: The Secret Trauma: Incest in the Lives of Girls and Women. New York, Basic Books, 1986

Russell GFM, Szmukler GI, Dare C, et al: An evaluation of family therapy in anorexia nervosa and bulimia nervosa. Arch Gen Psychiatry 44:1047–1056, 1987

Rusted L: Family adjustment to chronic disability in mid-life, in Chronic Illness and Disability Through the Life Span. Edited by Eisenberg MG, et al. New York, Springer, 1985

Rutter M: Protective factors in children's responses to stress and disadvantage, in Primary Prevention of Psychopathology: Social Competence in Children. Edited by Kent M, Rolf J. Hanover, NH, University Press of New England, 1979

Rutter M: Stress, coping, and development: some issues and some questions, in Stress, Coping, and Development in Children. Edited by Garmezy N, Rutter M. New York, McGraw-Hill, 1983, pp 1–42

Rutter M: Psychosocial resilience and protective mechanisms. Am J Orthopsychiatry 57: 316–331, 1987

Rutter M: Commentary: some focus and process considerations regarding effects of parental depression on children. Dev Psychol 26:60–67, 1990

Rutter M, Giller H: Juvenile Delinquency: Trends and Perspectives. New York, Penguin Books, 1983

Rutter M, Quinton D: Parental psychiatric disorder: effects on children. Psychol Med 14: 853–880, 1984

Rutter M, Tizard J, Whitmore K (eds): Education, Health and Behaviour. London, Longman, 1970

Rutter M, Cox A, Tupling C, et al: Attainment and adjustment in two geographical areas, I: the prevalence of psychiatric disorder. Br J Psychiatry 126:493–509, 1975

Rychtarik RG: Alcohol-related coping skills in spouses of alcoholics: assessment and implications in treatment, in Alcohol and the Family: Research and Clinical Perspectives. Edited by Collins RL, Leonard KE, et al. New York, Guilford, 1990, pp 356–379

Rychtarik RG, Tarnowski KJ, St Lawrence JS: Impact of social desirability response sets on the self-report of marital adjustment in alcoholics. J Stud Alcohol 50:24–29, 1989

Ryckoff I, Day J, Wynne L: Maintenance of stereotyped roles in the families of schizophrenics. Arch Gen Psychiatry 1:93–98, 1959

Sadock V: Normal human sexuality and sexual disorders, in Comprehensive Textbook of Psychiatry. Edited by Kaplan HI, Sadock BJ. Baltimore, MD, Williams & Wilkins, 1991

Sagar R, Wiseman KK: Understanding Organizations. Washington, DC, Georgetown Family Center, 1982

Sager CJ: Transference in compound treatment of married couples. Arch Gen Psychiatry 16:185–193, 1967

Sager C: Marriage Contracts and Couples Therapy. New York, Brunner/Mazel, 1976

Sager C: Couples therapy and marriage contracts, in Handbook of Family Therapy. Edited by Gurman AS, Kniskern DP. New York, Brunner/Mazel, 1981, pp 143–187

Sager CJ, Kaplan HS (eds): Progress in Group and Family Therapy. New York, Brunner/Mazel, 1972

Sager CJ, Brown HS, Crohn H, et al: Treating the Remarried Family. New York, Brunner/Mazel, 1983

Sailor WS: Family perception and its relation to personality and adjustment factors in the child. Unpublished master's thesis, University of Kansas, Lawrence, KS, 1963

Saltzer LP: Adoption after infertility, in Infertility Counseling: A Comprehensive Handbook for Clinicians. Edited by Burns LH, Covington SN. New York, Parthenon Publishing Group, 1999, pp 391–409

Salter MD: The role of the clinical psychologist in Canada. Can J Psychol 3:6–18, 1949

Santa-Barbara J, Woodward C, Levin S, et al: The McMaster Family Therapy Outcome Study: an overview of methods and results. International Journal of Family Therapy 16:304–423, 1979

Santisteban DA, Szapocznik J, Perez-Vidal A, et al: Efficacy of intervention for engaging youth and families into treatment and some variables that may contribute to differential effectiveness. Journal of Family Psychology 10:35–44, 1996

Santisteban DA, Coatsworth JD, Perez-Vidal A, et al: Brief structural/strategic family therapy with African American and Hispanic high-risk youth. J Community Psychol 25: 453–471, 1997

Santrock J, Sitterle K: The developmental world of children in divorced families, in Contemporary Marriage. Edited by Goldberg D. Homewood, IL, Dorsey Press, 1985, pp 166–214

Santrock JW, Warshak RA: Development of father custody relationships and legal/clinical considerations in father-custody families, in The Father's Role: Applied Perspectives. Edited by Lamb ME. New York, Wiley, 1986, pp 135–166

Sass L, Gunderson J, Singer M, et al: Parental communication deviance and forms of thinking in male schizophrenic offspring. J Nerv Ment Dis 172:513–520, 1984

Satin W, La Greca AM, Zigo MA, et al: Diabetes in adolescence: effects of multifamily group intervention and parent simulation of diabetes. J Pediatr Psychol 14:259–275, 1989

Satir V: Conjoint Family Therapy: A Guide to Theory and Technique. Palo Alto, CA, Science & Behavior Books, 1964

Satir V: Peoplemaking. Palo Alto, CA, Science & Behavior Books, 1972

Satterwhite B, Zweig S, Iker H, et al: The Family Functioning Index: five-year test-retest reliability and implications for use. Journal of Comparative Family Studies 7:111–116, 1976

Saxe BJ, Johnson SM: An empirical investigation of group treatment for a clinical population of adult female incest survivors. Journal of Child Sexual Abuse 8:67–88, 1999a

Saxe BJ, Johnson SM: Group therapy for a clinical population of adult incest survivors. Journal of Child Sexual Abuse 8:67–88, 1999b

Sayers SL, Baucom DH, Sher TG, et al: Constructive engagement, behavioral marital therapy and changes in marital satisfaction. Behavioral Assessment 13:25–49, 1991

Sayger TV, Horne AM, Walker JM, et al: Social learning family therapy with aggressive children: treatment outcome and maintenance. Journal of Family Psychology 1:261–285, 1988

Scarf M: Intimate Partners: Patterns in Love and Marriage. New York, Ballantine Books, 1987

Scarf M: Intimate Worlds: How Families Thrive and Why They Fail. New York, Ballantine Books, 1995

Scazufca M, Kuipers E: Stability of expressed emotion in relatives of those with schizophrenia and its relationship with burden of care and perception of patients' social functioning. Psychol Med 28:453–461, 1998

Schaefer ES, Bell RQ: Development of a parental attitude research instrument. Child Dev 29:339–361, 1958

Scharff D, Scharff J: Object Relations Family Therapy. Northvale, NJ, Jason Aronson, 1987

Scharff J: Psychoanalytic marital therapy, in Clinical Handbook of Couple Therapy, 2nd Edition. Edited by Jacobson N, Gurman A. New York, Guilford, 1995, pp 164–193

Scher J, Dix C: Preventing Miscarriage: The Good News. New York, Harper & Row, 1990

Schetky D: Child sexual abuse in mythology, religion and history, in A Handbook for Health Care and Legal Professionals. Edited by Schetky D, Green A. New York, Brunner/Mazel, 1981

Schiavi R: Interview, psychometric, and psychophysiologic strategies to assess sexual disorder etiology (monograph). J Clin Psychiatry 10(2):19–26, 1992a

Schiavi RC: Normal aging and the evaluation of sexual dysfunction. Psychiatr Med 10:217–225, 1992b

Schiavi RC, Schreiner-Engel P, White D, et al: Pituitary-gonadal function during sleep in men with hypoactive sexual desire and in normal controls. Psychosom Med 50:304–318, 1988

Schiavi R, Schreiner-Engel P, Mandeli J, et al: Healthy aging and male sexual function. Am J Psychiatry 147:766–771, 1990

Schindler L, Hohenberger-Sieber E, Hahlweg K: Observing client-therapist interaction in behaviour therapy: development and first application of an observational system. Br J Clin Psychol 28:213–226, 1990

Schmaling KB, Jacobson NS: Marital interaction and depression. J Abnorm Psychol 99:229–236, 1990

Schmidt D: When Is It Helpful to Convene the Family? Journal Fam Pract 16:967–973, 1983

Schmidt G: The outcome of different versions of partner-therapy of sexual dysfunctions: results of a controlled study. Paper presented at the Third Annual Meeting of the International Academy of Sex Research, Bloomington, IN, 1977

Schmidt SE, Liddle HA, Dakof G: Changes in parenting practices and adolescent drug abuse during multidimensional family therapy. Journal of Family Psychology 10:12–27, 1996

Schnarch DM: Constructing the Sexual Crucible: An Integration of Sexual and Marital Therapy. New York, WW Norton, 1991

Schnarch DM: Passionate Marriage: Love, Sex, and Intimacy in Emotionally Committed Relationships. New York, Henry Holt, 1998

Schoenfeld P, Halevy-Martini J, Hemley-Van der Velden E, et al: Network therapy: an outcome study of twelve social networks. J Community Psychol 13:281–287, 1985

Schooler N, Levine J, Severe J, et al: Prevention of relapse in schizophrenia: an evaluation of fluphenazine decanoate. Arch Gen Psychiatry 37:16–24, 1988

Schooler NR, Keith SJ, Severe JB, et al: Treatment strategies in schizophrenia: effects of dosage reduction and family management on outcome. Schizophr Res 9:260, 1993

Schooler NR, Keith SJ, Severe JB, et al: Relapse and rehospitalization during maintenance treatment of schizophrenia. Arch Gen Psychiatry 54:453–463, 1997

Schor JB: The Overworked American: The Unexpected Decline of Leisure. New York, Basic Books, 1991

Schover L: Sexual problems in chronic illness, in Principles and Practice of Sex Therapy: Update for the 1990s, 2nd Edition. Edited by Leiblum S, Rosen R. New York, Guilford, 1992

Schover L, Jensen S: Sexuality and Chronic Illness: A Comprehensive Approach. New York, Guilford, 1988

Schreiner-Engel P, Schiavi RC: Patterns of personal problems of adolescent girls. Journal of Educational Psychology 49:1–5, 1958

Schreiner-Engel P, Schiavi RC: Lifetime psychopathology in individuals with low sexual desire. J Nerv Ment Dis 174:646–651, 1986

Schreiner-Engel P, Schiavi RC, Vietorisz D, et al: The differential impact of diabetes type on female sexuality. J Psychosom Res 31:23–33, 1987

Schuckit M: Drug and Alcohol Abuse. New York, Plenum, 1979

Schwartz R: Narrative therapy expands and contracts family therapy's horizons. J Marital Fam Ther 25:263–267, 1999

Schwartzman J: Family ethnography: a tool for clinicians, in Cultural Perspectives in Family Therapy. Edited by Hansen JC, Falicov CJ. Rockville, MD, Aspen Systems, 1983, pp 137–149

Schwoeri L, Schwoeri F: Interactional and intrapsychic dynamics in a family with a borderline patient. Psychotherapy: Theory, Research, and Practice 19:198–204, 1982a

Schwoeri L, Schwoeri F: Some diagnostic treatment issues in the family treatment of borderline patients. International Journal of Family Psychiatry 2(2), 1982b

Schwoeri L, Sholevar G: Social learning family model of depression and aggression: focus on the single mother, in The Transmission of Depression in Families and Children: Assessment and Intervention. Edited by Sholevar GP, Schwoeri L. New York, Jason Aronson, 1994

Scoresby ES, Christensen B: Differences in interaction and environmental conditions of clinic and nonclinic families: implications for use. Journal of Marriage and Family Counseling 2:63–71, 1976

Scott R, Stone D: MMPI profile consultation in incest families. J Consult Clin Psychol 54: 364–368, 1986

Seeman MV: Gender differences in treatment response in schizophrenia, in Gender and Psychopathology. Edited by Seeman MV. Washington, DC, American Psychiatric Press, 1995, pp 227–251

Segraves RT: Drugs and desire, in Sexual Desire Disorders. Edited by Leiblum SR, Rosen RC. New York, Guilford, 1988, pp 313–347

Segraves R: Overview of sexual dysfunction implicating the treatment of depression (monograph). J Clin Psychiatry 10(2):4–10, 1992

Seifer D, Sameroff A: Multiple determinants of risk and invulnerability, in The Invulnerable Child. Edited by Anthony J, Cohler B. New York, Guilford, 1987

Selekman MD: Solution-Focused Therapy With Children. New York, Guilford, 1997

Seligman M: Helplessness: On Depression, Development and Death. San Francisco, CA, WH Freeman, 1975

Seltzer A, Roncari I, Garfinkel P: Effect of patient education on medication compliance. Can J Psychiatry 25:638–645, 1980

Selverstone R: Governance, psychology, education, and sexuality. Journal of Sex Education and Therapy 25:114–121, 2000

Selvini Palazzoli M: Self-Starvation: From Individual to Family Therapy in the Treatment of Anorexia Nervosa. New York, Jason Aronson, 1978

Selvini Palazzoli M, Boscolo L, Cecchin G, et al: Paradox and Counterparadox. New York, Jason Aronson, 1978

Selvini Palazzoli M, Cecchin G, Prata G, et al: Hypothesizing, circularity, neutrality: three guidelines for the conductor of the session. Fam Process 19:3–12, 1980

Selvini Palazzoli M, Cirillo SL, Selvini M, et al: Family Games. New York, WW Norton, 1989

Sexton SB, Glanville DN, Kaslow NJ: Attachment and depression: implications for family therapy. Child Adolesc Psychiatr Clin N Am 10(3):465–486, 2001

Sgroi S: Vulnerable Population: Sexual Abuse Treatment for Children, Adult Survivors, Offenders and Persons With Mental Retardation, Vol 2. Lexington, MA, DC Heath, 1982

Sgroi SM, Blick LC, Porter FS: A conceptual framework for child sexual abuse, in Handbook of Clinical Intervention in Child Sexual Abuse. Edited by Sgroi SM. Lexington, MA, DC Heath, 1982

Shadish WR, Montomery LM, Wilson P, et al: Effects of family and marital psychotherapies: a meta-analysis. J Consult Clin Psychol 61:992–1002, 1993

Shadish WR, Ragsdale K, Glaser RR, et al: The efficacy and effectiveness of marital and family therapy: a perspective from meta-analysis. J Marital Fam Ther 21:345–360, 1995

Shain M: Health promotion programs and the prevention of alcohol abuse: forging a link, in Alcohol Problem Intervention in the Workplace. Edited by Roman PM. New York, Quorum Books, 1990, pp 163–179

Shain M: Alternatives to drug testing, in Drug Testing in the Work Place (Research Advances in Alcohol and Drug Problems, Vol 11). Edited by McDonald S. New York, Plenum, 1994, pp 257–277

Shambaugh PW, Kanter SS: Spouses under stress: group meetings with spouses of patients on hemodialysis. Am J Psychiatry 125:928–936, 1969

Shanas E: The family as a social support system in old age. Gerontologist 19:169–174, 1979

Shapiro D: A family data base for the family oriented medical record. J Fam Pract 13:881–887, 1981

Shapiro RL: Adolescence and the psychology of the ego. Psychiatry Journal for the Study of Interpersonal Process 26:77–87, 1963
Shapiro RL: Identity and ego autonomy in adolescence, in Science and Psychoanalysis. Edited by Masserman JH. New York, Grune & Stratton, 1966, pp 16–24
Shapiro R: Psychodynamic approaches to family therapy, in Emotional Disorders in Children and Adolescents. Edited by Sholevar GP. Jamaica, NY, Spectrum, 1980
Shapiro T: The development and distortion of empathy. Psychoanal Q 43:4–25, 1974
Shaver P, Hazan C: Adult romantic attachment: theory and evidence, in Advances in Personal Relationships. Edited by Perlman D, Jones W. London, PA, Jessica Kingsley, 1994, pp 29–70
Shaw JA (ed): Sexual Aggression. Washington, DC, American Psychiatric Press, 1999
Shea M, Elkin I, Imber S, et al: Course of depressive symptoms over follow-up: findings from the National Institute of Mental Health Treatment of Depression Collaborative Research Program. Arch Gen Psychiatry 49:782–787, 1992
Shocket BR, Lisansky ET, Shuba AF, et al: Medical psychiatric study of patients with rheumatoid arthritis. Psychosomatics 10:271–278, 1969
Sholevar GP: A family therapist looks at the problem of incest. Bull Am Acad Psychiatry Law 3:25–31, 1975
Sholevar G: Psychosomatic disorders and family therapy, in Emotional Disorders in Children and Adolescents. Edited by Sholevar GP. New York, Pergamon, 1980, pp 343–351
Sholevar GP: Family therapy with hospitalized and disabled patients, in Family Therapy With Families With Problems. Edited by Trexler M. New York, Jason Aronson, 1983, pp 15–34
Sholevar GP: Marital assessment, in Contemporary Marriage. Edited by Goldberg DC. Homewood, IL, Dorsey, 1985, pp 290–311
Sholevar GP: Families of institutionalized children, in Emotional Disorders in Children and Adolescents. Edited by Sholevar GP. Jamaica, NY, Spectrum, 1986a, pp 181–190
Sholevar GP (ed): The Handbook of Marriage and Marital Therapy. New York, SP Medical & Scientific Books, 1986b
Sholevar GP: Psychosomatic disorders and family therapy, in Emotional Disorders in Children and Adolescents. Edited by Sholevar GP. Jamaica, NY, Spectrum, 1986c, pp 343–351
Sholevar GP (ed): Emotional Disorders in Children and Adolescents. Jamaica, NY, SP Medical & Scientific Books, 1986d
Sholevar GP: Resocialization of family therapy into psychiatry. Contemporary Psychiatry 8:242–245, 1989a
Sholevar GP: The birth of family psychiatry: an essay review of the book of Family and Marital Therapy, G Glick, J Clarkin (eds). Contemporary Psychiatry 8:187–190, 1989b
Sholevar GP: Family development and life cycle, in Psychiatry, Vol 2. Michels R (editor-in-chief). Philadelphia, PA, JB Lippincott, 1995, pp 1–9
Sholevar GP: Psychoanalytic marital therapy: a case presentation. Grand Rounds, Robert Wood Johnson Medical School at Camden, UMDNJ, October 1996
Sholevar GP: "Affect as process" and Affect, object and character structure": an essay review. Int J Psychoanal 78:1239–1245, 1997a
Sholevar GP: Initial and diagnostic family interviews, in Textbook of Child and Adolescent Psychiatry. Edited by Wiener JM. Washington, DC, American Psychiatric Press, 1997b, pp 103–115
Sholevar GP: Marital therapy with character disorders. Presented at scientific meeting of Philadelphia Psychoanalytic Society and Association, Philadelphia, PA, February 17, 2000
Sholevar GP: Family interventions in conduct disorders. Child Adolesc Psychiatr Clin N Am 10(3):501–518, 2001
Sholevar G, Brashear D: Structural family therapy in medicine. Contemporary Psychiatry 3(1):61–64, 1984

Sholevar GP, Lalli D: Why people obtain a second divorce. Med Aspects Hum Sex 19(7): 158–159, 1985

Sholevar GP, Perkel R: Family systems intervention and physical illness. Journal of Psychiatry 12:1–10, 1990

Sholevar GP, Sholevar EH: Conflict with in-laws. Med Aspects Hum Sex 18:168–169, 1984

Sholevar GP, Burland JA, John L, et al: Psychoanalytic treatment of children and adolescents. J Am Acad Child Adolesc Psychiatry 28:685–690, 1989

Shon SP, Ja DY: Asian families, in Ethnicity and Family Therapy. Edited by McGoldrick M, Pearce JK, Giordano J. New York, Guilford, 1982, pp 208–228

Shor-Posner G, Baldewicz T, Feaster D, et al: Psychological distress in HIV-1 disease in relationship to hypocholesterolemia. Int J Psychiatry Med 27:159–171, 1997

Silliman B, Schumm WR: Marriage preparation programs: a literature review. Family Journal: Counseling and Therapy for Couples and Families 8:133–142, 2000

Simon R: Family therapy, in Comprehensive Textbook of Psychiatry/IV, 4th Edition. Edited by Kaplan HI, Sadock BJ. Baltimore, MD, Williams & Wilkins, 1985, pp 1427–1432

Simoneau TL, Miklowitz DJ, Saleem R: Expressed emotion and interactional patterns in the families of bipolar patients. J Abnorm Psychol 107:497–507, 1998

Simoneau TL, Miklowitz DJ, Richards JA, et al: Bipolar disorder and family communication: effects of a psychoeducational treatment program. J Abnorm Psychol 108:588–597, 1999

Simpson J, Rholes W: Stress and secure base relationships in adulthood, in Attachment Processes in Adulthood. Edited by Bartholomew K, Perlman D. London, PA, Jessica Kingsley, 1994, pp 181–204

Singer GH, Irvin LK, Irvine B, et al: Evaluation of community-based support services for families of persons with developmental disabilities. Journal of the Association for Persons With Severe Handicaps 14:312–323, 1989

Singer M, Wynne L: Differentiating characteristics of parents of childhood schizophrenics, childhood neurotics, and young adult schizophrenics. Am J Psychiatry 120:234–243, 1963

Singer MT, Wynne LC: Thought disorder and family relations of schizophrenics, III: methodology using projective techniques. Arch Gen Psychiatry 12:187–200, 1965a

Singer MT, Wynne LC: Thought disorder and family relations of schizophrenics, IV: results and implications. Arch Gen Psychiatry 12:201–212, 1965b

Sisson RW, Azrin NJ: Family member involvement to initiate and promote treatment of problem drinkers. J Behav Ther Exp Psychiatry 17:15–21, 1986

Skelton M, Dominian J: Psychological stress in wives of patients with myocardial infarction. BMJ 2:101–103, 1973

Skinner BF: Science and Human Behavior. New York, Free Press, 1953

Skinner HA: Instruments for assessing alcohol and drug problems. Bulletin of the Society of Psychologists in Addictive Behaviors 3:21–33, 1984

Skinner H, Steinhauer P, Santa-Barbara J: The Family Assessment Measure. Journal of Family Therapy 22:190–210, 2000

Sluzki C: Migration and family conflict. Fam Process 18:379–390, 1979

Sluzki CE: In memoriam: Mara Selvini-Palazzoli, M.D. (1916–1999). Fam Process 38:391–392, 1999

Smilkstein G: The Family APGAR: a proposal for family function test and its use by physicians. J Fam Pract 6:1231–1239, 1978

Smith H, Israel E: Sibling incest: a study of the dynamics of 25 cases. Child Abuse Negl 17:101–108, 1987

Smith JV, Birchwood MJ: Relatives as partners in the management of schizophrenia: the development of a service model. Br J Psychiatry 156:654–660, 1990

Smith MD: Sociodemographic risk factors in wife abuse: result from a survey of Toronto women. Canadian Journal of Sociology 15:39–58, 1990

Smith R: Marriage and family enrichment: a new professional area. The Family Coordinator 28:87–93, 1979

Snow CE: Mothers' speech to children learning language. Child Dev 43:549–565, 1972

Snyder DK: Clinical and research applications of the Marital Satisfaction Inventory, in Marriage and Family Assessment: A Sourcebook for Family Therapy. Edited by Filsinger EE. Beverly Hills, CA, Sage, 1983, pp 169–189

Snyder D, Wills R: Behavioral versus insight oriented marital therapy: effects on individual and interspousal functioning. J Consult Clin Psychol 57:39–46, 1989

Snyder D, Wills R: Facilitating change in marital therapy and research. Journal of Family Psychology 4:426–435, 1991

Snyder D, Wills R, Grady-Fletcher A: Long-term effectiveness of behavioral versus insight oriented marital therapy. J Consult Clin Psychol 59:138–141, 1991

Sobel N, Sobel L: Problem Drinkers Guided Self-Change Treatment. New York, Guilford, 1993

Solnit A, Cohen D, Neubauer P: The Many Meanings of Play: A Psychoanalytic Perspective. New Haven, CT, Yale University Press, 1993

Solomon P: Moving from psychoeducation to family education for families of adults with serious mental illness. Psychiatr Serv 47:1364–1370, 1996

Solovey G, Duncan BL: Ethics and strategic therapy: a proposed ethical direction. J Marital Fam Ther 18:53–61, 1992

Sonne J: Transference considerations in marriage and marital therapy, in The Handbook of Marriage and Marital Therapy. Edited by Sholevar GP. New York, SP Medical & Scientific Books, 1981, pp 154–168

Sonne JC, Speck RV, Jungress J: The absent member maneuver as a resistance in family therapy of schizophrenia. Fam Process 1:44–62, 1962

Sonne JD: Triadic transferences of pathological family images. Contemporary Family Therapy: An International Journal 13:219–229, 1991

Spanier GB: Measuring dyadic adjustment: new scales for assessing the quality of marriage and similar dyads. Journal of Marriage and the Family 38:15–28, 1976

Spanier GB, Glick PC: Paths to remarriage. Journal of Divorce 3:283–298, 1980

Speck RV, Attneave CL: Social network intervention, in Changing Families. Edited by Haley J. New York, Grune & Stratton, 1971, pp 312–332

Speck RV, Attneave CL: Family Networks. New York, Pantheon Books, 1973

Speck RV, Rueveni U: Network therapy—a developing concept. Fam Process 8:182–191, 1969

Spector IP, Carey M: Incidence and prevalence of the sexual dysfunctions: a critical review of the empirical literature. Arch Sex Behav 19:389–408, 1990

Spencer J, Glick I, Haas G: A randomized clinical trial of inpatient family intervention, III: effects at 6-month and 18-month follow-ups. Am J Psychiatry 145:1115–1121, 1988

Spiegel D, Wissler T: Family environment as a predictor of psychiatric hospitalization. Am J Psychiatry 143:56–60, 1986

Spiegel J: Transactions: The Interplay Between Individual, Family, and Society. New York, Science House, 1971

Spitzer RL, Williams JBW, Gibbon M, et al: Structured Clinical Interview for DSM-III-R—Patient Version. New York, Biometric Research Department, New York State Psychiatric Institute, 1988

Sprenkle DH: Introduction: divorce therapy, in Divorce Therapy. Edited by Sprenkle DH. New York, Haworth, 1985

Sroufe LA: Wariness of strangers and the study of infant development. Child Dev 48:731–746, 1977

Sroufe LA: Attachment classification from the perspective of infant-caregiver relationships and infant temperament. Child Dev 56:1–14, 1985

Sroufe LA: Appraisal: Bowlby's contribution to psychoanalytic theory and developmental psychology. J Child Psychol Psychiatry 27:841–849, 1986

Sroufe LA: The role of infant caregiver attachment in development, in Clinical Aspects of Attachment. Edited by Belsky J, Nesworski T. Hillsdale, NJ, Lawrence Erlbaum, 1988

Stack C: All Our Kin: Strategies for Survival in a Black Community. New York, Harper & Row, 1975

Stanton MD: The addict as savior: heroin, death and the family. Fam Process 16:191–197, 1977

Stanton MD: Structural family therapy with heroin addicts, in The Family Therapy of Drug and Alcohol Abuse. Edited by Kaufman E, Kaufman P. New York, Gardner Press, 1979

Stanton M: Family therapy: systems approaches, in Emotional Disorders in Children and Adolescents. Edited by Sholevar GP. New York, SP Medical & Scientific Books, 1980, pp 159–173

Stanton MD: An integrated structural/strategic approach to family therapy. J Marital Fam Ther 7:427–439, 1981

Stanton MD: Systems approaches to family therapy, in Emotional Disorders in Children and Adolescents. Edited by Sholevar GP. Jamaica, NY, SP Medical & Scientific Books, 1986, pp 159–180

Stanton MD, Shadish WR: Outcome, attrition, and family-couples treatment for drug abuse: a meta-analysis. Psychological Bulletin 122:170–191, 1997

Stanton MD, Todd TC: Structural family therapy with drug addicts, in The Family Therapy of Drug and Alcohol Abuse. Edited by Kaufman E, Kaufman P. New York, Gardner Press, 1979, pp 55–69

Stanton MD, Todd T: Engaging "resistant" families in treatment. Fam Process 20:261–293, 1981

Stanton MD, Todd TC, and Associates: The Family Therapy of Drug Abuse and Addiction. New York, Guilford, 1982

Stayton D, Ainsworth MD: Individual differences in infant responses to brief, everyday separations as related to other infant and maternal behaviors. Developmental Psychology 9:226–235, 1973

Stayton D, Hogan R, Ainsworth MD: Infant obedience and maternal behavior: the origins of socialization reconsidered. Child Dev 42:1057–1069, 1971

Stayton D, Ainsworth MD, Main MB: Development and separation behavior in the first year of life: protest, following, and greeting. Developmental Psychology 9:213–225, 1973

Steinbock L: Nest-leaving: family systems of runaway adolescents. Unpublished doctoral dissertation, California School of Professional Psychology, San Diego, 1978 [Dissertation Abstracts International 38:4544B, 1978]

Steinglass P: Experimenting with family treatment approaches to alcoholism 1950–1975: a review. Fam Process 16:97–123, 1976

Steinglass P: The home observation assessment method (HOAM): real-time naturalistic observation of families in their homes. Fam Process 18:337–354, 1979

Steinglass P: A life history model of the alcoholic family. Fam Process 19:211–225, 1980

Steinglass P: The alcoholic family at home: patterns of interaction in dry, wet, and transitional stages of alcoholism. Arch Gen Psychiatry 38:578–584, 1981

Steinglass P: Family therapy, in Comprehensive Textbook of Psychiatry/VI, Sixth Edition. Edited by Kaplan HI, Sadock BJ. Baltimore, MD, Williams & Wilkins, 1995, pp 1838–1847

Steinglass P, Weiner S, Mendelson JH: A system approach to alcoholism: a model and its clinical application. Arch Gen Psychiatry 24:401–408, 1971

Steinglass P, Davis DI, Berensen D: Observations of conjointly hospitalized "alcoholic couples" during sobriety and intoxication: implications for theory and therapy. Fam Process 16:1–16, 1977

Steinglass P, Gonzalez J, Dosovitz I, et al: Discussion groups for chronic hemodialysis patients and their families. Gen Hosp Psychiatry 4:7–14, 1982

Steinglass P, Bennett L, Wolin S, et al: The Alcoholic Family. New York, Basic Books, 1987
Steinhauer PD: Assessing for parenting capacity. Am J Orthopsychiatry 53:468–481, 1983
Steinhauer PD, Santa-Barbara J, Skinner H: The process model of family functioning. Can J Psychiatry 29:77–88, 1984
Stern P: Stepfather families: integration around child discipline. Issues in Mental Health Nursing 1(2):50–56, 1978
Sternberg R: Love, sex, and intimacy. Psychol Rev 93:119–135, 1986
Sternberg R, Barnes M: The Psychology of Love. New Haven, CT, Yale University Press, 1988
Stierlin H: Separating Parents and Adolescents. New York, Quadrangle/New York Times Book Company, 1974
Stirling J, Tantam D, Thomas P, et al: Expressed emotion and early onset schizophrenia: a one year follow-up. Psychol Med 21:675–685, 1991
Stith S, Rosen K, McCollum E, et al: The voices of children: preadolescent children's experiences in family therapy. J Marital Fam Ther 22:69–86, 1996
Stoddard F, Wilbergere M, Olafson E: A case of functional urinary retention: the use of family play therapy. Fam Process 32:279–289, 1993
Stolorow RD, Brandchaft B, Atwood GE: Intersubjectivity in psychoanalytic treatment. Bull Menninger Clin 47:117–128, 1983
Stone M: Murder. Psychiatr Clin North Am 12:643–651, 1989
Stone M: The Fate of Borderlines. New York, Guilford, 1990
Stone M: Incest, Freud's seduction theory and borderline personality. J Am Acad Psychoanal 20:167–181, 1992
Stout R, McCrady B, Longabaugh R, et al: Marital therapy enhances the long term effectiveness of alcohol treatment (abstract). Alcohol Clin Exp Res 11:213, 1987
Stover L, Guerney J: The efficacy of training procedures for mothers in filial therapy. Psychotherapy: Theory, Research, and Practice 4:110–115, 1967
Strachan AM: Family intervention for the rehabilitation of schizophrenia: toward protection and coping. Schizophr Bull 12:678–698, 1986
Strachan A, Goldstein M, Miklowitz D: Do relatives express emotion?, in Treatment of Schizophrenia: Family Assessment and Intervention. Edited by Goldstein MJ, Hand I, Hahlweg K. Heidelberg, Springer-Verlag, 1986a
Strachan A, Leff J, Goldstein MJ, et al: Emotional attitudes and direct communication in the families of schizophrenics: a cross-national replication. Br J Psychiatry 149:279–287, 1986b
Strachan A, Feingold D, Goldstein M: Is expressed emotion an index of a transactional process? II: patient's coping style. Fam Process 28:169–181, 1989
Strachan T, Read AP: Human Molecular Genetics. New York, BioScientific Publishers, 1996
Straus MA: Communication, creativity, and problem-solving ability of middle-class families in three societies. American Journal of Sociology 73:417–430, 1968
Straus MA: Measuring intrafamily conflict and violence: the Conflict Tactics (CT) Scales. Journal of Marriage and the Family 41:75–88, 1979
Straus MA, Gelles RJ: Gender differences in reporting marital violence and psychological consequences, in Physical Violence in American Families: Risk Factors and Adaptation to Violence in 8145 Families. Edited by Straus MA, Gelles RJ. New Brunswick, NJ, Transaction Publishers, 1990, pp 227–244
Straus M, Sweet S: Verbal/symbolic aggression in couples: incidence rates and relationships to personal characteristics. Journal of Marriage and the Family 54:61, 1992
Straus MA, Tallman I: SIMFAM: a technique for observational measurement and experimental studies of families, in Family Problem Solving. Edited by Aldous J. Hinesdale, IL, Dryden Press, 1971, pp 381–438
Straus MA, Gelles RJ, Steinmetz SK: Behind Closed Doors: Violence in the American Family. Garden City, NY, Anchor, 1980

Straus MA, Hamby SL, Boney-McCoy S, et al: The Revised Conflict Tactics Scales (CTS2): development and preliminary psychometric data. Journal of Family Issues 17:283–316, 1996

Streit F: A test and procedure to identify secondary school children who have a high probability of drug abuse. Dissertation Abstracts International 34(10-B):5177, 1974

Streit F, Halsted DL, Pascale PJ: Differences among youthful users and nonusers of drugs based on their perceptions of parental behavior. International Journal of Addictions 9:749–768, 1974

Stromwall LK, Robinson AR: When a family member has a schizophrenic disorder: practice issues across the family life cycle. Am J Orthopsychiatry 68:580–589, 1998

Stuart RB: Operant-interpersonal treatment for marital discord. J Consult Clin Psychol 33:675–682, 1969

Stuart RB: Helping Couples Change: A Social Learning Approach to Marital Therapy. New York, Guilford, 1980

Stuart RB: Helping Clients Change. New York, Guilford, 1990

Stuart RB, Stuart F: Marital Precounseling Inventory, in Handbook of Family Measurement Techniques. Edited by Touliatos J, Perlmutter B, Straus M. Newbury Park, CA, Sage, 1990

Stuart RB, Jayaratne S, Tripodi T: Changing adolescent deviant behavior through reprogramming the behaviour of parents and teachers: an experimental evaluation. Canadian Journal of Behavioural Science 8:132–144, 1976

Sturgeon D, Turpin G, Berkowitz R: Psychophysiological responses of schizophrenic patients to high and low expressed emotion relatives: a follow-up study. Br J Psychiatry 145:62–69, 1984

Suarez SA, Flowers BJ, Garwood CS, et al: Biculturalism, differentness, loneliness, and alienation in Hispanic college students. Hispanic Journal of Behavioral Sciences 19:489–505, 1986

Sue DW, Sue D: Counseling the Culturally Different: Theory and Practice. New York, Wiley, 1990

Sullivan HS: The Interpersonal Theory of Psychiatry. New York, WW Norton, 1953

Summit R: The child sexual abuse accommodation syndrome. Child Abuse Negl 7:177–193, 1983

Summit R, Kryso J: Sexual abuse of children: a clinical spectrum. Am J Orthopsychiatry 48:236–251, 1978

Sunquist A: First-person account: family psychoeducation can change lives. Schizophr Bull 25:619–621, 1999

Sussett J, Tessier C, Wincze J, et al: Effect of yohimbine hydrochloride on erectile impotence: a double-blind study. J Urol 141:1360–1363, 1989

Sussman M: The isolated nuclear family; fact or fiction? Social Problems 6:333–340, 1959

Swan JH, Fox PJ, Estes CL: Community mental health services and the elderly: retrenchment or expansion? Community Ment Health J 22:275–285, 1986

Swann W, Predmore S: Intimates as agents of social support sources of consolation or despair. J Pers Soc Psychol 49:1609–1617, 1985

Swanson L, Biaggio M: Therapeutic perspectives on father-daughter incest. Am J Psychiatry 142:667–674, 1985

Szapocznik J, Kurtines W: Breakthroughs in Family Therapy With Drug Abusing and Problem Youth. New York, Springer, 1980

Szapocznik J, Rio A, Murray E, et al: Structural family therapy versus psychodynamic child therapy for problematic Hispanic boys. J Consult Clin Psychol 57:571–578, 1989a

Szapocznik J, Santisteban D, Rio A, et al: Family effectiveness training: an intervention to prevent drug abuse and problem behaviors in Hispanic adolescents. Hispanic Journal of Behavioral Sciences 11:4–27, 1989b

Szapocznik J, Kurtines W, Santisteban DA, et al: The evolution of structural ecosystemic theory for working with Latino families, in Psychological Interventions and Research With Latino Populations. Edited by Garcia JG, Zea MC. Needham Heights, MA, Allyn & Bacon, 1997, pp 166–190

Szasz TS: The myth of mental illness. Am Psychol 15:113–118, 1960

Szykula SA, Morris SB, Sudweeks C, et al: Child-focused behavior and strategic therapies: outcome comparisons. Psychotherapy 24:546–551, 1987

Taffel R: How to talk with kids. Family Therapy Networker 15(4):39–45, 1991

Talbott J: The Chronic Mental Patient: Five Years Later. New York, Grune & Stratton, 1984

Talbott J: Families of the chronically ill, in Marital and Family Therapy. Edited by Glick ID, Clarkin J, Kessler D. Orlando, FL, Grune & Stratton, 1987

Tanaka S, Mino Y, Inoue S: Expressed emotion and the course of schizophrenia in Japan. Br J Psychiatry 167:794–798, 1995

Tannen D: You Just Don't Understand: Women and Men in Conversation. New York, Ballantine Books, 1990

Tarrier N, Vaughn C, Lader M: Bodily reactions to people and events in schizophrenia. Arch Gen Psychiatry 36:311–315, 1979

Tarrier N, Barrowclough C, Porceddu K: The assessment of psychophysiological reactivity to the expressed emotion of the relatives of schizophrenic patients. Br J Psychiatry 152:618–624, 1988a

Tarrier N, Barrowclough C, Vaughn C, et al: The community management of schizophrenia: a controlled trial of a behavioral intervention with families to reduce relapse. Br J Psychiatry 153:532–542, 1988b

Tarrier N, Barrowclough C, Vaughn C, et al: Community management of schizophrenia: a two-year follow-up of a behavioral intervention with families. Br J Psychiatry 154:625–628, 1989

Tarrier N, Barrowclough C, Porceddu K, et al: The Salford Family Intervention Project: relapse rates of schizophrenia at five and eight years. Br J Psychiatry 165:829–832, 1994

Teitelbaum LM, Carey KB: Alcohol assessment in psychiatric patients. Clinical Psychology: Science and Practice 3:323–338, 1996

Telles C, Karno M, Mintz J, et al: Immigrant families coping with schizophrenia: behavioural family intervention v case management with a low-income Spanish-speaking population. Br J Psychiatry 167:473–479, 1995

Tennant C, Andrews G: The pathogenic quality of life event stress in neurotic impairment. Arch Gen Psychiatry 35:859–863, 1978

Terkelson KG: Toward a theory of the family life cycle, in The Family Life Cycle. Edited by Carter EA, McGoldrick M. New York, Gardner Press, 1980, pp 21-22

Terr L: Unchained Memories. New York, Basic Books, 1994

Tharp R, Wetzel R: Behavior Modification in the Natural Environment. New York, Academic Press, 1969

Thibaut JW, Kelley HH: The Social Psychology of Groups. New York, Wiley, 1959

Thomas A, Chess S: Temperament and Development. New York, Brunner/Mazel, 1979

Thompson RJ Jr, Armstrong FD, Kronenberger WG, et al: Family functioning, neurocognitive functioning, and behavior problems in children with sickle cell disease. J Pediatr Psychol 24:491–498, 1999

Thrower S, Bruce WE, Walton RF: The family circle method for integrating family systems concepts. Family Practice 15:451–457, 1982

Tiblier K: Intervening with families of young adults with AIDS, in Families and Life-Threatening Illness. Springhouse, PA, Springhouse, 1987

Tiefer L: Sex Is Not a Natural Act and Other Essays. Boulder, CO, Westview Press, 1995

Tienari P: Finnish adoptive family study of schizophrenics. Paper presented at the VIIIth Interactional Symposium on the Psychotherapy of Schizophrenia, Yale University, New Haven, CT, 1987

Tienari P, Lahti I, Naarald M: Biological mothers in the Finnish adoption study: alternative definitions of schizophrenia. Paper presented at the VIIth World Congress of Psychiatry, Vienna, Austria, June 1983

Tienari P, Lahti I, Sorri A, et al: The Finnish adoptive study of schizophrenia: possible joint effects of genetic vulnerability and family interaction, in Understanding Major Mental Disorder: The Contribution of Family Interaction Research. Edited by Hahlweg K, Goldstein M. New York, Family Process Press, 1987, pp 33–54

Todd T, Stanton M: Research on marital and family therapy, in Handbook of Family and Marital Therapy. Edited by Wolman B, Sticker B. New York, Plenum, 1983, pp 91–116

Tolan P, Mitchell M: Families and the therapy of antisocial and delinquent behavior. Journal of Psychotherapy and the Family 6:29–48, 1989

Tomm K: One perspective on the Milan systemic approach, Part I: overview of development, theory and practice. J Marital Fam Ther 10:113–125, 1984a

Tomm K: One perspective on the Milan systemic approach, Part II: description of session format, interviewing style and interventions. J Marital Fam Ther 10:253–271, 1984b

Trepper T, Barrett MJ: Treating Incest: A Multiple Systems Perspective. New York, Haworth, 1986

Trepper T, Barrett MJ: Systemic Treatment of Incest. New York, Brunner/Mazel, 1989

Trevarthan C: The foundations of intersubjectivity: development of interpersonal and cooperative understanding in infants, in The Social Foundation of Language and Thought. Edited by Olson DR. New York, WW Norton, 1980

Trevarthan C, Hubley P: Secondary intersubjectivity: confidence, confiders and act of meaning in the first year, in Action, Gesture and Symbol. Edited by Lock A. New York, Academic Press, 1978

Trimble D: A guide to the network therapies. Connections (Department of Sociology, Toronto) 3:9–21, 1980

Tseng W-S, McDermott J: Culture, Mind and Therapy: An Introduction to Cultural Psychiatry. New York, Brunner/Mazel, 1981

Turkewitz H, O'Leary K: A comparative outcome study of behavioral marital therapy and communication therapy. J Marital Fam Ther 7:159–169, 1981

Update on mood disorders, Part II. Harvard Mental Health Letter 7:1–17, 1965

U.S. Bureau of the Census, Department of Commerce: Single parent families 1970–1991, in World Almanac, 1992, pp 942–943

U.S. Census Bureau: Resident population of the United States by sex, race, and origin, 1999. Available at: www.census.gov/population/estimates/nation/intfile

U.S. Department of Labor, The Women's Bureau, Fair Pay Clearinghouse: Worth more than we earn: fair pay for working women. Washington, DC, U.S. Government Printing Office, 1996

U.S. Executive Office of the President, Office of National Drug Control Policy: National Drug Control Strategy, 1989 (Order from National Institute of Justice, NCJRS, Paper Reproduction Box 6000, Dept F, Rockville, MD 20849; Publ NCJ 119466)

Uzee E: Videotaped discussion of working with Asian-American families (Working With Minority Families). Symposium conducted at the 142nd annual meeting of the American Psychiatric Association, San Francisco, CA, May 6–11, 1989

Uzoka A: The myth of the nuclear family: historical background and clinical implications. Am Psychol 34:1095–1106, 1979

Vaillant GE, Milofsky ES: Natural history of male alcoholism: paths to recovery. Arch Gen Psychiatry 39:127–133, 1982

Valone K, Norton JP, Goldstein MJ, et al: Parental expressed emotion and affective style in an adolescent sample at risk for schizophrenia spectrum disorders. J Abnorm Psychol 92:399–407, 1983

van der Kolk B: Psychological Trauma. Washington, DC, American Psychiatric Press, 1987

van der Veen F: Family Concept Q Sort. Madison, WI, Dane County Mental Health Center, 1960

van der Veen F: Family Concept Inventory. Unpublished manuscript, Institute for Juvenile Research, Chicago, IL, 1969
van der Veen F, Novak AL: The family concept of the disturbed child: a replication study. Am J Orthopsychiatry 44:763–772, 1974
van der Veen F, Olson RE: Manual and Handbook for the Family Concept Assessment Method. Unpublished manuscript, Encintas, CA, 1983
van der Veen F, Waszak AL: Family Concept Assessment Method (abstract). Unpublished manuscript, Institute for Juvenile Research, Chicago, IL, 1975
van der Veen F, Huebner B, Jurgens B, et al: Relationships between the parent's concept of the family and the family adjustment. Am J Orthopsychiatry 34:45–55, 1964
van der Veen F, Howard KI, Austria AM: Stability and equivalence of scores based on three different response formats, in Proceedings of the 78th Annual Convention of the American Psychological Association. 1970, pp 99–100
Vanzetti NA, Notarius C: Relational efficacy: a summary of findings, in Weiss RL (chair), Taking a Broader View of Marital Cognitions: Symposium conducted at the 25th annual meeting of the Association for the Advancement of Behavior Therapy, New York, 1991
Vanzetti NA, Notarius CI, NeeSmith D: Specific and generalized expectancies in marital interaction. J Fam Psychol 6:1–13, 1992
Vaughan K, Doyle M, McConaghy N, et al: The relationship between relative's expressed emotion and schizophrenic relapse: an Australian replication. Soc Psychiatry Psychiatr Epidemiol 27:10–15, 1992
Vaughn C: Family factors in schizophrenic relapse: a replication. Schizophr Bull 8:425–426, 1982
Vaughn C, Leff J: The influence of family and social factors on the course of psychiatric illness: a comparison of schizophrenic and depressed neurotic patients. Br J Psychiatry 129:125–137, 1976
Vaughn CE, Leff JP: Patterns of emotional response in relatives of schizophrenic patients. Schizophr Bull 7:45–56, 1981
Vaughn C, Snyder K, Jones S: Family factors in schizophrenic relapse: replication in California of British research on expressed emotion. Arch Gen Psychiatry 41:1169–1177, 1984
Veach TA: Cognitive therapy techniques in treating incestuous fathers. Journal of Family Psychotherapy 8(4):1–20, 1997
Veach TA, Nicholas DR: Understanding families of adults with cancer: combining the clinical course of cancer and stages of family development. Journal of Counseling and Development 76:144–156, 1998
Velligan D, Funderburg L, Giesecke S, et al: Longitudinal analysis of communication deviance in the families of schizophrenic patients. Psychiatry: Interpersonal and Biological Processes 58:6–19, 1995
Velligan D, Miller A, Eckert S, et al: The relationship between parental communication deviance and relapse in schizophrenic patients in the 1 year period after hospital discharge. J Nerv Ment Dis 184:490–496, 1996
Veltro F, Magliano L, Falloon IRH, et al: Behavioural family therapy for patients with schizophrenia: a randomised controlled trial. Paper presented at the Congress of the World Association for Psychosocial Rehabilitation, Rotterdam, the Netherlands, May 1996
Verhulst F, Eussen M, Berden G, et al: Pathways of problem behaviors from childhood to adolescence. J Am Acad Child Adolesc Psychiatry 32:388–396, 1993
Veroff J, Kulka RA, Douvan E: Mental health in America: patterns of help seeking from 1957 to 1976. New York, Basic Books, 1981
Villeneuve C: The specific participation of the child in family therapy. Journal of the American Academy of Child Psychiatry 18:44–53, 1979
Villeneuve C, La Roche C: The child's participation in family therapy: a review and a model. Contemporary Family Therapy 15(2):105–119, 1993

Vincent J, Friedman L, Nugent J, et al: Demand characteristics in observations of marital interaction. J Consult Clin Psychol 47:557–566, 1979
Visher E, Visher J: Stepfamilies: A Guide to Working With Stepparents and Stepchildren. New York, Brunner/Mazel, 1979
Visher EB, Visher JS: How to Win as a Stepfamily. New York, Brunner/Mazel, 1982
Visher E, Visher J: Old Loyalties, New Ties: Therapeutic Strategies With Stepfamilies. New York, Brunner/Mazel, 1988
Visher E, Visher J: Parenting coalitions after remarriage: dynamics and therapeutic guidelines. Family Relations 38(1):65–70, 1989
Visher EB, Visher JS: Therapy With Stepfamilies. New York, Brunner/Mazel, 1996
Visher EB, Visher JS, Pasley K: Stepfamily therapy from the client's perspective. Marriage and Family Review 26(1/2):191–213, 1997
Vivian D, Heyman RE: Is there a place for conjoint treatment of couple violence? In Session 2:25–48, 1996
Vivian D, Malone J: Relationship factors and depressive symptomatology associated with mild and severe husband-to-wife physical aggression. Violence Vict 12:1–19, 1996
von Bertalanffy L: Robots, Men and Minds: Psychology in the Modern World. New York, George Braziller, 1967
von Bertalanffy L: General System Theory: Foundations, Development, Applications. New York, George Braziller, 1968
Wachtel P: Psychoanalysis and Behavior Therapy: Toward an Integration. New York, Basic Books, 1978
Wadsworth M: Roots of Delinquency: Infancy, Adolescence and Crime. New York, Barnes & Noble, 1979
Wagener D, Hogarty G, Goldstein M: Information processing and communication deviance in schizophrenic patients and their mothers. Psychiatry Res 18:365–377, 1986
Wagner BM, Reiss D: Family systems and developmental psychopathology: courtship, marriage, or divorce? in Developmental Psychopathology, Vol 1: Theory and Methods. Edited by Cicchetti D, Cohen DJ. New York, Wiley, 1995, pp 696–730
Wahlberg KE, Wynne L, Oja H, et al: Gene-environment interaction in vulnerability to schizophrenia: findings from the Finnish Family Study of Schizophrenia. Am J Psychiatry 154:355–362, 1997
Wahler RG, Dumas JE: Maintenance factors in coercive mother-child interactions: the compliance and predictability hypotheses. J Appl Behav Anal 19:13–22, 1986
Wahler RG, Dumas JE: Family factors in childhood psychopathology: a coercion neglect model, in Family Interaction and Psychopathology: Theories, Methods, and Findings. Edited by Jacob T. New York, Plenum, 1987, pp 581–627
Walker G: Checklist for interviewing/questioning children. NRCCSA News 3 (suppl 4):5, 1993
Walker L: Terrifying Love. New York, Harper & Row, 1989
Wallace CJ, Liberman RP: Social skills training for patients with schizophrenia: a controlled clinical trial. Psychiatry Res 15:239–247, 1985
Wallace H: Family Violence: Legal, Medical, and Social Perspectives. Boston, MA, Allyn & Bacon, 1999
Wallerstein JS: Children of divorce: the psychological tasks of the child. Am J Orthopsychiatry 53:230–243, 1983
Wallerstein JS: Children of divorce: preliminary report of a ten-year follow-up of older children and adolescents. Journal of the American Academy of Child Psychiatry 24:545–553, 1985
Wallerstein JS: Women after divorce. Am J Orthopsychiatry 56:65–77, 1986
Wallerstein JS: Children of divorce: report of a ten-year follow-up of early latency-age children. Am J Orthopsychiatry 57:199–211, 1987
Wallerstein JS: Transference and countertransference in clinical intervention with divorcing families. Am J Orthopsychiatry 60:337–345, 1990

Wallerstein JS, Blakeslee S: Second Chances. New York, Ticknor & Fields, 1989
Wallerstein JS, Corbin S: Daughters of divorce. Am J Orthopsychiatry 59:593–604, 1989
Wallerstein J, Kelly J: The effects of parental divorce: the adolescent experience, in The Child in His Family: Children at Psychiatric Risk, Vol 3. Edited by Anthony EJ, Koupernik C. New York, Wiley, 1974
Wallerstein J, Kelly J: The effects of parental divorce: the experiences of the preschool child. Journal of the American Academy of Child Psychiatry 14:600–616, 1975
Wallerstein J, Kelly J: Divorce and children, in Basic Handbook of Child Psychiatry, Vol 4. Noshpitz JD, Editor-in-Chief. New York, Basic Books, 1979, pp 345–416
Wallerstein JS, Kelly JB: Surviving the Breakup: How Children and Parents Cope With Divorce. New York, Basic Books, 1980
Wallerstein JS, Corbin SB, Lewis JM: Children of divorce: a ten-year study, in Impact of Divorce, Single-Parenting, and Step-Parenting on Children. Edited by Hetherington EM, Arasteh J. Hillsdale, NJ, Lawrence Erlbaum, 1988, pp 198–214
Walsh F (ed): Normal Family Processes. New York, Guilford, 1982
Walsh F: The concept of family resilience: crisis and challenge. Fam Process 35:261–281, 1996
Waring E, Chamberlaine C, McCrank E, et al: Dysthymia: a randomized study of cognitive marital therapy and antidepressants. Can J Psychiatry 33:96–99, 1988
Waring E, Stalker C, Carver C, et al: Waiting list controlled trial of cognitive marital therapy in severe marital discord. J Marital Fam Ther 17:243–256, 1991
Warner V, Weissman M, Fendrich M, et al: The course of major depression in the offspring of depressed parents: recurrence, and recovery. Arch Gen Psychiatry 49:795–801, 1992
Waslow M, Wikler L: Reflections on professionals' attitudes toward the severely mentally retarded and the chronically mentally ill: implications for parents. Family Therapy 10:229–307, 1983
Wasow M: Coping With Schizophrenia: A Survival Manual for Parents, Relatives and Friends. Palo Alto, CA, Science & Behavior Books, 1982
Wasow M, Lefley HP (eds): Helping Families With Mental Illness. New York, Gordon & Breach, 1994
Wattie B: Evaluating short-term casework in a family agency. Social Casework 54:609–616, 1973
Wattie B: The social worker's perception of client change. The Social Worker 42:309–314, 1974
Watzlawick P: A structured family interview. Fam Process 5:256–271, 1966
Watzlawick P, Beavin J, Jackson D: Pragmatics of Human Communication: A Study of Interactional Patterns, Pathways, and Paradoxes. New York, WW Norton, 1957
Watzlawick P, Weakland J, Fisch R: Change: Principles of Problem Formation and Problem Resolution. New York, WW Norton, 1974
Wayne L: Methodologic and conceptual issues in the study of schizophrenia and their families. J Psychiatr Res 6:185–199, 1968
Weakland J: Family somatics: a neglected edge. Fam Process 16:263–272, 1977
Weakland JH, Fisch R, Watzlawick P, et al: Brief therapy: focused problem resolution. Fam Process 13:141–176, 1974
Weber T, McKeever J, McDaniel SH: The beginner's guide to the problem-oriented first family interview. Fam Process 24:357–364, 1985
Webster's Seventh New Collegiate Dictionary. Springfield, MA, G & C Merriam, 1969
Webster-Stratton C, Dahl RW: Conduct disorder, in Advanced Abnormal Child Psychology. Edited by Hersen M, Ammerman R. Hillsdale, NJ, Lawrence Erlbaum, 1995, pp 333–352
Weddige RL: The hidden psychotherapeutic dilemma: spouse of the borderline. Am J Psychother 40:52–61, 1986
Weeks G, Hof L (eds): Integrating Sex and Marital Therapy. New York, Brunner/Mazel, 1987

Weiner H: Psychobiology and Human Disease. New York, Elsevier North Holland, 1977

Weinraub M, Wolf BM: Effects of stress and social supports on mother-child interactions in single- and two-parent families. Child Dev 54:1297–1311, 1983

Weisman AG, Nuechterlein KH, Goldstein MJ, et al: Expressed emotion, attributions, and schizophrenia symptom dimensions. J Abnorm Psychol 107:355–359, 1998

Weiss R: Marital Separation. New York, Basic Books, 1975

Weiss RL: The conceptualization of marriage from a behavioral perspective, in Marriage and Marital Therapy: Psychoanalytic, Behavioral and Systems Theory Perspectives. Edited by Paolino TJ, McCrady BS. New York, Brunner/Mazel, 1978

Weiss RL: Strategic behavioral marital therapy: toward a model for assessment and intervention, in Advances in Family Intervention, Assessment, and Theory, Vol 1. Edited by Vincent JP. Greenwich, CT, JAI Press, 1980

Weiss RL: The new kid on the block: behavioral systems approach, in Assessing Marriage: New Behavioral Approaches. Edited by Filsinger EE, Lewis RA. Beverly Hills, CA, Sage, 1981, pp 22–37

Weiss RL: Cognitive and strategic interventions in behavioral marital therapy, in Marital Interaction: Analysis and Modification. Edited by Hahlweg K, Jacobson NS. New York, Guilford, 1984, pp 337–355

Weiss RL, Cerreto MC: The Marital Status Inventory: development of a measure of dissolution potential. American Journal of Family Therapy 8:80–85, 1980

Weiss RL, Heyman RE: Marital distress, in International Handbook of Behavior Modification and Therapy, 2nd Edition. Edited by Bellack AS, Hersen M, Kazdin AE. New York, Plenum, 1990a, pp 475–501

Weiss RL, Heyman RE: Observation of marital interaction, in The Psychology of Marriage: Basic Issues and Applications. Edited by Fincham FD, Bradbury TN. New York, Guilford, 1990b, pp 87–117

Weiss RL, Perry BA: Assessment and Treatment of Marital Dysfunction. Eugene, Oregon Marital Studies Program, 1979

Weiss RL, Perry BA: The Spouse Observation Checklist: developments and clinical applications, in Marriage and Family Assessment: A Sourcebook for Family Therapy. Edited by Filsinger EE. Beverly Hills, CA, Sage, 1983, pp 65–84

Weiss RL, Weider GB: Marital distress, in International Handbook of Behavior Modification. Edited by Bellack AS, Hersen M, Kazdin AE. New York, Plenum, 1982, pp 767–809

Weiss RL, Hops H, Patterson GR: A framework for conceptualizing marital conflict: a technology for altering it, some data for evaluating it, in Behavior Change: Methodology Concepts and Practice. Edited by Handy LD, Mash EL. Champaign, IL, Research Press, 1973, pp 309–342

Weissman M: Psychopathology in the children of depressed parents: direct interview studies, in Relatives at Risk for Mental Disorder. Edited by Dunner DL, Gershon ES, Barrett JB. New York, Raven, 1988, pp 143–159

Weissman M, Paykel E: The Depressed Woman: A Study of Her Relationships. Chicago, IL, University of Chicago Press, 1974

Weissman M, Gammon D, Karen J: Children of depressed parents. Arch Gen Psychiatry 44: 847–853, 1984a

Weissman MM, Prusoff BA, Gammon GD, et al: Psychopathology in children (ages 6–18) of depressed and normal parents. Journal of the American Academy of Child Psychiatry 23:78–84, 1984b

Weissman M, Gammon G, John K, et al: Children of depressed parents: increased psychopathology and early onset of major depression. Arch Gen Psychiatry 44:847–853, 1987

Weissman M, Leaf P, Tischler G, et al: Affective disorders in five United States communities. Psychol Med 18:141–153, 1988

Weitzman L: The Unexpected Social and Economic Consequences for Women and Children in America. New York, Free Press, 1985
Weller E, Weller R, Visselman J: Depression in children and adolescents, in Transmission of Depression in Families and Children. Edited by Sholevar GP, Schwoeri L. Northvale, NJ, Jason Aronson, 1994, pp 58–99
Wells K, Egan J: Social learning and system family therapy for childhood oppositional disorder: comparative treatment outcome. Compr Psychiatry 29:138–146, 1988
Wertz R: Children of alcoholics. Chemical People Newsletter, November–December 1986, p 9
West D: Delinquency: Its Roots, Careers and Prospects. Cambridge, MA, Harvard University Press, 1982
West D, Farrington D: Who Becomes Delinquent? London, Heinemann, 1973
West ML, Sheldon-Keller AE: Patterns of Relating: An Adult Attachment Perspective. New York, Guilford, 1994
Westerink J, Giarratano L: The impact of posttraumatic stress disorder on partners and children of Australian Vietnam veterans. Aust N Z J Psychiatry 33:841–847, 1999
Wheeler D, Avis J, Miller L, et al: Rethinking family therapy training and supervision: a feminist model, in Women in Families: A Framework for Family Therapy. Edited by McGoldrick M, Walsh F. New York, WW Norton, 1988, pp 135–151
Whisman M, Jacobson N: Power, marital satisfaction and responses to marital therapy. Journal of Family Psychology 4:202–212, 1990
Whitaker CA: The symptomatic adolescent, in The Adolescent in Group and Family Therapy. Edited by Sugar M. New York, Brunner/Mazel, 1975, pp 205–215
Whitaker CA: Symbolic sex in family therapy, in Changing Sexual Values and the Family. Edited by Shoelvar GP. Springfield, IL, Charles C Thomas, 1976a, pp 136–143
Whitaker CA: The technique of family therapy, in Changing Sexual Values and the Family. Edited by Sholevar GP. Springfield, IL, Charles C Thomas, 1976b, pp 144–157
White D: Schizophrenics' perceptions of family relationship. Unpublished doctoral dissertation, Department of Education, St Louis, MO, St Louis University, 1978 [Dissertation Abstracts International 39:1451A, 1978]
White M: Pseudo-encopresis: from avalanche to victory, from vicious to virtuous cycles. Journal of Family Systems Medicine 2:150–160, 1984
White M: Negative explanation, restraint, and double description: a template for family therapy. Fam Process 25:169–184, 1986
White M: The externalizing of the problem. Dulwich Centre Newsletter, Summer 1989
White M: Re-Authoring Lives: Interviews and Essays. Adelaide, Australia, Dulwich Centre Publications, 1995
White M: Narratives of Therapists' Lives. Adelaide, Australia, Dulwich Centre Publications, 1997
White M, Epston D: Narrative Means to Therapeutic Ends. New York, WW Norton, 1990
White TB: A developmental sociolinguistic study of the doctor register. Unpublished doctoral dissertation, Boston College, Boston, MA, 1982
Whitfield W, Taylor C, Virgo N: Family care of schizophrenia. J R Soc Health 1:1–4, 1988
Widiger TA, Frances AJ, Pincus HA, et al: Toward an empirical classification for the DSM-IV. J Abnorm Psychol 100:280–288, 1991
Wiener N: The Human Use of Human Beings: Cybernetics and Society. New York, Avon Books, 1950
Wiener N: Cybernetics. Cambridge, MA, MIT Press, 1961
Williams A, Miller W: Evaluation and research on marital therapy, in The Handbook of Marriage and Marital Therapy. Edited by Sholevar GP. New York, SP Medical & Scientific Books, 1981, p 373
Williams CA: Patient education for people with schizophrenia. Perspectives in Psychiatric Care 25:14–21, 1989

Williams JBW: Psychiatric classification, in The American Psychiatric Press Textbook of Psychiatry. Edited by Talbott JA, Hales RE, Yudofsky SC. Washington, DC, American Psychiatric Press, 1988, pp 201–224
Williams J, Gold M: From delinquent behavior to official delinquency. Problems 20:209–229, 1972
Williams LM, Finkelhor D: The Characteristics of Incestuous Fathers. New York, Plenum, 1997
Wills TA, Weiss RL, Patterson GR: A behavioral analysis of the determinants of marital satisfaction. J Consult Clin Psychol 47:802–811, 1974
Wilson EO: Sociobiology. Cambridge, MA, Belknap Press of Harvard University, 1975
Wilson H: Parental supervision: a neglected aspect of delinquency. British Journal of Criminology 20:215–221, 1980
Wincze J, Carey M: Sexual Dysfunction: A Guide for Assessment and Treatment. New York, Guilford, 1991
Wing J, Brown G: Institutionalism-Schizophrenia. New York, Cambridge University Press, 1978
Winnicott DW: Collected Papers. New York, Basic Books, 1958
Winnicott D: The Maturational Process and the Facilitating Environment. New York, International Universities Press, 1965
Winnicott DW: Playing and Reality. London, Tavistock, 1971
Wise T: A model for the assessment of sexual dysfunction etiology (monograph). J Clin Psychiatry 10(2):11–18, 1992
Witt P, Greenfield D, Steinberg J: Evaluation and treatment of PTSD. N J Med 90:464–467, 1993
Wolf N: Fire With Fire. New York, Random House, 1993
Wolin S, Bennett L: Family rituals. Fam Process 23:401–420, 1984
Wolin SJ, Bennett LA, Noonan DL: Family rituals and the recurrence of alcoholism over generations. Am J Psychiatry 136(4B):589–593, 1979
Wolin SJ, Bennett LA, Noonan DL, et al: Disrupted family rituals: a factor in the intergenerational transmission of alcoholism. J Stud Alcohol 41:199–214, 1980
Wolin SJ, Bennett LA, Jacobs JS: Assessing family rituals in alcoholic families, in Rituals in Families and Family Therapy. Edited by Imber-Black E. New York, WW Norton, 1988, pp 143–167
Wolpe J: Psychotherapy by Reciprocal Inhibition. Stanford, CA, Stanford University Press, 1958
Woo S, Goldstein M, Nuechterlein K: Relatives' expressed emotion and non-verbal signs of subclinical psychopathology in schizophrenic patients. Br J Psychiatry 170:58–61, 1997
Wood JT: The part is not the whole: weaving diversity into the study of relationships. Journal of Social and Personal Relationships 12:563–567, 1995
Woodall M: Kinship care: blessing, burden. Philadelphia Inquirer, November 14, 1993, pp B1, B6
Woodward J, Goldstein M: Communication deviance in the families of schizophrenics: a comment on the misuse of analysis of covariance. Science 197:1096–1097, 1977
Wright L, Leahey M: Families and life-threatening illness: assumptions, assessment, and intervention, in Families and Life-Threatening Illness. Springhouse, PA, Springhouse, 1987
Wright RE: Disruptions to the intersect between individual and the family life cycle development due to Crohn's disease. Dissertation Abstracts 59(7-B), 1999
Wynne LC: Methodological and conceptual issues in the study of schizophrenics and their families. J Psychiatr Res 6:185–199, 1968
Wynne LC: Family variables in the University of Rochester, in Understanding Major Mental Disorder: The Contribution of Family Interaction Research. Edited by Hahlweg K, Goldstein J. New York, Family Process Press, 1987, pp 55–73
Wynne LC: The rationale for consultation with families of schizophrenic patients. Acta Psychiatr Scand Suppl 90:384–305, 1994

Wynne L: Family and marital therapy research: a retrospective and look ahead. Paper presented at the National Conference on Marital and Family Therapy Outcome and Process Research: State of the Science, Philadelphia, PA, 1995

Wynne L, Cole R: The Rochester Risk Research Program: a new look at parental diagnoses and family relationships, in Psychosocial Intervention in Schizophrenia: An International View. Edited by Stierlin H, Wynne LC, Wirsching M. Berlin, Springer-Verlag, 1983, pp 25–48

Wynne L, Singer M: Thought disorder and family relations of schizophrenics, I: a research strategy. Arch Gen Psychiatry 9:191–198, 1963

Wynne L, Ryckoff I, Day J, et al: Pseudomutuality in the family relations of schizophrenics. Psychiatry 21:205–220, 1958

Wynne L, Singer M, Toohey M: Communication of the adoptive parents of schizophrenics, in Schizophrenia 75: Psychotherapy, Family Studies, Research. Edited by Jorstad J, Ugelstad E. Oslo, Norway, Universitetsforlaget, 1976, pp 413–452

Wynne L, Singer M, Bartko J: Schizophrenics and their families: recent research on parental communication, in Developments in Psychiatric Research. Edited by Tanner JM. London, Hodder & Stoughton, 1977, pp 254–286

Wynne LC, Shields CG, Sirkin MI: Illness, family theory, and family therapy, I: conceptual issues. Fam Process 31:3–18, 1992

Wynne RD, McCrady B, Kahler C, et al: When addictions affect the family, in Understanding and Treating the Changing Family. Edited by Harway M. New York, Wiley (in press)

Xiang M, Ran M, Li S: A controlled evaluation of psychoeducational family intervention in a rural Chinese community. Br J Psychiatry 165:544–548, 1994

Xiong W, Phillips MR, Hu X, et al: Family based intervention for schizophrenic patients in China: a randomised controlled trial. Br J Psychiatry 165:239–247, 1994

Yolles S, Kramer: Vital statistics, in The Schizophrenic Syndrome. Edited by Bellack L, Loeb L. New York, Grune & Stratton, 1969, pp 66–113

Zanarini M, Gunderson J, Marino M: Childhood experience of borderline patients. Compr Psychiatry 30:18–25, 1989

Zaphiropoulos M: Harry Stack Sullivan, in Comprehensive Textbook of Psychiatry/IV, Fourth Edition, Vol 1. Edited by Kaplan HI, Sadock BJ. Baltimore, MD, Williams & Wilkins, 1985, pp 426–432

Zarit J: Predictors of burden and distress for caregivers of senile dementia patients. Unpublished doctoral dissertation, University of Southern California, 1982

Zarit JM, Zarit SH: Measurement of burden and social support. Paper presented at the meeting of the Gerontological Society of America, San Diego, CA, November 1982

Zarit SH: Aging and Mental Disorder. New York, Free Press, 1980

Zarit SH: Senile dementia, in Handbook of Behavioral Family Therapy. Edited by Falloon IRM. New York, Guilford, 1988, pp 372–395

Zarit SH, Zarit JM: Families under stress: interventions for caregivers of senile dementia patients. Psychotherapy; Theory, Research and Practice 19:461–471, 1982

Zarit SH, Orr NK, Zarit JM: The Hidden Victims of Alzheimer's Disease: Families Under Stress. New York, New York University Press, 1985

Zastowny TR, Lehman AF, Cole RA, et al: Family management of schizophrenia: a comparison of behavioral and supportive family treatment. Psychiatr Q 63:159–186, 1992

Zavala-Martinez I: Quien soy? Who am I? Identity issues for Puerto Rican adolescents, in Race, Ethnicity, and Self: Identity in Multicultural Perspective. Edited by Salette EP, Kaslow DR. Washington, DC, National Multicultural Institute, 1994

Zeanah CH, Anders TF, Seifer R, et al: Implications of research on infant development for psychodynamic theory and practice. J Am Acad Child Adolesc Psychiatry 28:657–668, 1989

Zhang M, Yan H: Effectiveness of psychoeducation of schizophrenic patients: a prospective cohort study in five cities of China. International Journal of Mental Health 22:47–59, 1993

Zhang M, Wang M, Li J, et al: Randomised-control trial of family intervention for 78 first-episode male schizophrenic patients: an 18-month study in Suzhou, Jiangsu. Br J Psychiatry 165 (suppl 24):96–102, 1994

Ziegler-Driscoll G: Family research study at Eagleville Hospital and Rehabilitation Center. Drug Abuse and the Family 16:175–189, 1977

Zilbach JJ: Family development, in Modern Psychoanalysis. Edited by Marmor J. New York, Basic Books, 1968, pp 335–368

Zilbach JJ: Family development and familial factors in etiology, in Basic Handbook of Child Psychiatry, Vol 2. Edited by Noshpitz JD, Call JD, Cohen RL, et al. New York, Basic Books, 1979, pp 62–87

Zilbach JJ: Young Children in Family Therapy. New York, Brunner/Mazel, 1986

Zilbach JJ: The family life cycle, in Children in Families: Ecological and Treatment Perspectives. Edited by Combrinck-Graham L. New York, Guilford, 1988, pp 46–66

Zilbach JJ: Children in Family Therapy: Treatment and Training. New York, Haworth, 1989a

Zilbach J: The family life cycle: framework for understanding children in family therapy, in Children in Family Context. Edited by Combrinck-Graham L. New York, Guilford, 1989b, pp 46–68

Zilbach JJ, Bergel E, Gass C: Role of the young child in family therapy, in Progress in Group and Family Therapy. Edited by Sager CJ, Kaplan HS. New York, Brunner/Mazel, 1972, pp 385–399

Zilbergeld B: The Male Sexuality. New York, Bantam, 1992a

Zilbergeld B: The man behind the broken penis, in Principles and Practice of Sex Therapy: Update for the 1990s. Edited by Leiblum S, Rosen R. New York, Guilford, 1992b, pp 27–51

Zimmer D: Does marital therapy enhance the effectiveness of treatment for research dysfunction? J Sex Marital Ther 13:193–203, 1987

Zimmerman J, Dickerson V: If Problems Talked: Adventures in Narrative Therapy. New York, Guilford, 1996

Zimpfer D: Marriage enrichment programs: a review. Journal for Specialists in Group Work 13:44–53, 1988

Zinner J: The implication of projective identification for marital interaction, in Contemporary Marriage. Edited by Grunebaum H, Christ J. Boston, MA, Little, Brown, 1976

Zinner J, Shapiro RL: Projective identification as a mode of perception and behaviour in families of adolescents. Int J Psychoanal 53:523–530, 1972

Zinner J, Shapiro RL: The family group as a single psychic entity: implications for acting out in adolescence. International Review of Psycho-Analysis 1:179–186, 1974

Zinner J, Shapiro ER: Splitting in families of borderline adolescents, in Borderline States in Psychiatry. Edited by Mack J. New York, Grune & Stratton, 1975, pp 103–122

Zubin J, Spring B: Vulnerability—a new view of schizophrenia. J Abnorm Psychol 86:103–126, 1977

Zuk G: Family Therapy: A Triadic-Based Approach. New York, Behavioral Publications, 1971

Zuniga M: Assessment issues with Chicanos: practice implications. Psychotherapy 25:288–293, 1988

Zweig MH: A view of mediation from the perspective of Bowen Family Systems Theory. Family Systems 3:160–165, 1996

Zweig-Frank H, Paris J: Parents' emotional neglect and overprotection according to recollections of patients with borderline personality disorder. Am J Psychiatry 148:648–651, 1991

Zwerling I, Scheflen A, Jackson D: Expanding Theory and Practice in Family Therapy. New York, Family Service Association, 1967

Index

*Page numbers printed in **boldface** type refer to tables or figures.*

Absent Member Maneuver, and inpatient family intervention, 647
Ackerman, Nathan, 5, 29, 81, 368
Acting-out behavior
  efficacy of family therapy for, 793
  family functioning and, 324
  incest and, 711
Action-oriented therapy, and parent-adolescent conflicts, 780
Activity patterns, and behavioral family therapy, 156
Actualization, and structural family therapy, 229
Acute medical problems, and medical family therapy, 758–759
Acute phase, of depression, 627
Adaptation, and family functioning, 320
Addiction Research Foundation (Canada), 689
Adequate families, 322
Adjustment, after divorce, 515
Adolescents. *See also* Children; Parents and parenting
  behavior problems and effects of family therapy, 775–777, 781–784
  borderline personality disorder and, 718
  conflicts with parents and family therapy, 779–781
  depression and, 625
  divorce and, 510–511
  inpatient family intervention and, 651–653
  Latino family and, 736
  multigenerational family systems theory with juvenile delinquents, 124
  nonshared environment and development of, 377
  parent management training and conduct disorders in, 405–407
  psychoeducational family intervention and depression in, 187–188
  separation-individuation process and, 371
  structural family therapy and, 47, 51–52
  substance abuse and, 686–691
  techniques for family therapy with, 17–18, 686–691
Adoption studies. *See also* Danish Adoption Study; Finnish Adoption Studies; Genetic factors; Iowa Adoption Studies; Swedish Adoption Studies
  alcoholism and, 675
  development of family psychiatry and, 18–19
  history of family therapy and, 8
Advocacy, and National Alliance for the Mentally Ill, 660

Affect. *See also* Affective disorders
multimodal therapy for depression and, 631
psychodynamic family therapy and, 240–241
schizophrenia and style of, 19–20, 586, 593–604, 615
Affection-based behavior, and incest, 708
Affective disorders. *See also* Depression
behavioral family therapy and, 167
research on efficacy of family therapy for, 790–791
substance abuse and, 672
African Americans
children and divorce, 507–508, 516
culture and characteristics of family, 728–731, 740–741
Aftercare research project, and psychoeducational family intervention, 178
Agency, and medical family therapy, 747
Aggression
domestic violence and, 483
incest and, 708, 709
Aging, and multigenerational family systems theory, 124
Agoraphobia
couples therapy and, 805
gender-sensitive family therapy and, 213
Aichorn, August, 404
Al-Anon, 693
Alcohol abuse and alcoholism
couples therapy and, 805
divorce and, 518
domestic violence and, 214
family factors in, 673–674
family intervention and, 22, 682–684, 794
genetic factors in, 672–673, 674–677
prevalence of, 671–672
psychological studies of families and, 677–682

therapeutic models and settings, 692–694
trauma patients and psychoeducational family intervention, 190
Alcoholics Anonymous (AA), 681, 693
Alexander, Franz, 129
Alliances, and structural family therapy, 48
Altruism
problem-solving therapy and, 60
relational ethics and, 140
Ambient stress, 150–151
Ambivalence, and dysfunctional family, 328
American Beauty (film), 539
American Institute of Family Relations, 418
American Psychiatric Association, 664. *See also Diagnostic and Statistical Manual of Mental Disorders*
Amnesia, and incest, 705
Amsterdam Family Intervention Study, 614
Anderson, C. M., 174, 177
Andragogy, and marital enrichment, 555
Anger, and differentiation levels, 121
Animal studies, and multigenerational family systems theory, 124–125, 126
Anorexia nervosa. *See also* Eating disorders
research on efficacy of family therapy for, 786
structural family therapy and, 35–36, 378
systemic family therapy and, 69
Anticipation, of future stressors, 644
Antidepressants. *See also* Medication
relapse of depression and, 629
sexual response and side effects of, 564, 569
Antihypertensive medications, and sexual response, 564

Index 909

Antiparkinsonian agents, and sexual response, 564
Antipsychotic medication, and psychoeducational approach to schizophrenia and mood disorders, 175, 176
Antisocial behavior. *See also* Antisocial personality disorder
  increase in studies of, 404
  ineffective discipline of children and, 408
  intergenerational transmission of, 81
  irritable behavior in families and children with, 405–406
Antisocial personality disorder, 405, 518, 672
Anxiety
  emotional system and multigenerational family systems theory, 108, 110, 111, 113, 114, 117
  gender-sensitive family therapy and, 213
Applied family intervention, and schizophrenia, 613
Areas of Change Questionnaire (AOC), 485
Arrests, for domestic violence, 215
Asian Americans, and family, 736–738, 743. *See also* Chinese Americans
Assembly social network intervention, 194, 195, 196–198
Assessment. *See also* Diagnosis; Evaluation
  behavioral couples therapy and, 481–486
  contextual therapy and, 136–140
  culture and, 728
  depression and family dysfunction, 625
  domestic violence and gender-sensitive therapy, 216–218
  evaluation scales and, 278–302
  of family relational disorders, 341–363
  incest and, 710
  initial and diagnostic interviews and, 257–275
  medical family therapy and, 753
  psychoeducational family intervention and, 186
  sex therapy and, 564
Assignments, and psychodynamic couples therapy, 450
Associated features, of family relational disorders, 355
Association of Couples for Marriage Enrichment (ACME), 541, **542**, 545, 546, 553, 554
Assortative mating, and marital dysfunction, 623
Assumptions, and cognition in marriage, 475
Asthma, and medical family therapy, 758
Ataque de nervios, 732
Attachment and attachment theory
  couples therapy and, 436, 801–802
  depression and, 621–622
  psychodynamic family therapy and, 89–90, 93
Attention-deficit/hyperactivity disorder (ADHD), 265–266, 376, 783
Attributions, and cognition in marriage, 475
Autonomy, and family functioning, 335–336
Aversive behaviors, and behavioral couples therapy, 463–464

Backdoor entry, into psychotherapy through network intervention, 195
Balance theory, 65
Baseline, and behavioral family therapy, 235
Bateson, Gregory, 36–37, 38, 55–56, 58–59, 74
Beardslee, William, 174, 185

Beavers-Timberlawn Family
  Evaluation Scale (BTFES),
  269–270, 280, **282–284, 298,** 753
Beck Depression Inventory (BDI), 565
Behavior. *See also* Aggression;
    Antisocial behavior
  behavioral contracting and, 468
  chronic illness and, 757
  depression and, 631
  diagnostic family interview and
    nonverbal, 260
  family functioning and observable
    patterns of, 331–337
  family of mentally ill patient and
    bothersome, 664
  family therapy and problems in
    children and adolescents,
    775–777, 781–784
  incest and, 705–706
  psychoanalytic theories of, 403
  stepfamily and emotions, 536
Behavioral couples therapy (BCT)
  alcohol or substance abuse and, 693
  basic concepts of, 462–467
  broadening of focus in 1980s,
    473–474
  clinical issues in, 495–499
  conceptualization using cognitive/
    behavioral perspective and,
    486–488
  depression and, 351–352
  early treatment applications,
    468–469
  empirical base for, 469–472
  future directions in, 500
  innovations of 1990s, 478–480
  outcome studies and cognitive
    additions to, 476–477
  relationship dysfunction and, 462
  research on efficacy of, 802–805,
    806, 807, 808, 812
  sexual dysfunctions and, 574–575
  specific intervention techniques for,
    488–495
  theory of, 427–429, 436

Behavioral-enactive model, and
  schizophrenia, 611–612
Behavioral family management (BFM),
  and schizophrenia, 609–610
Behavioral family therapy (BFT)
  adolescent behavior problems and
    delinquency, 782
  applications of, **162**
  clinical assessment and, 481–486
  depression and, 633
  effectiveness of, 252, 777
  family theory and, 32
  future directions in, 171–172
  history of, 5, 147–149
  methodology of, 154–162
  as model of family therapy, 14–15
  recent developments in, 167–171
  research on, 162–167, 777
  schizophrenia and, 788, 789, 790
  strategic family therapy compared
    with, 777
  techniques of, 234–237
  theory and, 149–154
Behavior management training, and
  attention-deficit/hyperactivity
  disorder, 783
Behavioral marital therapy (BMT). *See*
  Behavioral couples therapy
Beliefs. *See* Relationship Beliefs
  Inventory; Values; Worldview
Bell, John, 5, 368
Benzodiazepines, 564, 571
Bereavement, and family therapy,
  778–779. *See also* Loss
Bertalanffy, Ludwig von, 38
Beyond awareness marital contracts,
  425
Bibliotherapy
  cognitive-behavioral therapy and
    adolescents, 781
  remarriage and, 525
Binuclear family, 501, 505, 521
Biofeedback, and family theory, 124
Biological factors
  in depression, 621

psychoeducational family intervention and, 174, 178
Bion, Wilfred, 92
Biopsychosocial model, of illness, 748
Bipolar disorders
  behavioral family therapy and, 167
  expressed emotion and, 596, 603
  research on efficacy of family therapy for, 790
Blame and blaming. *See also* Shame
  gender-sensitive family therapy and, 212
  narcissistic personality disorder and, 719–720
Blended family, 312
Bloch, Donald, 747, 748
Bonding
  psychodynamic family therapy and, 89–90
  stepfamily couples and, 527
Borderline families, and family functioning, 324–325
Borderline personality disorder
  dysfunctional family members and, 325
  family and couples therapy with, 716–719
  incest and, 706
  psychodynamic family therapy and, 11
Boscolo, Luigi, 70
Boszormenyi-Nagy, Ivan, 12, 127–132, 138
Boundaries
  diffusion of between family members, 225
  family functioning and, 333–334
  incest and, 707, 711
  multigenerational family system therapy and formation of, 243
  structural family therapy and, 13, 40, 47, 228
Bowen, Gary, 549
Bowen, Murray, 5–6, 12, 29, 81, 103, 104–106, 426, 763

Bowlby, John, 5, 429
Brain, and animal studies of multigenerational family systems theory, 125, 126. *See also* Neurological disorders
Breakthrough phase, of social network therapy, 199
Brief Psychiatric Rating Scale (BPRS), 163
Brief strategic/interactional therapy, theory and techniques of, 61–64
Brown, George, 177
Buber, Martin, 129, 130, 134
Buckingham Early Intervention Project, 166–167
Buddhism, 737

Calvo, Father Gabriel, 540
Camberwell Interview, 598, 600
Canada, and adolescent substance abuse, 689
Canadian Occupational Therapy Association Social Network Therapy Program, 201
Cancellation, of initial family interview, 262
Cancer, and psychoeducational family intervention with children, 188
Card Sorting Procedure, 270
Caregivers and caregiving
  behavioral family therapy and, 169
  National Alliance for the Mentally Ill and families as, 662
Caring days, and behavioral family therapy, 236
Caring Family: Living With Chronic Mental Illness, The (Bernheim 1982), 651
Carlson, Jon, 541, 546
Cartooning, and dysfunctional family, 336
Case examples
  of communication with young children, 383
  of contextual therapy, 142–145

Case examples *(continued)*
  of cultural issues in family therapy, 741, 742–743
  of diagnostic or initial family interview, 270–274
  of family life cycle, 312–316
  of family therapy with children, 388–390, 392, 393, 394, 397–399, 402
  of gender-sensitive family therapy, 210, 213
  of inpatient family intervention, 650, 652–653
  of parent management training, 409–411
  of phases of marital relationships, 443, 445–446
  of psychodynamic couples therapy, 450, 451, 452–453, 455
  of sex therapy, 577–580
  of social network therapy, 199–200
  of stepfamily integration, 533, 535
  of transferences and narcissistic personality disorder, 721–722
Case management, and structural family therapy, 50–51
Catastrophic thinking, and cognitive interventions, 493
Catch a Person Pleasing You exercise, 490, 493
Causality
  of domestic violence, 219
  of incest, 698–699
Cecchin, Gianfranca, 70
Center for Substance Abuse Prevention (CSAP), 692
Centrifugal pull, and medical family therapy, 757
Centrifugal style, of family functioning, 320, 323–324, 324–325, 325–326, 762
Centripetal style, of family functioning, 320, 323, 324, 325
Chicano, use of term, 732. *See also* Latinos

Child abuse and neglect, and family therapy, 777. *See also* Sexual abuse
Childcare, and African-American family, 730
Child custody, and divorce, 517
Child guidance movement, 4
Childhood's Future (Luov 1990), 50
Child psychiatry, 17–18
Children. *See also* Adolescents; Child abuse; Childcare; Child custody; Development; Family; Parents and parenting; Siblings
  African-American family and, 730–731
  behavior problems and impact of family therapy, 755–777
  contextual therapy and, 141–142
  of depressed parents, 21, 185–187, 625–627
  divorce and, 503, 507–511, 513–514, 515–516, 517, 518, 519, 520
  family life cycle and, 307
  inpatient family intervention and, 651–654
  Latino family and, 736
  medical family therapy and, 758
  model for engagement of family and, 381–402
  multigenerational family systems theory and, 119
  psychoeducational family intervention and, 187–188
  psychological impact of incest, 699
  research on family therapy and, 775–777, 778–779, 793
  solution-focused therapy and, 65, 66–67
  sex play and, 698
  stepfamily and parent-child relationship, 527–528
  structural family therapy and individual psychodynamic therapy for, 51–52
  techniques for family therapy with, 17–18, 367–369

Children and Families (Zilbach 1988), 312
Children in Family Therapy: Treatment and Training (Zilbach 1989), 312
Children Who Hate: The Disorganization and Breakdown of Behavior Controls (Redl and Wineman 1951), 404
Child Welfare League of America, 730
China, and family-based interventions for schizophrenia, 612
Chinese Americans, and family life cycle, 311. *See also* Asian Americans
Chodorow, Nancy, 206
Chronic illness. *See* Illness; Medical family therapy
Circularity, and gender-sensitive family therapy, 207–208
Circular questioning, and strategic family therapy, 231
Circumplex Model/Family Adaptability Scale, 550
Class, socioeconomic and domestic violence, 214
Classic couples, 352
Classification
  historical methods of for families, 347–350, 352–361
  of marital disorders, 429–431
  of sexual dysfunction, 564–573
  use of term, 343
Classification System of Relational Disorders (CORD), 357, 359
Client-centered family groups, 782
Closeness, in relationships, 209, 478
Closure, of diagnostic family interview, 264
Coaching
  behavioral family therapy and, 236
  multigenerational family system therapy and, 241
Coalition formation, and family boundaries, 225
Cocaine use disorder, 784–785

Codependency, and alcoholism or substance abuse, 674
Coercion, and behavior therapy, 235, 428, 464
Coercive Family Processes (Patterson 1982), 404
Coercive family process theory, 405–407
Coercive parent-child processes
  family-based dysfunctions and, **358**
  family therapy with childhood disorders and, 373
Cognition. *See also* Cognitive interventions
  mediation and behavioral couples therapy, 466
  models of in marriage and behavioral couples therapy, 474–477, 487
  modes of relationships and, 242
  multimodal therapy for depression and, 632
  psychoeducational family interventions and, 186
  structural family therapy and constructions of, 230
Cognitive-behavioral therapy
  adolescent behavior problems and delinquency, 781–784
  behavioral family therapy and techniques of, 160
  couples therapy and, 428–429
  marriages and depression, 351–352
  research on efficacy of, 791–792
  sexual dysfunction and, 570
Cognitive interventions
  behavioral couples therapy and, 492–493
  incest and, 696
Cohesion Evaluation Scale, 550
Cohesive self, 91
Cohort approach, and divorce rate, 502
Collaboration, and strategic family therapy, 14

Collaborative conversations, and narrative therapy, 234, 427
Collaborative model, of family therapy, 657–669
Collaborative relationship, with therapist, 248, 458
Collaborative set, and behavioral couples therapy, 496
Collusion
　family boundaries and, 225
　phases of marital relationships and, 442, 444
Columbia University, 664
Combined couples therapy, 423
Combrinck-Graham, Lee, 304
Communication. *See also* Communication deviance; Communication disorders; Communication skills training
　adolescent substance abuse and, 689
　Asian-American family and, 738
　contingency management techniques and, 776
　couples therapy and, 420, 426–427, 432
　defensive interactions in parent-child and parent-parent, 374
　development and barriers to, 383
　family theory and, 29–30
　incest and, 709
　sexual dysfunction and, 569
　structural family therapy and, 36
　systems approach to family therapy and, 13
Communication deviance (CD), and schizophrenia, 6, 19–20, 348–349, **358**, 585, 587–593, 615
Communication disorders, criteria for spousal, **355, 356**
Communication skills training. *See also* Communication
　attention-deficit/hyperactivity disorder and, 783
　behavioral couples therapy and, 491
　behavioral family therapy and, 159
　marital enrichment and, 546–547
Community, and marital enrichment, 545. *See also* Community reentry; Community reinforcement approach; Therapeutic community
Community Mental Health Centers Act (1963), 659
Community reentry, and psychoeducational family intervention, 184
Community reinforcement approach, to alcohol or substance abuse, 693, 785, 793–794
Community Resource Specialist (CRS), 52–53
Compadrazgo, 734
Companionate marriage, 506, 520
Compensatory needs, and couples therapy, 424
Competence
　personality types and couples therapy, 431
　structural family therapy and, 44–45
　styles of family functioning and, 319, 338
Complementarity
　of gender roles and gender-sensitive family therapy, 208
　sexuality and, 332
　structural family therapy and, 48–49
Complementary midrange disorders, 248
Complementary needs satisfaction, model of marriage, 419
Compliance
　inpatient family intervention and medication, 654
　medical family therapy and, 759–760
Concurrent couples therapy, 422
Concurrent validation, of standardized tests, 279

Index

Conduct disorders
  family therapy with children and, 373–376
  incest and, 705
  inpatient family intervention and children of divorced parents, 654
  parent management training and, 405–407
Conductor type, of therapist, 227, 720
Confidentiality, and inpatient family intervention, 647
Configuration, and family dimension of medical disorders, 349
Conflict-habituated marriages, 351, 430
Conflicts
  couples therapy and, 424, 431, 433, 477, 548
  divorce and, 513–514
  family functioning and, 337
  multigenerational family systems theory and emotional, 112
  parents and adolescents, 779–781
  psychodynamic family therapy and, 31, 79, 94
Conflict Tactics Scale (CTS), 483–484
Confucianism, 737
Conjoint therapy
  couples therapy and, 421, 422
  domestic violence and, 220
Conroy, Pat, 458
Constructions, of new interpretive frameworks and structural family therapy, 45–46
Constructive entitlement, and contextual therapy, 131, 134, 139
Construct-related validity, and standardized tests, 279
Consultants, and social network therapy, 196
Consultation model, of medical family therapy, 749
Consumer action, and National Alliance for the Mentally Ill, 660

Content dimensions, of marital enrichment, 541
Content-related validity, of standardized tests, 278–279
Context. *See also* Social context
  definition of cultural, 727
  of stepfamily, 530–531
Contextual therapy
  applicability of, 142
  basis of, 132–133
  case example of, 142–145
  effectiveness of, 253
  family theory and, 32
  history of, 128–132
  introduction to concepts of, 127–128
  as model of family therapy, 12
  multidirected partiality and, 128, 130, 141–142
  relational ethics and, 133–134
  strategies of, 136–140
  techniques of, 243–244
  therapeutic contract and, 140
  transgenerational dynamics and, 134–136
Contextual transference, 85
Contingency contracting, and behavioral family therapy, 148
Contingency management techniques, and family communication, 776
Continuity, and psychodynamic family therapy, 92–93
Continuum, of family functioning, 319
Contracting. *See also* Contingency contracting; Marital contract theory; Therapeutic contract
  behavioral family therapy and, 235
  family therapy with children and, 393
Contraindications, to family therapy, 9
Control/responsibility, and integrative couples therapy, 478
Convener, and social network therapy, 196, 197

Conventionality/unconventionality, and integrative couples therapy, 478
Cooperative orientation, and behavioral couples therapy, 496
Coordination, and medical family therapy, 349, 749
Co-parenting, and divorce, 517, 519–520
Coping
  depression and, 635
  divorce and, 515
  psychoeducational family interventions and, 32, 179, **181–182**
  stress and, 151
Coping With Schizophrenia: A Survival Manual for Parents, Relatives and Friends (Wasow 1982), 651
Core affective exchanges, 239
Cornell Medical Center, 787, 790
Corrective mourning, 647. *See also* Loss
Cost-benefit analysis, and behavioral couples therapy, 482
Co-therapy, and inpatient family intervention, 646
Counseling, for couples, 419–420
Counterconditioning, and behavioral family therapy, 237
Countertransference. *See also* Transference
  couples therapy and, 449, 456
  domestic violence and, 220
  incest and, 712
  psychodynamic family therapy and, 86–87
Couple Communication Program (CCP), 541, **542**, 550, **552**, 553, 554, 556
Couples therapy. *See also* Divorce; Marriage
  behavior therapy and, 427–429, 461–500
  classification of marital disorders and, 429–431

common problems in, 432–433
definition of, 419–420
future directions for, 435–437
history of, 418–419
indications and contraindications for, 420–421
marital enrichment and, 539–557
present status of, 417–418
psychodynamic approach to, 439–458
remarriage and, 523–538
research on, 23, 435, 797–814
sex therapy and, 559–581
theories of, 423–427
types of, 421–423
Coupling, and family life cycle, 307
Covert behaviors, and communication theory, 29–30
Covert family problems, 8
Crisis intervention
  alcohol or substance abuse and, 692
  behavioral family therapy and, 161
  incest and, 711
Crisis theory, of divorce, 507
Criterion-related validity, of standardized tests, 279
Critical events paradigm, and couples therapy, 810
Croce, Mauro, 201
Cross-cultural adaptations, of family-based treatment for schizophrenia, 612
Crossover, and antisocial behavior in children, 406
Culture. *See also* Social context
  changing structure of society and, 725
  characteristics of families and, 728–743
  children and stepfamilies, 529
  definition of, 726
  diagnosis and, 346–347, 726–728
  domestic violence and, 214
  family-based treatment for schizophrenia and, 612

Index

family and cultural masks, 728, 745
family life cycle and, 311
functional and dysfunctional families, 338
gender roles and, 205, 209, 332, 338
marital enrichment and, 550
motherhood and, 210
Parent management training and, 413
structural family therapy and, 40
training of therapists and, 744
Curander and *Curanderos*, 727
Cut-offs, and remarriage family, 526
Cybernetics, 58, 107

Daily Checklist of Marital Activities (DCMA), 482
Daily Record of Dysfunctional Thoughts, 493
Danish Adoption Study, 675–676
Dark, children and fear of, 778
Day treatment programs, for alcohol or substance abuse, 692
Decency, and family functioning, 327–328
Decomposition, in family of hospitalized patient, 647, 655
Deconstruction, and narrative therapy, 72, 73
Deductive approach, to marital enrichment, 541
Defenses. *See also* Denial
  psychodynamic family therapy and, 31, 376
  sex therapy and, 576
Defensive affects, and emotionally focused therapy, 93
Defensive forces, and psychodynamic family therapy, 79
Defensive interactions, in parent-child and parent-parent communication, 374
Defiance, and paradoxical interventions in structural family therapy, 46

Derogatis Sexual Functioning Inventory, 566
Deinstitutionalization, impact of on mentally ill, 657–658, 659, 662, 668
Delayed closure, and medical disorders, 350
Delegation, and separation-individuation of adolescent, 371
Delinquency, and adolescent behavior problems, 781–784
Demand/withdraw patterns, and behavioral couples therapy, 470, 478
Denial. *See also* Defenses
  of conflict and couples therapy, 431
  of disease onset, 757
  of incest, 705–706, 707
  trauma patients and psychoeducational family intervention, 189, 190
Denial couples, and depression, 352
Dependent members, of family, 307
Depression. *See also* Affective disorders
  behavioral family therapy and, 165–167
  children of parents with, 185–187
  classification of marriages and, 351–352
  couples therapy and, 431, 433, 452–453, 806
  divorce and, 518
  expressed emotion and, 596
  family functioning and, 622–630
  family interventions and, 21, 630–635, 649, 790
  incest and, 705
  lifetime risk of, 619–620
  measurement of family and marital functioning and, 629–630
  psychoeducational family intervention and, 177–187
  substance abuse and, 672
  vulnerability to, 620–622

Depression and Bipolar Support
  Alliance, 817
Depression-resistance, and social
  network therapy, 198–199
Desire, and sex therapy, 560. *See also*
  Sexual desire disorders
Destructive entitlement, and
  contextual therapy, 134, 139
Destructive family roles, and inpatient
  family intervention, 647
Detoxification, and alcoholism, 683
Detriangulation, and multigenerational family system therapy, 242
Development. *See also* Children
  barriers to communication and, 383
  children in divorced families and,
    508–511
  contextual therapy and delays in,
    143–145
  diagnostic family interview and,
    265–266
  gender roles and, 205
  nonshared environment and
    adolescent, 377
  of personality, 715
Devitalized marriages, 351, 430
Diabetes, and sexual dysfunction, 562
Diagnosis. *See also* Assessment;
    Evaluation
  of alcoholism, 683
  culture and, 726–728
  problem-solving therapy and
    categories of, 59–60
  psychodynamic couples therapy
    and, 447–448
  relation of individual to family
    diagnoses, 357, **358**
  schizophrenia and, 587–588
  structural family therapy and
    nosology of, 40
  use of term, 343
*Diagnostic and Statistical Manual of
  Mental Disorders* (American Psychiatric Association), 22, 341, 342,
  346, 353, 359, 360, 361–362, 567

Dialectic view, of relationships, 132
Diathesis-stress theory
  family psychiatry and, 18
  inpatient family intervention and,
    640, 655
  psychoeducational family therapy
    and, 15
Dicks, Henry, 80, 86
Differences, and marital enrichment,
  549–550
Differentiation
  borderline personality disorder and,
    719
  family therapy and concept of, 6, 12,
    17
  multigenerational family systems
    theory and, 32, 110–118,
    120–122, 123–124, 241
Dimensions, of family functioning, 350
Dinkmeyer, Don, 541, 546
Direct observation, and behavioral
  couples therapy, 481–482
Directed play, 387
Directives
  problem-solving therapy and, 61
  strategic family therapy and, 231
Disadvantaged families, and structural
  family therapy, 52–53
Discharge planning, family
  involvement in, 663
Discipline, characteristics of effective,
  408
Disclosure, and incest, 706
Discontinuity, and psychodynamic
  family therapy, 92–93
Discriminative stimuli
  behavioral couples therapy and,
    466
  behavioral family therapy and, 237
Discussion area, and family therapy
  with children, 385
Disempowerment, and gender-
  sensitive family therapy, 212–213
Disengaged family, and structural
  family therapy, 40

Disintegration, and family of
    hospitalized persons, 647
Displaced homemaker, 512
Dissociation, and incest, 705
Distance, in relationships, 209, 478
Distanced play, 386–387
Distress-maintaining attributions, and
    couples therapy, 475, 798–802
Divorce. *See also* Couples therapy;
    Marriage; Remarriage; Single-
    parent families
  changing family structures and, 204
  child custody and, 517
  children and, 503, 507–511, 513–514,
    515–516, 517, 518, 519, 520
  couples and divorce therapy,
    433–435
  family life cycle and, 312
  family process and, 513–516
  gender-sensitive family therapy and
    child support after, 211–212
  inpatient family intervention and
    children, 653–654
  mediation and, 518–520
  as normative process, 501–502
  process and stages of, 503–506
  psychopathology and, 517–518
  rise in rate of, 418, 502–503, 520,
    523
  social networks and, 511–512
  special syndromes in parents and,
    512
  theories of, 506–507
Domestic violence
  couples therapy and, 431, 483–484,
    813
  gender roles and, 207–208
  gender-sensitive family therapy and,
    213–222
Dominant personality type, and
    couples therapy, 431
Dominant-submissive emotional
    patterns, 112–113
Double-bind interaction, and
    schizophrenia, 7, 36–37, 661

Drawings, and family therapy with
    children, 388
Dreams, and experiential family
    therapy, 246
Dropout rate, and family therapy for
    substance abuse, 686
DSM-IV. *See Diagnostic and Statistical
    Manual of Mental Disorders*
Duration. *See also* Timing
  of behavioral family therapy, 169
  of family relational disorder, 355
  of marital enrichment, 553–554
Dyadic Adjustment Scale (DAS), 484,
    630
Dyadic relationships, and stepfamily,
    535
Dyer, Preston and Jeannie, 541, 546
Dysfunctional family. *See also*
    Functional family
  conduct-disordered youth and,
    405–407
  definition of, 318
  depression and, 624–625
  family model and, 318–326
  future directions for study of,
    337–338
  identification of, 326–327
  media and, 540
  severe type of, 325–326
Dyspareunia, 572
Dysthymia, and recurrence of
    depression, 628

Early childhood, and impact of divorce
    on development, 509
Eastern Pennsylvania Psychiatric
    Institute, 129
Eating disorders. *See also* Anorexia
    nervosa
  expressed emotion and, 596
  research on efficacy of family
    therapy for, 786
  structural family therapy and, 52
Eclectic-dynamic approach groups,
    782

Ecological matrix, and family interactions, 407
Education. *See also* Psychoeducational family intervention
  behavioral family therapy and, 158–159
  domestic violence and, 222
  family of mentally ill patient and, 664
  schizophrenia and family interventions, 608
  sex therapy and, 561
  stepfamily therapy and, 532–533
  structural family therapy and, 47
Efficacy expectancies, and behavioral couples therapy, 466–467, 475
Ego psychology, 5, 79
Ellis, Havelock, 560
Emergency Network Center (Sweden), 201
Emotionally focused therapy (EFT)
  couples therapy and, 429, 436, 803–804, 806, 807, 809, 812
  psychodynamic family therapy and, 93, 241
Emotions. *See also* Expressed emotion; Feelings
  couples therapy and, 477, 812–813
  emotional conflict and, 112
  emotional cutoff and, 241–242, 719
  emotional desert and alcoholism, 683–684
  emotional distance, 111–112
  emotional divorce, 242, 347, 504
  emotional economy in couples, 447
  emotional expressiveness training and, 491–492
  emotional modes in relationships, 242
  emotional objectivity and, 108
  emotional overinvolvement and schizophrenia, 602
  emotional system and multigenerational family systems theory, 107–108
  gender-sensitive family therapy for domestic violence and, 220
  patterns of functioning and multigenerational family systems theory, 111–114
  stepfamily and behavior, 536
Empathy
  behavioral couples therapy and, 478–479
  narcissistic personality disorder and, 718
  psychodynamic family therapy and, 97–98, 240
Employee assistance programs (EAPs), 65
Employment. *See* Unemployment
Empowerment, and gender-sensitive family therapy, 212–213, 219, 222
Empty nest, 308
Enactive style, and inpatient family intervention, 648
Enactment
  goal enactment in family therapy with children and, 396–399
  structural family therapy and, 41–42, 52, 229
Encopresis, 398–399
Endings, and family life cycle, 309–310
Engagement, and psychoeducational family intervention, 179, 182, 183
Engagement as usual (EAU), and substance abuse, 686–687
Engel, George, 748
English, as second language and structural family therapy, 52
Enmeshed family, and structural family therapy, 40, 228
ENRICH measure, 549
Entrances, and family life cycle, 307–308
Entremundos, 742
Environment, and depression, 178, **181**
Epidemiologic Catchment Area (ECA) study, 671

Equality. *See also* Power
  cultural definitions of, 332
  problem-solving therapy and, 60
Erickson, Milton, 5, 55, 56, 57–58, 74
Erotic exchange behavior, and incest, 708, 709
Escape conditioning model, and behavioral couples therapy, 464
Esperanto, and developmental issues in communication, 383
Espiritistas, 733
Ethics, contextual therapy and relational, 32, 133–134, 139–140
Ethnicity. *See also* African Americans; Asian Americans; Latinos
  changing nature of society, 725
  diagnosis of, 726
  intermarriage and, 726
Evaluation. *See also* Assessment; Diagnosis
  inpatient family intervention and, 642
  medical family therapy and, 752–755
  psychodynamic couples therapy and, 449
  substance abuse and, 691
Evaluation scales. *See* Standardized tests
Everyday activities, and family functions, 310
Evolutionary theory, and multigenerational family systems theory, 125
Exchange interventions, and behavioral family therapy, 235
Exchange theory, and adult love, 801
Existential philosophy, 129, 130
Exits, and family life cycle, 308
Expansion, and family life cycle, 308
Expectancy concept, and behavioral couples therapy, 472
Expectations
  cognition in marriage and, 475
  marital enrichment and, 549
  stepfamily and, 526–527, 532

Experience, and structural family therapy, 41. *See also* Life events
Experiential family therapy
  as model of family therapy, 11
  techniques of, 245–246
Exploration, of family structure in diagnostic family interview, 260
Exploratory family therapy, 83
Expressed beliefs, and family functioning, 326–327
Expressed emotion (EE), and schizophrenia, 19–20, 348–349, 585, 593–604, 615
Extended family. *See also* Grandparents
  culture and, 734–735
  divorce and, 507, 516
  incest and, 703
Extinction
  behavioral couples therapy and, 465
  behavioral family therapy and, 237
Extrafamilial processes, 311
Extramarital affairs, and couples therapy, 420, 432

Facts, and contextual therapy, 136–137
Factual play, 387–388
Fairness, and contextual therapy, 32, 139–140
False self, 90
Families and Family Therapy (Minuchin 1974), 38
Familismo, 733
Family. *See also* Children; Dysfunctional family; Extended family; Family history; Family relational disorders; Family therapy; Functional family; Life cycle; Parents and parenting; Siblings; Single-parent family; Stepfamily
  as behavioral system, 152–153
  borderline personality disorder and, 716–717
  changing structure of, 203–207, 501, 507

Family *(continued)*
  chronic illness and implications of, 759–760
  classification and diagnosis, 22, 343–344
  cohesiveness of, 530
  culture and structure or behavior of, 728–745
  definition of, 153–154, 317, 304–306
  depression and functioning of, 622–627
  gender issues in evaluation of, 222
  incest and configurations of, 707
  management of stress and, 151–152
  model of functioning, 318–326
  risk factors for incest, 699
  roles of women in, 203–207
  somatoform disorders and, 762–765
Family Adaptability and Cohesion Evaluation Scales (FACES), 270, 280–281, **282–284**, 286, **298**, 753
Family albums and pictures, and experiential family therapy, 246
Family APGAR, 754
Family Approach to Psychiatric Disorders, A (Perlmutter 1996), 762
Family Assessment Device (FAD), 270, **282–284**, 286–287, **298**, 629, 753
Family Assessment Measure (FAM), 287–288, **298**
Family choreography, and experiential family therapy, 245
Family circle method, and medical family therapy, 754
Family Concept Assessment Method (FCAM), 288–289, **299**
Family Concept Inventory (FCI), 288
Family Concept Q Sort (FCQS), 288
Family coordination, and conduct disorders in children, 375
Family database, and medical family therapy, 755
Family discussion, and psychoeducational family intervention, 187

Family drawing, and experiential family therapy, 246
Family Effectiveness Training (FET), 780
Family Environment Scale (FES), 270, 290–293, **299**, 301, 630, 753
Family Evaluation Form (FEF), 289–290, **299**
Family Functioning Index (FFI), 293–294, **299**
Family game, and systemic family therapy, 69
Family history. *See also* Patient history
  of alcoholism, 675
  changes in family structures and, 204
  depression and, 621
  diagnostic family interview and, 264–265
  psychodynamic family therapy and, 96–97, 240
  stepfamily and, 534
  strategic family therapy and, 233
Family image, and psychodynamic family therapy, 88–89
Family Interaction Coding System (FCIS), 412, 413
Family mapping, and structural family therapy, 229
Family medicine, as medical specialty, 748
Family mental disorder, 342
Family physicians, and medical family therapy, 750–752
Family Process (journal), 55
Family projection process, and multigenerational family system therapy, 243
Family psychiatry
  development of, 18–22
  future of family therapy and, 819
  medical family therapy and, 749–750, 751–752

Family relational disorders
  advantages and disadvantages of diagnosing families, 343–344, 345–347, 362
  assumptions of family-based typologies, 344–345
  classification of distressed marriages and, 350–352
  definition of mental disorders, 342
  future directions in, 361–362
  historical methods of family classification, 347–350, 352–361
  introduction to concepts of, 341–342
Family Research Center (Washington, DC), 672–673
Family Ritual Interview, 678
Family and Social Network (Bott 1957), 194
Family Systems Medicine (journal), 747, 748
Family systems theory. *See also* Family theory; Systems theory
  family intervention with alcoholism and, 682
  inpatient family intervention and, 640–641
  models of family therapy and, 12
Family theory. *See also* Family systems theory
  definitions of terms, 3–4
  family life cycle and, 16–17
  future of family therapy and, 819
  introduction to, 29–33
Family therapy. *See also* Adolescents; Children; Family; Goals; Guidelines; History; Research
  alcohol and substance abuse, 671–694
  behavioral techniques, 234–237
  contextual techniques, 243–244
  contraindications to, 9
  culture and ethnicity as issues in, 725–745
  depression and, 619–636
  experiential techniques, 245–246
  future directions in, 819–820
  goals of, 4
  history of, 4–8, 24–25
  incest and, 695–714
  indications for, 8–9
  inpatient family intervention and, 637–655
  medical family therapy and, 747–766
  medication and, 249
  models of, 9–16
  multigenerational family systems and techniques, 241–243
  National Alliance for the Mentally Ill and, 657–669
  narrative techniques, 234
  personality disorders and, 715–723
  psychiatric hospitals and, 22–23
  psychodynamic and object relations techniques, 238–241
  psychoeducational techniques, 246–247
  schizophrenia and, 585–617
  strategic, systemic, and triadic-based techniques, 230–234
  structural therapy techniques, 228–230
  summary of findings on, 815–819
  therapist styles, 226–228
  types of interventions, 225–226
Family Therapy Techniques (Minuchin and Fishman 1981), 38, 42
Fantasies
  experiential family therapy and, 246
  psychodynamic family therapy and, 79
Favors, and behavioral couples therapy, 489
Fear
  diagnostic family interview and, 262
  family therapy with children and, 400, 778
Feelings, and emotional system, 108. *See also* Emotions

Female orgasmic disorder, 570–571
Female sexual arousal disorder, 569
Feminism
   criticism of structural family
      therapy and, 53
   critiques of therapeutic circularity
      and neutrality, 76
   functional and dysfunctional
      families, 317
   gender-sensitive family therapy and,
      15–16, 32–33
   therapy for incest and, 712
Field of participation, and
   psychodynamic family therapy,
   239
Field trials, of behavioral family
   therapy, 169–170
Filial piety, and Chinese-American
   family, 311
Films, and experiential family therapy,
   246
Finances, and gender-sensitive family
   therapy, 210
Finnish Adoption Studies, 8, 18–19,
   590, 668. *See also* Adoption studies
FIRO model, and lifestyle disorders,
   760–761
First International Marriage
   Enrichment Conference (1988),
   541
First-wave behavioral couples therapy
   programs, 468–469, 473
Fission, psychodynamic family therapy
   and unconscious assumptions, 92
Five-minute speech sample (FMSS),
   600
Floating family, 204
Fluphenazine, 166
Focused transference, 85
Folk beliefs, about illness, 732–733
Follow-up, and marital enrichment,
   554
Forehand-McMahon Parent Training
   Program, 411–412
Forgiving, and incest, 713

Formula tasks, and solution-focused
   therapy, 67
Forsberg, Gunnar, 201
Foster family, and social network
   therapy, 193
Foucault, Michel, 71
Fragmented self, 91
Free drawing, 388
Freud, Anna, 403
Freud, Sigmund, 36, 83, 104, 132, 137,
   330, 403, 406, 441, 560, 697
Fromm-Reichmann, Frieda, 5, 661
Functional analysis
   behavioral couples therapy and,
      465–466
   behavioral family therapy and,
      157–162, 236–237
Functional family. *See also*
   Dysfunctional family; Functional
   family therapy
   definition of, 318
   future directions for study of,
      337–338
   identification of, 326–327
Functional family therapy, 24, 374,
   688–689, 784. *See also* Functional
   family
Functional impairment, and family
   relational disorders, 355
Funneling, through therapist, 228, 720
Fusion
   multigenerational family systems
      theory and, 32, 110–118
   psychodynamic family therapy and
      unconscious assumptions, 92

Gacic, Branko, 201
Gender. *See also* Gender-sensitive
   family therapy; Women
   couples therapy and, 799
   culture and roles, 735, 737–738
   impact of divorce on child
      development and, 510
   marital enrichment and differences
      of, 550

misapplication of gender-sensitive family therapy and roles, 207–209
Gender-sensitive family therapy. *See also* Feminism; Gender
development of, 203–204
domestic violence and, 213–222
family theory and, 32–33
misapplication of basic concepts of, 207–209
as model of family therapy, 15–16
technical application of, 209–213
training in gender issues and, 222
views of women in families and, 204–207
Generalizability, of standardized tests, 278
General systems theory, 107
Genetic factors. *See also* Adoption studies; Twin studies
alcoholism and, 672–673, 674–677
psychoeducational family intervention and, 174, 178
Genogram, of family, 12, 244, 533–534, 755. See also Sexual genogram
Georgetown University School of Medicine (Washington, DC), 105–106, 125
George Washington University, 672–673
Gestalt therapy, and enactment, 41
Gilligan, Carol, 206
Global Assessment of Relational Functioning (GARF) Scale, 359–361
Goals. *See also* Guidelines
of behavioral family therapy, 169
of diagnostic family interview, 258, 263–264
of family therapy, 4
of family therapy with children, 394–400
of inpatient family intervention, 642, 643–645

of psychodynamic family therapy, 93–94
of psychoeducational family intervention, 174
of structural family therapy, 43
of treatment for narcissistic personality disorder, 720
Go-between, and strategic family therapy, 233–234
Goldstein Crisis Intervention Model, 605, 608
Good divorce, 433, 502
Good faith contract, 235
Gordon, Lori, 541, 549
Gottman, John, 429, 798–802
Gottman Institute, 547
Grandiosity, and defenses, 376
Grandparents, and African-American families, 516, 730, 731. *See also* Extended family
Grieving, and family life cycle, 309. *See also* Loss
Group for Advancement of Psychiatry (GAP), 22, 357, 359, 361, 639, 641–643
Groups, multigenerational family systems theory and functioning of nonfamily, 123. *See also* Subgroups; Support groups
Group therapy. *See also* Support groups
adolescent behavior problems and delinquency, 781
adolescent substance abuse and, 691
couples therapy and, 423
history of family therapy and, 5
incest and, 711–712
marital enrichment and, 545, 551, 553
multifamily behavioral family therapy and, 170–171
multifamily psychoeducational model and, 180, 182–185
schizophrenia and, 789
Growing Together program, 541, 542, 550, **552**, 553, 554

Growth in Marriage for Newlyweds program, 541, **542**, 550
Gruppo Abele (network of therapists), 201
Guarded alliance, and family patient relationship, 663
Guerney, Bernard, 541
Guidelines. *See also* Goals; Manuals; Standards
  for assessment of domestic violence, 218
  for family assessment, 263
  for family therapy with children, 384
  for medical family therapy, 756
  for sex therapy, 575–577
Gyarfas, Kalman, 128

Haley, Jay, 7, 59, 61
Halfway house, and social network therapy, 201
Hamilton Rating Scale for Depression (Ham-D), 565
Healing, kinds of, 194
Healing letters, and incest, 712
Health care. *See also* Illness; Managed care
  domestic violence and, 221–222
  incest and medical consultation, 710
Helplessness
  problem-solving therapy and, 60
  stepfamily and, 533
Help-seeking, and culture, 727–728
Hierarchy, and problem-solving therapy, 60
Hispanic American, use of term, 732. *See also* Latinos
History
  of behavioral family therapy, 147–149
  of contextual therapy, 128–132
  of couples therapy, 418–419
  of family classification, 347–350
  of family therapy, 4–8, 24–25
  of family therapy with children, 368–369

  of incest, 696–697
  of inpatient family intervention, 638–639
  of medical family therapy, 748–749
  of multigenerational family systems theory, 104–106
  of National Alliance for the Mentally Ill, 658–660
  of psychodynamic family therapy, 80–83
  of psychoeducational family intervention, 175
  of structural family therapy, 36–38
Holding environment, and psychodynamic family therapy, 11, 89, 239, 268
Holistic health therapy (HHT), 787
Homeostasis, and structural family therapy, 39
Homeostatic maintainer (HM), and intensive structural therapy, 49–50
Homework
  behavioral couples therapy and, 498
  brief strategic/interactional therapy and, 64
  Parent management training and, 412
  problem-solving therapy and, 61
Homogeneity, of standardized tests, 278
Horizontal dimension, and social network therapy, 195
Hospitalization. *See also* Inpatient family intervention; Staffing
  alcoholism and substance abuse, 683, 692
  family involvement in discharge planning and, 663
Hostility, and problem-solving therapy, 60
Household, and coupling, 307
Housing, and family life cycle, 313
Human Sexual Inadequacy (Masters and Johnson 1970), 559

Huntington's disease, and medical family therapy, 757, 758
Hypoactive sexual desire disorder, 566–567
Hysteria, and couples therapy, 430

Ideology. *See also* Values; Worldview
 cultural issues in diagnosis and, 726
 gender-sensitive family therapy and, 222
Illness. *See also* Health care; Medical family therapy
 culture and beliefs about etiology of, 732–733
 family dimensions of, 349–350
 family life cycle and, 311
 psychoeducational interventions with family of child with, 21
 sex therapy and, 562–563
 stress responses to, 150
Imaginative play, 387–388
Immigration, and structure of family, 736
Implied beliefs, and family functioning, 326–327
Inadequate-overadequate marriage, and couples therapy, 431
Incest. *See also* Sexual abuse
 causality of, 698–699
 definition of, 695, 697–698
 detection and identification of behavior, 705–706, 708–710
 family configurations and, 707
 family intervention strategies with, 710–713
 history of, 696–697
 incidence and prevalence of, 703–705
 interviews with victim of, 708
 psychological impact of, 699
 types of, 700–703
Incongruent cycles, and stepfamilies, 525–526
Index patient
 diagnostic family interview and, 259, 263–264
 first session of family therapy with children and, 390–391
Individual psychology, and contextual therapy, 137–138. *See also* Psychology
Individual supportive therapy (IST), efficacy of compared with behavioral family therapy, 163
Individual therapy
 of intrafamilial sexual abuse, 696, 712
 of marital disorders, 421–422
Inductive approach, to marital enrichment, 541
Infants, and impact of divorce on development, 509, 519
Infertility, and sex therapy, 563
Informational statement, and psychodynamic couples therapy, 451
Inhibited female orgasm, 571–572
Inhibited male orgasm, 571
Inpatient family intervention (IFI). *See also* Hospitalization; Psychopathology
 acute, recurrent, and chronic disorders and, 648–650
 children and adolescents, 651–653
 definition of, 639
 families of chronically ill patients and, 650–651
 family systems theory and, 640–641
 goals of 642, 643–645
 history of, 638–639
 model of, 23
 results of, 641–643, 654–655
 schizophrenia and, 634–635
 strategies and techniques of, 645–648, 664–665
 theory of, 640–641
Insight oriented marital therapy (IOMT), 473, 499, 804
Instincts, Freud's theory of, 137
Institutional marriage, 506
Institutional support, for stepfamilies, 529–530. *See also* Social services

Integration
  sex therapy and, 561–562
  of stepfamilies, 525
  view of medical family therapy and, 763–764
Integrative couples therapy, 429, 436, 478–479, 480, 494–495
Integrity, and Latino culture, 734
Intellectualization, and concepts of true and false self, 90
Intellectual system, and multigenerational family systems theory, 108, 120–121
Intensified family interactional technique, 227–228
Intensity, and structural family therapy, 44, 230
Intensive structural therapy, 49–50
Interactional diagnosis, 268–269
Interactive markers, and case management in structural family therapy, 50–51
Intergenerational aspects, of narcissistic personality disorder, 720–721
Intergenerational systems theory, 426
Interlocking neuroses, and marital relationships, 80, 502, 723
Interlocking psychopathologies, and schizophrenia, 602
Interlocking transferences, 84
Internalizing discourses, and narrative therapy, 72, 234
Internet, and marital enrichment, 557
Interpersonal context, of psychoeducational family intervention, 174
Interpersonal therapy, and depression, 630–631, 636, 806
Interpretation, and psychodynamic family therapy, 98–99, 239
Intersubjectivity, and empathy of therapist, 98
Interviews, initial and diagnostic
  assessment and diagnosis, 260–264
  basic concepts and, 257–258
  establishment of therapeutic system and joining operations, 266–274
  family history and, 264–265
  family life cycle and developmental issues, 265–266
  goals of, 258
  stages of, 258–260
Intimacy, and power differences, 331
Invariant prescription, and systemic approach, 31
Inventory of Rewarding Activities (IRA), 483
Invisible loyalties, and contextual therapy, 135–136
Involved play, 386–387
Iowa Adoption Studies, 675
Isomorphism, and intensive structural therapy, 49–50
"I stand" position, and multigenerational family system therapy, 243

Johnson, Susan, 81, 100
Joining
  behavioral couples therapy and, 478–479
  diagnostic family interview and, 266–274
  family life cycle and, 307, 310
  family therapy with children and, 393–394
  psychoeducational family intervention and, 182, 183
  structural family therapy and, 43–44, 228–229
Joint Commission on the Accreditation of Healthcare Organizations (JCAHO), 682
Joint Commission on Mental Illness and Health, 659
Jones, Maxwell, 129
Journal of Marital and Family Therapy, 55
Journal of Strategic and Systemic Therapies, 55

Kerr, Michael E., 106
Kinship bonds, and culture, 729, 734–735
Kliman, Jodi, 200–201

Language, and therapy with stepfamily, 537
Latinos
    culture and characteristics of family, 732–736, 742–743
    family life cycle and, 311
Launching, and families with mentally retarded or schizophrenic members, 311
Lawyers, and divorce, 434
Layout, of therapeutic environment for family therapy with children, 385
Leadership
    marital enrichment and, 555
    psychoeducational family intervention and, 184–185
Learning theory
    history of family therapy and, 5
    marital enrichment and, 554
Leaving Home: The Therapy of Disturbed Young People (Haley 1980), 685
Legal issues, and treatment of sexual abuse, 696, 710
Levy, David, 5
Liberman, Robert, 148–149
Lidz, Theodore, 6, 82
Life cycle, of family. *See also* Family
    alcoholic family and, 679–682
    basic family functions and, 310–312
    clinical case examples of, 312–316
    diagnostic family interview and, 265–266
    family theory and, 16–17
    family unit and, 305
    introduction to concepts of, 303–304
    marital enrichment and, 550–551
    sex therapy and, 563–564
    stages of, 307–310
Life events, and stress, 151, 631. *See*

also Experience
Life forces, and multigenerational family systems theory, 110–118
Life sciences, and research on multigenerational family systems theory, 125
Lifestyle disorders, and medical family therapy, 760–761
Limpias, 733
Listening and Loving program, 541, **543, 552,** 554
Listening skills, and marital enrichment, 546
Living family history, 265, 272
Locke-Wallace Marital Adjustment Test (MAT), 485
Locus of control, and medical family therapy, 750
Loss. *See also* Bereavement; Corrective mourning; Grieving; Operational mourning
    depression and, 621–622
    divorce and, 512
    stepfamilies and, 525, 532
Love
    problem-solving therapy and, 60
    theory of adult, 800, 801–802
Love (loving) days
    and behavioral couples therapy, 489
    and behavioral family therapy, 236
Loyalty, and contextual therapy, 130–131, 135–136, 244
Luov, Richard, 50
Lutheran Social Services (LSS), 675

Mace, David and Vera, 539, 540, 541, 546
Machismo, 735
Madanes, Cloe, 59, 61
Mahler, Margaret, 90–91
Maintenance, and joining operation, 267
Male erectile disorder, 567–569
Malinowski, Bronislaw, 697
Mal puesto and *Mal de ojo*, 733

Managed care. *See also* Health care
 interactive markers and structural family therapy, 50–51
 medical family therapy and, 765–766
Manuals, for family therapy, 773. *See also* Guidelines; Standards
Marianismo, 735
Marital Agendas Protocol (MAP), 484–485
Marital Attitude Survey (MAS), 484
Marital contract theory, 425
Marital enrichment. *See also* Couples therapy; Marriage
 cautions and limitations, 555
 definition and background of, 539–541
 focus of, 541, 545
 implementation considerations, 551–555
 Internet and, 557
 outcome research on, 556
 programs and, 541, **542–544**
Marital neurosis, 424, 723
Marital satisfaction, and behavioral couples therapy, 477, 485–486
Marital Satisfaction Inventory (MSI), 485
Marital schism and marital skew, 347
Marital Tensions (Dicks 1967), 80
Marital therapy. *See* Couples therapy
Markey, Barbara, 541
Markman, Howard, 541, 546, 548, 549
Marriage. *See also* Couples therapy; Divorce; Marital enrichment; Marriage counseling; Remarriage
 African-American family and, 731
 borderline personality disorder and, 716–717, 718
 changing functions of, 506
 classification of distressed, 350–352
 depression and, 21, 623–624, 632
 ethnicity and, 726
 family life cycle and, 16–17
 interlocking neuroses and, 80
 models of cognition in, 474–476
 narcissistic personality disorder and, 719–720
 normative concept of, 502
 phases of, 442–446
 psychodynamic family therapy and, 78
Marriage Consultation Center (NY), 418
Marriage Council of Philadelphia, 418
Marriage counseling, 4, 420
Marriage Encounter (ME), **543**, 545, 547, 556
Marriage Enrichment: Preparation, Mentoring and Outreach (Hunt et al. 1998), 556
Massachusetts General Hospital, 221
MATE measure, 549
McMaster Model of Family Functioning (MMFF), 286
Mead, Margaret, 697
Meaning
 of chronic illness, 757
 of family functioning, 330
Measurement instruments. *See* Standardized tests
Media, and dysfunctional family, 540
Mediation, and divorce, 434, 518–520
Medical College of Virginia, 125
Medical disorders. *See* Illness
Medical family therapy. *See also* Health care; Illness
 acute medical problems and, 758–759
 children and, 758
 chronic medical illness and, 756–757
 definition of, 747
 evaluation and, 752–755
 family dimension of medical disorders and, 349–50
 family physicians and, 750–752
 history of, 748–749
 lifestyle disorders and, 760–761
 managed care and, 765–766

model of, 749–750
neurological disorders and, 757–758
referrals and, 755–756
somatoform disorders and, 761–765
treatment adherence and compliance, 759–760
Medication. *See also* Antidepressants
Asian culture and, 739
depression and combined therapy, 633–634
inpatient family intervention and, 640, 654, 655
sexual dysfunction and, 564
Meetings, and social network therapy, 196–198
Memory, and incest, 710
Memory board, and marital enrichment, 546
Menninger Clinic (Kansas), 81, 104, 105
Menopause, and sex therapy, 563–564
Mental disorders, definition of, 342. *See also* Psychopathology
Mental Research Institute (MRI), 7, 14, 30
Mental retardation, and sexual abuse, 698
Meta-analysis, of family intervention, 792–793
Metaphorical sequences, and problem-solving therapy, 60
Michael, Phyllis, 541
Midelfort, Christian, 80–81
Midrange family dysfunction, 248, 322–324
Migration, and family structure and behavior, 735–736, 738
Milan School of Family Therapy, 7, 68–71, 75
Miller, Sherod, 540–541
Mimesis
diagnostic family interview and, 266–267
structural family therapy and, 229

Mindreading, and cognitive interventions, 493
Minnesota Multiphasic Personality Inventory (MMPI), 405, 565
Minuchin, Salvador, 7, 13, 37–38, 368–369
Mirroring, and narcissistic personality disorder, 721
Mittleman, Bela, 80, 419
Mixed families, and family functioning, 324
Mobilization, and social network therapy, 198
Models
of family functioning, 318–326
of family therapy, 9–16
for first session of family therapy with children, 390–402
modeling and behavioral family therapy, 236
Monoamine oxidase (MAO) inhibitors, 564
Moreno, J. L., 82
Motivational forces, and psychodynamic family therapy, 79
Mount Tom Institute (Massachusetts), 200
Multidimensional approach, to family therapy, 24, 690–691
Multidimensional inquiry, and diagnostic family interview, 259–260
Multidirectional partiality
contextual therapy and, 128, 130, 141–142, 243–244
empathy of therapist and, 98
Multifaceted self, structural family therapy and concept of, 45
Multifamily therapy
behavioral family therapy and, 170–171
psychoeducational family intervention and, 180, 182–185, 190–191
Multigenerational emotional process, 116–118

Multigenerational family system
theory. *See also* Systems theory
  applicability of, 122–124
  future directions in, 126
  history of, 104–106
  incest and, 707
  introduction to concepts of, 29, 31–32, 103–104
  medical family therapy and, 763
  methodology of, 118–122
  research on, 124–125
  techniques of, 241–243
  theoretical concepts and, 106–109
Multigenerational loyalty, and borderline personality disorder, 719
Multimodal therapy
  for depression, 631–632
  for sexual dysfunction, 571
Multiple-family education groups, and schizophrenia, 613
Multiple family therapy, and psychoeducational family intervention, 176
Multiple Impact Therapy (MIT) group (Texas), 8, 373
Multisystemic therapy (MST)
  child abuse or neglect and, 777
  conduct disorders in children and, 375–376
  substance abuse and, 689–690, 785
Mutually dependent marriage, and couples therapy, 431
Mutual projection, and couples therapy, 444, 446, 450–451
Myers-Briggs Type Indicator, 550

Naive trusting, and family patient relationship, 663
Narcissism
  borderline personality disorder and marriage, 717–718
  couples therapy and personality type, 430
  psychodynamic family therapy and, 11, 376
Narcissistic personality disorder
  divorce and family therapy and, 719–721
  self psychology theory and, 91–92
Narrative therapy
  couples therapy and, 427
  effectiveness of, 252
  incest and, 713
  medical family therapy and, 760
  strategic interventions and, 14
  techniques of, 73–74, 234
  theory of, 71–73
National Alliance for the Mentally Ill (NAMI), 185, 651, 657–699, 817
National Center for Health Statistics, 756
National Child Abuse Prevention Act of 1974, 710
National Comorbidity Survey, 619–620, 671, 672
National Depressive and Manic-Depressive Association, 817
National Institute on Drug Abuse (NIDA), 214, 687
National Institute of Mental Health (NIMH), 105, 165–166, 214, 659, 672, 704, 789
National Library of Medicine, 125
National Resource Center on Child Sexual Abuse (NRCCSA), 704
Nattering, and coercive behavior in parents, 406, 408
Natural sciences, and systems thinking, 107
Navigating the Marital Journey (Bowen 1991), 549
Need-templates, and self-delineation, 133
Negative affective communication, and schizophrenia, 593, 596–597
Negative affective expression, and couple-based dysfunctions, **358**
Negative attributions, and couple-based dysfunctions, **358**, 799–800

Negative explanation, and narrative therapy, 72
Negative interaction, and behavioral couples therapy, 490–491
Negative reciprocity
 couples therapy and, 357, 464–465, 467
 schizophrenia and, 603
Negative reinforcement, and behavior therapy, 235, 428, 463, 486
Neglect, and irritable behavior in parents, 407
Negligence, and treatment of sexual abuse, 696
Negotiation
 family functioning and, 337
 stepfamily and, 536
Nesting stage, of remarriage, 526
Networking Families in Crisis (Rueveni 1979), 199
Network-mapping inventory, 200
Network therapy, and multifamily psychoeducational model, 180. *See also* Social network therapy
Neuroleptics, interactions between family interventions and, 165–166
Neurological disorders, and medical family therapy, 757–758
Neurophysiology, of depression, 632
Neurosis
 contextual therapy and, 142
 couples therapy and personality types, 431
 marriage of interlocked neurotic spouses and, 424, 723
Neutrality, degree of emotional, 121
New Sex Therapy, The (Kaplan 1974), 560
New-wave behavioral couples therapy, 469
Nondirected play, 387
Nonshared environment, in adolescent development, 377
Normative model, and structural family therapy, 40

Normative process, divorce as, 501–502
Nurses, and inpatient family intervention, 646

Oberndorf, Clarence P., 80, 418–419
Obesity, and lifestyle disorders, 761
Object relations
 borderline personality disorder and, 717
 contextual therapy and, 132
 history of family therapy and, 7
 psychodynamic family therapy and, 11, 79, 91, 238–241
Observable patterns, of family behavior, 331–337
Observational learning, and behavioral couples therapy, 466
Observation area, and family therapy with children, 385
Obsessive-compulsive disorder, and couples therapy, 430
Official image, and diagnostic family interview, 259
Olson, David, 549
Omnipresence, of family, 303
Operant conditioning, and couples therapy, 427–428, 462–463, 469–470
Operational mourning, 647
Optimal families, 322
Optimal Treatment Project (OTP), 172
Ordeal Therapy (Haley 1984), 61
Oregon Marital Studies Program model, 468
Oregon Social Learning Center (OSLC), 404, 408–409, 413
Organismic model, of structural family therapy, 36, 37
Orgasmic disorders, 570–572
Orientation, and family therapy with children, 391–392
Other, and contextual therapy, 133–134

Outcome expectancies, and behavioral couples therapy, 467, 475
Outcome studies. *See also* Research
  behavioral couples therapy and, 473, 476–477
  behavioral family therapy and, 167
  integrative couples therapy and, 480
  marital enrichment and, 556
  medical family therapy and, 765
  parent management training and, 413
  psychoeducational family intervention and, 191
  self-regulatory couple therapy and, 480
  sex therapy and, 435
  therapist relationship skills and therapeutic alliance, 75
Outpatient treatment, for alcoholism or substance abuse, 683, 692
Overfunction, of emotional system, 112–113
Overgeneralization, and behavioral couples therapy, 492–493
Overinvolvement
  inpatient family intervention and, 649
  of parent with child, 113–114
  schizophrenia and emotional, 602
  within family system, 228

Papaverine, 569
Paradoxical interventions
  brief strategic/interactional therapy and, 64
  couples therapy and, 427
  strategic family therapy and, 13–14, 46
Parallel contract, 235
Paranoid personality type, and couples therapy, 431
Paranoid predators, and distressed marriages, 350, 351
Parent Adolescent Relationship Development (PARD), 541
Parental psychopathology model, of schizophrenia, 592
Parent Communication Project (Canada), 689
Parent Daily Report (PDR), 412
Parent Effectiveness Training (PET), 689, 780
Parentification, and contextual therapy, 131
Parent management training (PMT)
  case examples of, 409–411
  coercive family processes and, 373–374
  conduct-disordered youth and, 405–407
  definition of, 407
  development of, 405, 408
  measurement indices for, 412–413
  methodology and techniques of, 408–409, 411–412
  outcome studies of, 413
  research on, 23–24, 778
Parents and parenting. *See also* Adolescents; Children; Parent Effectiveness Training; Parentification; Parent management training; Single-parent families
  adolescents and conflicts with, 779–781
  adolescent substance abuse and, 690
  African Americans and culture, 730
  borderline personality disorder and, 717, 718
  coalitions and, 528, 532–533
  culture and views of motherhood, 210
  depression and, 622, 624, 625–627
  divorce and, 510, 512, 516, 519–520
  family life cycle and, 309
  family therapy and difficulties in, 777–778
  first session of family therapy with young children, 390–391
  gender-sensitive family therapy and, 211

incest and, 707
multigenerational emotional process and, 116–118
overinvolvement with child and, 113–114
overprotectiveness of, **358**
schizophrenia and, 661
stepfamily and absent biological, 528–529
stepfamily and parent-child relationship, 527–528
therapeutic mismanagement of family therapy with children and, 372

Passive-congenital marriages, 351

Passive-dependent personality, and couples therapy, 431

Pathogenic relating, and triadic-based go-between technique, 233

Patient history, and behavioral couples therapy, 487–488. *See also* Family history

Patient preselection, and medical family therapy, 757

Patterson, Gerald, 148, 405

Pattison Psychosocial Kinship Inventory, 200

Pedophilia, and incest, 700

Peer groups, and adolescent substance abuse, 691

Peer relationships. *See also* Relationships; Social network
depression and, 626
divorce and, 516

Penile injection treatment, 569

Penn State University, 541

Perceptions, couples therapy and distorted, 442–443, 446–447

Performance anxiety, and sexuality, 332, 574

Persistence, and coercive behavior by parents, 406

Personae, and spousal roles, 475. *See also* Self

Personal gain, and problem-solving therapy, 60

Personalismo, 733, 734

Personality disorders. *See also* Personality types
contextual therapy and, 142
divorce and, 518
incest and, 700
psychoeducational family intervention and, 190

Personality types. *See also* Personality disorders
classification systems for marital disorders and, 430–431
life experiences and formation of, 715–716
marital enrichment and, 550
social adaptation and, 722

Person-to-person relationship, and multigenerational family system therapy, 243

Philadelphia Child Guidance Clinic, 7

Phobias, and sex therapy, 576

Physically disabled, and sexual abuse, 698–699

Physicians, and domestic violence, 221–222

Physiological changes, in schizophrenia, 599–600

Planning
future stressors and, 644
treatment for incest and, 708

Play. *See also* Toys
family therapy with children and, 385, 386–390
psychodynamic family therapy and, 82, 239–240

Point of view, and family functioning, 328–330

Polarization
couples therapy and, 423, 478
social network therapy and, 197–198

Police, and domestic violence, 218, 221

Positioning, and strategic family therapy, 232
Positive associations, and therapy for incest, 713
Positive connotation
  strategic family therapy and, 233
  systemic approach and, 31, 69
Positive event scheduling, 489
Positive feelings, family functioning and sharing of, 337
Positive Feelings Questionnaire (PFQ), 486
Positive interaction, and behavioral couples therapy, 488–490
Positive reinforcement
  behavioral couples therapy and, 427–428, 463, 469
  behavioral family therapy and, 235
Postmodernism, and strategic marital therapy, 427
Posttraumatic stress disorder (PTSD). *See also* Trauma and traumatic events
  culture and, 727
  incest and sexual abuse, 699, 712
Powell, Gleam, 541
Power
  couples therapy and, 799
  family functioning and overt differences in, 331–333
  gender-sensitive family therapy and, 210, 218
  problem-solving therapy and, 60
  stepfamilies and issues of, 531
Practical Application of Intimate Relationship Skills (PAIRS), 541, **543**, 549, 550, 553, 554
Predictive index, and schizophrenia, 593, 596–597
Predictive validity, of standardized tests, 279
Preexisting conditions, in trauma patients, 190
Preferred provider organizations (PPOs), 765

Premarital Relationship Enhancement Program (PREP), 541, 546
Premature ejaculation, 571
Preoccupied couples, and narcissistic personality disorder, 720
Prepare-Enrich measure, 549, 566
Preschoolers, and impact of divorce on development, 509
Present, family functioning and operation in, 334–335
Presenting problem, and diagnostic family interview, 257
Pre-separation, and divorce, 504
Pretending, and strategic family therapy, 232–233
Prevalence, of domestic violence, 215–216
Prevention
  behavioral couples therapy and, 473
  of depression in children of depressed parents, 21, 185
  family physicians and, 751
  inpatient family intervention and relapse, 644–645
Prevention and Relationship Enhancement Program (PREP), **543**, 546, 548, 549, 550, **552**, 553, 554
Primary care specialists, and medical family therapy, 748, 751
Primary intrafamilial processes, 311
Primary prevention, of depression, 185
Primary relationship disorders, and family interactional diagnosis, 268
Primary residence, and definition of stepfamily, 524
Prince of Tides (Conroy), 458
Problem exploration, and family therapy with children, 396, 400–401
Problem-solving, and couple-based dysfunctions, **358**
Problem-solving family therapy
  culture and, 728
  theory of, 59–61

Index 937

Problem-solving training (PSST)
  attention-deficit/hyperactivity disorder and, 783
  behavioral couples therapy and, 491
  behavioral family therapy and, 159–160
  domestic violence and, 219
  marital enrichment and, 547–548
  parenting difficulties and, 777–778
Problem story, and narrative therapy, 234
Process dimensions, of marital enrichment, 541
Process Model of Family Functioning, 287
Professional relationships, and abuse of power, 218
Project on Child Abuse and Neglect (Michigan), 704
Projective identification
  borderline personality disorder and, 717
  family therapy with children and adolescents, 17
  psychodynamic couples therapy and, 423–424, 444, 446–447, 450–451
  psychodynamic family therapy and, 88
Propranolol, 564
Prostatitis, and sexual dysfunction, 562
Prosthetic penile implants, 569
Protection, and sexual abuse, 710–711
Protective factors, and divorce, 514
Pseudomutuality
  couples therapy and, 431
  schizophrenia and, 6, 83, 347–348
Psychiatric hospitals
  family intervention in, 22–23
  hospitalization of children and family disintegration, 370–371
Psychiatry, and Asian culture, 739
Psychic divorce, 434

Psychoanalysis and psychoanalytic theory
  history of family therapy and, 5
  incest and, 712
  as model of structural family therapy, 36
  psychodynamic family therapy and, 77
  theories of behavior and, 403
Psychoanalytic Study of the Family (Flugel 1921), 80
Psychodynamic couples therapy
  clinical and technical interventions and, 449–456
  diagnosis and, 447–448, 449
  relational circumstances of, 440
  theory and, 423–425, 436, 440–447
  therapeutic considerations and, 448–449
Psychodynamic family data, and diagnostic family interview, 267–268
Psychodynamic family therapy
  applicability and methodology of, 94–100
  conduct disorders in children and, 376
  definition of, 78–79
  depression and, 632–633
  development of, 77–78
  effectiveness of, 252–253, 791–792
  family life cycle and, 17
  family theory and, 31
  goals of, 93–94
  history of, 80–83
  medical family therapy and, 762
  as model for family therapy, 10–11
  techniques of, 238–241
  theory of, 83–93
Psychoeducational family intervention. *See also* Education
  children and, 187–188
  definition of, 173
  depression and, **181–182,** 635
  description of approach, 173–174

Psychoeducational family intervention
    (continued)
    effectiveness of, 192, 253
    family theory and, 32
    history of, 175–176
    illness in children and, 21
    inpatient family intervention and,
      651, 655, 665
    medical family therapy and, 749
    as model for family therapy, 9, 15
    outcome data on, 191
    phases of, 186–187
    research on, 177–185
    schizophrenia and, 610–611, 789
    structure of approach to, 190–191
    techniques of, 246–247
    trauma patients and, 188–190
Psychology. *See also* Individual
    psychology
    impact on incest and, 699
    studies of alcoholic families,
      677–682
Psychopathology. *See also*
    Hospitalization; *specific disorders*
    couples therapy and, 805–807
    depression and comorbidity, 620
    divorce and, 517–518
    inpatient family intervention and,
      637–655
    sexual dysfunctions and
      comorbidity, 565
    substance abuse and comorbidity,
      672
Psychopharmacology. *See* Medication
Psychosexual therapy, 577
Psychosis
    behavioral family therapy and,
      168
    contextual therapy and, 142
    inpatient family intervention and,
      645
Psychosocial factors, in chronic illness,
    753–754
Psychosocial transmission model, of
    schizophrenia, 588–590

Psychosomatic avoiders, and distressed
    marriages, 350–351
Psychosomatic complaints, and incest,
    705
Psychosomatic Families (Minuchin et al.
    1978), 38
Psychosomatic family, 7, 38, 52
Psychosomatic medicine, 762
Puerto Rico, influence of culture on
    family, 734, 736
Punishment
    behavioral couples therapy and,
      428, 463
    behavioral family therapy and, 235
    coercive behavior by parents and,
      406

Quasi-experimental developmental
    studies, of divorce, 508
Quid pro quo contract, 235

Race. *See* African Americans; Asian
    Americans; Ethnicity; Latinos
Rage behavior, and incest, 708, 709
Randomized studies, and research on
    family therapy, 773, 775, 776, 780,
    781, 782, 783, 786
Rapprochement, and separation-
    individuation process, 91
Reactive statement, and
    psychodynamic couples therapy,
    451
Reactivity model, of schizophrenia,
    590–591, 597
Reactor type, of therapist, 227
Reality, and phases of marital
    relationships, 444
Reciprocity
    behavioral couples therapy and, 428
    behavioral family therapy and, 148,
      152, 236, 237, 777
    phases of marital relationships and,
      442
Recognition, of stressful family
    patterns, 644

Index

Recommendations, for family therapy with children, 401–402
Reconstruction, and forms of interpretation, 99
Recovery, from depression, 628
Recovery of Hope program, **544**
Recurrent disorders, and inpatient family intervention, 649
Referrals
  family life cycle and, 315–316
  family therapy with children, 391
  medical family therapy and, 751–752, 755–756
Reframing
  brief strategic/interactional therapy and, 64
  gender-sensitive family therapy and, 220
  psychoeducational family intervention and, 179
  stepfamily and, 536–537
  strategic family therapy and, 233
  structural family therapy and, 230
Rehabilitation, and inpatient family intervention, 665
Rehabilitative phase, of psychoeducational family intervention, 184–185
Reid, John, 148
Reinforcement survey, and behavioral family therapy, 156
Reiss, David, 749
Relabeling
  strategic family therapy and, 233
  structural family therapy and, 230
Relapse
  of depression, 628–629, 632
  inpatient family intervention and, 644–645, 649
  of schizophrenia, 191, **594–595**
Relationship Attribution Measure, 484
Relationship Beliefs Inventory (RBI), 484
Relationship Code, The (Reiss et al. 2000), 820

Relationship Enhancement (RE), and couples therapy, 475, 541, **544,** 548, 550, 553, 554, 556
Relationship Enrichment Facilitating Open Communication, Understanding, and Study (REFOCUS), 541, **543,** 545, **552,** 554
Relationships. *See also* Extramarital affairs; Peer relationships
  Asian-American families and, 743
  behavioral couples therapy and dysfunctions of, 462
  cognitive and emotional modes of, 242
  contextual therapy and dialectic view of, 132
  depression and, 620, 623–624, 632
  gender-sensitive family therapy and closeness or distance in, 209
  person-to-person and multigenerational family systems therapy, 243
  psychodynamic theory and, 441
  sex therapy and, 562
  therapeutic alliance and, 95
Reliability, of standardized tests, 278
Religion
  culture and family, 731, 737, 740
  institutions and marital enrichment, 540
Remarriage. *See also* Divorce; Marriage; Stepfamily
  changes in family structure and, 501, 523
  divorce and, 503, 506
  family life cycle and, 312
  psychodynamic couples therapy and, 440
  rate of, 523
Remission, of depression, 627–628, 631
Repetition compulsion defense, and psychodynamic couples therapy, 441–442, 450–451

Repetitive cycling, and alcoholic
family, 680
Reporting, of sexual abuse, 710
Research. *See also* Adoption studies;
Outcome studies
on adolescent substance abuse,
687–688
on behavioral family therapy,
162–167
on couples therapy, 23, 435,
797–814
current status of on family therapy,
771–794
on family competence, 338
on family therapy with children,
378–379
history of family therapy and, 23–24
on multigenerational family systems
theory, 124–125
on psychoeducational family
intervention, 177–185
on schizophrenia and family
intervention, 605–615
on sex therapy, 560
on social network therapy, 200–201
on stepfamily, 537–538
Residential treatment programs, for
alcohol or substance abuse,
692
Resistance
behavioral couples therapy and,
498–499
diagnostic family interview and, 259
Erickson's ideas on family therapy
and, 58
family therapy with children and,
372
psychodynamic family therapy and,
87–88
solution-focused therapy and, 65
strategic approach to family therapy
and, 30
Respeto, 734
Responsiveness, level of in treatment
modalities, 23

Restraints
narrative therapy and, 72
strategic family therapy and, 232
Retribalization, and social network
therapy, 198
Rewards, and functional family, 328
Risk factors
for chronic disease, 760
for family dysfunction, 624
for incest, 699
Rituals
alcoholism and family, 22, 678–679
Latino family and, 734
stepfamilies and, 536
strategic family therapy and, 233
Role conflicts, and depression, 631. *See
also* Gender
Role-playing
experiential family therapy and, 245
family therapy with children and,
388–390, 396–400
Rolland, John, 749
Rorschach exam, 587, 591

Safety, and domestic violence, 21
Satir, Virginia, 7, 11
Scapegoating
diagnostic family interview and, 260
inpatient family intervention and,
647
Scharff, David and Jill, 8, 369
Schizophrenia
behavioral family therapy and,
163–164, 165–167, 168
communication deviance and, 6,
19–20, 348–349, **358**, 585,
587–593
contextual therapy and, 142
family classification and studies of,
347–349
family intervention studies and,
605–615
family variables in, 19–20
future directions in family
interventions for, 615–617

history of family therapy and, 6
inpatient family intervention and, 649
intergenerational transmission of, 82
National Alliance for the Mentally Ill and, 661
negative affective communication variables and, 593–604
psychoeducational family intervention and, 174, 175–176, 180, 191
research on effectiveness of family therapy for, 24, 786–790, 793, 794
risk indicators for, 585–586
structural family therapy and, 36–37
vulnerability-stress model of, 586–587
School-age children, and impact of divorce on development, 510
Schools, and divorce, 516
Screening, for marital enrichment, 555
Searchlights on Delinquency: New Psychoanalytic Studies (Eissler 1949), 404
Secondary prevention, of depression, 185
Secrets
  couples therapy and, 421, 425
  incest and, 707
Selective attention, and cognition in marriage, 474
Selective serotonin reuptake inhibitors (SSRIs), 571
Self. *See also* Personae; Self-esteem; Self-image; Self-validation
  couples therapy and concept of, 813
  depression and concept of, 626
  narrative therapy and, 73
  psychodynamic family therapy and, 90, 93
  structural family therapy and, 42, 45
Self-confrontation, and experiential family therapy, 245

Self-delineation, and contextual therapy, 132–133
Self-destructive behavior, and incest, 705
Self-disclosure, and couple-based dysfunctions, **358**
Self-esteem
  domestic violence and, 217
  stepfamilies and, 532
Self-help
  alcoholic family and, 681
  National Alliance for the Mentally Ill and, 660
Self-image, and borderline personality disorder, 717
Selfobject, and self psychology theory, 91–92
Self psychology, 79, 91–92
Self-regulatory couple therapy (SRCT), 478, 479–480, 495
Self-regulatory structure, and self psychology theory, 91
Self-validation, and contextual therapy, 133
Selvini Palazzoli, Mara, 7, 68, 69, 70–71
Sensation, and multimodal therapy for depression, 631
Separation, as transitional stage in divorce, 504–505
Separation-individuation
  borderline personality disorder and, 717
  family therapy with adolescents and, 371
  psychodynamic family therapy and theory of, 90–91
Separations, and family life cycle, 310
Separation studies, and alcoholism, 675
Sequences, and positive reinforcement, 469–470
Setting, for family therapy with children, 384–385
Setting events, and coercive processes, 407

Sex therapy. *See also* Sexuality
  assessment and, 564
  case examples of, 577–580
  changing views on treatment of
    sexual dysfunction and,
    560–564
  classification of sexual dysfunctions
    and, 564–573
  couples therapy and, 434–435,
    453–454, 807
  development of, 559–560
  intervention techniques for,
    573–577
Sexual abuse. *See also* Child abuse and
    neglect; Incest; Sexual violence
  legal issues in treatment of, 696
  prevalence of, 704
  substance abuse and, 672
Sexual arousal disorders, 567–569
Sexual desire disorders, 566–567
Sexual genogram, 566
Sexual harassment, 218
Sexual Interaction Inventory, 566
Sexuality. *See also* Sex therapy
  power differences and, 332
  psychological impact of incest and,
    699
Sexual pain disorders, 572–573
Sexual status examination, 566
Sexual violence, and gender roles,
  207–208
Shame, and Asian-American family,
  738, 739, 743. *See also* Blame and
  blaming
Shaping, and behavior therapy, 237,
  465
Shared contextual transference, 85
Shared vulnerability model, of
  schizophrenia, 591–592
Shelters, and domestic violence,
  213–214, 219
Short-term intervention, for alcohol or
  substance abuse, 692
Shrunken family, 308
Siblings. *See also* Family; Parents and
  parenting
  divorce and, 515–516
  family structure and, 309
  incest and, 701–703, 707
Simulated Family Activity Measure
  (SIMFAM), 280, **285**, 295–296,
  300, 301
Single-parent families. *See also*
  Divorce; Parents and parenting
  adolescent behavior problems and
    delinquency, 781–782
  family functioning and, 320
  family life cycle and, 307
  task overload and, 511
Skewed marriage, 431
Skills-training (ST) group, and parent-
  adolescent conflicts, 780
Skin conductance fluctuation rate
  (SCR), and schizophrenia,
  599–600
Smith, Leon and Antoinette, 540
Smoking, and lifestyle disorders, 761
Social cognitive theory, and behavioral
  couples therapy, 466
Social constructionist family therapy,
  427
Social context. *See also* Context;
  Culture
  of multigenerational family systems
    theory, 123–124
  of structural family therapy, 39
Social exchange, and behavioral
  couples therapy, 467, 472
Social Intervention Program, 608–609
Socialization. *See also* Social skills
  extrafamilial processes and, 311
  gender roles and, 209
  sex therapy and, 561
Social learning family therapy,
  776–777
Social learning theory
  behavioral couples therapy and,
    466, 471–472
  behavioral family therapy and, 15,
    32, 148, 153

development of, 404
divorce and, 506–507
Socially shared psychopathology, and psychodynamic family therapy, 88
Social networks. *See also* Peer relationships; Relationships; Social network therapy; Social support
  behavioral family therapy and concept of, 154
  divorce and, 511–512
  inpatient family intervention and, 649–650
  psychoeducational family intervention and, 185, 191
Social network therapy. *See also* Social networks
  effectiveness of, 253
  family theory and, 32
  introduction to concepts of, 193–194
  as model of family therapy, 16
  research on, 200–201
  techniques of, 196–200
  theory of, 194–195
Social psychology, and literature on couples therapy, 800
Social skills. *See also* Socialization
  behavioral family therapy and, 170–171
  schizophrenia and, 787
Social stage, of diagnostic family interview, 258–259
Social support. *See also* Social networks; Support services
  behavioral couples therapy and transactions, 472
  contextual therapy and social disintegration, 131–132
  depression in one member of couple and, 352
  marital enrichment and, 545
  psychoeducational family intervention and, 176
  stepfamily and, 529–530

Sociobiology, 125
Sociology
  development of family therapy and, 5
  theories of divorce and, 507–508
Solomon Four Group Design, 780
Solution-focused therapy
  couples therapy and, 427
  medical family therapy and, 765–766
  strategic interventions and, 14
  techniques of, 66–68
  theory of, 64–66
Somatization, and Asian culture, 739
Somatoform disorders, and medical family therapy, 761–765
Spanier Dyadic Adjustment Scale, 565
Speck, Ross, 16
Spectatoring, and sexuality, 332
Spiritism, and Latino culture, 734
Spousal psychopathology, 502
Spouse Observation Checklist (SOC), 472, 482
Stability, of standardized tests, 278
Stabilizing factors, in alcoholic families, 677
Stable-satisfactory marriages and stable-unsatisfactory marriages, 350, 431
Staffing, and inpatient family intervention, 645–646, 663. *See also* Hospitalization
Standardized tests, for family assessment
  comparison of instruments, 296–301
  depression and, 629–630
  descriptions of specific instruments, 280–296
  diagnostic family interview and, 269–274
  of marital adjustment and marital satisfaction, 485–486
  parent management training and, 412–413

Standardized tests, for family
assessment *(continued)*
sexual dysfunctions and, 565–566
test construction and, 278–279
Standards. *See also* Goals; Manuals
cognition in marriage and, 475–476
research on treatment development and, 772–774
Stepfamilies Stepping Ahead (Stepfamily Association of America), 535
Stepfamily. *See also* Divorce; Remarriage
changing structure of family and, 501, 523
characteristics of, 524–530
contextual considerations, 530–531
definition of, 524
incest and, 698, 701, 704
research on, 537–538
stepchildren and family life cycle, 312
therapeutic interventions for, 531–537
Stepfamily Association of America, 525, 535
Stepping Together: Creating Strong Stepfamilies (Stepfamily Association of America), 535
Stereoscopic therapy, 441
Stereotypes
of family, 153, 523
gender roles and, 799
Stern, Daniel, 98
Stierlin, Helm, 371
Strategic family therapy. *See also* structural-strategic family therapy
behavioral family therapy compared with, 777
depression and, 632
effectiveness of, 251–252, 791–792
as model of family therapy, 13–14
resistance and, 30
techniques of, 230–233
theory of, 59–61

Stress
coping and, 151
definition and measurement of family, **586**
depression and, 433, 620, 631
divorce and, 513–514
inpatient family intervention and, 643–644
Stress-diathesis theory
inpatient family intervention and, 640
psychoeducational family interventions and, 32
Stress-vulnerability model
behavioral family therapy and, 149–153, 169
psychoeducational family intervention and, 176
schizophrenia and, 586–587
Structural Family Interaction Scale (SFIS), 294–295, **300**
Structural family therapy (SFT). *See also* Structural-strategic family therapy
anorexia nervosa and, 35–36, 69, 378
applications of, 49–53
attention-deficit/hyperactivity disorder and, 783
basic concepts of, 35–36
effectiveness of, 53–54, 251, 791–792
family as system and, 30
history of family therapy and, 7, 36–38
medical family therapy and, 763
as model of family therapy, 13
parent-adolescent conflicts and, 780
recent developments in, 53
techniques of, 40–49, 228–230
theoretical concepts and, 38–40
Structural Profile (BASIC-ID), 550
Structural-strategic family therapy, and substance abuse, 684–685, 785

Structural strategic systems
    engagement (SSSE), 686–687
Structure, structural family therapy
    and concept of, 39–40
Structured Behavioral Exchange
    Contracting (SBE), 553
Structured Enrichment (SE), **544**
Stuart, Richard, 148
Stuck situation, and narrative therapy
    for couples, 427
Subgroups, and diagnostic family
    interview, 262
Subjective reality, and family
    functioning, 326–327
Substance abuse
    comorbidity of with
        psychopathology, 672
    divorce and, 518
    domestic violence and, 214
    family factors in, 673–674
    family therapy with adolescents and,
        686–691
    family therapy with adults and,
        684–686
    prevalence of, 671
    research on efficacy of family
        therapy for, 784–786
    suicide attempts and, 672
    therapeutic models and settings,
        692–694
    trauma patients and
        psychoeducational family
        intervention, 190
Substance Abuse Subtle Screening
    Inventory (SASSI), 565
Subsystems, family boundaries and
    structural family therapy, 47
Successive approximation, and
    behavioral family therapy,
    237
Suicide and suicidal ideation
    depression and, 629
    incest and, 711
    neurological disorders and,
        757–758

psychoeducational family
    intervention and, 180, 188
schizophrenia and, 788
substance abuse and, 672
Sullivan, Harry Stack, 5, 630–631
Summarizing self syndrome, 432
Support groups. *See also* Group
    therapy; Self-help
    for children in remarriage, 525
    schizophrenia and
        psychoeducational, 789
Supportive family intervention, and
    schizophrenia, 613
Support services. *See also* Institutional
    support; Social support
    domestic violence and, 219
    marital enrichment and, 553
    social context of family and, 50
    structural family therapy for
        disadvantaged and, 52–53
Supra-family system, 530
Survival-skills workshops, and
    schizophrenia, 788
Susto, 727
Swedish Adoption Studies, 675, 676
Symbolic Family Model, and
    schizophrenia, 611–612
Symmetrical midrange dysfunctions,
    248
Symmetrical relationships, and
    relational ethics, 139
Symptom Checklist–90—Revised
    (SCL-90-R), 565
Symptom prescription, and strategic
    family therapy, 232
Systemic couples, and depression, 352
Systemic family therapy, 68–71
Systems approach, to family therapy,
    12–13, 31
Systems theory. *See also* Family systems
    theory; Multigenerational family
    systems theory; Systemic family
    therapy
    couples therapy and, 426–427
    gender roles and, 205

Systems theory *(continued)*
    psychodynamic family therapy and, 78
    structural family therapy and, 38, 48–49
Szasz, Thomas, 129

Task overload, in single parents, 511
Tavistock Clinic (England), 80
Taylor-Johnson Temperament Analysis (T-ITA), 565
Termination
    of psychodynamic family therapy, 100
    of social network therapy, 199
Tertiary prevention, of depression, 185
Testosterone, and sexuality, 564
Textbook of Family Therapy and Family Medicine (Doherty and Baird 1983), 748
Thematic Apperception Test (TAT), 35, 588, 589, 591
Theory. *See also* Multigenerational family systems theory
    behavioral family therapy, 149–154
    brief strategic/interactional therapy and, 61–63
    couples therapy and, 423–427
    family therapy with children and, 369–371, 382
    inpatient family intervention and, 640
    models of family therapy and, 10
    narrative therapy and, 71–73
    psychodynamic couples therapy and, 423–425, 436, 440–447
    psychodynamic family therapy and, 83–93
    self psychology and, 91–92
    social network therapy and, 194–195
    solution-focused therapy and, 64–66
    strategic/problem-solving therapy and, 59–61

Therapeutic alliance
    behavioral family therapy and, 154–155
    family therapy with children and, 382–383
    positive strength of and outcome of family therapy, 75
    psychodynamic family therapy and, 95–96, 240
Therapeutic community. *See also* Community
    alcohol or substance abuse and, 692
    contextual therapy and, 129
Therapeutic contract. *See also* Contracting
    contextual therapy and, 140, 244
    diagnostic family interview and, 269
    family therapy with children and, 383–384
Therapeutic environment, and family therapy with children, 384–386
Therapeutic frame, of psychodynamic family therapy, 239
Therapeutic paradox, and strategic family therapy, 231–232
Therapeutic staff support (TSS), 193
Therapeutic system, diagnostic family interview and establishment of, 266–274
Therapeutic voyages, and multigenerational family system therapy, 242
Therapists. *See also* Training
    behavioral family therapy and concerns of, 161
    collaborative relationship with, 248, 458
    relationship skills of and outcome of family therapy, 75
    styles of, 226–228
Thresholds, diagnostic, 346
Time-limited programs, for marital enrichment, 553–554
Time-outs, and behavior therapy, 237, 428

Timing, of inpatient family intervention, 645. *See also* Duration
Tiu Lien, 738
Token economy, and behavioral family therapy, 236
Tolerance building, and integrative couples therapy, 479
Total Aversive Behavior (TAB) index, 412, 413
Total marriage, 351
Toys, and family therapy with children, 385–386. *See also* Play
Tracking
   definition of, 267
   structural family therapy and, 229
Traditions, and family rituals, 678–679
Training. *See also* Therapists
   in couples therapy, 418
   in cultural diversity, 744
   in gender-sensitive family therapy, 222
   National Alliance for the Mentally Ill and mental health professionals, 667–668
Training in Marriage Enrichment (TIME), 541, **544**, 546, **552**, 553, 554
Transactional model, of schizophrenia, 587, 597, 602, 603
Transactions, and contextual therapy, 138
Transference. *See also* Countertransference
   narcissistic personality disorder and, 721–722
   psychodynamic couples therapy and, 455, 457, 458
   psychodynamic family therapy and, 83–86, 94
Transgenerational dynamics, and contextual therapy, 134–136
Transitional objects, 86
Transitional stages, of divorce, 504–506
Transmission, of alcoholism in families, 678–679

Trauma and traumatic events. *See also* Posttraumatic stress disorder
   family therapy with children and adolescents, 17
   psychodynamic family therapy and, 79
   psychoeducational family intervention and, 174, 188–190
Treatment of Families in Crisis project (Colorado), 638–639
Treatment Strategies in Schizophrenia study (TSS), 613–614
Triadic-based go-between technique, and strategic family therapy, 233–234
Triangle, emotional system and multigenerational family systems theory, 111, 122
Triangulation, and family boundaries, 225
Trimble, David, 200–201
True self, 90
Truth
   family functioning and, 326–327
   interventions for incest and, 713
   structural family therapy and, 46
Twin studies. *See also* Genetic factors
   adolescent development and nonshared environment, 19
   in alcoholism, 676–677
   history of family therapy and, 8
   nonshared environment and adolescent development, 377

Unbalancing, and structural family therapy, 48, 230
Unconscious assumptions, and psychodynamic family therapy, 92
Underfunction, of emotional system, 112–113
Unemployment
   family and social changes, 50
   trauma patients and psychoeducational family intervention, 190

Unified detachment, and integrative couples therapy, 479
Unilateral view, of therapeutic contract, 140
University of California at Los Angeles (UCLA), 603
University of Southern California (USC), 165
Unstable-unsatisfactory marriages, 350

Vaginismus, 572–573
Valency, of unconscious assumptions, 92
Validity, of standardized tests, 278–279
Value Behavior Congruency Model, 549
Values. *See also* Ideology; Worldview
 countertransference and, 87
 cultural issues in diagnosis and, 726
 culture and family, 733, 735, 736, 741
 domestic violence and, 220
 marital enrichment and, 546
Venn diagram, 781
Verbalized contract, and marriage, 425
Vertical element, and social network therapy, 195
Veterans Administration, 610, 789
Victimization, and incest, 701
Victimizers, and diagnostic family interview, 260
Videotaping, and experiential family therapy, 245–246
Violence. *See also* Domestic violence; Sexual violence
Vital marriage, 351, 430
Voluntary behavior, and problem-solving therapy, 60

Vulnerability
 depression and, 620–622
 divorce and, 513–514
Vulnerability-stress model, of schizophrenia. *See* Stress-vulnerability model

Waiting room, and family therapy with children, 385
Wayward Youth (Aichorn 1935), 404
Weakland, John, 74–75
Whitaker, Carl, 7, 11, 81–82, 368
White, Michael, 71–72
Wiener, Norbert, 38
Wiltwyck School for Boys (New York), 37
Women. *See also* Feminism; Gender
 changing social roles of, 203–207, 338
 domestic violence and, 215–216
 family functioning and power differences, 332
Working through, and psychodynamic family therapy, 99–100
Workshop phase, of psychoeducational family intervention, 179–180, 183–184
Worldview, and structural family therapy, 44. *See also* Ideology; Values
Writing, of healing letters as therapy for incest, 712
Wynne, Lyman, 6, 82–83

Yocon (yohimbine), 569
Yohimbine (Yocon), 569
Young Children in Family Therapy (Zilbach 1986), 312

Zilbach, Joan, 8, 312, 369